Oxford Medical Publications

A Life Course Approach to Chronic Disease Epidemiology

Contents

A Life Course Approach to Chronic Disease Epidemiology

SECOND EDITION

Edited by

Diana Kuh

Medical Research Council National Survey of Health and Development, Department of Epidemiology and Public Health, Royal Free and University College London Medical School, UK

and

Yoav Ben-Shlomo

Department of Social Medicine, University of Bristol, UK

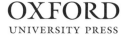
OXFORD
UNIVERSITY PRESS

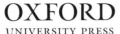

UNIVERSITY PRESS

Great Clarendon Street, Oxford OX2 6DP

Oxford University Press is a department of the University of Oxford.
It furthers the University's objective of excellence in research, scholarship,
and education by publishing worldwide in

Oxford New York
Auckland Cape Town Dar es Salaam Hong Kong Karachi
Kuala Lumpur Madrid Melbourne Mexico City Nairobi
New Delhi Shanghai Taipei Toronto

With offices in

Argentina Austria Brazil Chile Czech Republic Frnace Greece
Guatemala Hungary Italy Japan South Korea Poland Portugal
Singapore Switzerland Thailand Turkey Ukraine Vietnam

Oxford is a registered trade mark of Oxford University Press
in the UK and in certain other countries

Published in the United States
by Oxford University Press Inc., New York

© Oxford University Press 2004

The moral rights of the author have been asserted
Database right Oxford University Press (maker)

First published 2004
Reprinted 2005

A catalogue record for this title is available from the British Library

ISBN 0 19 857815 6 (Pbk)

10 9 8 7 6 5 4 3 2

Typeset by Cepha Imaging Pvt Ltd., Bangalore, India
Printed in Great Britain
on acid-free paper by
Ashford Colour Press Ltd, Gosport, Hampshire

Foreword: The seven ages of man

All the world's a stage,
And all the men and women merely players;
They have their exits and their entrances,
And one man in his time plays many parts,
His acts being seven ages. At first, the infant,
Mewling and puking in the nurse's arms.
Then the whining schoolboy, with his satchel
And shining morning face, creeping like snail
Unwillingly to school. And then the lover
Sighing like furnace, with a woeful ballad
Made to his mistress' eyebrow. Then a soldier,
Full of strange oaths and bearded like the pard,
Jealous in honour, sudden and quick in quarrel,
Seeking the bubble reputation
Even in the canon's mouth. And then the justice,
In fair round belly with good capon lined,
With eyes severe and beard of formal cut,
Full of wise saws and modern instances;
And so he plays his part. The sixth age shifts
Into the lean and slippered pantaloon
With spectacles on nose and pouch on side;
His youthful hose, well saved, a world too wide
For his shrunk shank, and his big manly voice,
Turning again toward childish treble, pipes
And whistles in his sound. Last scene of all,
That ends this strange eventful history,
Is second childishness and mere oblivion,
Sans teeth, sans eyes, sans taste, sans everything.

As You Like It, 2.7 139–167
William Shakespeare

Like Jacques in *As you like it*, epidemiologists today are thinking across the stages of life. Life course epidemiologists extend Jacques' perspective in several respects. They begin at conception rather than birth, with growing awareness that events before birth can set the stage for what transpires from birth until death. They also consider the ways in which the experience of one generation can be transmitted to the next.

The growth of "life course epidemiology", and indeed the term itself, owes much to the first edition of this book. While the first edition put forth a still novel and incomplete perspective, this second edition reflects the rapid maturing of the field, both in theory and in empirical findings. Life course studies have become a significant part of epidemiology. The current text provides a sophisticated and compelling schema for guiding future work. It is therefore timely to locate this development within the broader context of the evolution of the discipline.

Epidemiology is in a healthy state of flux. The study of individual behaviours and other risk factors in adult life, which was predominant from the 1950s up to the end of the twentieth century, is now being subsumed within a broader framework. We venture a perspective on what is emerging, with a slant toward what we wish to happen in future.

We see epidemiology changing along four lines in parallel. All are nascent rather than established practices. These changes are nonetheless quite evident in epidemiology journals and ongoing research. They are also well reflected in the chapters of this book.

First, epidemiologists increasingly are examining multiple levels of causation. The causes of health outcomes in populations can be sought at macro levels, such as in the distribution of wealth in a society; at the individual level, such as in individual behaviour; and at micro levels, such as in the cellular and molecular processes that generate cancers. Different approaches are required to study these levels of causation. Although ultimately, a disease outcome is always expressed in the individual, its causes may be sought in the society, the individual, and the cells within the individual. One epidemiological task is to explore and assemble these different levels of causation, and to draw from them the implications for public health.

Second, epidemiologists are investigating the interplay between genetic and environmental factors. The discipline is in a strategic position to do so. As a central science of public health, it encompasses all the causes of population health that have implications for preventive action. Today these undoubtedly include genetic as well as non-genetic factors. In the simplest scenario, some environmental exposures may take effect only in the presence of genetic factors that are now measurable. A current hypothesis, for example, is that low prenatal folate intake may cause neural tube defects only in the presence of genetic mutations, some of which have been identified and others of which are yet to be.

Third, epidemiologists are in the process of reversing a trend toward fragmentation into subspecialties, and bringing closer together the domains of epidemiology. Until recently, for example, infectious and chronic disease epidemiology were diverging. Investigators are now demonstrating that methods developed for infectious diseases—such as modelling transmission of epidemics across and within populations—are relevant for non-infectious diseases. Conversely, methods developed for the study of chronic diseases—such as risk factor designs—are relevant for infectious disease epidemiology. Another example of convergence pertains to physical and mental disorders. The resulting cross-fertilization is having a perceptible, and in some respects a notable, impact. The more comprehensive view enables the discipline to assume a position at the forefront of investigation in many disease areas.

Fourth, the new edition of this book shows that epidemiologists have begun to recognize the enrichment that follows from examining health and illness over the life course. We have far to go. We have still to apply life course epidemiology systematically to devastating communicable diseases of low income countries such as tuberculosis, malaria, and HIV/AIDS. Three quarters of a century has gone by since Wayde Hampton Frost and V.H. Springett independently showed how illuminating studies of tuberculosis over successive generations could be. This approach could contribute much to understanding the onset and expression of these diseases and to developing preventive actions. Also, we have still to tap the great potential of the life course approach in genetic epidemiology. As we progress from genomics to the study of gene expression, we will need to determine whether genes can be "turned on and off" in response to experiences or interventions across the life span. Likewise, as we turn our attention to relating the vast number of identified genotypes to a smaller number of well-defined phenotypes, we will need to know how these phenotypes vary over the stages of life, so elegantly described by Shakespeare five centuries ago.

Finally, life course studies have still to extend across the full life span. As the members of existing birth cohorts assembled for various studies age, we shall acquire the means to connect prenatal experience to late life outcomes, including diseases such as Alzheimer's dementia, and impairments in sensory and motor capacities. Also needed are more studies that cross generations. The unexplored territory makes it a safe bet that life course epidemiology will play a central role in the discipline in coming decades. It may well be that the most intriguing relationships are yet to be discovered.

To describe a structure embracing all the elements of this emergent way of thinking, we have proposed the term "eco-epidemiology". Whether or not the name proves durable, the endeavour of integration is essential. An integrated approach to investigating disease and its prevention will have necessarily to subsume levels of causation, kinds of causes, and types of diseases. Equally important, it will have to be embedded in a life course perspective.

Professor Ezra Susser and
Professor Mervyn Susser

Preface

At the beginning of the twenty-first century, adult chronic disease has become not only a major public health problem of industrialized countries but also of developing countries. The prevailing aetiological model that predominantly emphasized adult lifestyle, such as smoking, diet, and lack of physical exercise has been successfully challenged, by growing international evidence that impaired early growth and development, childhood infection and poor nutrition, and socioeconomic or psychosocial disadvantage across the life course, affect chronic disease risk. The study of these exposures and the life course pathways through which they have their effects lies at the heart of life course epidemiology. Initially applied to cardiovascular disease, diabetes, and chronic bronchitis, life course epidemiology is now seen to be relevant for a broader range of diseases, disorders, and aspects of adult function, as reflected in the new content for the second edition. This broader scope has revived and extended connections with researchers in other disciplines who have a more longstanding tradition of taking a life course perspective. In this new edition we have paid more attention to life course explanations for the development of unequal health, for time trends in specific diseases, and to policies and interventions that spring from a focus on life course. These are all rapidly growing areas of life course epidemiology.

A small interdisciplinary group of 16 mainly London-based research scientists was responsible for the first edition of this book in 1997 that coined the term 'life course epidemiology'. The 36 contributors to this second edition, from North America as well as the UK, reflect the rapid growth of this field. Life course epidemiology is now recognized as an established area of epidemiological research. It has been an exciting privilege to play our part in its development. Along the way we have made many friends and established new collaborations.

We remain committed to an approach that studies individual and cohort experience from conception to death and does not draw false dichotomies between adult lifestyle and early life influences, or between biological and social risk processes. The contributors to this book offer a comprehensive and fully updated review of epidemiological, biological, and sociological evidence relating to influences on disease risk in both early and later life. They discuss whether early experiences 'programme' particular body systems during critical periods of growth and development with long-term direct consequences for adult chronic disease, cause damage to body systems which steadily accumulates with continuing exposure to adverse circumstances, or trigger a chain of events that ultimately raise disease risk. These processes are not mutually exclusive and operate interactively with genetic processes. As editors, we have tried to maintain the common life course framework across all chapters of this extended volume and test the usefulness of conceptual developments in life course epidemiology.

After the publication of the first edition, some researchers argued that 'life course epidemiology' was merely re-badging what epidemiologists had always traditionally undertaken using the 'black-box' approach. While the idea of early life influences on adult disease is far from new, the current revival of a life course approach in epidemiology benefits from a number of new developments. These include the emergence of clear theoretical models, novel biological mechanisms, greater understanding of lifetime social processes, and good quality empirical data for testing life course hypotheses. This makes the second edition timely, capturing the findings of an explosion of publications in the last few years and making them more accessible. It remains an invaluable resource for epidemiologists, social scientists, clinicians, and public health physicians, and of interest to other medical researchers, policy makers, students, and the interested lay reader. It assumes no prior epidemiological knowledge, although some basic understanding of human biology is expected.

We would like to thank everybody who has made this second edition a reality. As before, we have learnt an enormous amount from our fellow contributors. Diana would like to thank Professor Mike Wadsworth, the director of the National Survey of Health and Development, and other members of the research team for their support. Rachel Cooper, one of a new generation of life course epidemiologists, proof read the manuscript and constructed the index. Jill Skehan and Suzie Butterworth provided administrative expertise. Our families have borne our dedication to this project with their usual good grace and humour.

Diana Kuh and Yoav Ben-Shlomo
January 2004

Acknowledgements

The authors would like to thank the following for permission to reproduce published material: Figs1.1 and 1.2 reproduced from Ben-Shlomo Y, Kuh D. A life course approach to chronic disease epidemiology: conceptual models, empirical challenges and interdisciplinary perspectives. *Int J Epidemiol* 2002,**31**:285–93, with permission of Oxford University Press; Fig. 1.3 from Kuh D, Ben-Shlomo Y, Lynch J, Hallqvist J, Power C. Glossary for life course epidemiology. *J Epidemiol Commun Health* 2003;**57**:778–83, with permission of Oxford University Press; Figs 2.1 and 2.3 updated from Kuh D, Davey Smith G. When is mortality risk determined? Historical insights into a current debate. *Soc Hist Med* 1993;**6**:101–23, by permission of Oxford University Press; Fig. 4.2 reproduced from Szreter S. The population health approach in historical perspective. *Am J Pub Health* 2002;**93**:421–31, reprinted with permission from the American Public Health Association; Fig. 8.3 from Willett WC, Dietz WH, Colditz GA. Guidelines for healthy weight. *N Engl J Med* 1999;**341**:427–34, Copyright © 1999 Massachusetts Medical Society, reprinted with permission of the Massachusetts Medical Society; Fig.8.4 reproduced from Kim S, Popkin BM. The nutrition transition in South Korea. *Am J Clin Nutr* 2000;**71**:44–53, reproduced with permission by the *American Journal of Clinical Nutrition*. Copyright © *Am J Clin Nutr*. American Society for Clinical Nutrition; Fig. 8.7 Copyright © American Diabetes Association 1991, reprinted with permission of The American Diabetes Association; Fig. 8.8 from Dabelea D, Hanson RL, Lindsay RS, Pettitt DJ, Imperatore G, Gabir MM, *et al.* Intrauterine exposure to diabetes conveys risks for type 2 diabetes and obesity: a study of discordant sibships. *Diabetes* 2000;**49**:2208–11, Copyright © American Diabetes Association 2000, reprinted with permission of The American Diabetes Association; Fig. 8.10 reproduced from Dietz WH. "Adiposity rebound": reality or epiphenomenon? *Lancet* 2000;**356**:2027–8, reprinted with permission from Elsevier; Figs. 12.1, 12.4, 12.8 from Swerdlow A, Dos Santos Silva I, Doll R. *Cancer incidence and mortality in England and Wales: trends and risk factors* (2001), reproduced by permission of Oxford University Press; Fig. 12.5 from LaVecchia C, Negri E, Levi F, Decarli A. Age, cohort-of-birth, and period-of-death trends in breast cancer mortality in Europe. *J Natl Cancer Inst* 1997;**89**:732–3, reproduced by permission of Oxford University Press; Fig. 12.6 from Tarone RE, Chu KC, Gandetta LA. Birth cohort and calendar period trends in breast cancer mortality in the United States and Canada. *J Natl Cancer Inst* 1997;**89**: 251–6, reproduced by permission of Oxford University Press; Fig. 12.9 from Bergström R, Adami H-O, Möhner M, Zatonski W, Storm H, Exbom A *et al.* Increase in testicular cancer incidence on sex European countries: a birth cohort phenomenon. *J Natl Cancer*

Inst 1996;**88**:727–33, reproduced by permission of Oxford University Press; Table 13.1 reprinted from Sayer AA, Cooper C, Evans JR, Rauf A, Wormald RPL, Osmond C *et al.* Are rates of ageing determined *in utero*? *Age Ageing* 1998;**27**:579–83, with permission of Oxford University Press; Fig.13.2 reproduced from Aihie Sayer A, Cooper C. Early undernutrition: good or bad for longevity? In Watson RR, ed. *Handbook of nutrition in the aged.* CRC Press, 2000:97–106, with permission of CRC Press; Fig. 13.3 reproduced from Aihie Sayer A, Dunn R, Langley-Evans S, Cooper C. Prenatal exposure to a maternal low protein diet shortens life span in rats. *Gerontology* 2001;**47**:9–14, © Karger, Basel with permission of Karger, Basel; Fig. 13.5 reproduced from Gale CR, Martyn CN, Kellingray S, Eastell R, Cooper C. Intrauterine programming of adult body composition. *J Clin Endocrinol Metab* 2001;**86**:267–72, © The Endocrine Society with permission of the Endocrine Society; Figs. 15.2 and 15.3 reproduced from Wilcox AJ. On the importance—and the unimportance—of birthweight. *Int J Epidemiol* 2001;**30**:1233–41, with permission of Oxford University Press.

To our partners (Jeannette and Peter), our children (Elie and Eva, Nick and Ellie) and Diana's grandson Finn.

Contributors

Dr Avan Aihie Sayer
Medical Research Council Clinical Scientist
and Honorary Senior Lecturer in
Geriatric Medicine
Medical Research Council Resource Centre,
University of Southampton, UK

Professor Mel Bartley
Professor of Medical Sociology
Department of Epidemiology and Public
Health, Royal Free and University College
London Medical School, UK

Dr Yoav Ben-Shlomo
Senior Lecturer in Clinical Epidemiology
Department of Social Medicine, University of
Bristol, UK

Dr David Blane
Reader in Medical Sociology
Department of Social Science and Medicine,
Imperial College, London, UK

Professor W. Thomas Boyce
Professor of Epidemiology and
Child Development
Division of Community Health and Human
Development, School of Public Health and
Institute of Human Development, University
of California, Berkeley, USA

Professor Derek G. Cook
Professor of Epidemiology
St George's Hospital Medical School,
London, UK

Professor Cyrus Cooper
Professor of Rheumatology and Director
Medical Research Council Resource Centre,
University of Southampton, UK

Professor George Davey Smith
Professor of Clinical Epidemiology
Department of Social Medicine, University of
Bristol, UK

Professor Jonathan Elford
Professor in Evidence-Based Health Care
Institute of Health Sciences, City University,
London, UK

Professor Pam Factor-Litvak
Associate Professor of Clinical
Epidemiology
Mailman School of Public Health,
Columbia University, New York, USA

Dr Nita Forouhi
Specialist Registrar
Public Health Department, Brent Primary
Care Trust, London, UK

Dr Johanna M. Geleijnse
Senior Research Scientist
Division of Nutrition, Wageningen University,
the Netherlands

Professor Matthew W. Gillman
Associate Professor of Ambulatory Care and
Prevention
Harvard Medical School and Harvard Pilgrim
Health Care, and Harvard School of Public
Health, USA

Dr Elizabeth Hall
Clinical Research Fellow
Epidemiology Unit, Department of
Epidemiology and Population Sciences,
London School of Hygiene and Tropical
Medicine, UK

Dr Rebecca Hardy
Medical Statistician* and Honorary
Senior Lecturer†
*Medical Research Council National Survey
of Health and Development and
†Department of Epidemiology and Public
Health, Royal Free and University College
London Medical School, UK

Professor KS Joseph
Associate Professor of Obstetrics and
Gynaecology, Paediatrics and Community
Health and Epidemiology
Perinatal Epidemiology Research Unit,
Dalhousie University and the IWK Health
Centre, Halifax, Nova Scotia, Canada

Professor Daniel P. Keating
Professor of Human Development and
Applied Psychology
University of Toronto, Canada

Professor Michael S. Kramer
Departments of Epidemiology and
Biostatistics and of Pediatrics, McGill
University Faculty of Medicine, Montreal,
Canada

Professor Diana Kuh
Senior Research Scientist* and Professor of
Life Course Epidemiology†
*Medical Research Council National Survey
of Health and Development and
†Department of Epidemiology and Public
Health, Royal Free and University College
London Medical School, UK

Dr Debbie A. Lawlor
Senior Lecturer in Epidemiology and Public
Health Medicine
Department of Social Medicine, University of
Bristol, UK

Professor David A. Leon
Professor of Epidemiology
Department of Epidemiology and Public
Health, London School of Hygiene and
Tropical Medicine, UK

Professor L.H. Lumey
Associate Professor of Clinical
Epidemiology
Department of Epidemiology, Mailman School
of Public Health, Columbia University, USA

Professor John Lynch
Associate Professor of Epidemiology
Department of Epidemiology, School of
Public Health, University of Michigan. USA

Professor Paul McKeigue
Professor of Metabolic and Genetic
Epidemiology
Epidemiology Unit, London School of
Hygiene and Tropical Medicine, UK

Dr Clive Osmond
Medical Research Council Senior Scientist
and Reader in Medical Statistics
Medical Research Council Environmental
Epidemiology Unit, University of
Southampton, UK

Professor Ivan J. Perry
Professor of Public Health
Department of Epidemiology and Public
Health, University College Cork, Ireland

Dr Nancy Potischman
Nutritional Epidemiologist
Applied Research Program, Division of Cancer
Control and Population Sciences, National
Cancer Institute, Bethesda, Maryland, USA

Professor Chris Power
Professor of Epidemiology and Public Health,
Centre for Epidemiology and Biostatistics,
Institute of Child Health, Royal Free and
University College Medical School,
London, UK

Dr Isabel dos Santos Silva
Senior Lecturer in Epidemiology
Non-Communicable Disease Epidemiology
Unit, Department of Epidemiology and
Population Health, London School of
Hygiene and Tropical Medicine, UK

Professor Aziz Sheikh
Professor of Primary Care Research and
Development
Division of Community Health Sciences:
GP Section, University of Edinburgh,
Edinburgh, UK

Professor David P. Strachan
Professor in Epidemiology
Department of Public Health Sciences,
St George's Hospital Medical School,
London, UK

Professor Mervyn Susser
Emeritus Professor of Epidemiology and
Director of the Sergievsky Centre
Sergievsky Centre, Columbia,
New York, USA

Professor Ezra Susser
Professor of Epidemiology and Psychiatry Chair
Department of Epidemiology, Mailman
School of Public Health, Columbia University,
New York, USA

Professor Rebecca Troisi
Epidemiologist
Division of Cancer Epidemiology and
Genetics, National Cancer Institute, National
Institutes of Health, and Department of
Community and Family Medicine, Dartmouth
Medical School, New Hampshire, USA

Professor Lars Vatten
Professor of Epidemiology
Department of Community Medicine and
General Practice School of Medicine,
Norwegian University of Science and
Technology, Trondheim, Norway

Professor Peter H. Whincup
Professor of Cardiovascular
Epidemiology,
St George's Hospital Medical School,
London, UK

Part I

Background

Chapter 1

Introduction

Diana Kuh and Yoav Ben-Shlomo

Life course epidemiology is the study of long-term biological, behavioural, and psychosocial processes that link adult health and disease risk to physical or social exposures acting during gestation, childhood, adolescence, earlier in adult life, or across generations. Life course epidemiology grew out of research in the 1980s and 1990s showing that factors early in life, such as poor growth and development or adverse childhood environmental conditions, are associated with a raised risk of adult chronic disease. This research challenged the prevailing twentieth century aetiological model for adult disease that emphasized adult risk factors, particularly aspects of adult lifestyle. Since we reviewed the scientific evidence in the first edition of this book (published in 1997) there has been a dramatic increase in the number of life course studies and a parallel development in the application of life course conceptual models in chronic disease epidemiology. One life course model hypothesizes that adult chronic disease and many of its adult risk factors are biologically 'programmed' during critical periods of growth and development *in utero* or early infancy. The extent to which these effects can be modified by later experience is a key question in life course epidemiology. An alternative model hypothesizes that adult chronic disease reflects cumulative differential lifetime exposure to damaging physical and social environments. Risk factors for chronic disease often cluster together because many are related to socioeconomic position. They may also be linked in a temporal sequence to form a chain of risk. These life course models are not mutually exclusive, may operate simultaneously and can be difficult to distinguish empirically. Contributors to this book take a broad life course approach, reviewing the epidemiological, social, and biological evidence to see which experiences at different stages of the life course may contribute to the development of chronic disease and other aspects of adult health.

1.1 Adult risk factors and chronic disease

In the second half of the twentieth century, adult chronic disease became the main public health problem of industrialized countries. Figures from the World Health Organization show that by the end of the century, non-communicable conditions were responsible for between 83 and 89% of deaths in the very-low-mortality countries of the European and Western Pacific regions and the Americas.[1] Cardiovascular disease, cancers, chronic obstructive lung disease and diabetes have now become a major and growing public health problem worldwide, accounting for 50% of the global mortality burden. The contribution from low- and middle-income countries already accounts for almost three-quarters of this global burden.[2]

The prevailing aetiological model for adult chronic disease during the twentieth century emphasized adult risk factors. Post-war cohort studies were successful at identifying both a number of bodily attributes that predispose individuals to specific chronic diseases and various personal behaviours, associated with adult lifestyle, which affect underlying biological processes. For example, cigarette smoking is the classic risk factor for lung cancer and chronic bronchitis and contributes to the risk of coronary heart disease along with the other conventional risk factors including hypertension, raised blood cholesterol, diabetes, obesity, and physical inactivity. This evidence was used to support government health education strategies that encourage adults to adopt healthier lifestyles.

The extent to which classic risk factors account for the occurrence of chronic disease and the striking and well-documented social and geographical inequalities in the distribution of chronic disease are matters of long-term lively academic debate.[3,4] This has stimulated further research into genetic markers, other adult risk factors to do with the psychosocial environment, more detailed assessment of adult dietary intake and childhood risk factors.[5]

1.2 *In utero*, childhood and adolescent risk factors for adult chronic disease

Initially, interest in childhood in relation to adult chronic disease was stimulated by research findings (discussed in Chapters 2 and 3) that suggested that the process of atherosclerosis begins in early life. For example, the arteries of young children contain fatty streaks. Blood pressure and cholesterol levels in individuals 'track' from childhood to early adult life. Overweight children are at greater risk of becoming overweight adults. Life-long smoking, dietary, and exercise habits are acquired in childhood and adolescence. The lifestyle model, which arose from the study of those in mid-life, was gradually extended beyond adulthood as it was increasingly recognized that the establishment of healthy lifestyles, in terms of the classic risk factors, had to begin in childhood.

A second line of research emphasized the importance of deprivation rather than affluence in childhood for adult chronic disease and challenged the lifestyle model. This research investigated environmental conditions and experiences during prenatal life, infancy, childhood, and adolescence associated with poverty, illness, and poor early growth, which may make individuals more susceptible to developing adult chronic disease, either independently or in combination with adult risk factors. This research built on ecological studies in the 1970s and 1980s that found strong correlations between rates of past infant mortality and current adult mortality from various chronic diseases within the same geographical areas. More extensive studies of this type revealed that mortality rates from coronary heart disease, stroke, obstructive lung disease and lung cancer were differentially correlated with neonatal mortality, postneonatal mortality, mortality from respiratory and enteric disease, maternal mortality, and mean height (see Chapter 6).

These ecological studies were interpreted by David Barker and colleagues at the Medical Research Council Environmental Epidemiology Unit at Southampton University as indicating the importance of prenatal or infant exposures. In a series of imaginative historical cohort studies in the UK, Barker's team traced the whereabouts of hundreds of adults for whom birth records from health visitors and hospitals were available. Various markers of prenatal and infant growth (such as birthweight, thinness or shortness at birth, weight at 1 year and the ratio of placental weight to birthweight) were found to be inversely associated with coronary heart disease, stroke, diabetes, and respiratory disease and their associated risk factors (such as high blood pressure, insulin resistance, and poor lung function). Barker generated a number of hypotheses to explain how undernutrition *in utero* or in early postnatal life programmes an individual's risk of a number of adult chronic diseases. For example, in the case of coronary heart disease it was hypothesized that fetal undernutrition during middle to late gestation leads to disproportionate fetal growth and raises the risk of coronary heart disease by programming blood pressure, cholesterol metabolism, blood coagulation, and hormonal settings.[6,7] This research stimulated a large number of similar investigations in other developed and developing countries.

Other researchers with a particular interest in social epidemiology interpreted infant mortality as a marker of childhood living conditions.[8,9] It was shown that for some causes of death but not others, the ecological associations between past infant mortality and current adult mortality were strongly attenuated after adjustment for markers of adult deprivation or current infant mortality,[9,10] suggesting in these cases that the association was due to continuity in living conditions over the life course. A plethora of studies in the 1990s investigated markers of childhood socioeconomic position in relation to cardiovascular disease and other health outcomes in a number of cohorts (reviewed in Chapters 4 and 16). They generally found an effect of childhood socioeconomic position that was additional to the effect of adult risk factors and socioeconomic position. These studies suggest that socially patterned exposures in childhood have important influences on adult health and chronic disease.

Researchers investigating either the fetal origins or the childhood social origins of adult chronic disease share a common interest in the underlying biological processes involved and both groups of researchers are now concerned with understanding the role of postnatal growth and development, childhood illness, and intergenerational influences on adult chronic disease. The first edition of this book in 1997 coined the term life course epidemiology. It reflected an attempt to demonstrate the common interests of these various strands of early life research in cardiovascular and respiratory epidemiology and to link them to research in cancer epidemiology where there has been a longstanding interest in long-term latent effects. By giving consideration to underlying early social as well as biological processes and how they co-evolve and then interact with adult exposures, our vision of life course epidemiology did not draw false dichotomies between biological and social or between early and later influences on chronic disease risk.

1.3 The growth of life course epidemiology and the aims of this book

Life course epidemiology is the study of long-term effects on later health and disease risk of physical or social exposures during gestation, childhood, adolescence, young adulthood, and later adult life.[11,12] The aim is to elucidate the underlying biological, behavioural, and psychosocial processes that operate across an individual's life course or across generations. Life course epidemiology represents a revival of a longstanding epidemiological and public health interest in the childhood origins of adult health, eclipsed in the middle of the twentieth century by the adult lifestyle model of chronic disease. It is part of a growing body of research emanating from a variety of scientific disciplines that appreciates the importance of a life course perspective for studying variation in human development and ageing (see Chapter 2).

Time is a fundamental concept in life course epidemiology, not just in terms of lifetime (as indexed by the chronological age of individuals) but also in terms of historical time at the population level (as indexed by membership of a birth cohort). Changing individuals should be studied in a changing environment and these contextual factors affect exposure to risk and the individual's response strategies. Thus life course explanations for disease occurrence, temporal trends and differentials in disease risk between social groups in a population are likely to be time and place dependent.

Since the first edition of this book was published in 1997 there has been increasing interest in conceptualizing chronic disease aetiology (and other aspects of health) within a life course framework.[11,12] The life course perspective has become a central part of the World Health Organization's programme on non-communicable disease prevention and health promotion.[13] Grant-giving bodies such as the European Science Foundation, the UK Medical Research Council, and the UK Economic and Social Research Council have funded programmes of life course research. Oxford University Press has set up a book series on the life course and adult health, of which this is the second volume. The number of researchers involved in life course epidemiology has grown rapidly and is reflected in the increased number of contributors to this second edition and to the first book in the series on women's health.[14] Beyond the traditional life course focus on cardiovascular and respiratory diseases and diabetes, the life course approach is now being more systematically applied to the study of biological ageing and musculoskeletal function (see Chapter 13 and Reference 15), health behaviours and other risk factors (see Chapters 4 and 8 and References 16–18), reproductive health,[19,20] and the development of cancers (see Chapters 11 and 12 and Reference 21).

In the last few years many new findings have been published in the scientific literature, utilizing existing and revitalized cohort studies to investigate exposures acting and interacting across the whole life course on later health and disease risk. More use has also been made of other study designs, for example, using twin and sibling studies to try to disentangle environmental and genetic effects or control for confounding (see Chapters 3). There have been numerous animal studies designed to test biological mechanisms hypothesized to underlie fetal programming (see, for example, Reference 22). There is growing evidence that several hormonal axes, such as the hypothalamic–pituitary–adrenal axis, are programmed in early life.[23] Findings from randomized controlled trials of early nutritional interventions in humans followed into adolescence have now been published[24,25] and do not always show the same results as the observational studies.[25] More attention has been paid to the social and biological factors at each stage of the life course that drive temporal disease trends in various populations or explain differences in disease risk between social groups within a population.[26] Finally there is a growing interest in the public health and policy implications of life course research (see Chapters 17 and 18 and References 13, 27, and 28).

Therefore the first aim of this revised second edition is to review this new evidence. As well as updating and extending the original chapters on cardiovascular disease, diabetes, blood pressure, respiratory disease, and cancer, we have added chapters on obesity, biological ageing, and neuropsychiatric disorders (where there is a strong tradition of research on childhood origins).

We have also changed the structure of the book to reflect the fact that a life course perspective is increasingly being used to investigate social and geographical variations in disease across time and place as well as the occurrence of disease within a population. Davey Smith and Lynch in Chapter 4 argue convincingly that associations between exposures acting at different stages of the life course and adult chronic disease are dynamic in relation to time and place. A fuller interpretation of these associations is possible if we draw inferences across population studies of individual risk, time trends and group differences with respect to particular disease outcomes. We have therefore discarded the somewhat false dichotomy that was drawn between these types of studies in the first edition. Rather chapters are grouped together according to their main disease outcome or associated proximal risk factors. For example, the chapters that focus on life course influences on cardiovascular disease, its time trends and its socioeconomic differentials are clustered together. A new chapter on cancer trends complements the new chapter on life course influences on cancer epidemiology. Trends in respiratory disease are incorporated into the updated chapter on respiratory and allergic diseases.

We have kept and expanded the two chapters that explore possible risk mechanisms: one examines the role of nutrition and intergenerational factors on fetal growth and development; the other examines the evidence for social processes acting throughout life that affect adult disease risk by ameliorating or exacerbating biological factors.

Epidemiological theories that propose an important role for early life factors in relation to adult chronic disease present a direct challenge to the contemporary wisdom of health education strategies that focus on adult health behaviour and lifestyle. The two chapters in the final section of the book are concerned with the policy implications of these theories. Chapter 17 assesses the evidence from intervention studies that have attempted to improve the nutritional state of young women or alter fetal and infant growth and survival. It asks whether there would be a positive change in the nation's health if current health promotion strategies shifted towards an emphasis on early life-risk factors facing the next generation of mothers and babies. Chapter 18, which is new to this edition of the book, assesses the evidence to support interventions to improve childhood circumstances as a way of improving population health. In the final chapter we draw together the conclusions of the various chapters to highlight the emerging research themes in life course epidemiology and their implications for public health and policy.

1.4 Life course conceptual models

In parallel with the strong growth of epidemiological interest in life course studies, attention has been paid to the clarification of key concepts and ideas and the development of life course conceptual models.[11,12,29,30] These models postulate pathways linking exposures across the life course to later life health and disease. Some of the

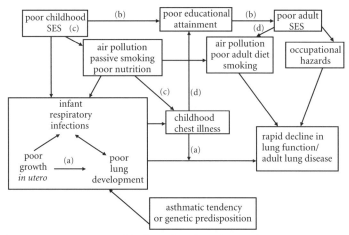

Fig. 1.1 Schematic representation of biological and psychosocial exposures acting across the life course that may influence lung function or respiratory disease.[11]

concepts and terms have been adapted from scientific disciplines such as psychology, biology, demography, anthropology, and sociology where a life course perspective is often seen as an integral part of the study of development or ageing (see Chapter 2).

A life course approach to epidemiology is more than the collection of longitudinal data or the use of a particular study design or analytical method. Rather it is a theoretical model where the temporal ordering of exposure variables and their inter-relationships with respect to a particular health or disease outcome are specified and then tested using life course data. An example of a conceptual model linking early childhood exposures (such as childhood socioeconomic circumstances or poor *in utero* growth) with respect to respiratory disease and impaired lung function illustrates many possible pathways with potential mediating or confounding factors (Fig. 1.1). Path (a) represents a predominantly biological pathway whereby impaired fetal and infant lung development is associated with future respiratory insults from infectious agents and greater susceptibility to impaired lung function in adulthood or chronic obstructive airways disease. Path (b) represents a predominantly social pathway whereby adverse childhood socioeconomic position increases the risk of adverse childhood exposures as well as adult socioeconomic position and smoking behaviour. Path (c) represents a sociobiological pathway whereby adverse childhood socioeconomic position is associated with poor postnatal lung function and subsequently with poor adult lung function through its effects on immune function and the likelihood of exposure to infectious agents. Path (d) represents a biosocial pathway where repeated childhood infection results in adverse educational attainment and lower adult socioeconomic position. Even such a crude model highlights the complex interrelationships and rather arbitrary differentiation between biological and social mechanisms.

Life course epidemiology requires some understanding of the development, maintenance, and ageing of normal biological systems. This is diagrammatically represented for lung function by line A in Fig. 1.2, although it could equally apply to many other continuous physiological measures, such as muscle strength and cognitive function.

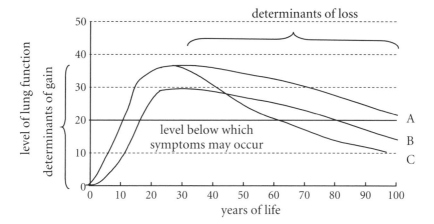

A=normal development and decline; B=exposure in early life reducing lung function potential; C=exposure acting in mid to later life accelerating age related decline

Fig. 1.2 Relative importance of exposures acting across different life course time windows in terms of the natural history of lung function.[11] Modified from Strachan (1997).

Later-acting exposures acting after the developmental period can only affect the timing and rate of decline. An exposure acting in early life may adversely affect lung function during the development period resulting in a diminished physiological reserve without having any appreciable effect on the rate of decline (line B). Alternatively, damage to function from early exposures may not be manifested until they interact with fundamental or pathogenic ageing processes to accelerate decline in function (line C). Early-life exposures may only have a long-term effect on function or disease if they act during a critical period of development, when there are rapid and usually irreversible intrinsic changes toward greater complexity taking place. Sensitive periods are also times of rapid change but in this case there is more scope to modify or even reverse the changes outside the developmental time window.

Given the wide range of exposures over the life course and the potential importance of timing and duration, exposures may affect disease risk in a variety of ways. We have identified four broad models.[11] The 'critical period model' is when an exposure acting during a specific period has lasting or lifelong effects on the structure or function of organs, tissues, and body systems that are not modified in any dramatic way by later experience. This process precipitates the development of chronic disease later in life. It is also known as 'biological programming' or a 'latency model'[31] and is the basis of the 'fetal origins of adult disease' hypothesis.[7] Exposures acting in later life may interact with exposures in early life either to enhance the effects on chronic disease ('synergism') or diminish them ('antagonism'). The second model, called a 'critical period model with later effect modifers', is an extension of the first.

In contrast to the first two models, the 'accumulation of risk model' assumes that risks to health gradually accumulate over the life course although this does not preclude factors acting at sensitive developmental periods having a greater impact. As the number, duration, and severity of exposures increase, there is cumulative damage

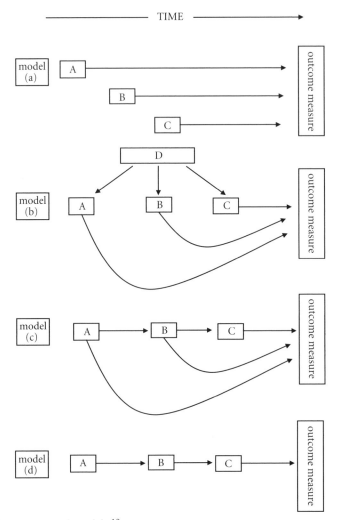

Fig. 1.3 Life course causal models.[12]

to biological systems. Risk exposures may be independent (Fig. 1.3(a)) or clustered (Fig. 1.3(b)); the latter is known as an 'accumulation model with risk clustering'. A common reason for clustering is where exposures all relate to an individual's or family's socioeconomic position in society. Low childhood socioeconomic position is associated, for example, with low birthweight, fewer educational opportunities, more family stress, inadequate diet, and passive smoke exposure.

   A 'chain of risk' model is a special version of the accumulation model and refers to a sequence of linked exposures that lead to impaired function and increased disease risk because one bad experience or exposure leads to another and so on. This has also been described as a 'pathway model'.[31,32] Each exposure in a chain of risk may not only increase the risk of a subsequent exposure (in a probabilistic rather than deterministic way), but may also have an independent 'additive effect' on later function or disease (Fig. 1.3(c)). Alternatively, a 'trigger effect' describes a chain of risk where it is only the final link in the chain that has any marked effect (Fig.1.3(d)).

The life course models described above are not mutually exclusive and may operate simultaneously. It may not be easy to distinguish these models empirically, nor to develop standardized and acceptable methods of combining cumulative exposures. These are just two of a number of complex methodological problems encountered in life course studies.

1.5 Methodological challenges encountered in studying the life course

Longitudinal designs are most appropriate for the study of accumulation of risk particularly where the effects of exposures in later life vary among individuals according to past experience and development. Studies that collect data repeatedly provide the most accurate time sequences of events and intra-individual change over time necessary to test causal hypotheses and to study 'escape' from risk. But longitudinal studies are expensive and do not yield quick returns unless the appropriate prospective data have already been collected. Historical cohort studies, where new data are collected on a population for whom data were collected earlier (perhaps for another purpose), are more cost effective but the detail on early life factors is often restricted to routine data and any information on the intervening years has to be recalled. In any type of study, reliance on recall data is not possible for many exposures of interest (for example, where measurements are needed), memory is often unreliable and details of the timing or duration of exposures are limited.

Testing of life course models presents many methodological challenges beyond study design. Losses to follow-up are an inevitable feature of longitudinal and historical cohort studies and raise the possibility of selection bias, especially if migrants are not traced or have a higher loss rate. If sufficient data have been collected before loss occurs some account may be taken of the likely effects of this bias. There are also analytical challenges associated with modelling repeat observations, hierarchical data, latent exposures, and multiple interactive or small effects. Multilevel,[33] latent growth,[34] Markov, and graphical chain models[35] are some of the techniques being used to deal with these problems. A forthcoming book in this series will address some of these theoretical and methodological challenges and the practicalities of setting up and running life course studies.[36]

A long intervening period between the exposure and outcome raises the distinct possibility that any association may be due to confounding by a third factor. For example, low birthweight may be associated with heart disease, because small babies are more likely to smoke as adults. Birthweight, in this case, may be acting as a surrogate marker for smoking behaviour. Multivariable statistical methods enable the adjustment of risk estimates so that the size of any effect is independent of the confounding factor but are limited if the exposure and confounder are very closely correlated[37] or if there is a difference in the measurement error ('misclassification')[38] of exposure and confounder.[39] The latter may be particularly likely to occur in studies where early life experiences are collected retrospectively whereas current ones are measured or more detailed or in longitudinal studies when better measurement techniques are available at the later follow-ups. One strategy is to break the confounding by testing the association between exposure and disease in a population where the confounding variable is not related to the exposure.[40]

Studying the relationship between exposure and disease is further complicated because of variation in the time between exposure and initiation of the disease process (induction period) or between disease initiation and detection (latency period).[41] This variability makes it difficult to detect the true causal agents and the strength of the association between an exposure and a disease can be diluted or missed if the wrong time frame is measured.[42] Similarly if an exposure has a long latency period, its public health importance will vary according to when in the life course one is exposed. Hence a 30-year induction is important if an individual is young but may be irrelevant if the individual is over 80 years old.

1.6 Conclusions

Research findings on the biological and social risks and protective factors that have long-term effects on adult health and disease risk are scattered throughout the scientific press. The growing number of publications on this research topic necessitated this second edition and reflects the dynamic and rapid development of the field of life course epidemiology. It is our hope that making this important and varied scientific work more accessible will encourage further development of this field and more cross-fertilization with other disciplines that share a life course perspective. The growth of empirical data on fetal and childhood risk factors and interest in life course conceptual models are mutually reinforcing and should lead to the better use of existing life course data and clearer rationales for the collection of new data. Some of the most exciting new work involves the integration of social and biological risk processes, searching for the ways in which social factors leave enduring biological imprints and shape subsequent behaviour. It also includes a growing number of studies investigating the transmission of intergenerational risk. The integration of genetics and developmental biology is a blossoming area of interdisciplinary research. Finally, the closer integration of research and policy should encourage the translation of evidence into action when this may benefit public health. With this in mind, we hope the overview of the evidence given in the following chapters proves stimulating to policy makers as well as scientists and to interested lay readers with a general interest in understanding the health of populations and the pathways to successful ageing and disease prevention.

References

Those marked with an asterisk are especially recommended for further reading.

1 **World Health Organization.** *The World Health Report 2000. Health systems: improving performance.* Geneva: World Health Organization, 2000.

2 **Yusuf S, Reddy S, Ounpuu S, Anand S.** Global burden of cardiovascular diseases. Part I: general considerations, the epidemiologic transition, risk factors, and the impact of urbanization. *Circulation* 2001;**104**:2746–53.

3 **Syme LS.** Rethinking disease: where do we go from here? *Ann Epidemiol* 1996;**6**:463–8.

4 **Magnus P, Beaglehole R, Rodgers A, Bennett S.** The real contribution of the major risk factors to the coronary epidemics—time to end the "only-50%" myth. *Arch Int Med* 2001;**161**:2657–60.

5 **Marmot M, Elliot P.** *Coronary heart disease epidemiology: from aetiology to public health.* Oxford: Oxford Medical Publications, Oxford University Press, 1992.

6 **Barker DJP.** Fetal origins of coronary heart disease. *Br Med J* 1995;**311**:171–4.

*7 **Barker DJP.** *Mothers, babies and health in later life.* Edinburgh: Churchill Livingstone, 1998.

*8 **Forsdahl A.** Momenter til belysning ar den høye dødelighet; Finnmark Fylke. *Tidsskr Nor Lægeforen* 1973;**93**:661–7. Translated and reprinted as Observations throwing light on the high mortality in the county of Finnmark. Is the high mortality today a late effect of very poor living conditions in childhood and adolescence? *Int J Epidemiol* 2002;**31**:302–7.

*9 **Leon DA, Davey Smith G.** Infant mortality, stomach cancer, stroke, and coronary heart disease: ecological analysis. *Br Med J* 2000;**320**:1705–6.

10 **Ben-Shlomo Y, Davey Smith G.** Deprivation in infancy or adult life: which is more important for mortality risk? *Lancet* 1991;**337**:530–4.

*11 **Ben-Shlomo Y, Kuh D.** A life course approach to chronic disease epidemiology: conceptual models, empirical challenges, and interdisciplinary perspectives. *Int J Epidemiol* 2002;**31**:285–93.

*12 **Kuh D, Ben-Shlomo Y, Lynch J, Hallqvist J, Power C.** A glossary for life course epidemiology. *J Epidemiol Community Health* 2003;**57**:778–83.

13 **Aboderin I, Kalache A, Ben-Shlomo Y, Lynch JW, Yajnik CS, Kuh D** *et al.* *Life course perspectives on coronary heart disease, stroke and diabetes: key issues and implications for policy and research.* Geneva: World Health Organization, 2002.

*14 **Kuh D, Hardy R.** *A life course approach to women's health.* Oxford: Oxford University Press, 2002.

15 **Bassey EJ, Aihie Sayer A, Cooper C.** Musculoskeletal ageing: muscle strength, osteoporosis and osteoarthritis. In Kuh D, Hardy R, eds. *A life course approach to women's health*, Oxford: Oxford University Press, 2002:141–60.

16 **Schooling M, Kuh D.** A life course perspective on women's health behaviours. In Kuh D, Hardy R, eds. *A life course approach to women's health*, Oxford: Oxford University Press, 2002:279–303.

17 **Marks NF, Ashleman K.** Life course influences on women's social relationships at midlife. In Kuh D, Hardy R, eds. *A life course approach to women's health*. Oxford: Oxford University Press, 2002:255–78.

18 **Power C, Parsons T.** Overweight and obesity from a life course perspective. In Kuh D, Hardy R, eds. *A life course approach to women's health*. Oxford: Oxford University Press, 2002:304–38.

19 **Rich-Edwards J.** A life course approach to women's reproductive health. In Kuh D, Hardy R, eds. *A life course approach to women's health.* Oxford: Oxford University Press, 2002:23–43.

20 **Hardy R, Kuh D.** Menopause and gynaecological disorders: a life course perspective. In Kuh D, Hardy R, eds. *A life course approach to women's health.* Oxford: Oxford University Press, 2002:64–85.

21 **dos Santos Silva I, De Stavola B.** Breast cancer aetiology: where do we go from here? In Kuh D, Hardy R, eds. *A life course approach to women's health.* Oxford: Oxford University Press, 2002:44–63.

22 **Kwong WY, Wild AE, Roberts P, Willis AC, Fleming TP.** Maternal undernutrition during the preimplantation period of rat development causes blastocyst abnormalities and programming of postnatal hypertension. *Development* 2000;**127**:4195–202.

*23 **Seckl J.** Physiologic programming of the fetus. *Emerging Concepts Perinat Endocrinol* 1998;**25**:939–62.

24 **Singhal A, Cole TJ, Lucas A.** Early nutrition in preterm infants and later blood pressure: two cohorts after randomised trials. *Lancet* 2001;**357**:413–19.

25 **Singhal A, Fewtrell M, Cole T, Lucas A.** Low nutrient intake and early growth for later insulin resistance in adolescents born preterm. *Lancet* 2003;**361**:1089–97.

*26 Leon D, Walt G. Poverty, inequality and health: an international perspective. Oxford: Oxford University Press, 2001.

27 **Independent Inquiry into Inequalities in Health.** *Report of the independent inquiry into inequalities in health.* London: The Stationery Office, 1998.

28 Halfon N, Hochstein M. Life course health development: an integrated framework for developing health, policy, and research. *Milbank Q* 2002;**80**:433–79.

29 Hallqvist J, Lynch J, Bartley M, Blance D. Accumulation, critical periods and social mobility: evidence from SHEEP study. *Soc Sci Med* (in press).

30 Hertzman C. The biological embedding of early experience and its effects on health in adulthood. *Ann NY Acad Sci* 1995;**896**:85–95.

31 Hertzman C, Power C, Matthews S, Manor O. Using an interactive framework of society and life course to explain self-rated health in early adulthood. *Soc Sci Med* 2001;**53**:1575–85.

*32 Keating D, Hertzman C. *Developmental health and the wealth of nations: social, biological and educational dynamics.* New York: Guilford Press, 1999.

33 Goldstein H. *Multilevel statistical models.* London: Edward Arnold, 1995.

34 Muthen B. Latent variable mixture modeling. In Marcoulides G, Schumacker R, eds. *New developments and techniques in structural equation modeling.* Mahwah NJ: Lawrence Erlbaum, 2001:1–33.

35 Whittaker J. *Graphical models in applied multivariate statistics.* Chichester: Wiley, 1990.

36 Pickles A, Maughan B, Wadsworth MEJ. *Methods, theory and analysis in life course research.* Oxford: Oxford University Press, (in preparation).

37 Davey Smith G, Phillips A. Declaring independence: why we should be cautious. *J Epidemiol Community Health* 1990;**44**:257–8.

38 Leon DA. Failed or misleading adjustment for confounding. *Lancet* 1993;**342**:479–81.

39 Phillips AN, Davey Smith G. How independent are "independent" effects? Relative risk estimation when correlated exposures are measured imprecisely. *J Clin Epidemiol* 1991;**44**:1223–31.

40 Davey Smith G. Confounding in epidemiological studies: why 'independent effects' may not be all they seem. *Br Med J* 1992;**305**:757–9.

41 Rothman KJ. *Epidemiology. An introduction.* Oxford: Oxford University Press, 2002.

42 Rothman KJ. Induction and latent periods. *Am J Epidemiol* 1981;**114**:253–9.

Chapter 2

The life course and adult chronic disease: an historical perspective with particular reference to coronary heart disease

Diana Kuh and George Davey Smith

In the first half of the twentieth century there was considerable public health and epidemiological interest in the idea that early life experiences influenced adult vitality and mortality risk. This was complementary to ideas that emerged in the biological and psychological sciences at that time. A key feature of the scientific debate was the relative contribution of the early environment compared with heredity. During the inter-war period the 'epidemics' of coronary heart disease and lung cancer shifted attention to the aetiology of specific chronic diseases. The potential of the environment at different life stages to modify an individual's constitution and disease susceptibility was recognized but interest grew in the possible effects of adult physiological function and habits and the socioeconomic environment on the development of chronic disease.

In the early postwar period adult risk factors were emphasized because of the natural interests of the cardiologists and physiologists who initiated cardiovascular epidemiology, the use of the prospective cohort to study disease incidence and the need to develop preventive strategies to a pressing public health problem. The re-emergence of interest in early life factors from the 1970s stemmed first from the need to understand the natural history of these adult risk factors and secondly, and more importantly, from the inability of the lifestyle model to explain social and geographical variations in chronic disease risk. Epidemiological research is increasingly concerned with the independent and combined effects of early life and later life influences on chronic disease risk within the broad context of a revival in interdisciplinary developmental science.

2.1 Introduction

This chapter traces the twentieth century development of the idea that experiences early in the life course may have long-term effects on the development of chronic disease. This may be either because they occur at some critical period of development or because they contribute to a more gradual process of risk accumulation (see Chapter 1). Why, in postwar chronic disease epidemiology, were these ideas eclipsed by the adult lifestyle model and why have they re-emerged recently in epidemiology and related disciplines?

2.2 Child health, adult vitality, and mortality risk: the 'generation effect'

Between 1851 and 1940 there was a dramatic decline in all-cause mortality rates of children and young adults under 45 years of age in the UK, mainly due to the decline in mortality from infectious diseases that were common at younger ages. Despite these improvements the widespread concern at the beginning of the twentieth century about a possible deterioration in national fitness, which might impede economic or military success, focused public health attention on infant mortality, which had shown no signs of improvement during the nineteenth century.[1,2] While bacteriological research dominated public health in the first four decades of this century[3] the idea that early life conditions and experiences affected adult health was a component of the prevailing public health model in the UK and USA.[4] To UK public health officials it was evident that fitness and general vitality depended on the development of a stock of good health in early life, itself dependent on adequate care and nutrition in childhood. According to George Newman writing in 1914 when he was Chief Medical Officer to the Board of Education, 'recent progess has shown a) that the health of the adult is dependent upon the health of the child ... [and] ... b) that the health of the child is dependent upon the health of the infant and its mother' (p. 16).[5]

These ideas and the research studies that were undertaken to support them, discussed in more detail elsewhere,[6–9] lay behind the development of infant and child health services in the UK and USA. These social reforms were seen as misguided by the eugenicists such as Karl Pearson who believed that good health was inherited rather than nurtured by a good environment. He argued that interfering with natural selection by adapting the environment to man would lead to a British race of 'degenerate and feeble stock' (p. 29).[10]

Early cohort analysis, applied to the age-specific UK death rates for the period 1841–1925, revealed the existence of a 'generation effect',[11,12] in that the mortality risk of each successive generation was found to be lower at all ages (see Fig. 2.1). The medical scientists who published the later paper[12] interpreted the generation effect as evidence of the importance of early environmental factors for adult health and used it to refute Pearson's concern about national degeneration. To Kermack and his colleagues, their findings suggested that 'the expectation of life was determined by the conditions which existed during a child's earlier years' and that 'a good environment in childhood builds up a stronger constitution and raises the standard of physique' (p. 703)[12] and that this had a decisive effect at all later ages.

Kermack and colleagues also detected a cohort effect using Scottish and Swedish mortality data but the relative mortalities for Sweden did not show the same simple regularities as those for the other countries. The generation effect was discussed widely in the 1930s although other medical scientists were more cautious about the overwhelming importance of the childhood years. For example, Major Greenwood, in his valedictory address for Pearson, argued that 'persons over the age of 40 need not abandon hope that social and hygienic betterments introduced after their school days may

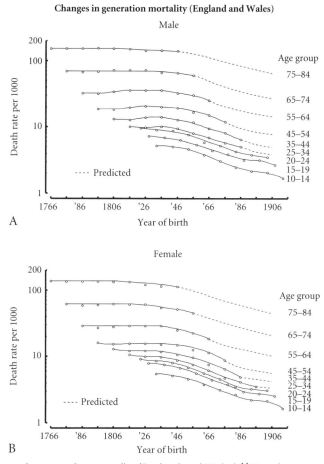

Fig. 2.1 Changes in generation mortality (England and Wales).[11] Based on age-specific death rates 1841–1925.

increase their expectations of life' (p. 706). In the discussion George Yule commented that the more interesting question was the 'relative influences on the mortality of any age group of a) the conditions to which they had been earlier subjected, especially at the beginning of life and of b) the contemporaneous conditions' (p. 710).[13]

2.3 Developmental critical periods and the early origins of constitution

The notion that early life factors affected adult health by modifying the constitution and altering vitality clearly underlay the studies of child nutrition[14] and child health[15] in the 1930s, with the emphasis on the accumulation of environmental effects on health throughout childhood. It informed the development of paediatric epidemiology, with Dugald Baird and colleagues in Aberdeen[16–18] recognizing the importance of early life development for the reproductive success of women. Meanwhile, in the biological sciences,[19–22] psychoanalysis,[23] and behavioural psychology[24,25] the idea of developmental critical periods was gaining ground, that is, environmental insults or lack of appropriate stimuli during critical periods at the embryonic stage,[19,21,22,26–28] or during infancy[23–25,29,30] could have long-term effects on physical or mental development. Developmental scientists in the inter-war period generally saw development as an invariant sequence of developmental stages.[31] Change was cumulative and usually irreversible. The role of the environment was to provide the initial stimuli and appropriate opportunities for growth and maturation to unfold. Once maturity was reached systems were unable to be manipulated.

Charles Stockard, Professor of Anatomy at Cornell University Medical College and an experimental embryologist, studied how growth and development, particularly in the prenatal period, could be modified by a change in environmental conditions. From his animal experiments he concluded in 1927 that there are 'critical moments in the origin and development of organs when they suffer acutely from an unfavourable change in developmental conditions, and there are somewhat passive periods when the given organ may be only slightly affected by the same unfavourable conditions' (pp. 27–8).[21] He went on to argue that 'the prenatal period is probably the most important in determining all later constitutional conditions since at this time the actual gross body form and structure is being laid down and any environmental peculiarity may exert a marked influence on the course of development … The prenatal stage, although … the one on which all subsequent life stages depend, has been largely neglected and is almost unknown to the majority of physicians' (p. 157).[26] In the early postwar period, the idea of a developmental critical period became a central concept in research into animal behaviour,[32,33] growth,[34–36] and psychosocial development.[37–39]

The reference by Kermack and his colleagues to constitution and physique was part of a wider revival of interest in these subjects in the inter-war period.[40–44] The notion of constitution was accorded many different meanings but, in essence, it referred to the total nature of the organism and, in particular, to those intrinsic characteristics that determined an individual's reaction, successful or unsuccessful, to the stress of the environment. Some, like Pearson, maintained that a person's constitution was dependent solely on genetic factors.[43] Others took what we would now describe as a life course approach.[40,44] For example, George Draper divided the lifespan into five great epochs: fetal life, infancy, childhood, the central span of adult life (marked by the two main dividing points, puberty and the climacteric), and the final stage of life. 'It is probable', speculated Draper, 'that the results of an individual's reaction to environment in one phase of growth has an important bearing on the next. This is especially true of the first, second and third stages during which the skeleton is forming and solidifying in its fixed condition' (p. 27).

Raymond Pearl, referring to the work of the early embryologists,[45] saw constitution as the outcome of an interaction between an individual's genetic make-up and environmental forces acting 'during development primarily, but also in some degree throughout the duration of the life of the individual' (p. 36). Thus the constitution of the individual at any given moment is in part the resultant of his past history—the diseases he has had, the vicissitudes of embryonic development through which he has passed, and so on' (p. 34).[44] Concern about the health of army recruits in the Second World War caused Anthony Ciocco and colleagues to compare information on over 200 men from the records of school physical examinations and the medical information available from local Draft Boards in Washington County, Maryland. They commented that 'disease in adulthood is often brought about by the cumulative effects over a long period of time of many pathological conditions, many incidents, some of which take place and are even perceived in infancy' (p. 2374).[46]

The idea that disease episodes left permanent scars was not new, the long-term heart sequelae of rheumatic fever, for example, were already recognized.[47,48] There was also interest in whether other infectious diseases predisposed sufferers to the subsequent development of arteriosclerosis,[49,50] presaging the more recent debate on the role of infectious diseases in coronary heart disease.[51] In 1921, Ophuls,[50] a pathologist at Stanford University Medical School, building on ideas of French clinicians in the nineteenth century, had linked the development of arteriosclerosis in 500 necropsies to chronic streptococcal infections recorded in clinical records. The first recorded infection usually dated back to childhood or early adult life. 'At that time,' he commented, 'the body as a whole and the arteries in particular appear most susceptible to the influence of infections of this character' (p. 36). Analysis of mortality statistics led others to suggest a link between tuberculosis and the later development of cancer[52] or to stress the importance of diseases in childhood on later ageing. [53,54]

In a number of studies of constitution and disease, detailed measurements of body build were taken in order to classify the somatological variations into broad categories and to examine their relationship with different disease types.[40,43,55–59] Pearl and Ciccio, in a study of somatological differences associated with heart disease[55] published a photograph in 1934 to illustrate the differences between the cardiac and the non-cardiac individual (Fig. 2.2). In fact, this study found that the most significant differences were the greater body weight and functional deficiency of the chest in the

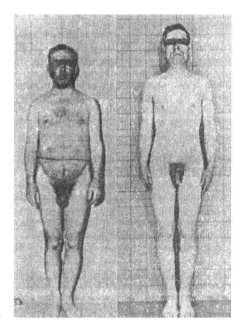

Fig. 2.2 Cardiac and non-cardiac individual.

cardiac group compared with the non-cardiac group and the authors concluded that these were 'not innate constitutional differences ... but rather due to accumulation of body fat from relative over-eating and lack of physical exercise' (p. 711).[55] The relationships of various chronic diseases to overweightness and short stature were also being revealed by studies of life insurance data.[60–63] The relative importance attached to adult lifestyle and constitution (genetic or acquired in early life) was beginning to change.

2.4 The waning of the generation effect and the growing interest in adult lifestyle and chronic disease

Public health interest in early life determinants of susceptibility to adult disease waned as attention was drawn to the poor health of adults that occurred despite the improvements in child health. Predictions by Derrick[11] made on the basis of the 'generation effect' (see Fig. 2.1) suggested that death rates in middle-age would begin to fall sharply as the cohorts who had experienced dramatic improvements in survival during childhood reached this age. These predictions failed to be confirmed (see Fig. 2.3) and concern in the UK and USA at the lack of improvements in middle-age life expectancy, raised during the 1920s and 1930s,[64,65] became a major focus of social medicine and public health. Increases in the numbers of deaths attributed to heart disease and cancer were observed. While some of this increase was the inevitable result of an ageing population, this could not explain the upward trends in age-specific rates.[66–76] The degree to which these increases were real or due to changes in cause-of-death coding, changing diagnostic fashions, or improved diagnostic methods, was, and still is, much discussed.[77–83] The reversal of declining mortality rates among the middle-aged population that occurred between 1920 and 1940 convinced contemporary[84] and later[85] observers that real increases in some causes of death did occur. For those influenced by Pearson's arguments the worsening trends in the middle-age death rates were a sign of reduced vitality of the population caused by genetically weaker members of the population surviving childhood. Newman, by then Chief Medical Officer at the Ministry of Health, denied there was any evidence of national deterioration[82] and continued to emphasize the key role of infant and child health. In contrast, the establishment of the American Society for the Control of Cancer as early as 1913 and the American Heart Association in 1922 reflected widespread concern in the USA about the threat posed by these diseases.[65] Calls for preventive programmes of 'adult hygiene' were voiced.[86]

The 'epidemics' of coronary heart disease and lung cancer shifted attention away from acute infectious disease[87] and gave impetus to the concept of host, environment, and agent, as it was already apparent that interacting factors influenced chronic disease risk. Demonstration of differential mortality risks by social class and sex[88,89] and geographical region[90] suggested that potentially modifiable environmental factors were responsible for the increased death rates.[65] Early research suggested that the physical labour of working men shortened life expectancy[91] and increased the risk of coronary thrombosis[92] and arteriosclerosis[93] through blood pressure elevation. Tobacco and alcohol consumption also shortened life expectancy[94,95] and had adverse effects on physiological function in ways that might cause long-term damage to the heart or its arteries.[96,97] Many were unconvinced of the harmful effects of tobacco[73,98] or alcohol and the research debate was clouded with moral overtones.[96,99] Those involved in

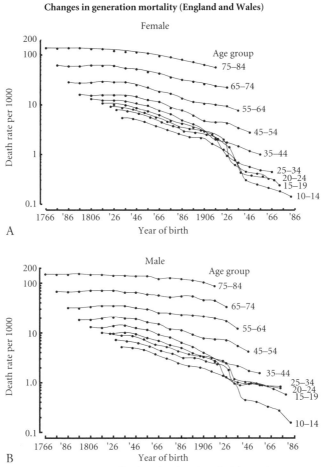

Fig. 2.3 Changes in generation mortality (England and Wales). Based on age-specific death rates 1841–2000.[219]

the development of social medicine, such as John Ryle, were particularly interested in aspects of the social and economic environment associated with chronic disease.[100] Some blamed the stress of living and working in the modern era for the rising rates of heart disease.[65,101] Generally attention focused on the contemporary environment although several observers who speculated that the considerable hardships suffered by recruits during the First World War might have caused the subsequent increase in heart disease were more concerned with the life course.[102,103]

2.5 Atherosclerosis and the emergence of coronary heart disease

When the dominant view of arteriosclerosis as an intrinsic process of ageing came under attack in the 1940s,[93,104] the possible importance of earlier infections was reported but not followed up. Rather the search for aetiological factors focused on the adult environment. A review of chemical, experimental, and pathologic studies of atherosclerosis in 1934 concluded that 'the pathogenesis of atherosclerosis of the aorta is principally dependent on age, cholesterol metabolism and blood pressure' (p. 684).[105] This consideration of the possible role of cholesterol metabolism in humans built on the knowledge gained from animal experiments regarding diet and atherosclerosis, which had been ongoing from the turn of the century.[106] Rosenthal reported that evidence from 28 studies of the relationship of diet and blood pressure to atherosclerosis undertaken all over the world among different ethnic and racial groups showed that 'in no race for which a high cholesterol intake (in the form of eggs, butter and milk) and fat intake are recorded is atherosclerosis absent' (pp. 493–4).[105] Early clinical investigations showed that those with diseases associated with serious lipid disorders, such as diabetes and hypothyroidism, had a higher risk of atherosclerosis and coronary thrombosis.[104,107]

The emergence of coronary heart disease as an important cause of death in middle-aged men helped to define the territory of a new specialty of cardiology.[108] Before the twentieth century myocardial infarction and coronary thrombosis were generally seen as terminal events[106] and reports of their occurrence were rare. Clinicians' interest in coronary thrombosis was stimulated by the work of James Herrick, a Chicago physician, which linked the physiological properties of the living heart (as measured by the newly invented electrocardiograph) to various clinical symptoms, such as chest pain and breathlessness and, subsequently, to underlying organic disorder.[109,110]

Paul Dudley White and Samuel Levine, two of the first US cardiologists, used their detailed clinical records as a basis for some of the first aetiological studies of coronary thrombosis.[92,111] The importance of hypertension, a natural candidate for investigation because it was already recognized as a marker of underlying arterial or renal disease, was demonstrated by the early clinical studies. This supported observations from life insurance companies showing that even moderate elevations of blood pressure raised disease risk. It was succeeded by a series of follow-up studies of army personnel by White and colleagues, which showed the prognostic importance of transient hypertension for cardiovascular risk (see, for example, Reference 112). Early clinical studies also implicated lack of exercise in the development of coronary disease risk.[111] Findings were contradictory with respect to smoking and alcohol consumption.[111,113,114]

In keeping with the theories of the day, some of the early studies also investigated the role of early life factors in the development of coronary thrombosis. Muscular mesomorphs were found to be prone to coronary heart disease,[92,111] pointing to a role for constitution. However, there were no indications that those who suffered poor growth or infections in childhood had a raised risk. Indeed, early clinical studies found that coronary heart disease patients reported fewer of the common infectious diseases[92,111] and a study of the armed services suggested that young men destined to die from coronary heart disease had, compared with their controls, been physically early developers and had mothers who had been in better condition during pregnancy.[115]

2.5.1 Early postwar cohort studies of coronary heart disease

The early cardiologists like White sowed the seeds of a new epidemiological approach to the study of heart disease, which used the new cardiac technology and biochemical tests of the laboratory to measure the prevalence, incidence, and causes of heart disease in the general population.[116] The Second World War delayed putting this idea into practice but the international and national institutions that were put into place after the war served an important function in the organization and funding of large epidemiological studies. The creation of the World Health Organization in 1948 marked a new era in international cooperation and made worldwide research collaboration more possible. In the USA, the reorganization of the National Institutes of Health (NIH)[117] and of public voluntary health organizations, such as the American Heart Association,[118] encouraged greater emphasis on chronic disease and large-scale funding of preventive medical research. After the Second World War adult chronic diseases became a major public health concern because of the ageing of the population, the general public insistence that efforts should made to prevent all forms of illness and disability and the fact that mortality rates from cancer and coronary heart disease rose rapidly after the war, particularly among men during the most productive stage of their working life.[71,119] They were now seen as a preventable problem and there was widespread belief in the power of medical research to deal as successfully with the new diseases of affluence as it had done with the infectious diseases. The decline in the latter and the obvious improvement in child health also encouraged more emphasis to be placed on adult chronic disease.

The clinicians, such as White and Levine, and laboratory scientists, such as Ancel Keys, who initiated American cardiovascular epidemiology were the driving forces behind the postwar cohort studies of heart disease in populations of healthy men in the USA[120–125] and elsewhere.[126] They were naturally more interested in the pathological precursors to coronary thrombosis rather than the social and occupational factors that might underlie them. This was reflected in a strong attachment to the lipid theory of coronary heart disease, extensively reviewed in the 1950s[107,127] and systematically developed by Keys, Director of the Laboratory of Physiological Hygiene at the University of Minnesota, in the postwar period.[128,129] Drawing on the aetiological clues from the inter-war studies, the Framingham study[122] investigated the importance of various diseases (such as diabetes and hypothyroidism), hypertension, overweight, a number of personal habits (dietary intake, alcohol consumption, smoking and physical activity), and physique as sources of risk for coronary heart disease. Framingham was chosen as the location for the classic prospective coronary heart disease study because a successful prospective community-based investigation of tuberculosis had been carried out there in the early part of the twentieth century.[130] Because tuberculosis was a disease in which the adult illness was often seen as the outcome of infection in childhood, long latency periods were involved and many factors related to susceptibility were seen as key in the expression of the actual disease. Thus the methods of chronic disease epidemiology were developed with respect to a disease of clear infectious origin.[131]

In the UK, clinical awareness of coronary thrombosis investment occurred later than in the USA and funding of population studies, usually by the Medical Research Council (MRC), was more modest. Richard Doll and Bradford Hill's prospective study of 40 000 doctors,[132–134] showed that smoking was a risk factor for lung cancer, coronary heart disease, and chronic bronchitis. This study gave great impetus both to the prospective study as a powerful epidemiological tool and to the possibility that ways of life, modifiable by changes in personal behaviour, might be behind the poor health of middle-aged men and women. An analysis by Jerry Morris of a long series of post-mortem records from the London hospital revealed no increase in coronary atheroma over the previous 40 years, while there had been an apparent increase in coronary thrombosis.[72,84] This caused him to question the traditional view that atheroma underlay thrombosis and coronary occlusion and directed his attention to the thrombotic processes that precipitated the disease. As a strong supporter of social medicine he was particularly interested in the social and economic factors that might have caused the rise in disease and less interested in the more proximal factors, which he called the 'pathological precursors', such as cholesterol and blood pressure. The occupational studies by Morris and his colleagues confirmed that coronary heart disease was on the increase.[135–137] Contrary to the findings of earlier studies, they showed that men in jobs that demanded more physical activity (bus conductors and postmen) had a lower incidence of coronary heart disease and a lower early-case fatality than those in less active occupations (bus drivers and civil servants in sedentary grades). At the same time other UK investigators expanded their community surveys of respiratory disease to include studies of coronary heart disease and from the late 1960s the MRC and other bodies provided more extensive funding of prospective cohorts.[138–142]

The Framingham Study and the Doll and Hill study have been described as the two 'intellectual levers' of modern epidemiology.[143] Despite initial differences in approach among UK and US researchers, a general consensus gradually emerged about the classic risk factors connected with adult lifestyle that raised individual risk and in some cases population risk, of the most common adult chronic diseases.[144]

2.6 Changing role of early life factors as explanations for adult health and chronic disease in the postwar period

In the first 25 years after the war, little attention was given to early life factors or to a consideration of the life course in the aetiology of coronary heart disease. Although a full appraisal of physique was carried out on most members of the Framingham study, few interesting results emerged[145] and it was adult body weight, rather than the more long-term aspects of body build that later became a classic risk factor. Sidney Abraham and his colleagues at the Public Health Service had the foresight to investigate whether the effects of overweight differed if it was lifelong or acquired in adult life. In their follow-up of children who participated in the morbidity studies in Haggerston, Maryland, in the 1920s,[146] the highest rates for hypertensive vascular disease and cardiovascular renal disease were among overweight adults who were below-average weight children.

In the UK, Morris[72,147] did consider the importance of intergenerational influences, programming, and childhood precursors of adult disease. There was a possibility that new cohorts reaching middle-age might be qualitatively different from their predecessors in that 'they have survived, or been preserved through, hazards that would have previously been mortal. Consequently they may be in some way constitutionally more liable than their coevals of forty years ago to succumb to diseases that are prevalent, including coronary heart-disease' (p. 72).[72] A decade later Geoffrey Rose echoed the same theme after a small study of familial patterns in ischaemic heart disease revealed that those who in adult life suffered from the disease came from families who had experienced excess mortality, particularly in infancy. One interpretation discussed by Rose was that these individuals came from 'a constitutionally weaker stock, more liable to succumb to a variety of diseases.' (p. 80)[148]

Morris[72] suggested that methodological problems inherent in life course research hindered development of this approach. Nevertheless, well-designed life course studies were conducted on other aspects of adult health, shedding light, for example, on the long-term effects of famine exposure *in utero* on mental performance[149] and infant respiratory illness on adult respiratory morbidity (see below). Contextual factors also inhibited investigation of a possible link between childhood experience and adult disease. For example, in the UK a number of organizational and administrative changes in state health and welfare services broke the pre-war public health connection between child and adult health. Coronary heart disease appeared more prevalent at the time among the upper social groups whose early experiences were likely to have been more favourable than those of their lower social class peers. Lower child mortality had been accompanied by evidence of better child health and reductions in social inequalities, of which Morris and others were well aware,[82,150] and did not suggest that the origins of adult disease lay in early life. On a practical level, individual prospective studies could not be applied to the whole life course without an unacceptable time lag; even the adult studies had to plan a long follow-up to get sufficient cases for analysis.

2.6.1 The natural history of chronic disease and its risk factors

The difficulties in changing adult risk factors and questions about the natural history of respiratory and cardiovascular diseases and cancers from the late 1950s caused researchers to look again at the childhood years. In his presidential address to the Royal Society of Medicine in 1969, Donald Reid suggested that 'the true beginnings' of chronic bronchitis lay in early life, that 'the bronchitic child is father to the bronchitic man' (p. 315).[151] His hypothesis, based on earlier retrospective research[152,153] and cohort mortality trends in lower respiratory illness, stimulated longitudinal research. This included a follow-up study of the 1946 UK birth cohort that showed respiratory symptoms in early adult life were associated with respiratory illness before the age of 2 years.[154,155] In cancer epidemiology, birth characteristics were linked to childhood cancers[156] and cohort effects[157] and long-term latent effects of early reproductive[158] or occupational exposures on adult cancers were recognized. Even so, it was not until 1990 that Trichopoulos[159] hypothesized that the origins of breast cancer lay *in utero*.

Increasing attention was paid to atherosclerosis in young people after it was found that over three-quarters of young soldiers killed in the Korean war had gross evidence of coronary disease.[160] Fatty streaks were present in the aortas of three year olds[161] and appeared in the coronary arteries in the second decade of life[162] and in a later study these were found to relate to measures of cholesterol taken before death.[163] Longitudinal research revealed that blood pressure and serum cholesterol 'tracked' through childhood and adolescence, in that children maintained their percentile position in the distribution (see, for example, References 164–168). Atherosclerosis from a paediatric perspective[169] meant the encouragement of healthy lifestyles in childhood, such as lower fat consumption, which might directly inhibit early atherosclerosis and, to the extent that behaviours were maintained throughout life, indirectly reduce adult risk by improving adult risk-factor profile. In more directly pathological terms, Osborn[170] argued that artificial infant feeding led to arterial damage but these ideas were not taken up at the time.[8]

2.6.2 Early deprivation and adult chronic disease

The inability of the lifestyle model to explain social and geographical variations in chronic disease risk also encouraged others to consider the possible effects of early deprivation on adult disease. Since the late 1970s and 1980s there has been a growing body of evidence, discussed in later chapters, to suggest that poor living conditions in early life, and more specifically, poor growth, undernutrition, and infectious disease, increase the risk of adult cardiovascular and respiratory diseases. This work originated mainly from David Barker and his research team at the MRC Environmental Epidemiology Unit (reviewed in References 171–174), but also from the Norwegian researcher Anders Forsdahl,[175–178] the maturing UK cohorts,[154,155,179–181] and studies of adult height and chronic disease.[182–186]

Forsdahl argued that 'whereas the weaker of the cohort die in infancy, the fit survive and carry with them a lifelong vunerability' and suggested that 'various types of injury to health may add up so as to cause an increased risk of early ageing and death' (p. 95).[176] He thereby emphasized the accumulation of risk over the life course. In contrast, Barker's model of biological programming *in utero* and infancy (see Chapters 1 and 15), which he tested on a series of imaginative follow-ups of historical cohorts, is a development of the longstanding concept of critical periods in the biological sciences. In emphasizing the role of fetal undernutrition and studying body proportions[173] Barker drew on the findings of earlier postwar research on nutrition and growth, which had been previously neglected by those studying chronic adult disease.[34,35] Others, drawing on similar material,[36] emphasized the role of childhood nutrition.[187]

2.7 Revival of a life course perspective in understanding disease patterns

The epidemiological revival of interest in the childhood origins of adult disease began with ecological analyses of official mortality statistics. Although reminiscent of early cohort analysis in the 1930s, the focus was on correlations between adult mortality rates and infant rather than child mortality rates. Further application of a life course perspective to understand variations in disease risk in populations over time, across countries, and between social groups revives the traditional epidemiological concern with population trends and differences in specific diseases.[188,189] Demographers have continued to investigate whether cohorts exposed during childhood or adolescence to high death rates or harsh conditions in Sweden,[190,191] Italy,[192] Germany,[193] France,[194,195] the USA,[196,197] and Japan[198] subsequently experienced a mortality advantage or disadvantage. Similarly, research has investigated the relationships between adult mortality and height[199] and body size[200] in historical populations. This body of work has placed the research by Kermack and his colleagues in its long-term context and emphasized the importance of historical and geographical specificity. For example, the US studies have drawn attention to the changing impact across successive cohorts of growing up in urban and rural areas on later mortality risk.[196,197] The Swedish studies[190,191] provide support for the early disease environment rather than the standard of nutrition being the major mechanism linking early conditions to later mortality.[201] Studies that link infant mortality to old-age mortality[191] and childhood mortality to mortality in early rather than late adult life[192] may give clues to the timing of causal factors and their underlying mechanisms. The study of population disease trends and differences will be furthered by interdisciplinary research of specific diseases within their historical, cultural, and social context, modelling the effects of changing risk factors simultaneously rather than looking at each one in turn.

2.8 Revival of interdisciplinary developmental science

In contrast to chronic disease epidemiology, which was dominated by the adult lifestyle model in the postwar period, the early life paradigm dominated postwar psychology and was not seriously questioned until the 1960s.[39] Some effects of early life experiences were found to be reversible or at least more modifiable than early theories assumed and dependent on the nature of the subsequent environment. A lifespan perspective in developmental psychology emerged in the 1970s, partly as a response to this controversy, encouraging some to study developmental processes and adaptations to environmental challenges in middle- and old-age.[202] Others, like Rutter,[203] maintained their interest in continuity between childhood and adult life but argued that 'simplistic concepts of immutable effects need to be put aside and replaced by more dynamic notions of the continuing interplay over time between intrinsic and extrinsic influences on individual development' (p. 24). The modern revival of the life course perspective in human biology[204,205] and anthropology[206] links early development to ageing and emphasizes how early environmental factors (as well as later factors) influence human form and function at every age.

In recent years developmental scientists have called for an integrated, unified framework for the study of development,[207] bringing together psychological, cognitive, and biological research on developmental processes from conception to death.[208] The emphasis has shifted from ideas of homogeneity, continuity, and universality of developmental processes prevalent in the 1930s to heterogeneity, discontinuity, and context-specific development. The search is for the range of plasticity and its age-associated changes and constraints.[209] The focus is now more on variability in human development—its extent, its causes and its long-term consequences for function, disease, and ageing.[210] The maturing birth cohorts in the UK[211] and New Zealand,[212] the US child developmental studies,[213–216] and the revitalization of many historical cohorts allow us to test empirically early life and life course hypotheses about the development of adult health and disease on individuals with a variety of experiences and exposures.

2.9 Conclusions

In the first half of the twentieth century the importance of the life course in health and disease was generally recognized through the notion of constitution; controversy centred on the relative influence of nurture and nature. Pearson attributed long-term constitutional vulnerability to hereditary factors because social reforms prevented the weak from dying in infancy, whereas others attributed such vulnerability to both genetic and environmental factors. In the modern revival of interest in constitution it was the early environmental conditions that were seen to determine constitutional susceptibility to adult disease. In the more recent debate Forsdahl emphasized poor childhood living conditions, particularly if followed by later affluence, as leading to an accumulation of disease risk; for Barker undernutrition during critical periods of development remains the most important environmental risk factor. This chapter has shown that both ideas, risk accumulation over the life course and developmental critical periods were discussed in the scientific literature throughout the twentieth century. The novel development in the current debate has been Barker's biological programming hypothesis, which links differential development during critical periods to adult chronic disease risk. Barker's hypothesis on the fetal origins of cardiovascular disease was presented as a direct challenge to the adult lifestyle model of chronic disease. It acted as a catalyst to the revival of a life course approach in chronic disease epidemiology[217] and public health. This approach shares Barker's interest in fetal influences but emphasized from the start the importance of the postnatal social and physical environment, the psychological as well as physical developmental processes, and their interaction with later life social and biological factors in the development of disease risk. Increasingly the role of genetic factors and the interaction of genetic and environmental factors on developmental processes associated with adult chronic disease risk are being investigated. Conceptually, a life course approach is broad enough to encompass genetic, early life, and later life risk factors although operationalizing and testing life course hypotheses is challenging.[218] It remains to be seen whether the recent revival of a life course perspective in epidemiology will help avoid polarizations, for example, of nature versus nurture, fetal growth versus adult lifestyle, social versus biological factors and materialist versus psychosocial explanations, that beset the investigation of models of chronic disease causation over the twentieth century.

References

Those marked with an asterisk are especially recommended for further reading.

1 **Great Britain Parliamentary Papers.** *Report of the Inter-departmental Committee on Physical Deterioration. Vol. I: Report and appendix Cmnd. 2175; Vol. II: List of witnesses and minutes of evidence, Cmnd. 2210; Vol. III: Appendix and general index, Cmnd. 2186.* London: His Majesty's Stationery Office, 1904.

2 **Newman G.** *Infant mortality: a social problem.* London: Methuen, 1906.

3 **Rosen G.** *A history of public health.* New York: MD Publications, 1958.

4 **Fisher I.** *Report on national vitality, its wastes and conservation.* National Conservation Commission, Bulletin 30 of the Committee of One Hundred on National Health. Washington: Government Printing Office, 1909.

5 **Newman G.** *Annual report for 1913 of Chief Medical Officer of the Board of Education, Cmnd 7330.* London: His Majesty's Stationery Office, 1914.

6 **Kuh DJL.** *Assessing the influence of early life on adult health.* Unpublished PhD thesis, University of London, 1993.

*7 **Kuh D, Davey Smith G.** When is mortality risk determined? Historical insights into a current debate. *Soc Hist Med* 1993;**6**:101–23.

8 **Davey Smith G, Kuh D.** Does early nutrition affect later health? Views from the 1930s and 1980s. In Smith D, ed. *The history of nutrition in the twentieth century. Studies in the social history of medicine.* London: Routledge, 1997:214–237.

9 **Davey Smith G, Kuh D.** William Ogilvy Kermack and the childhood origins of adult health and disease. *Int J Epidemiol* 2001;**30**:696–703.

10 **Pearson K.** *Darwinism, medical progress and eugenics. The Cavendish Lecture.* London: Eugenics Laboratory Lecture Series IX, 1912.

11 **Derrick VPA.** Observations on (1) errors on age on the population statistics of England and Wales and (2) the changes in mortality indicated by the national records. *J Inst Actuaries* 1927;**58**:117–59.

*12 **Kermack WO, McKendrick AG, McKinlay PL.** Death rates in Great Britain and Sweden: some general regularities and their significance. *Lancet* 1934;**226**:698–703. Reprinted in *Int J Epidemiol* 2001;**30**:678–83.

13 **Greenwood M.** English death-rates, past, present and future. A valedictory address. *J R Stat Soc* 1936;**99**:674–713.

14 **Boyd Orr J.** *Food health and income.* London: Macmillan, 1937.

15 **M'Gonigle GCM, Kurby J.** *Poverty and public health.* London: V Gollancz, 1936.

16 **Baird D, Illsley R.** Environment and child bearing. *Proc R Soc Med* 1952;**56**:53–64.

17 **Baird D.** Environmental and obstetrical actors of prematurity, special reference to experience at Aberdeen. *WHO Bull* 1962;**26**:291–5.

18 **Drillien CM.** The social and economic factors affecting the incidence of premature birth. *J Obstet Gynaecol Br Empire* 1957;**64**:161–84.

19 **Stockard CR.** Developmental rate and structural expression: an experimental study of twins, "double monsters" and single deformities and their interaction among embryonic organs during their origins and development. *Am J Anat* 1921;**28**:115–225.

20 **Stockard CR.** Human types and growth reactions. *Am J Anat* 1923;**31**:261.

21 **Stockard CR.** *Hormones and structural development. The Beaumont Foundation Lecture, Series 6.* Detroit: Wayne County Medical Society, 1927.

22 **Speman H.** *Embryonic development and induction.* New Haven: Yale University Press, 1938.

23 **Freud S.** The claims of psycho-analysis to scientific interest: the interest of psycho-analysis from a developmental point of view (1913). In Strachey J, ed. *The complete psychological works of Sigmund Freud, Vol. XIII.* London: Hogarth Press, 1955:182–4.

24 **Watson JB.** *Psychological care of infant and child.* New York: Norton, 1928.

25 **Watson JB.** *Behaviorism.* Chicago: University of Chicago Press, 1930.

26 **Stockard CR.** *Constitution and type in relation to disease. De Lamar lectures* 1925–26. Baltimore: Williams and Wilkins, 1927.

27 **Child CM.** *The origin and development of the nervous system.* Chicago: University of Chicago Press, 1921.

28 **Gregg NM.** Congenital cataract following German measles in the mother. *Trans Opthal Soc Aust* 1941;**3**:35–46.

29 **Lorenz K.** The establishment of the instinct concept. In Lorenz K, ed. *Studies in animal and human behaviour* (Vol. I) (R. Martin trans). Cambridge, Massachusetts: Harvard University Press, 1971.

30 **Hess EH.** *Imprinting: early experience and the developmental psychology of attachments.* New York: Van Nostrand Reinhold, 1973.

31 **Cravens H.** Behaviorism revisited: developmental science, the maturation theory, and the biological basis of the human mind, 1920s–1950s. In Benson KR, Maienschein J,

Rainger R, eds. *The expansion of American biology*. New Brunswick: Rutgers University Press, 1991:133–63.

32 **Beach FA, Jaynes JA.** Effects of early experience upon the behavior of animals. *Psychol Bull* 1954;**51**:239–63.

33 **Henderson ND.** Effects of early experience upon the behavior of animals: the second twenty five years of research. In Simmel EC, Baker G, eds. *Early experiences and early behavior: implications for social development*. New York: Academic Press, 1980:45–77.

34 **McCance RA.** Food, growth, and time. *Lancet* 1962;**ii**:621–6 and 671–5.

*35 **McCance RA, Widdowson EM.** The determinants of growth and form. *Proc R Soc Lond* 1974;**185**:1–17.

36 **Leitch I.** Growth and health. *Br J Nutr* 1951;**5**:142–51. Reprinted in *Int J Epidemiol* 2001;**30**:212–5.

37 **Bowlby J.** *Maternal care and mental health, World Health Organization Monograph Series 2*. Geneva: World Health Organization, 1951.

38 **Bowlby J.** *Child care and the growth of love*. Harmondsworth: Penguin, 1953.

39 **Clarke AM, Clarke ADB.** The formative years? In Clarke AM, Clarke ADB, eds. *Early experience: myth and evidence*. New York: Free Press, 1976:3–24.

*40 **Draper G.** *Human constitution: a consideration of its relationship to disease*. Philadelphia and London: Saunders, 1924.

41 **Petersen WF.** Constitution and disease. *Physiol Rev* 1932;**12**:283–308.

42 **Ciocco A.** The historical background of the modern study of constitution. *Bull Hist Med* 1936;**4**:23–38.

43 **Bauer J.** *Constitution and disease*. New York: Grune and Stratton, 1943.

44 **Pearl R.** *Constitution and disease*. London: Kegan Paul, Trench, Trubner, 1933.

45 **Stockard CR.** *The physical basis of personality*. London: George Allen and Unwin, 1931.

46 **Ciocco A, Klein H, Palmer CE.** Child health and the selective service physical standards. *Pub Health Rep* 1941;**56**:2365–75.

47 **White PD.** *Heart disease*. New York: Macmillan, 1931.

48 **Wilson MG, Lubschez R.** Longevity in rheumatic fever. *J Am Med Assoc* 1948;**138**:794–8.

49 **Thayer WS.** On the late effects of typhoid fever in the heart and vessels. *Am J Med Sci* 1904;**127**:391–415.

50 **Ophuls W.** Arteriosclerosis, cardiovascular disease: their relation to infectious diseases. In *Medical Sciences*. Stamford: Stamford University Publications, 1921;**1**:5–102.

51 **Nieto FJ.** Infections and atherosclerosis: new clues from an old hypothesis? *Am J Epidemiol* 1998; **148**:937–48.

52 **Cherry T.** Cancer and acquired resistance to tuberculosis. *Med J Aust* 1924;**2**:372–8.

53 **Jones HB.** A special consideration of the ageing process, disease, and life expectancy. *Adv Biolog Med Phys* 1956;**4**:281–337.

54 **Jones HB.** The relation of human health to age, place, and time. In Birren JE, ed. *Handbook of aging and the individual*. Chicago: University of Chicago Press, 1959:336–63.

55 **Pearl R, Ciocco A.** Studies in constitution II. Somatological differences associated with disease of the heart in white males. *Hum Biol* 1934;**6**:650–713.

56 **Reed LJ, Love AG.** Biometric studies on US army officers—somatological norms in disease. *Hum Biol* **2**:61–93.

57 **Pearl R.** An index of body build. *Am J Physical Anthropol* 1940;**26**:315–48.

58 **Sheldon WH, Stevens SS, Tucker WB.** The varieties of human physique. New York: Harper, 1940.

59 Draper G, Dupertuis CW, Caughey JL. *Human constitution in clinical medicine.* New York: Paul B Hoeber, 1944.

60 Du Bray ES. Comments on body weight in relation to health and disease. *Am J Med Sci* 1925;564.

61 Dublin LI. The influence of weight on certain causes. *Hum Biol* 1930;**II**:159–83.

62 Dublin LI, Marks HH. The weight standard and mortality of very tall men. *Proc Assoc Life Ins Dirs Am* 1937;**23**:153–81.

63 Dublin LI, Marks HH. Mortality of women according to build—experience in substandard issues. *Proc Assoc Life Ins Dirs Am* 1938;**22**:203–36.

64 Ministry of Health. *Report of the Chief Medical Officer for 1921.* London: HMSO, 1921.

*65 Sydenstricker E. *Health and environment.* New York and London: McGraw-Hill, 1933.

66 Registrar General. *Eightieth Annual Report (1917).* London: HMSO, 1919.

67 Wiehl DG. Some recent changes in the mortality among adults. *J Prev Med* 1930;**4**:215–37.

68 Dublin LI, Armstrong DB. *Favorable aspects of heart disease with special reference to the health officer.* New York: Metropolitan Life Insurance Company, 1933.

69 Greenwood M. *Epidemics and crowd diseases. An introduction to the study of epidemiology.* New York: MacMillan, 1935.

70 Woolsey TD, Moriyama IM. Statistical studies of heart diseases. II. Important factors in heart disease mortality trends. *Pub Health Rep* 1948;**63**:1247–73.

71 Moriyama IM, Woolsey TD. Statistical studies of heart disease. *Pub Health Rep* 1951;**66**:355–68.

*72 Morris JN. Recent history of coronary heart disease. *Lancet* 1951;**257(1–7)**:69–73.

73 Ryle JA, Russell WT. The natural history of coronary disease. *Br Heart J* 1949;**XI**:370–204.

*74 Gertler MM, White PD. *Coronary heart disease in young adults.* Cambridge, Massachusetts: Harvard University Press, 1954.

75 Acheson RM. The etiology of coronary heart disease: a review from the epidemiological standpoint. *Yale J Biol Med* 1962;**35**:143–70.

76 Case RAM. Cohort analysis of cancer mortality in England and Wales, 1911–1954 by site and sex. *Br J Prev Soc Med* 1956;**10**:172–99.

77 Bolduan CF, Bolduan NW. Is the "appalling increase" in heart disease real? *J Prev Med* 1932;**6**:321–33.

78 Levy RL, Bruenn HG, Kurtz D. Facts on disease of the coronary arteries, based on a survey of the clinical and pathologic records of 762 cases. *Am J Med Sci* 1934;**187**:376–90.

79 Lew AE. Some implications of mortality statistics relating to coronary artery disease. *J Chron Dis* 1957;**6**:192–209.

80 Campbell M. Death rate from diseases of the heart: 1876 to 1959. *Br Med J* 1963;**August 31**: 528–35.

81 Robb-Smith AHT. *The enigma of coronary heart disease.* Chicago: Year Book of Medical Publishers, 1967.

*82 Bartley M. Coronary heart disease and the public health 1850–1983. *Sociol Health Illness* 1985;**7**:289–313.

83 Stehbens WE. An appraisal of the epidemic rise of coronary heart disease and its decline. *Lancet* 1987;**ii**:606–10.

84 Morris JN. Epidemiology and cardiovascular disease of middle age: part I. *Mod Concepts Cardiovasc Dis* 1960;**29**:625–32.

85 Davey Smith G, Marmot M. Trends in mortality in Britain 1920–1986. *Ann Nutr Med* 1991; **35(suppl 1)**:53–63.

86 Bigelow GH, Lombard HL. *Cancer and other chronic diseases in Massachusetts*. Cambridge: River Side Press, 1933.

87 Gordon JE. Epidemiology—old and new. *J Mich St Med Soc* 1950;**49**:194–9.

88 Stevenson THC. The social distribution of mortality from different causes in England and Wales 1910–12. *Biometrika* 1923;**15**:382–400.

89 Stocks P. The effects of occupation and its accompanying environment on mortality. *J R Stat Assoc* 1938;**101**:690.

90 Askanazy M, ed. *Deuxième conférence internationale de pathologie géographique, Utrecht*. Utrecht: Oosthoek, 1934.

91 Pearl R. *Studies in human biology*. Baltimore: Williams and Wilkins, 1924.

92 Levine SA, Brown CL. Coronary thrombosis: its various clinical features. *Medicine* 1929;**8**:245–418.

*93 Hueper F. Arteriosclerosis. *Arch Pathol* 1945;**39**:187–216.

94 Pearl R. *Alcohol and longevity*. New York: Knopf, 1926.

95 Pearl R. Tobacco smoking and longevity. *Science* 1938;**87**:216–17.

96 Burnham JC. American physicians and tobacco use: two surgeon generals, 1929 and 1964. *Bull Hist Med* 1989;**63**:1–31.

97 Grollman A. The action of alcohol, caffeine, and tobacco, on the cardiac output (and its related functions) of normal man. *J Pharmacol Exp Ther* 1930;**39**:313–27.

98 Cassidy SM. Coronary heart disease: the Harveian Oration of 1946. *Lancet* 1946;**ii**:587–90.

99 Weeks CC. *Alcohol and human life*. London: Lewis, 1938.

100 Ryle JA. *Changing disciplines*. London: Oxford University Press, 1948.

101 Stewart IMcDG. Coronary disease and modern stress. *Lancet* 1950;**ii**:867–70. Reprinted in *Int J Epidemiol* 2002;**31**:1103–7.

102 Ministry of Health. *Report of the Chief Medical Officer for 1939*. London: HMSO.

103 Stocks P. The mortality of men between the ages of 50 and 65. *Lancet* 1943;**i**:543–9.

*104 Hueper F. Arteriosclerosis. *Arch Pathol* 1945;**38**:162–81.

*105 Rosenthal SR. Studies in atherosclerosis: chemical, experimental and morphologic. *Arch Pathol* 1934;**18**:473–506, 660–98, 827–42.

106 Acierno LJ. *The history of cardiology*. London: Parthenon, 1994.

107 Katz LN, Stamler J. *Experimental atherosclerosis*. Illinois: Charles C. Thomas, 1953.

108 Lawrence C. "Definite and material": coronary thrombosis and cardiologists in the 1920s. In Rosenberg CE, Golden J, eds. *Framing disease*. New Brunswick: Rutgers University Press, 1992.

109 Herrick JB. Clinical features of sudden obstruction of the coronary arteries. *J Am Med Assoc* 1912;**59**:2015–20.

110 Herrick JB, Nuzum FR. Angina pectoris, clinical experience with two hundred cases. *J Am Med Assoc* 1918;**70**:67–70.

111 Glendy RE, Levine SA, White PD. Coronary disease in youth. *J Am Med Assoc* 1937;**109**:1775–81.

112 Levy RL, White PD, Stroud WD, Hillman CC. Sustained hypertension, predisposing factors and causes of disability and death. *J Am Med Assoc* 1947;**135**:77–80.

113 White D, Sharber T. Tobacco, alcohol and angina pectoris. *J Am Med Assoc* 1934;**102**:655–7.

114 English JP, Willius FA, Berkson J. Tobacco and coronary disease. *J Am Med Assoc* 1940;**115**:1327–8.

115 Yater WM, Traum AH, Spring S, Brown WG, Fitzgerald RP, Geisler MA *et al.* Coronary artery disease in men eighteen to thirty-nine years of age. *Am Heart J* 1948;**36**:334–722.

*116 White PD. Heart disease, a world problem. *Bull NY Acad Med* 1940;**16**:431.

117 Williams RC. *The United States public health service 1798–1950.* Washington DC: Commissioned Officers Association of the United States Public Health Service, 1951.

118 Blackburn H, Epstein FH. History of the Council on Epidemiology and Prevention, American Heart Association. *Circulation* 1995;**91**:1253–62.

119 Kaiser RF. Why cancer "control"? *Pub Health Rep* 1950;**65**:1203–8.

120 Keys A, Longstreet Taylor HL, Blackburn H, Brozek J, Anderson JT, Simonson E. Coronary heart disease among Minnesota business and professional men followed fifteen years. *Circulation* 1963;**28**:381–95.

121 Keys A, Taylor HL, Blackburn H, Borzek J, Anderson JT, Simonson E. Mortality and coronary heart disease among men studied for 23 years. *Arch Intern Med* 1971;**128**:201–14.

*122 Dawber TR. *The Framingham study. The epidemiology of atherosclerotic disease.* London: Harvard University Press, 1980.

123 Doyle JT, Heslin AS, Hilleboe HE, Formel PF, Korns RF. A prospective study of degenerative cardiovascular disease in Albany: report of three years' experience—1. Ischemic heart disease. *Am J Pub Health* 1957;**47(suppl)**:25–32.

124 Chapman JM, Goerke LS, Dixon W, Loveland DB, Phillips E. The clinical status of a population group in Los Angeles under observation for two to three years. *Am J Pub Health* 1957;**47(suppl)**:33–42.

125 Stamler J, Lindberg HA, Berkson DM, Shaffer A, Miller W, Poindexter A *et al.* Prevalence and incidence of coronary heart disease in strata of the labor force of a Chicago industrial corporation. *J Chron Dis* 1960;**11**:405–20.

*126 Keys A. *Seven countries: a multivariate analysis of death and coronary heart disease.* London: Harvard University Press, 1980.

127 Katz LN, Stamler J, Pick R. *Nutrition and atherosclerosis.* London: Henry Kimpton, 1959.

128 Keys A. Atherosclerosis: a problem in newer public health. *J Mt Sinai Hospital* 1953;**20**:118–39.

129 Keys A. Prediction and possible prevention of coronary disease. *Am J Pub Health* 1953;**43**:1399–407.

130 Armstrong DB. The medical aspects of the Framingham community health in tuberculosis demonstration. *Am Rev Tuberculosis* 1918;**2**:24–7.

131 Ness AR, Rynolds LA, Tansey EM. *Field epidemiology in South Wales: from tuberculosis to non-communicable disease.* Wellcome Witness to Twentieth Century Medicine No. 13. London: Wellcome Trust, 2002;**13**.

132 Doll R, Hill AB. Mortality in relation to smoking: 10 years of observations on male British doctors. *Br Med J* 1964;**1**:1399–460.

133 Doll R, Peto R. Mortality in relation to smoking: 20 years' observations on male British doctors. *Br Med J* 1976;**2**:1525–36.

134 Doll R, Peto R, Wheatley K, Gray R, Sutherland I. Mortality in relation to smoking: 40 years' observations on male British doctors. *Br Med J* 1994;**309**:901–11.

135 Morris JN, Heady JA, Barley RG. Coronary heart disease in medical practitioners. *Br Med J* 1952;**1**:503–20.

136 Morris JN, Heady HA, Raffle PAB, Roberts CG, Parks JW. Coronary heart-disease and physical activity of work. *Lancet* 1953;**ii**:1052–1057, 1111–20.

137 Morris JN, Kagan A, Pattison DC, Gardner MJ, Raffle PAB. Incidence and prediction of ischemic heart disease in London busmen. *Lancet* 1966;**ii**:553–9.

138 Reid DD, Brett GZ, Hamilton PJS, Keen H, Jarrett RJ, Rose G. Cardiorespiratory disease and diabetes among middle-aged male civil servants. *Lancet* 1974;**i**:469–73.

139 Shaper AG, Pocock SJ, Walker M, Cohen NM, Wale CJ, Thomson AG. British regional heart study: cardiovascular risk factors in middle-aged men in 24 towns. *Br Med J* 1981;**283**:179–86.

140 Meade TW, North WRS, Chakrabarti R, Stirling Y, Haines AP, Thompson SG *et al.* Haemostatic function and cardiovascular death: early results of a perspective study. *Lancet* 1980;**i**:1050–4.

141 Thomas AJ, Cochrane AL, Higgins ITT. The measurement of the prevalence of ischaemic heart-disease. *Lancet* 1958;**ii**:540–4.

142 Higgins ITT, Cochrane AL, Thomas AJ. Epidemiological studies of coronary disease. *Br J Prev Soc Med* 1963;**17**:153–65.

*143 Susser M. Epidemiology in the United States after World War II: the evaluation of technique. *Epidemiol Rev* 1985;**7**:147–77.

144 Kannel WB. An overview of the risk factors for cardiovascular disease. In Buck C, Llopis A, Najera E, Terris M, eds. *The challenge of epidemiology: issues and selected readings*, Pan American Health Organization, Scientific Publication No. 505. Washington: World Health Organization, 1988:699–718.

145 Damon A, Damon ST, Harpending HC, Kannel WB. Predicting coronary heart disease from body measurements of Framingham males. *J Chron Dis* 1969;**21**:781–802.

*146 Abraham S, Collins G, Nordsieck M. Relationship of childhood weight status to morbidity in adults. *HSMHA Health Rep* 1971;**86**:273–84.

147 Morris JN. *Uses of epidemiology*. London: Churchill Livingstone, 1964.

148 Rose G. Familial patterns in ischaemic heart disease. *Br J Prev Soc Med* 1964;**18**:75–80.

*149 Stein S, Susser M, Saenger G, Marolla F. *Famine and human development: the Dutch hunger winter of 1944–45*. New York: Oxford University Press, 1975.

150 Anon. Health and social class. *Lancet* 1959;**i**:303–5.

*151 Reid DD. The beginnings of bronchitis. *Proc R Soc Med* 1969;**62**:311–6.

152 Reid DD, Fairbairn AS. The natural history of chronic bronchitis. *Lancet* 1958;**i**:1147–52.

153 Oswald WC, Harold JT, Martin WJ. Clinical pattern of chronic bronchitis. *Lancet* 1953;**ii**:639–43.

154 Colley JRT, Douglas JWB, Reid DD. Respiratory disease in young adults; influence of early childhood lower respiratory tract illness, social class, air pollution, and smoking. *Br Med J* 1973;**2**:195–8.

155 Kiernan KE, Colley JRT, Douglas JWB, Reid DD. Chronic cough in young adults in relation to smoking habits, childhood environment and chest illness. *Respiration* 1976;**33**:236–44.

156 MacMahon B, Newill VA. Birth characteristics of children dying of malignant neoplasms. *J Natl Cancer Inst* 1962;**28**:231–44.

157 MacMahon B. Breast cancer at menopausal ages: an explanation of observed incidence changes. *Cancer* 1957;**10**:1037–44.

158 Cole P, MacMahon B. Oestrogen fractions during early reproductive life in the aetiology of breast cancer. *Lancet* 1969;**i**:604–6.

159 Trichopoulos D. Hypothesis:does breast cancer originate *in utero*? *Lancet* 1990;**335**:939–40.

160 Enos WF, Holmes RH, Beyer J. Coronary disease among United States soldiers killed in action in Korea. *J Am Med Assoc* 1953;**152**:1090–3.

161 Holman KL, McGill HC, Strong JP, Geer JC. The natural history of atherosclerosis: the early aortic lesions as seen in New Orleans in the middle of the 20th century. *Am J Pathol* 1958;**35**:209–35.

162 Strong JP, McGill HC. The natural history of coronary atherosclerosis. *Am J Pathol* 1962;**40**:37–49.

163 Newman WP, Freedman DS, Voors AW, Gard PD, Srinivasan SR, Cresanta JL *et al*. Relation of serum lipoprotein levels and systolic blood pressure to early atherosclerosis. *N Engl J Med* 1986;**314**:138–44.

164 Lauer RM, Clarke WR, Rames LK. Blood pressure and its significance in childhood. *Postgrad Med J* 1978;**54**:206–10.

165 Strasser T. Prevention in childhood of major cardiovascular diseases of adults. In Falkner F, ed. *Prevention in childhood of health problems in adult life*. Geneva: World Health Organization, 1980.

166 de Swiet M. The epidemiology of hypertension in children. *Br Med Bull* 1986;**42**:172–5.

167 Cresanta JL, Borke GL. Determinants of blood pressure levels in children and adolescents. In Berenson GS, ed. *Causation of cardiovascular risk factors in children*. New York: Raven Press, 1986:157–89.

168 Webber LS, Freedman DS, Cresanta JL. Tracking of cardiovascular disease risk factor variables in school-age children. In Berenson GS, ed. *Causation of cardiovascular risk factors in children*. New York: Raven Press, 1986:42–64.

169 Subbiah R. *Atherosclerosis: a pediatric perspective*. Florida: CRC Press Inc, 1989.

170 Osborn GR. Stages in development of coronary disease observed from 1,500 young subjects. Relationship of hypotension and infant feeding to aetiology. *Coll Int Centre National Rech Scient* 1967;**169**:93–139.

171 Barker DJP. *Fetal and infant origins of adult disease*. London: British Medical Publishing, 1992.

172 Barker DJP. *Mothers, babies and health in later life*. Edinburgh: Churchill Livingstone, 1998.

173 Barker DJP. Fetal origins of coronary heart disease. *Br Med J* 1995;**311**:171–4.

174 Barker DJP. The Wellcome Foundation lecture, 1994. The fetal origins of adult disease. *Proc R Soc London* 1995;**262**:37–43.

*175 Forsdahl A. Momenter til belysning ar den høye dødelighet; Finnmark Fylke. *Tidsskr Nor Lægeforen* 1973;**93**:661–7. Translated and reprinted as Observations throwing light on the high mortality in the county of Finnmark. Is the high mortality today a late effect of very poor living conditions in childhood and adolescence? *Int J Epidemiol* 2002;**31**:302–7.

176 Forsdahl A. Living conditions in childhood and adolescence and important risk factor for arteriosclerotic heart disease? *Br J Prev Soc Med* 1977;**31**:91–5.

177 Forsdahl A. Living conditions in childhood and subsequent development of risk factors for arteriosclerotic heart disease. *J Epidemiol Commun Health* 1978;**32**:34–7.

178 Arnesen E, Forsdahl A. The Tromso heart study: coronary risk factors and their association with living conditions during childhood. *J Epidemiol Commun Health* 1985;**39**:210–14.

179 Britten N, Davies JMC, Colley JRT. Early respiratory experience and subsequent cough and peak expiratory flow rate in 36 year old men and women. *Br Med J* 1987;**294**:1317–20.

180 Strachan DP, Anderson HR, Bland JM, Peckham C. Asthma as a link between chest illness in childhood and chronic cough and phlegm in young adults. *Br Med J* 1988;**296**:890–3.

181 Wadsworth MEJ, Cripps HA, Midwinter RA, Colley JRT. Blood pressure at age 36 years and social and familial factors, cigarette smoking and body mass in a national birth cohort. *Br Med J* 1985;**291**:1534–8.

182 Notkola V, Punsar S, Karvonen MJ, Haapokoski J. Socioeconomic conditions in childhood and mortality and morbidity caused by coronary heart disease in adulthood in rural Finland. *Soc Sci Med* 1985;**21**:517–23.

183 **Marmot MG, Rose GA, Shipley MJ, Hamilton PJS.** Employment grade and coronary heart disease in British civil servants. *J Epidemiol Commun Health* 1978;**32**:244–9.

184 **Waaler HTH.** Height, weight and mortality. The Norwegian experience. *Acta Med Scand Suppl 1984*; **679**:1–56.

185 **Yarnell JWG, Limb ES, Layzell JM, Baker IA.** Height: a risk marker for ischaemic heart disease: prospective results from the Caerphilly and Speedwell heart disease studies. *Eur Heart J* 1992;**13**:1602–5.

186 **Leon D, Davey Smith G, Shipley M, Strachan D.** Height and mortality in London: early life influences, socioeconomic confounding or shrinkage? *J Epidemiol Commun Health* 1995;**49**:5–9.

187 **Gunnell DJ, Davey Smith G, Frankel SJ, Nanchqhal K, Braddon FEM, Peters TJ.** Childhood leg length and adult mortality—follow up of the Carnegie survey of diet and growth in pre-war Britain. *J Epidemiol Commun Health* 1998;**52**:142–52.

188 **Leon DA.** Common threads: underlying components of inequalities in mortality between and within countries. In Leon DA, Walt G, eds. *Poverty, inequality and health: an international perspective.* Oxford: Oxford University Press, 2001:58–87.

189 **Davey Smith G, Gunnell D, Ben-Shlomo Y.** Life-course approaches to socioeconomic differentials in cause-specific adult mortality. In Leon D, Walt G, eds. *Poverty, inequality and health: an international perspective.* Oxford: Oxford University Press, 2001:88–124.

190 **Fridlizius G.** The deformation of cohorts: nineteenth-century mortality decline in a generational perspective. *Scand Econ Hist Rev Econom Soc* 1989;**37**:3–17.

*191 **Bengtsson T, Lindstrom M.** Childhood misery and disease in later life: the effects of mortality in old age of hazards experienced in early life, southern Sweden, 1760–1894. *Pop Stud* 2000;**54**:263–77.

192 **Caselli G, Capocaccia R.** Age, period, cohort and early mortality: an analysis of adult mortality in Italy. *Pop Stud* 1989;**43**:133–53.

193 **Horiuchi S.** The long-term impact of war on mortality: old-age mortality of the First World War survivors in the Federal Republic of Germany. *UN Pop Bull* 1983;**5**:80–92.

194 **Preston SH, Van de Walle E.** Urban French mortality in the nineteenth century. *Pop Stud* 1978;**32**:275–97.

195 **Caselli G.** The influence of cohort effects on differentials and trends in mortality. In Vallin J, Dsouza S, Palloni A, eds. *Measurement and analysis of mortality-new approaches.* Clarendon Press: Oxford, 1990:229–49.

196 **Preston SH, Haines MR.** *Fatal years. Child mortality in late nineteenth century America.* Princeton: Princeton University Press, 1991.

197 **Preston SH, Hill ME, Drevenstedt GL.** Childhood conditions that predict survival to advanced ages among African-Americans. *Soc Sci Med* 1998;**47**:1231–46.

198 **Okubo M.** Increase in mortality of middle-aged males in Japan. *NUPRI Res Pap Ser 3* 1981;1–21.

199 **Floud R, Wachter K, Gregory A.** Height, health and history. Cambridge studies in population; economy and society in past time. Nutritional status in the United Kingdom 1750–1980. Cambridge: Cambridge University Press, 1990.

200 **Costa D, Steckel R.** Long-term trends in health, welfare and economic growth in the United States. In Steckl R, Floud R, eds. *Health and welfare during industrialization.* Chicago: University of Chicago Press, 1997:47–90.

201 **Harris B.** Commentary: 'The child is father of the man'. The relationship between child health and adult mortality in the 19th and 20th centuries. *Int J Epidemiol* 2001;**30**:688–96.

202 **Baltes PB, Lindenberger U, Staudinger UM.** Life-span theory in developmental psychology. In Damon W, Lerner RM, eds. *Handbook of child psychology Volume 1: Theoretical models of human development.* New York: John Wiley, 1998:1029–143.

*203 **Rutter M.** Pathways from childhood to adult life. *J Child Psychol Psychiat* 1989; **30**:25–51.

204 **Henry CJK, Ulijaszek SJ.** *Long-term consequences of early environment: growth, development and the lifespan perspective.* Oxford: Oxford University Press, 1996.

205 **Leidy LE.** Lifespan approach to the study of human biology: an introductory overview. *Am J Hum Biol* 1996;**8**:699–702.

206 **Panter-Brick C, Worthman CM.** *Hormones, health and behavior.* Cambridge: Cambridge University Press, 1999.

207 **Magnusson D.** *The lifespan development of individuals: behavioral, neurobiological and psychosocial perspectives.* Cambridge: Cambridge University Press, 1996.

208 **Cairns RB, Elder GH, Costello EJ.** *Developmental science.* Cambridge: Cambridge University Press, 1996.

209 **Sherrod LR, Brim OG Jr.** Epilogue: retrospective and prospective views of life-course research on human development. In Sorensen AB, Weinert FE, Sherrod LR, eds. *Human development and the life course: multidisciplinary perspectives.* Hillsdale, New Jersey: Lawrence Erlbaum Associates, 1986:557–80.

210 **Worthman CM.** Epidemiology of human development. In Panter-Brick C, Worthman CM, eds. *Hormones, health and behavior.* Cambridge: Cambridge University Press, 1999:47–104.

211 **Ferri E, Bynner J, Wadsworth MEJ.** *Changing Britain: changing lives. Three generations at the turn of the century.* London: Bedford Way Press, 2003.

212 **Poulton R, Caspi A, Milne BJ, Thomson WM, Taylor A, Sears MR et al.** Association between children's experience of socioeconomic disadvantage and adult health: a life-course study. *Lancet* 2002;**360**:1640–5.

213 **Must A, Willett WC, Dietz WH.** Remote recall of childhood height, weight, and body build by elderly subjects. *Am J Epidemiol* 1993;**138**:56–64.

214 **Must A, Jacques PF, Dallal GE, Bajema CJ, Dietz WH.** Long-term morbidity and mortality of overweight adolescents. A follow-up of the Harvard Growth Study of 1922 to 1935. *N Engl J Med* 1992;**327**:1350–5.

215 **Jones CJ, Meredith W.** Developmental paths of psychological health from early adolescence to later adulthood. *Psychol Aging* 2000;**15**:351–60.

216 **Schwartz JE, Friedman HS, Tucker JS, Tomlinson-Keasey C, Wingard DL, Criqui MH.** Sociodemographic and psychosocial factors in childhood as predictors of adult mortality. *Am J Pub Health* 1995;**85**:1237–45.

217 **Kuh D, Ben-Shlomo Y.** *A life course approach to chronic disease epidemiology; tracing the origins of ill-health from early to adult life.* Oxford: Oxford University Press, 1997.

218 **Ben-Shlomo Y, Kuh D.** A life course approach to chronic disease epidemiology: conceptual models, empirical challenges, and interdisciplinary perspectives. *Int J Epidemiol* 2002; **31**:285–93.

Part II

Life course influences on adult chronic disease

Chapter 3

Pre-adult influences on cardiovascular disease

Debbie A. Lawlor, Yoav Ben-Shlomo, and David A. Leon

Recent evidence suggests that factors acting across the life course, rather than just adulthood, are important in determining the risk of cardiovascular disease. Consistent evidence, from different settings, demonstrates an inverse association between birth size and coronary heart disease (CHD). Fewer studies have assessed stroke as an outcome, but here also there appears to be an inverse association with birth size. These relationships do not appear to be explained by bias or confounding factors such as socioeconomic status and do not appear to be mediated by conventional cardiovascular disease risk factors. The interpretation of these associations is controversial and is compatible with fetal programming and a genetic mechanism. Other childhood exposures, including accelerated postnatal growth, bottle feeding in infancy and childhood infection, may also increase risk. The empirical data are consistent with several life course models including a critical period model with effect modification, a risk clustering accumulation model, or the possibility of an additive chain of risk. Such models have distinct implications for intervention and prevention strategies, which will need to be considered in future public health policy. Despite the fact that the effects of pre-adult exposures on cardiovascular disease risk are likely to be felt most in developing countries over future decades very little research has been conducted in these countries. Future research needs to establish causal pathways and examine the effects in developing countries.

3.1 Introduction

Cardiovascular disease accounts for the majority of deaths in the developed world. For example, over the 5-year time period from 1995 to 1999 CHD and stroke (ICD 9 codes 410–414 and 430–438) together accounted for 34% of the deaths that occurred in men and 32% of the deaths that occurred in women aged 30 years and older in England and Wales.[1] The incidence and prevalence of cardiovascular disease in developing countries is increasing and worldwide these diseases are currently responsible for approximately 10 million of the 56 million total deaths per year.[2] CHD and stroke are rare until middle-age and over half of deaths due to these causes occur over the age of 70 years. Until recently,[3] most of our knowledge concerning aetiological risk factors focused on factors acting in adult life such as diet, smoking, physical activity, hypertension, and adult obesity.[4] Some have argued that these major adult risk factors explain most of the geographical and secular variations and that there is no need to seek further aetiological risk factors.[5,6] However, the pathophysiological process of atherosclerosis, which ultimately leads to CHD and ischaemic strokes, begins in childhood and young adulthood.[7–9] Cardiovascular risk factors, such as high blood pressure, obesity, dyslipidaemia, and insulin resistance are present in childhood, associated with atherosclerosis and endothelial dysfunction and track into adulthood.[10–14] If one could shift the distribution of these risk factors to the left so that mean levels were reduced in childhood, one would expect public health benefits in later life. For example, detection, treatment, and control of hypertension in adulthood, whilst effective,[15] does not reduce risk to that of normotensive levels.[16]

A growing body of research has highlighted the potential role of pre-adult influences that may operate through various different life course models.[17] Until recently, much of this evidence has been relatively weak and indirect, using either ecological or proxy measures, such as adult height. However both prospective[18] and historical cohort[19] studies have now provided far more rigorous evidence to test associations between circumstances and outcomes many decades apart. This chapter will review this evidence in terms of its association with CHD and stroke. Most emphasis will be given to the association between birth size and CHD. This is not because we feel birth size is necessarily the most important pre-adult determinant or that CHD is a more important outcome than stroke, but rather because it reflects the larger body of available research on this association. A considerable emphasis is also placed on the evidence concerned with potential biological pathways linking birth size with cardiovascular disease risk because the mechanisms that explain these associations are likely to have important public health policy implications.

3.2 Indirect evidence concerning the importance of early life influences

A number of indirect sources indicate the potential role of early life factors on cardiovascular disease risk (see Table 3.1). Ecological studies have noted strong positive correlations between infant mortality in the past and subsequent adult mortality from heart disease (see Chapter 6).[20–22] These associations have also been seen with height so that areas with lower mean adult or child height have been noted to have higher rates of CHD.[23–25] Studies of geographical and social mobility also suggest the importance of the childhood environment over and above that experienced in adulthood and studies of socioeconomic circumstances at different stages in the life course have found that CHD risk is associated with parental, hence childhood, socioeconomic position (see Chapter 4).[26] These studies suggest that both early and later environmental conditions may have independent influences on the risk of CHD in adult life.

3.3 Intrauterine growth

Demonstrating an association between birthweight and cardiovascular disease outcomes is arguably of greater importance than simply showing that size at birth is related to adult blood pressure (see Chapter 9) or insulin resistance (see Chapter 7).

Table 3.1 Evidence for pre-adult influences on adult disease

Type or source of information on early-life	How information is used to infer pre-adult influences on adult disease risk	Examples	Strengths and limitations
Recalled events or behaviour	Information on events or behaviour in pre-adult life obtained from adults in case–control or cohort studies. These early risk factors analysed in same way as adult risk factors.	Childhood socio-economic position and CVD. Recalled birthweight and CVD. Age at menarche and CVD.	Validity of recalled information may be questionable. Mainly limited to events and habits in childhood. For some exposures e.g. measures of socio-economic position may ask for information at a particular age or a non-specific question about childhood in general.
Infant mortality rates by geographic area	Infant mortality rates (IMR) taken as proxy measure of conditions in prenatal life and infancy. Early-life effects inferred from association of IMR for defined geographic areas in the past correlate with adult mortality rates in the same areas decades later.	IMR by area in England and Wales in first part of century correlated with current CHD mortality. (See Section 3.2.)	Design cannot exclude possibility that correlation is due to socio-economic confounding, e.g., areas with high IMR in past were deprived, and because of continued deprivation have high adult mortality today.
Social or geographic mobility studies	Place of birth or residence or socio-economic circumstances in pre-adult life used as indirect measures of exposure. Association with adult disease risk examined controlling for adult place of residence or socio-economic circumstances.	Socio-economic position in childhood and CHD. Place of residence in childhood and cardiovacular mortality. (See Chapter 4.)	Only provides the most general and non-specific indication of independent effects of circumstances at different points in the life course.
Adult height and components of adult height	Taken as a cumulative measure of nutritional status, history of infection in, and other exposures in childhood that may be correlated with adult outcomes. Leg-length is the specific component of adult height most influenced by pre-pubertal exposures.	Inverse association of adult height, and in some studies specifically leg-length with CHD (See Section 3.7.1)	Adult height and components of height are a relatively indelible measure of processes that occurred in childhood (acting together with genes).

Table 3.1 (*Cont.*)

Type or source of information on early-life	How information is used to infer pre-adult influences on adult disease risk	Examples	Strengths and limitations
Anthropometric studies in childhood	Anthropometric data collected in special studies of children often initially designed to obtain information on growth for its own sake. Related to occurrence of CVD events in adult life usually by retrospective collection of event data.	Carnegie/Boyd-Orr study. (See Section 3.2.4.)	Depends upon identifying individual records from growth studies from at least 40–50 years ago, which may be linked to subsequent occurrence of disease in the study subjects.
Prenatal exposures and/or nutrition	Information on size at birth, gestational age, complications of pregnancy etc., from obstetric records related to occurrence of CVD events in adult life usually by retrospective collection of event data.	Hertfordshire (UK) birth cohort and mortality from CHD. (See Section 3.3.)	Depends upon identifying historical series of obstetric records from at least 40–50 years ago, which may be linked to subsequent occurrence of disease in the study subjects.
Natural history studies from birth or childhood	Cohorts of subjects from birth or childhood examined and data collected on range of cardiovascular risk factors that are correlated with risk factor profiles in adult life and (more importantly) with markers of early CVD (e.g. evidence of lesions in coronary arteries).	British 1946 Birth Cohort Study. Bogalusa Heart Study and Muscatine Studies.	Available cohorts are still below the age at which sufficient numbers of CVD events occur.

These latter continuous outcomes are of importance insofar as they may mediate the association between exposures (such as intrauterine nutrition) and subsequent cardiovascular events and therefore may form a 'chain of risk'.

3.3.1 Birth size and coronary heart disease

Eleven studies have assessed the association between birth size and CHD risk in later life and most have found an inverse association across the distribution of 'normal' birthweight (see Table 3.2).[19,27–39] Much of the early evidence came from historical midwifery data from a large cohort of women and men born in Hertfordshire, UK between 1911 and 1930 and rediscovered by Professor David Barker and colleagues.[19,27,40–43] They were able to extract data on maternal characteristics, birthweight, and progress through the infant's first 12 months, including weight at 1 year. From the 37 000 live singleton births originally identified, Barker's team were able to trace the mortality (1951–1992) experience of 16 000 (43%). Results from the Hertfordshire cohort revealed a decline in mortality risk from CHD with increasing weight at birth in women and men.[19] Although the investigators were unable to control for potential confounding factors such as socioeconomic position and smoking there was a specific association between birthweight and cardiovascular disease, with other causes showing no clear pattern of association. In particular, there was no association between birthweight and lung cancer which one would have expected had the association between birthweight and CHD been largely explained by confounding due to smoking and socioeconomic position.

Since Barker and colleague's pioneering work, results from a number of historical and prospective studies, mostly from Europe and North America, but also one from India,[31] have largely replicated their findings (see Table 3.2). These results are seen both for self-reported birthweight and recorded birthweight. Whilst an inverse association between birthweight dimensions and CHD risk is generally consistent, the strength of this association with other anthropometric measures at birth is not. Some studies find the strongest association with birthweight whilst in others it is birth length or ponderal index. However both the Uppsala and Helsinki cohorts indicate that growth rate rather than actual birth size is the important risk marker.[35–38] In the Uppsala cohort, when both birthweight and birthweight relative to gestational age were simultaneously included in the same regression model, only birthweight for gestational age remained associated with cardiovascular disease outcomes.[35] Similarly in the Helsinki cohort adjustment for gestational age tended to strengthen inverse associations.[36–38]

3.3.1.1 Non-linear associations between birth size and coronary heart disease

In some of the studies there is a suggestion of a reverse 'J'-shaped or even a 'U'-shaped association, with risk increasing among those in the highest birthweight categories. In the Hertfordshire cohort small numbers in the highest birthweight category make detailed assessment of the nature of the association difficult to establish with confidence.[19] However, in the Uppsala cohort, among men, CHD risk decreased with increasing birthweight across the first three-quarters of the birthweight distribution and then increased in the last quarter (see Fig. 3.1).[35] Detailed analyses were not presented for women. This pattern was also seen in an Icelandic cohort, which noted only

Table 3.2 Cohort studies assessing the association between birth size and coronary heart disease

Study	Number (% of eligible)	Period of birth	Source of information on birth size	Outcome	Number of cases/deaths	Age at death or follow-up (years)	Main results	Comments
Hertfordshire, UK[19]	Women: 5585 (40) Men: 10141 (54)	Women: 1923–1930 Men: 1911–1930	Medical records	CHD mortality	Women: 88 Men: 853	Women: 20–74 Men: 20–81	Trend of falling SMRs with increasing birthweight.	Suggestion of a reverse 'J' shaped association with mortality increasing in those in the highest sixth of birthweight compared to the penultimate category, but based on just two CHD deaths in this highest category.
Hertfordshire, UK[28]	Men only: 290 (29)	1920–1930	Medical records	CHD prevalence	42	Mean age: 69	Weak inverse trend over first four categories of birthweight (P for trend = 0.9).	Weight at 1 year was more strongly inversely associated with CHD prevalence (P = 0.03) and this association remained when stratified by smoking status and SEP. Small numbers may have meant insufficient power.
Sheffield, UK[29]	Men only: 1586 (48)	1907–1924	Medical records	Total CVD mortality	316	27–83	Inverse trend birthweight (P = 0.06), head circumference (P = 0.02), PI (P = 0.05).	No adjustment for potential confounding factors. Results not affected when stratified by gestational age.
Gothenburg, Sweden[29]	Men only: 855 (not stated)	1913	Medical records	MI	Not stated	50–75	Positive association (P = 0.05)	No information on completeness of case ascertainment.

Study	Birth years	Ascertainment	Outcome	Cases	Cohort (%)	Age range	Findings	Comments
Mysore, India[31]	1934–1951	Medical records	CHD prevalence (Rose angina, ECG or clinical diagnosis)	52 Women: 27 Men: 25	517 (29) Women: 251 Men: 266	38–60	Inverse trend with birthweight ($P = 0.09$), birth length ($P = 0.03$), head circumference ($P = 0.08$) (results for both sexes combined).	Authors stated no sex difference. With adjustment for wide range of CHD risk factors (some of which may be on causal pathway) only association with birth length remained 'statistically significant'. Suggestion of reverse 'J'-shape across six categories of birthweight.
Caerphilly, Wales[32,33]	1920–1938	Self-report	Fatal CHD and non-fatal MI	137	Men only: 1258 (50)	45–69	Inverse association with birthweight ($P = 0.0005$) *only* among those in the highest third of BMI as adults.	Adjusted for SEP in childhood and adulthood, smoking, and other adult risk factors. Interaction between birthweight and adult BMI suggesting that low birthweight only increased CHD in those who were obese as adults.
Nurses' Health Study, USA[34]	1921–1946	Self-report	Non-fatal CHD events	889	Women only: 79 297 (61)	30–71	Percentage decrease in risk for every 454 g increase in birthweight 5% (0–9%).	Adjusted for a large number of potential confounding (and possible mediating) factors. Accuracy of self-report assessed in a subgroup and found to be 'reasonably' accurate.

Table 3.2 (*Cont.*)

Study	Number (% of eligible)	Period of birth	Source of information on birth size	Outcome	Number of cases/deaths	Age at death or follow-up (years)	Main results	Comments
Uppsala, Sweden[35]	Women: 6351 Men: 7012 (97.3 of total for both sexes)	Women: 1915–1929 Men: 1915–1929	Medical records	CHD mortality	Women: 187 Men: 679	29–80	RR for 1000 g increase in birthweight Women: 0.83 (0.62–1.10) Men: 0.77 (0.67–0.90)	Adjustment for adult and childhood SEP. Reverse 'J'-shaped association across quarters of birthweight. Mutual adjustment for birthweight and birthweight for gestational age showed the latter to be inversely associated with CHD but not the former.
Helsinki 1, Finland[36,37]	Women: 3447 (93) Men: 3641 (92)	1924–1933	Medical records	Fatal and non-fatal CHD events	279	38–71	Women: inverse trend birthweight (P = 0.01) and length (P = 0.001), no association with PI (P = 0.41). Men: inverse trend birthweight (P = 0.05) and PI (P <0.001).	Adjusted for age and gestational age. Effects of low birthweight greatest in those with accelerated postnatal growth. In women, associations with birthweight and length strengthened with additional adjustment for placental weight. Relatively homogenous group with respect to childhood SEP with 85% of fathers being labourers.

Helsinki 2, Finland[38]	Men only: 4630 (84)	1934–1944	Medical records	Fatal and non-fatal CHD events	357	27–63	Inverse trend birthweight (P = 0.006) and PI (P = 0.0006).	Adjusted for age only. Low weight and PI age 1 also associated with increased risk and accelerated growth between age 1 and 12 associated with increased risk.
Reykjavik, Iceland[39]	Women: 2376 Men: 2399 (78)	1914–1935	Medical records	Hospital admission with MI or fatal CHD	Women: 134 Men: 440	Women (mean age): 65 Men (mean age): 50	Women: 'U'-shaped association with birthweight, birth length, and PI Men: inverse trend with birthweight (P = 0.09) and length (P = 0.03).	Icelanders are a population who have high birthweights and are relatively genetically homogenous.

CHD, coronary heart disease; SMR, standardized mortality ratio; CVD, cardiovascular disease (= coronary heart disease and stroke in this study); PI, ponderal index; MI, myocardial infarction; ECG, electrocardiogram; BMI, body mass index; RR, rate ratio; SEP, socioeconomic position.

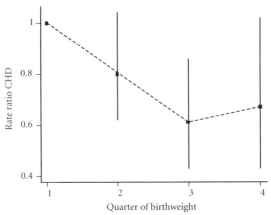

Fig. 3.1 Reverse 'J' shaped association between birthweight and CHD risk among Swedish men.[34]

a weak linear inverse association between birth size and CHD in men and a 'U'-shaped association among women.[39] Non-linear associations may be due to several competing influences. Babies who experience intrauterine growth retardation may have increased CHD risk through a nutritional programming or genetic effect (see Section 3.4). However, maternal diabetes that results in heavier offspring[44] may also result in increased insulin resistance and thence CHD risk in later life among these heavier offspring.[45] These competing influences may not act uniformly on babies of all birthweight categories. It is therefore plausible that a linear model is not an adequate representation of the association between birthweight and CHD.

3.3.2 **Birth size and stroke**

Four studies have assessed the association between birth size and stroke and have again found an inverse association in women and men (see Table 3.3).[34,35,43,46,47] In the Uppsala and Helsinki cohorts the separate associations between birthweight and stroke sub-types (based on routine death certificate and hospital discharge data) were assessed. In the Uppsala study the association was stronger for haemorrhagic than occlusive stokes.[46] The stronger association between birthweight and cerebral haemorrhage than between birthweight and occlusive arterial disease (stroke and CHD), may be explained by a stronger association of hypertension with haemorrhagic disease. In the largest study of stroke incidence to date (9.5 million person years) the relative risk of occlusive stroke per 20 mm Hg increase in systolic blood pressure was 2.27 (1.17, 2.33), whilst that for haemorrhagic stroke was 3.23 (3.03, 3.33), P for interaction <0.001.[48] Low birthweight is associated with raised blood pressure[49] and there have been important reductions in the population distribution of blood pressure over the last century in industrialized countries, most likely as a result of improvements in early life environmental conditions.[50] In the Helsinki cohort the magnitude of the associations of birthweight (and length) with each stroke sub-type were similar in models with adjustment for adult socioeconomic position and income. However, with additional adjustment for head circumference and birth a marked difference in the magnitudes of the

Table 3.3 Cohort studies assessing the association between birth size and stroke

Study	Number (% of eligible)	Period of birth	Source of information on birth size	Outcome	Number of cases/deaths	Age at death or follow-up (years)	Main results	Comments
Hertfordshire and Sheffield, UK[43]	Men only: 13 249 (44)	1907–1930	Medical records	Stroke mortality	230	20–83	12% (1–22%) fall in SMR across categories of approximate fifths of increasing birthweight, $P_{trend} = 0.01$.	Weight at 1 year also associated with increased stroke mortality. Inverse association remained when stratified by gestational age. No adjustment for other potential confounders.
Nurses' Health Study, USA[34]	Women only: 79 297 (61)	1921–1946	Self-report	Non-fatal stroke events	364	30–71	Percentage decrease in risk for every 454 g increase in birthweight 11% (5–18%).	Adjusted for a large number of potential confounding and mediating factors.
Uppsala, Sweden[35] Analysis of all stroke mortality stratified by sex	Women: 6351 Men: 7012 (97.3 of total of both sexes)	Women: 1915–1929 Men: 1915–1929	Medical records	Stroke mortality	Women: 105 Men: 113	29–80	RR for 1000 g increase in birthweight Women: 0.84 (0.62–1.10) Men: 0.71 (0.49–1.03).	Adjustment for age and adult and childhood SEP.

Table 3.3 (Cont.)

Study	Number (% of eligible)	Period of birth	Source of information on birth size	Outcome	Number of cases/deaths	Age at death or follow-up (years)	Main results	Comments
Uppsala, Sweden[46] Analysis by stroke sub-type, results for both sexes combined	Women and men: 10 853 (96)	1915–1929	Medical records	Fatal and non-fatal stroke incidence	Haemorrhagic stroke: 156 Occlusive stroke: 775 Ill defined: 60	29–80	HR for 1000 g increase in birthweight Haemorrhagic: 0.59 (0.43, 0.83) Occlusive: 0.93 (0.80, 1.09).	Adjustment for sex, period of birth, age, and adult and childhood SEP. Additional adjustment for gestational age had no substantive effect.
Helsinki 1, Finland[47]	Men only: 3639 (92)	1924–1933	Medical records	Fatal and non-fatal stroke incidence	331 62 diagnosed as haemorrhagic, 247 as occlusive	38–71	Linear inverse trend of all strokes with birthweight (P = 0.04), birth length (P = 0.05).	Adjusted for adult SEP and income. Associations with both birthweight and birth length were strengthened with additional adjustment for head circumference. Associations between birth size and each stroke sub-type were similar until additional adjustment for head-circumference. Associations of birthweight and birth length adjusted for head circumference were stronger for haemorrhagic than occlusive strokes.

SMR, standardized mortality ratio; RR, rate ratio; SEP, socioeconomic position; HR, hazard ratio.

associations became apparent with a stronger inverse association between birthweight (or length) adjusted for head circumference and haemorrhagic stroke. The investigators suggested this differential was most likely explained by haemorrhagic strokes being influenced more by 'brain sparing' (diversion of blood flow to the developing brain under circumstances of under-nutrition) than occlusive strokes.[47] However, in the Uppsala cohort there was a pronounced association between birthweight and haemorrhagic stroke (and a weak association with occlusive stroke) without adjustment for head circumference.[46] In that study additional adjustment for both head circumference and birth length strengthened the association with haemorrhagic stroke and the authors concluded that their data did not support a special role for birthweight relative to head size. They suggested that the risk of haemorrhagic stroke was related to impaired growth of soft tissue mass relative to bone growth.[46] Subgroup analyses need to be treated with caution and the use of routine data to differentiate stroke sub-types in both the Helsinki and Uppsala cohorts may have resulted in misclassification of these outcomes. However, the suggestion in two large prospective studies that birthweight may be differentially associated with haemorrhagic and occlusive stroke warrants further investigation because it may provide insights into mechanisms relating birthweight to cardiovascular disease.

In the Hertfordshire cohort and a Sheffield (UK) cohort there appeared to be some differences in the associations of patterns of birth size, placental size, and maternal pelvic dimensions with stroke and CHD risk.[43] These differences led the authors to conclude that the associations between low birth size and CHD and stroke mortality were most likely mediated via different mechanisms. They suggested that poor nutrition during a mother's own early childhood leads to increased stroke risk in her offspring via an effect on her bony pelvic growth, which results in an inability to sustain normal placental and fetal growth in her subsequent pregnancies.[43] It was suggested that CHD, on the other hand, most likely resulted from adaptations made by the fetus to intrauterine nutritional deprivation resulting from reasons other than a failure of placental growth.[43] In other studies, however, placental size has not been found to have important influences on associations with CHD or stroke.[35]

3.3.3 Birth size and atherosclerosis

In addition to the studies that have investigated the association between birth size and CHD and stroke events, three studies have assessed the association between birth size and carotid atherosclerosis.[51–54] Carotid atherosclerosis, determined by ultrasound measurement of intima-media thickness (IMT), is associated with both CHD and stroke incidence.[55,56] One might, therefore, expect birthweight to be inversely associated with atherosclerosis.

In one study of 346 women and men aged 49 to 51 years from the north of England, early life factors, which included both birthweight and socioeconomic position in childhood, accounted for only 2.0% of the variation in carotid IMT in women and 2.2% in men.[51] However, these results were adjusted for adult risk factors including blood pressure and lipids, which may represent over-adjustment because these may be intermediaries on the causal pathway between birthweight and CHD risk. In a study of 181 (8.1% eligible) older women and men from Sheffield the odds of clinically important carotid stenosis were greater in those whose birthweight was <6.5 lb than in those whose birthweight was >7.5 lb (odds ratio, 5.3; 95% confidence interval (CI), 2.0–14.0).[52] Further tracing of the cohort noted a weaker association (odds ratio, 1.8; 95% CI, 1.0–3.3)[53] when 389 participants (17.4%) were measured, suggesting some selection bias in the original results. By far the largest study to date to assess this association is an analysis of 9817 participants in the Atherosclerosis Risk in Communities (ARIC) study. In this study there was no association between birthweight and carotid IMT: a 1 kg greater birthweight was associated with a 0.004 mm higher IMT (95% CI, −0.002–0.012).[54] The use of self-reported birthweight may have biased the results towards the null due to misclassification, however one might have expected some indication of an inverse association in a study of such size if it truly existed.

The failure to note an inverse association with carotid atherosclerosis is surprising given the evidence for CHD and stroke. This might be explained if the relevant exposures that affect birth size and cardiovascular disease risk do so by increasing insulin resistance and causing high triglyceride/low high-density lipoprotein-cholesterol dyslipidaemia. This dyslipidaemia may have a role in the transition from atherosclerosis to atherothrombosis, rather than being associated with atherosclerosis formation *per se*.[57] In this way factors associated with reduced birth size may play a role in the progression of sub-clinical pathology to clinical disease end-points.

3.4 Possible interpretations for the association between birth size and coronary heart disease

3.4.1 Bias and confounding

The reason for the inverse association between birthweight and cardiovascular disease remains the subject of much debate. It has been suggested that the association is due to bias or residual confounding.[58] Losses to follow-up in some of the retrospective cohort studies were substantial.[58] However, large prospective studies with little loss to follow-up have found inverse associations between birthweight and cardiovascular disease suggesting that the selection bias is unlikely to explain much of this association.[34–38]

The possibility of residual confounding explaining the association between birth size and cardiovascular disease has been suggested.[58] Many studies of the association between birthweight and cardiovascular disease have not been able to adjust for socioeconomic position and smoking. However, among those that have adjusted for both of these potential confounding factors, the inverse association persists,[32–34] even after adjustment for both childhood and adulthood socioeconomic position[35] (see Table 3.2). Further, in the Hertfordshire and Uppsala cohorts, the association is specific for cardiovascular disease outcomes and in particular is not found for lung cancer,[19,35] suggesting that it is not explained by confounding due to smoking and socioeconomic position. To date no study has been able to examine the effect of maternal smoking during pregnancy on the association between birth size and later CVD. This may act as an important explanatory variable if intrauterine exposure to maternal smoking, which is known to cause low birthweight, programmes adult disease. The consistency of the association precludes chance as an explanation and it is unlikely that either bias or confounding could fully explain these findings.

3.4.2 The role of adult size and mediating factors

It has been suggested that the inverse association between birthweight and blood pressure is either an artefact or reflects postnatal growth because in several studies the association is only found, or its magnitude increased, with adjustment for contemporary size.[59,60] This criticism cannot be levelled at the inverse association between birth size and cardiovascular disease outcomes in which strong and consistent associations are found without adjustment for contemporary size.

The fetal origins hypothesis suggests that poor intrauterine nutrition leads not only to small birth size but also, depending upon the timing (or critical period), it 'programmes' selective changes in body composition, cell size and number, hormonal axes, and metabolism (see Section 3.4.3).[61] Programmed changes in insulin-mediated carbohydrate and lipid metabolism, the thrifty phenotype hypothesis, may be particularly important.[62] Similarly, the fetal insulin hypothesis (see Section 3.4.4) suggests that insulin resistance is an important mediating factor in the association between birth size and cardiovascular disease. However, those studies that have been able to control for these potential mediating factors (including lipids, blood pressure, and indicators of insulin-mediated glucose metabolism) still show an apparent 'independent' effect of birthweight on CHD risk.[32–34,63] Single cross-sectional measures of these potential mediating factors may be insufficient to take into account exposures over the life span of an individual. In addition, poor fetal growth may programme other pathways, such as prothrombotic risk factors and structural changes to the coronary vessels or myocardium.

3.4.3 Fetal and maternal nutrition

Fetal growth is determined by both maternal and fetal nutrition. Chapter 15 highlights the importance of distinguishing between maternal nutrition across the mother's life course before pregnancy, maternal nutritional status and diet during pregnancy, and fetal nutrition (that is, the net supply of metabolic substrate to the fetus).[64] With respect to explaining the association between birthweight and cardiovascular disease, much of the direct evidence for the effect of maternal pregnancy diet and fetal nutrition has come from animal studies, where experimental manipulation during pregnancy is possible resulting in intrauterine growth retardation of the offspring. Most animal work to date has focused on cardiovascular risk factors, such as hypertension and dyslipidaemia, though in some evidence of atherosclerosis or CHD has been assessed at autopsy.[64–66] Whilst such studies have found a direct effect of maternal pregnancy dietary manipulation and reduced fetal nutrition on both fetal growth and risk of cardiovascular disease, the generalizability of their findings as well as the extreme nature of some of the manipulations, for example, ligation of umbilical vessels, makes interpreting these results with respect to humans problematic.[64]

The effect of maternal pregnancy diet has been assessed in humans using two natural experiments, where pregnant women experienced extreme nutritional deprivation during the Second World War.[67–72] However, results from these studies have been inconsistent and in terms of disease events are based on very small numbers. Children born during the Dutch famine of 1944 and whose mothers were under-nourished during pregnancy had increased glucose tolerance and an atherogenic lipid profile but normal blood pressure when compared to those born immediately before or after the famine.[67–69] Of particular note, adults who experienced the famine in the last trimester of pregnancy were more insulin resistant than those not experiencing famine, consistent with a nutritional pregnancy programming hypothesis.[69] However, CHD prevalence was highest in those exposed to famine in the first trimester of pregnancy compared to those not exposed to famine (8.8% versus 3.2%), being no different in those born. In the third trimester compared to those unexposed it should be noted that these results are based on just 24 CHD cases across all four categories of first, second, and third trimester exposure, and unexposed.[70] In yet another publication from this study, all-cause adult mortality (between the ages of 18 and 50 years) was not associated with exposure to famine at any time during pregnancy.[71] Individuals born during the 1941 siege of Leningrad had similar fasting and post-challenge glucose and insulin levels and similar lipid and blood pressure levels to those born outside of the siege.[72] On-going follow-up studies of past randomized controlled trials in pregnancy will be important to further test the role of maternal nutrition in pregnancy on the association of birth size with CVD.[73]

3.4.4 A common genetic mechanism

Genetic polymorphisms with pleiotropic effects may determine both fetal development and hence birthweight and subsequent risk of insulin resistance and hence adult CHD (the fetal insulin hypothesis).[74–76] Definitive proof of the fetal insulin hypothesis requires the identification of candidate genes that are associated with birthweight and insulin resistance or cardiovascular disease. A mutation in the glucokinase gene, which results in an increased risk of type 2 diabetes, has been shown to be associated with low birthweight.[77] Though this provides evidence supporting the concept, this mutation is rare and could not explain the association between low birthweight, insulin resistance, and cardiovascular disease risk in the general population. The associations of a number of candidate genes involved in insulin metabolism with birth size have been examined but with inconsistent results,[78–81] and to date genetic factors that could explain this association in the general population have not been established.

3.4.5 Distinguishing genetic and environmental factors

3.4.5.1 Twin studies

A traditional approach to distinguish genetic from environmental influences is the use of twin studies. Twins, compared to singletons, experience intrauterine growth retardation and have on average birthweights that are 900 g lower than those of singletons. Though there may be some weak association between higher socioeconomic position and occurrence of dizygotic (DZ) twins, the likelihood of having a monozygotic (MZ) twin pregnancy is not influenced by socioeconomic position or maternal cigarette smoking. Therefore, if the intrauterine nutritional deprivation experienced by twins occurs through similar processes to that experienced by the general population, one would expect twins to be at greater risk of CHD and that such an association was unlikely to be confounded by social class or smoking. In one study, mortality from CHD among 8174 female and 6612 male twins (both MZ and DZ combined) was no greater than that among the general population, suggesting that the intrauterine growth retardation experienced by twins was not associated with increased CHD risk.[82] These results were confirmed in a second study of nearly 20 000 twins in which all-cause and cardiovascular disease mortality were found to be similar among MZ twins, DZ twins and the general population.[83,84] In addition, twins do not appear to have higher blood pressure than the general population or than their non-twin siblings[85,86] and being a twin is not importantly associated with other cardiovascular disease risk factors.[87] Divergence in fetal growth rates between twins and singletons may occur early in gestation, whereas intrauterine growth retardation in the population as a whole tends to occur in later gestation, as the rapidly increasing nutritional demands of the fetus exceed supply.[87–89] In addition there may be other important differences in the pathophysiological processes involved in growth retardation of twins compared to singletons. Thus the finding that twins have similar cardiovascular disease mortality to the general population may be consistent with a fetal programming hypothesis in which the 'critical period' of poor intrauterine nutrition for increasing CHD risk, or the underlying mechanisms, are not related to growth retardation in twins.[61,87]

A particularly powerful twin study design is to examine whether variation in size at birth specifically *within* MZ pairs is associated with differences in adult cardiovascular disease within these pairs. A logical progression in these studies is first to treat all of the twins as individuals and simply assess the association between birthweight and cardiovascular disease in the twin population (*between*-twin study). If an inverse association between birthweight and cardiovascular disease is found between twins this suggests that twins *per se* do not differ from the general populations in which this association has been demonstrated. A *within*-twin pair analysis is then equivalent to matching on factors that are identical within twin pairs. If there is no association within MZ pairs between birthweight and cardiovascular disease (that is, MZ twins with disease compared to their co-twins without disease do not differ from each other with respect to birthweight) but the inverse association is seen in DZ twins then this suggests that factors that are identical in MZ twins (but not DZ twins) explain the association. Because MZ twins are genetically identical, fetal genes would be the most obvious explanation. However, approximately two-thirds of MZ twins share a placenta, therefore the lack of an association specifically within MZ twins may also be consistent with non-genetic placental factors.[90] If there is no association within both MZ and DZ (that is, when the analysis is undertaken with matching on factors that are identical within either MZ or DZ twin pairs), but there is a between-pairs association then the association between birthweight and disease must be explained by fixed maternal factors that are identical for both twins in both MZ and DZ pairs. These factors would include maternal socioeconomic circumstances and environmental exposures in the mother's early life, maternal birth characteristics and growth across the mother's life, smoking, and maternal age. If the within-twin pair associations for both MZ and DZ pairs are similar to the between-twin association then this suggests that fetal nutrition (which varies within both twin types) or any other factor that is not identical within twin pairs explains the association.

Only two within-twin analyses have looked at the association of birthweight with CHD risk[91,92] and none have looked at the association with stroke risk. The following studies were undertaken by the same research group on two independent samples of Swedish twins. In the first study, there was no association between birthweight, birth length, ponderal index or head circumference, and acute myocardial infarction within 118 same-sex twin pairs (MZ and DZ), although low birthweight was associated with increased myocardial infarction between twins in the whole cohort, suggesting that either genetic or fixed maternal factors explained the association.[91] In the second study there was an association between low self-reported birthweight and increased risk of angina between 4594 same-sex twins and also within 55 pairs of same-sex DZ twins who were selected to be discordant for self-reported angina. However, within 37 MZ twin pairs, discordant for angina, there was no association with birthweight. Self-reported birthweight was validated in a subgroup of the study and found to be accurate.[92] These findings suggest that genetic factors or other factors that are uniquely shared within MZ twin pairs explain the low birthweight–CHD association. However, further studies based on larger numbers of twin pairs are necessary to be certain that these results are not due to chance.

3.4.5.2 Transgenerational studies

Another approach to distinguish between genetic and environmental factors is to study the cardiovascular disease risk of parents in relation to their offspring's birthweight ('transgenerational transmission of risk'). If the birthweight–cardiovascular disease association seen within individuals is due to a genetic mechanism from both maternal and paternal genes, then one would predict that offspring birthweight would be inversely associated with cardiovascular disease in both mothers and fathers. Offspring birthweight has been found to be inversely associated with increased risk of parental cardiovascular disease events and atherosclerosis in transgenerational studies (see Table 3.4).[93–98] These studies show that both maternal and paternal risk is increased, though the former to a greater degree. The association between offspring birthweight and maternal cardiovascular disease may reflect maternal/fetal nutritional factors and intrauterine programming, as women who themselves had poor fetal growth and low birthweight tend to have offspring who are small for their gestational age.[99,100] This effect may be mediated via maternal pelvic restriction, poor placental growth and hence a programming effect of intrauterine nutrition or via shared environmental exposures, for example, cigarette smoking, across generations.[43] The spousal correlation for birthweights is remarkably low (0.02)[101] so that despite the possibility of assortative mating, it is unlikely that any observed increased risk for fathers reflects paternal low birthweight or paternal characteristics being a proxy for maternal (their partner's) birth characteristics. Shared environmental factors between fathers and offspring (smoking and socioeconomic position) is another possible reason for fathers showing an increased risk with offspring birthweight. However, this association is independent of paternal smoking and other adult risk factors for cardiovascular disease, including socioeconomic position,[93,96,97] excluding the possibility of shared environmental exposures between parents as the sole explanation. The fetal insulin/shared genes hypothesis would also predict offspring birthweight to be associated with parental insulin resistance in later adulthood. Four studies have shown that offspring birthweight is associated with diabetes or insulin resistance in mothers and fathers.[102–105]

These observations provide support for a genetic explanation. The differential strength of the association between maternal and paternal risk in CHD risk with offspring birthweight is, however, somewhat problematic for the genetic model. This may

Table 3.4 Transgenerational studies of the association between parental cardiovascular disease risk and offspring birthweight

Study	Population	Outcome	Number of cases	Main results	Adjusted for
Davey Smith et al. (1997)[93]	794 married couples from west of Scotland	CVD mortality	Mothers: 17 Fathers: 28	HR for 1 kg decrease in offspring birthweight Mothers: 2.00 (1.18, 3.33) Fathers: 1.52 (1.03, 2.17)	Offspring: sex Parental: age, blood pressure, cholesterol, body mass index, smoking, social class, area deprivation, lung function, bronchitis, angina, ECG evidence CHD
Davey Smith et al, (2000)[94]	3706 women from Helsinki, Finland	CVD mortality	114	HR for 1 SD (584 g) increase in birthweight 0.77 (0.65, 0.90) 1 SD (2.8 cm) increase in birth length 0.85 (0.73, 0.99)	Offspring: sex Maternal: age, height, marital status, use of private health care during pregnancy, use of hormones during pregnancy
Davey Smith et al. (2000)[95]	44 813 women from England and Wales	CVD mortality	41	HR for 1 kg decrease in offspring birthweight 2.22 (1.46, 3.38)	Offspring: sex Maternal: age, socioeconomic position, and marital status
Rasmussen et al. (2001)[97]	573 437 women and 563 008 men from Sweden	CVD mortality	Mothers: 1349 Fathers: 6339	HR for a 1 kg increase in offspring birthweight Mothers: 0.58 (0.51, 0.66) Fathers: 0.85 (0.80, 0.90)	Offspring: sex, gestational age Parental: age, education Smoking at age 18 years was also taken into account in a sub-sample (n = 21 686) of fathers only and this adjustment did not alter the findings

Table 3.4 (*Cont.*)

Study	Population	Outcome	Number of cases	Main results	Adjusted for
Smith GCS et al. 2001[98]	129 920 women from Scotland	CHD mortality and acute hospital admissions for CHD	43 deaths 313 admissions	HR for CHD mortality comparing lowest fifth of offspring birthweight with highest four-fifths 2.4 (1.3, 4.4), HR for CHD mortality or admission 1.9 (1.5, 2.4)	Offspring: sex, pre-term delivery Maternal: age, height, social class, pre-eclampsia
Lawlor et al. 2003[96]	268 women and 221 men from two English towns	Carotid intima-media thickness		Percentage change in intima-media thickness for a 1 SD (0.52 kg) increase in offspring birthweight Women: −4% (−13, 5) Men: −3% (−12, 7)	Offspring: sex Parental: age, social class, smoking, body mass index

CVD, cardiovascular disease; HR, hazard ratio; ECG, electrocardiogram; CHD, coronary heart disease; SD, standard deviation.

reflect chance but consistent results (see Table 3.4) make this unlikely. Possible explanations include paternal misclassification (as some fathers in these studies will not be the biological parent and this would be expected to dilute the paternal association), poor maternal nutrition in the mother's childhood resulting in her own reduced vitality and therefore increased CHD risk and low offspring birthweight (resulting in stronger associations in mothers due to both environmental and genetic factors), maternal imprinting (imprinting refers to gamete-of-origin-dependent modification of the phenotype, that is, the phenotype resulting from a particular gene locus is differentially modified by the sex of the parent contributing that particular allele), or other epigenetic effects (epigenetic effects are a change in the outcome of a gene that is controlled by non-genetic factors, that is, the phenotype resulting from a particular gene is modified by environmental exposures).[106]

3.5 Accelerated postnatal growth

Accelerated growth, also referred to as 'catch-up growth', is defined as a period of accelerated growth occurring after a period of retardation ends, when favourable conditions are restored, and the children return to the original growth trajectory.[107] Tanner's original description referred to accelerated growth following infant (infectious) diseases, but recently it has been suggested that the inverse association between birthweight and cardiovascular disease may reflect accelerated postnatal growth following intrauterine growth restriction.[60] In developed countries most infants who are small for their gestational age catch up with respect to their growth during the first 2 years of their lives, with most of this catch-up occurring in the first 6 months of life.[108,109] In general this catch-up growth is beneficial because it is associated with reduced childhood morbidity and mortality[110] and for girls it may be associated with reduced risk of their offspring being born small for gestational age.[99] However, it is possible that this period of accelerated growth, rather than or in addition to any intrauterine mechanism, programmes later adult disease risk. To determine the effect of accelerated postnatal growth one needs infant growth data, yet most reported studies only have a measure of growth later in childhood or adulthood. This distinction is important as such studies cannot differentiate between accelerated growth within the first 2 years of life, from subsequent pubertal growth changes.

The most important studies with respect to examining the effects of accelerated postnatal growth are the Helsinki cohorts (see Table 3.2). In the first of these, birth size data were available on women and men born between 1924 and 1933 and in addition anthropometric measurements during school years (aged 6–15) were available.[36,37] In the second Helsinki cohort study, men born between 1934 and 1944 additionally had anthropometric measurements between birth and aged 6 obtained from childhood welfare clinics.[38] Both birthweight and weight at 1 year were inversely associated with risk of CHD morbidity or mortality for men in the Helsinki 2 cohort (there were no women in this study) as noted in the Hertfordshire cohort for men but not women.[41] The hazard ratios reported for the Helsinki 2 cohort, after simultaneous adjustment, were 0.94 (95% CI, 0.83–1.06) and 0.84 (95% CI, 0.75–0.94) for a 1 standard deviation increase in birthweight and weight at 1 year respectively.[111] Plotting the growth trajectories (Z-scores) of participants who later developed CHD standardized to the whole cohort revealed that CHD cases showed downward centile crossing in the first year of life but subsequently showed marked growth acceleration so that by 12 years their body mass index was almost identical to the rest of the cohort, though they remained slightly shorter. Significant interactions were reported for ponderal index at birth and body mass index after 2 years so that the greatest risk was observed amongst thin babies who were in the upper body mass index distribution in childhood. This is analogous to the results seen in the Caerphilly cohort where an interaction between birthweight and adult body mass index was observed.[32] The interaction between early and later growth highlights the potential role of an accumulation model of risk across the pre-adult period.

A recent follow-up of two randomized trials of postnatal growth using different infant feeds provides informative data on the possible role of accelerated postnatal growth on insulin resistance.[112] Babies who were randomized to a nutrient-enriched diet showed raised fasting-insulin at ages 13–16 years, regardless of birthweight. Using the data observationally, children who showed marked weight gain, particularly in the first 2 weeks of life, had even more raised 32–33 split pro-insulin levels, an indication of insulin resistance.[112] These data provide further support for postnatal as well as intrauterine mechanisms. However, the adverse effect on markers of insulin resistance of accelerated weight gain in the first 2 weeks of life in this study contradicts the findings from the much larger Helsinki 2 study which found that poor weight gain in the first year of life and subsequent accelerated growth was associated with increased CHD risk (see above).

3.6 Infant feeding and cardiovascular disease

A beneficial association between breastfeeding in infancy and cardiovascular disease risk was first proposed in the 1960s following post-mortem evidence of atherosclerosis in children who had been wholly artificially fed.[113] This observation was not confirmed in subsequent studies.[114,115] Investigators of the Hertfordshire historical cohort have reported that standardized mortality ratios for cardiovascular disease before the age of 65 were greater among those who were exclusively bottle fed than among those who were breastfed during the first year of life in both women and men.[19,27] However, these findings were not confirmed in a Californian cohort of children followed up for 65 years from 1922.[116]

In both historical and contemporary cohorts, breastfeeding in infancy has been shown to be associated with favourable lipid profiles, lower levels of glucose and lower blood pressure in later childhood or adulthood,[117,118] and reduced obesity.[119] A recent study of blood pressure in 13–16 year olds who had been born prematurely and were involved in a randomized controlled trial of different feeding interventions at birth found that the 66 children who had been assigned banked breast milk had a mean arterial blood pressure that was 4 mm Hg less than the 64 who were assigned pre-term formula milk.[120] Paradoxically, prolonged breastfeeding beyond 4 months has been reported to be associated with brachial arterial stiffness in both sexes.[121] However, this observation may have been a chance finding as there was no a priori hypothesis.

Breastfeeding may be associated with lower blood pressure through a hormonal effect or may be related to lower levels of sodium in breast milk or a protective effect of long-chain polyunsaturated fatty acids. Among adults, salt reduction is associated with small reductions in blood pressure.[122] However, in a Dutch study in which infants were randomized to a low or a normal sodium diet for the first 6 months of life, blood pressure was markedly lower after 15 years in those allocated to the low sodium diet, suggesting that sodium restriction in infancy may have even greater effects on later blood pressure than salt reductions in adulthood.[123] Long-chain polyunsaturated fatty acids are present in breast milk, but not in most formula feeds and these may be important in normal health and development of the infant.[124] A recent follow-up of a randomized controlled trial found that blood pressure at age 6 was lower (mean difference of systolic blood pressure, −3.0 mm Hg (95% CI, −5.4 to−0.5) and of diastolic blood pressure, −3.6 mm Hg (95% CI, −6.5 to −0.6)) among formula-fed children who had been randomized to a formula supplemented with a long-chain polyunsaturated fatty acid than among those randomized to an unsaturated formula.[125] The blood pressure among the supplemented group was similar to that among 6 year olds whose mothers had breastfed them.

3.7 Childhood exposures and cardiovascular disease

There is an established body of evidence that suggests that atherosclerosis (the process whereby arteries become narrowed and damaged by deposition of fatty material) starts in childhood.[126,127] Autopsy studies have found widespread macroscopic evidence of arteriosclerosis in adolescents and young adults[79,128] and have demonstrated that the prevalence and extent of fatty streaks in the aorta of children under the age of 10 years are correlated with a variety of cardiovascular risk factors (including total cholesterol and blood pressure) measured prior to their death.[129] Similarly results from a subset of participants in the Muscatine study found that calcification of the coronary arteries,[130,131] an established correlate of atherosclerotic disease,[132] was positively associated with childhood weight, body mass index, and waist–hip ratio, independently of risk factors measured at subsequent examinations.[133] The Bogalusa Heart Study[134] of a multi-ethnic population of approximately 8000 children has demonstrated tracking[135,136] and clustering[137] of cardiovascular risk factor levels, such as blood pressure and lipids, between childhood and young adult life.

3.7.1 Anthropometric measures as indicators of childhood exposures

Adult height across the population distribution is inversely associated with cardiovascular disease risk, independently of socioeconomic position or smoking behaviour.[138–140] Several plausible explanations exist for this association. First, genetic factors that determine growth patterns may be associated with cardiovascular disease risk. Second, coronary and cerebral artery vessel diameters increase with height and vessels with smaller diameters may result in clinical disease outcomes, due to occlusion, with relatively smaller amounts of atherosclerosis.[139] Third, adult height 'shrinks' with age and also with general ill-health and immobility and it has been suggested that 'shrinkage' may occur in the early (pre-diagnosis) stages of illness and so the height–cardiovascular disease association may really be one of reverse causation.[141] Fourth, the association between height and cardiovascular disease may simply be a reflection of the established birthweight–cardiovascular disease association.[61] Lastly, factors affecting childhood growth, such as infant feeding, childhood infections, childhood diet, and parental smoking, may also influence cardiovascular disease risk and hence explain the link between height and cardiovascular disease association.[142]

Recently it has been proposed that one way of further exploring the height–cardiovascular disease association is to look at the specific associations of the components of height (leg length and trunk length) with disease outcomes.[142] Leg length, in particular (as opposed to trunk length), may be a useful biomarker of pre-pubertal environmental influences on childhood growth, because up until puberty most increase in total height is due to increases in leg length.[142,143] Further, the dramatic increases in height in industrialized countries over the last century appear to arise more from increases in leg length than trunk growth.[144] These trends have occurred as result of improvements in childhood circumstances—in particular improvements in nutrition and reductions in serious infections.

Few studies have assessed the association between components of height and cardiovascular disease. In one study of middle-aged men, leg length was the component of height that was responsible for the height–CHD association.[145] In a second study, leg length measured in childhood (boys and girls aged 2–14 years) was also found to be inversely associated with CHD mortality over 52 years of follow-up.[146] Leg length has also been found to be specifically associated with insulin resistance and type 2 diabetes, with individuals with shorter legs being more insulin resistant and having a greater prevalence of diabetes.[145,147] In a cross-sectional analysis of the British Women's Heart and Health study leg length and trunk length were both inversely associated with prevalent CHD in simple age-adjusted models.[148] The association between trunk length and CHD was fully explained by the confounding effects of smoking. The leg length–CHD association was not explained by the confounding effects of smoking or other confounders.

The specific association of leg length with CHD is not supportive of the height–CHD association being due to increased vessel diameter in taller individuals or differential shrinkage because both of these explanations would have similar effects, or even stronger effects, on the trunk–CHD association. The effect is unlikely to be a reflection of the birthweight–CHD association because birthweight is similarly associated with both leg length and trunk length[145] and therefore if birthweight explained the height–CHD association one would not expect a specific leg length–CHD association. Findings from a study with adult anthropometric data on two generations suggest that genetic factors were not important in the associations between components of height and CHD risk factors (blood pressure and cholesterol), because adjustment for parental height had very little effect on these associations.[149]

A specific association between leg length and CHD most likely reflects an association between adverse pre-pubertal environmental factors that affect growth and result in an increase CHD risk in later life. Leg length appears to be a biomarker for factors acting specifically in the pre-pubertal period. Breastfeeding, high-energy diets at age 2, and affluent social circumstances are all specifically associated with longer leg length.[150,151,152] Further, childhood growth is stunted amongst those whose parents smoke.[153–155] Thus these factors—poor infant and childhood nutrition and parental smoking—may be important early life risk factors for CHD.

In the Helsinki 1 cohort, growth around the time of puberty has been assessed and it was found that men who subsequently died of CHD were of the same height between ages 7 and 15 as the whole cohort,[36] whilst for women those with CHD were shorter, as one might have predicted, though by 15 years they had almost caught up.[37] A significant interaction between length at birth and height at 7 years was observed for women so that the greatest risk of CHD was seen amongst women who were short at birth but tall at 7 years. Additional sex differences were observed so that whilst birth length and centile crossing for height were important for women, thinness at birth and centile crossing for body mass index were more important for CHD risk in men. These different associations were interpreted as demonstrating physiological sex differences in response to intrauterine growth retardation followed by childhood nutritional influences. However, such subgroup analyses need to be interpreted with caution.[156]

3.7.2 Infections in childhood

The notion that infection may play a role in the pathogenesis of atherosclerosis has existed since the beginning of this century.[157] However, results have been inconsistent (see Chapter 2, Section 2.4). Recent studies have largely focused on two specific infections with several case–control and cross-sectional studies finding elevated serum antibody levels specifically for *Chlamydia pneumoniae*, a respiratory pathogen and *Helicobacter pylori*, an enteric pathogen among adults with CHD.[158–166] Most of these studies have relied on measuring immunological markers of infection on cases with existing heart disease, hence infection could occur after disease onset or as a consequence due to reactivation (reverse causality). However, some studies have been able to measure levels on stored adult blood samples and demonstrate that elevation preceded clinical heart disease.[160,165,166] Results from the Helsinki Heart study found associations between *Chlamydia pneumoniae* and incident CHD were stronger for IgA rather than IgG titres indicating chronic persistent (from earlier in the life course) rather than acute infection.[160] However, a large prospective study combined with a meta-analysis of all previous studies found that neither IgA nor IgG titres were strongly predictive of CHD risk.[167]

Helicobacter pylori is likely to be acquired in childhood, with a quarter of current children under the age of 6 being positive for infection, rising to over 50% by the age of 12 or older.[168,169] Children in the past are more likely to have experienced infection with *Helicobacter pylori*, as exposure is associated with poor housing conditions, overcrowding, and sharing a bed with parents.[168,169] An earlier ecological study noted that areas with high levels of infant mortality from diarrhoea and enteritis, as opposed to pneumonia, were more likely to have high levels of CHD in later years.[170] Several biological mechanisms have been proposed to causally link *Helicobacter pylori* with CHD. Seropositivity has been associated with increases in fibrinogen, total leucocyte count, and C-reactive protein,[161,171] although one other study has failed to demonstrate raised fibrinogen.[162] However, the association between chronic inflammation and CHD may be unrelated to infections.[172] It is also plausible that the nutritional disruption of an enteric infection, such as *Helicobacter pylori*, or of any childhood infection affecting appetite, if it occurs during critical periods of organ, hormonal, or metabolic development during infancy, may programme future disease. Despite the evidence from a number of case–control studies and plausible mechanisms linking *Helicobacter pylori* to CHD a systematic review found that prospective studies found weaker associations than did case–control studies, suggesting the possibility of survivor effects,[173] reverse causality, or publication bias.

Childhood infections may mediate the association between poor childhood socioe-conomic circumstances and increased CHD risk.[157] Or indeed childhood infections may be a proxy indicator of poor childhood socioeconomic circumstances rather than having a direct effect. *Helicobacter pylori* infection is associated with diminished child-hood growth and may therefore explain the association between height and CHD (see Section 3.6.1).[174] However, the Helsinki 2 cohort failed to find an association between childhood overcrowding, a proxy for infection hazard and female CHD risk, despite demonstrating a strong inverse association with height.

3.8 Interpreting the empirical evidence within a life course perspective

This overview has demonstrated that pre-adult exposures clearly have some role in the aetiology of CHD and that these associations cannot merely be explained by con-founding with adult risk factors. The exact mechanisms for these exposures remain unclear and therefore limit our ability to conclude which life course model(s) (see Chapter 1) is operating. The most traditional explanation would favour an accumula-tion of risk model with 'risk clustering'. Exposures such as birthweight, breastfeeding, and childhood growth and adult risk factors such as obesity, smoking, and exercise are correlated with each other as they cluster under the broader exposure of adverse cumulative socioeconomic conditions from childhood to adult life (see Chapter 4). Improving such conditions would reduce CHD risk, though not abolish it, as some, but not all, exposures may be prevented.

A simple critical period model for fetal programming seems less likely as more evidence is produced highlighting how the risk associated with birth characteristics is modified by subsequent growth and development. For both the Caerphilly and Helsinki cohorts, birthweight and ponderal index are not associated with increased risk amongst thin men or boys at age 6 years respectively. A critical period model is still plausible with the inclusion of effect modifiers, though whether these observations reflect genetic mecha-nisms or environmental programming remains debatable. A 'chain of risk model' (see Chapter 1) is also feasible as fetal programming may directly lead to some of the observed later exposures. For example, growth retardation may programme the hypothalamic pitu-itary axis so that small babies have a greater cortisol response both to acute and chronic stressors resulting in childhood obesity, which in turn produces insulin resistance, leading to CHD. However, the relative lack of attenuation in statistical models that have included components of the chain makes this model less likely. It is possible that by aggregating participants who have developed CHD through different pathways, we may be masking this effect, which may only occur in a subgroup of the total population.

3.9 Policy implications

The greatest risk to public health, of the associations described in this chapter, are likely to be seen in developing countries where the effects of extreme poverty in early life and in earlier generations are increasingly combined with adverse Western diets and lifestyles in adulthood.[175] Despite this, very little of the research presented in this chapter has been conducted in the developing world. Work (from developed countries) suggesting that accelerated postnatal growth is detrimental to future cardiovascular disease health is a particularly important example of the need to extend this area of research into developing countries. As Victora has pointed out, few would disagree with the suggestion that late weight catch-up in stunted infants or children resulting in the 'stunted-(centrally) obese' adult is harmful to health. However, the short-term benefits of catch-up growth for small newborns, particularly in developing countries with continued exposures to infectious diseases and adverse environments, may outweigh any possible long-term detrimental effects.[176] A body of work is underway in developing countries, but studies to date are on relatively young populations on whom cardiovascular disease risk factors but not disease outcomes have been assessed.[175,177] Continued funding for detailed follow-up of the individuals in these studies, as they develop cardiovascular disease, is essential.

From a public health policy perspective, understanding the mechanisms and models that underlie the association between early life risk factors and cardiovascular disease is important. As Frayling and Hattersley have said 'this is not just a sterile intellectual debate, but will give fundamental insights into the aetiology of adult disease and the most appropriate prevention strategies.'[76] If intrauterine undernutrition of the fetus is important then improvements in the diets and general health of young girls and women or interventions that ensure optimal fetal nutrition may be important for cardiovascular disease prevention. If low birthweight is an indicator of genetic factors associated with both insulin-mediated fetal growth and insulin resistance and thence cardiovascular disease risk, it may be possible to identify individuals who have increased susceptibility to cardiovascular disease very early in their lives and ensure that all other known risk factors across their life course are minimized. If accelerated postnatal growth, which is generally seen as something positive and therefore promoted by health professionals, is detrimental to future adult health then current international policy concerning the early life nutritional management of infants who are growth retarded at birth may need re-thinking.[176] However, if accelerated growth, or infant growth in general, of girls reduces cardiovascular disease risk across generations,[43] then promoting this growth may be important rather than detrimental.

Over the next few years, more firmly based public health conclusions on pre-adult risk factors for cardiovascular disease, relevant to both developed and developing countries, are likely to appear . What is already clear is that giving credence to pre-adult factors should not be regarded as undermining the importance of the classic adult risk factors.[178] There is already evidence that for blood pressure,[179] non-insulin dependent diabetes,[180] and CHD,[132] adult risk factors such as obesity may exacerbate the susceptibilities that are established in early life. A framework that places accumulation of life course exposures and possible early life–adult interactions at its centre is likely to be the most fruitful.

References

Those marked with an asterisk are especially recommended for further reading.

1 **Office for National Statistics electronic data.** *ONS 20ᵗʰ Century Mortality (England and Wales 1901–1999).*

2 **World Health Organization.** *The world health report 2000. Health systems: improving performance.* Geneva: World Health Organization, 2000.

3 **Elo IT, Preston SH**. Effects of early-life conditions on adult mortality: a review. *Pop Ind* 1992;**58**:186–212.

4 **Marmot M, Elliott P**. *Coronary heart disease epidemiology: from aetiology to public health.* Oxford: Oxford University Press, 1992.

5 **Magnus P, Beaglehole R**. The real contribution of the major risk factors to the coronary epidemics: time to end the "only-50%" myth. *Arch Intern Med* 2001;**161**:2657–60.

6 **Beaglehole R, Magnus P**. The search for new risk factors for coronary heart disease: occupational therapy for epidemiologists? *Int J Epidemiol* 2002;**31**:1117–22.

7 **Enos MW, Holmes LCR, Beyer CJ**. Coronary disease among United States soldiers killed in action in Korea. *J Am Med Assoc* 1953;**152**:1090–3.

8 **McNamara JJ, Molot MA, Stremple JF, Cutting RT**. Coronary artery disease in combat casualties in Vietnam. *J Am Med Assoc* 1971;**216**:1185–7.

9 **Strong JP, Malcom GT, McMahan CA, Tracey RE, Newman WP, HerderickEE** *et al.* Prevalence and extent of atherosclerosis in adolescents and young adults. Implications for prevention from the pathobiological determinants of Atherosclerosis in Youth Study. *J Am Med Assoc* 1999;**281**:727–35.

10 **Ebbeling CB, Pawlak DB, Ludwig DS**. Childhood obesity: public-health crisis, common sense cure. *Lancet* 2002;**360**:473–81.

11 **McCarthy HD, Ellis SM, Cole TJ**. Central overweight and obesity in British youth aged 11–16 years: cross sectional surveys of waist circumference. *Br Med J* 2003;**326**:624.

12 **Freedman DS, Dietz WH, Srinivasan SR, Berenson GS**. The relation of overweight to cardiovascular risk factors among children and adolescents: The Bogalusa Heart Study. *Pediatrics* 1999;**103**:1175–82.

13 **Tounian P, Aggoun Y, Dubern B, Varille V, Guy-Grand B, Sidi D** *et al.* Presence of increased stiffness of the common carotid artery and endothelial dysfunction in severely obese children: a prospective study. *Lancet* 2001;**358**:1400–4.

14 **Fagot-Campagna A, Pettitt DJ, Engelgau MM** *et al.* Type 2 diabetes among North American children and adolescents: an epidemiologic review and a public health perspective. *J Pediat* 2000;**136**:664–72.

15 **Collins R, Peto R, MacMahon S** *et al.* Blood pressure, stroke, and coronary heart disease. Part 2, short-term reductions in blood pressure: overview of randomised drug trials in their epidemiological context. *Lancet* 1990;**335**:827–38.

16 **Andersson OK, Almgren T, Persson B, Samuelsson O, Hedner T, Wilhelmsen L**. Survival in treated hypertension: follow up study after two decades. *Br Med J* 1998;**317**:167–71.

17 **Ben-Shlomo Y, Kuh D**. A life course approach to chronic disease epidemiology: conceptual models, empirical challenges and interdisciplinary perspectives. *Int J Epidemiol* 2002;**31**:285–93.

18 **Wadsworth MEJ**. *The imprint of time: childhood, history and adult life.* Oxford: Clarendon Press, 1991.

*19 **Osmond C, Barker DJ, Winter PD, Fall CH, Simmonds SJ**. Early growth and death from cardiovascular disease in women. *Br Med J* 1993;**307**:1519–24.

20 **Forsdahl A**. Are poor living conditions in childhood and adolescence an important risk factor for arteriosclerotic heart disease? *Br J Prev Soc Med* 1977;**31**:91–5.

21 **Williams DRR, Roberts SJ, Davies TW**. Deaths from ischaemic heart disease and infant mortality in England and Wales. *J Epidemiol Commun Health* 1979;**33**:199–202.

22 **Barker DJP, Osmond C**. Infant mortality, childhood nutrition, and ischaemic heart disease in England and Wales. *Lancet* 1986;**i**:1077–81.

23 **Barker DJP, Osmond C, Golding J**. Height and mortality in the counties of England and Wales. *Ann Hum Biol* 1990;**17**:1–6.

24 Barker DJ, Osmond C, Golding J, Kuh D, Wadsworth ME. Growth *in utero*, blood pressure in childhood and adult life, and mortality from cardiovascular disease. *Br Med J* 1989;**298**:564–7.

25 Whincup PH, Cook DG, Adshead F, Taylor S, Papacosta O, Walker M *et al.* Cardiovascular risk factors in British children from towns with widely differing adult cardiovascular mortality. *Br Med J* 1996;**313**:79–84.

26 Davey Smith G, Ben-Shlomo Y, Lynch J. Life course approaches to inequalities in coronary heart disease risk. In Stansfeld S, Marmot M, eds. *Stress and the heart*. London: BMJ Books, 2002:20–49.

*27 Barker DJ, Winter PD, Osmond C, Margetts B, Simmonds SJ. Weight in infancy and death from ischaemic heart disease. *Lancet* 1989;**2**:577–80.

28 Fall CH, Vijayakumar M, Barker DJ, Osmond C, Duggleby S. Weight in infancy and prevalence of coronary heart disease in adult life. *Br Med J* 1995;**310**:17–9.

29 Barker DJ, Osmond C, Simmonds SJ, Wield GA. The relation of small head circumference and thinness at birth to death from cardiovascular disease in adult life. *Br Med J* 1993;**306**:422–6.

30 Eriksson M, Tibblin G, Cnattingius S. Low birthweight and ischaemic heart disease. *Lancet* 1994; **343**:731.

31 Stein CE, Fall CH, Kumaran K, Osmond C, Cox V, Barker DJ. Fetal growth and coronary heart disease in south India. *Lancet* 1996;**348**:1269–73.

*32 Frankel S, Elwood P, Sweetnam P, Yarnell J, Davey Smith G. Birthweight, body-mass index in middle age, and incident coronary heart disease. *Lancet* 1996;**348**:1478–80.

33 Frankel S, Elwood P, Sweetnam P, Yarnell J, Davey Smith G. Birthweight, adult risk factors and incident coronary heart disease: the Caerphilly Study. *Pub Health* 1996;**110**:139–43.

34 Rich-Edwards JW, Stampfer MJ, Manson JE, Rosner B, Hankinson SE, Colditz GA *et al.* Birthweight and risk of cardiovascular disease in a cohort of women followed up since 1976. *Br Med J* 1997;**315**:396–400.

*35 Leon DA, Lithell HO, Vagero D, Koupilova I, Mohsen R, Berglund L *et al.* Reduced fetal growth rate and increased risk of death from ischaemic heart disease: cohort study of 15 000 Swedish men and women born 1915–29. *Br Med J* 1998;**317**:241–5.

*36 Eriksson JG, Forsen T, Tuomilehto J, Winter PD, Osmond C, Barker DJ. Catch-up growth in childhood and death from coronary heart disease: longitudinal study. *Br Med J* 1999;**318**:427–31.

37 Forsen T, Eriksson JG, Tuomilehto J, Osmond C, Barker DJ. Growth *in utero* and during childhood among women who develop coronary heart disease: longitudinal study. *Br Med J* 1999;**319**:1403–7.

*38 Eriksson JG, Forsen T, Tuomilehto J, Osmond C, Barker DJ. Early growth and coronary heart disease in later life: longitudinal study. *Br Med J* 2001;**322**:949–53.

39 Gunnarsdottir I, Birgistottir BE, Thorsdottir I, Gudnason V, Bebediktsson R. Size at birth and coronary artery disease in a population with high birthweight. *Am J Clin Nutr* 2002;**76**:1290–4.

40 Fall CH, Barker DJ, Osmond C, Winter PD, Clark PM, Hales CN. Relation of infant feeding to adult serum cholesterol concentration and death from ischaemic heart disease. *Br Med J* 1992; **304**:801–5.

41 Fall CHD, Osmond C, Barker DJP, Clark PMS, Hales CN, Stirling Y *et al.* Fetal and infant growth and cardiovascular risk factors in women. *Br Med J* 1995;**310**:428–32.

42 Vijayakumar M, Fall CH, Osmond C, Barker DJ. Birthweight, weight at one year, and left ventricular mass in adult life. *Br Heart J* 1995;**73**:363–7.

43 Martyn CN, Barker DJ, Osmond C. Mothers' pelvic size, fetal growth, and death from stroke and coronary heart disease in men in the UK. *Lancet* 1996;**348**:1264–8.

44 Scholl TO, Sowers M, Chen X, Lenders C. Maternal glucose concentration influences fetal growth, gestation, and pregnancy complications. *Am J Epidemiol* 2001;**154**:514–20.

45 Reusens B, Remacle C. Intergenerational effect of an adverse intrauterine environment on perturbation of glucose metabolism. *Twin Res* 2001;**4**:406–11.

*46 Hypponen E, Leon DA, Kenward MG, Lithell H. Prenatal growth and risk of occlusive and haemorrhagic stroke in Swedish men and women born 1915–29: historical cohort study. *Br Med J* 2001;**323**:1033–4.

47 Eriksson JG, Forsen T, Tuomilehto J, Osmond C, Barker DJ. Early growth, adult income, and risk of stroke. *Stroke* 2000;**31**:869–74.

48 Song Y-M, Sung J, Lawlor DA, Davey Smith G, Shin Y, Ebrahim S. Blood pressure, haemorrhagic and ischaemic stroke: the Korean National Health System Study. *BMJ* 2003 (in press).

49 Huxley RR, Shiell AW, Law CM. The role of size at birth and postnatal catch-up growth in determining systolic blood pressure: a systematic review of the literature. *J Hypertens* 2000;**18**:815–31.

50 McCarron P, Davey Smith G, Okasha M. Secular changes in blood pressure in childhood, adolescence and young adulthood: systematic review of trends from 1948 to 1998. *J Hum Hypertens* 2002;**16**:677–89.

51 Lamont D, Parker L, White M, Unwin N, Bennett SMA, Cohen M *et al.* Risk of cardiovascular disease measured by carotid intima-media thickness at age 49–51: lifecourse study. *Br Med J* 2000;**320**:273–8.

52 Martyn CN, Gale CR, Jespersen S, Sherriff SB. Impaired fetal growth and atherosclerosis of carotid and peripheral arteries. *Lancet* 1998;**352**:173–8.

53 Gale CR, Ashurst HE, Hall NF, MacCallum PK, Martyn CN. Size at birth and carotid atherosclerosis in later life. *Atherosclerosis* 2002;**163**:141–7.

54 Tilling K, Davey Smith G, Chambless L *et al.* The relationship between birthweight and intima-media thickness in middle age: The ARIC study. *Epidemiology* 2003; (In press).

55 Chambless LE, Heiss G, Folsom AR, Rosamund W, Szklo M, Sharrett AR, *et al.* Association of Coronary Heart Disease Incidence with Carotid Arterial Wall Thickness and Major Risk Factors: The Atherosclerosis Risk in Communities (ARIC) Study, 1987–1993. *Am J Epidemiol* 1997;**146**:483–94.

56 Chambless LE, Folsom AR, Clegg LX, Sharrett AR, Shahar E, Nieto FJ *et al.* Carotid wall thickness is predictive of incident clinical stroke: the Atherosclerosis Risk in Communities (ARIC) study. *Am J Epidemiol* 2000;**151**:478–87.

57 Sharrett AR, Sorlie PD, Chambless LE, Folsom AR, Hutchinson RG, Heiss G *et al.* Relative importance of various risk factors for asymptomatic carotid atherosclerosis versus coronary heart disease incidence: the Atherosclerosis Risk in Communities Study. *Am J Epidemiol* 1999;**149**:843–52.

58 Joseph KS, Kramer MS. Review of the evidence on fetal and early childhood antecedents of adult chronic disease. *Epidemiol Rev* 1996;**18**:158–74.

59 Huxley R, Neil A, Collins R. Unravelling the "fetal origins" hypothesis: is there really an inverse association between birthweight and future blood pressure? *Lancet* 2002;**360**:659–65.

60 Lucas A, Fewtrell MS, Cole TJ. Fetal origins of adult disease—the hypothesis revisited. *Br Med J* 1999;**319**:245–9.

61 Barker DJP. *Mothers, babies and health in later life.* London: Churchill Livingstone, 1998.

62 Hales CN, Barker DJ. The thrifty phenotype hypothesis. *Br Med Bull* 2001;**60**:5–20.

63 Koupilova I, Leon DA, McKeigue PM, Lithell HO. Is the effect of low birthweight on cardiovascular mortality mediated through high blood pressure? *J Hypertens* 1999;**17**:19–25.

*64 Harding JE. The nutritional basis of the fetal origins of adult disease. *Int J Epidemiol* 2001;**30**:15–23.

65 Langley-Evans SC, Gardner DS, Welham SJ. Intrauterine programming of cardiovascular disease by maternal nutritional status. *Nutrition* 1998;**14**:39–47.

66 Petry CJ, Hales CN. Long-term effects on offspring of intrauterine exposure to deficits in nutrition. *Hum Reprod Update* 2000;**6**:578–86.

67 Roseboom TJ, van der Meulen JH, Ravelli AC, Van Montfrans GA, Osmond C, Barker DJP *et al.* Blood pressure in adults after prenatal exposure to famine. *J Hypertens* 1999;**17**:325–30.

68 Roseboom TJ, van der Meulen JHP, Osmond C, Barker DJP, Ravelli ACJ, Bleker OP. Plasma lipid profiles in adults after prenatal exposure to the Dutch famine. *Am J Clin Nutr* 2000;**72**:1101–6.

69 Ravelli AC, van der Meulen JH, Michels RP, Osmond C, Barker DJP, Hales CN. Glucose tolerance in adults after prenatal exposure to famine. *Lancet* 1998;**351**:173–7.

70 Roseboom TJ, van der Meulen JH, Osmond C, Barker DJP, Ravelli ACJ, Schroeder-Tanka JM *et al.* Coronary heart disease after prenatal exposure to the Dutch famine, 1944–45. *Heart* 2000;**84**:595–8.

71 Roseboom TJ, van der Meulen JH, Osmond C, Barker DJ, Ravelli AC, Bleker OP. Adult survival after prenatal exposure to the Dutch famine 1944–45. *Paediat Perinat Epidemiol* 2001;**15**:220–5.

72 Stanner SA, Bulmer K, Andres C, Lantsava OE, Borodina V, Poteer VV *et al.* Does malnutrition *in utero* determine diabetes and coronary heart disease in adulthood? Results from the Leningrad siege study, a cross sectional study. *Br Med J* 1997;**315**:1342–8.

73 Belizan JM, Villar J, Bergel E, del Pino A, Di Fulvio S, Galliano SV. Long-term effect of calcium supplementation during pregnancy on the blood pressure of offspring: follow up of a randomised controlled trial. *Br Med J* 1997;**315**:281–5.

74 McKeigue P. Diabetes and insulin action. In Kuh D, Ben-Shlomo Y, eds. *A life course approach to chronic disease epidemiology*. Oxford: Oxford University Press, 1997:78–100.

*75 Hattersley AT, Tooke JE. The fetal insulin hypothesis: an alternative explanation of the association of low birthweight with diabetes and vascular disease. *Lancet* 1999;**353**:1789–92.

76 Frayling TM, Hattersley AT. The role of genetic susceptibility in the association of low birthweight with type 2 diabetes. *Br Med Bull* 2001;**60**:89–101.

77 Hattersley AT, Beards F, Ballantyne E, Appleton M, Harvey R, Ellard S. Mutations in the glucokinase gene of the fetus result in reduced birthweight. *Nat Genet* 1998;**19**:268–70.

78 Dunger DB, Ong KL, Huxtable SJ *et al.* Association of the INS VTNR with size at birth. *Nat Genet* 1998;**19**:98–100.

79 Ong KK, Phillips DI, Fall C *et al.* The insulin gene VNTR, type 2 diabetes and birthweight. *Nat Genet* 1999;**21**:262–3.

80 Lindsay RS, Hanson RL, Wiedrich C, Knowler WC, Bennett PH, Baier LJ. The insulin gene variable number tandem repeat class I/III polymorphism is in linkage disequilibrium with birthweight but not Type 2 diabetes in the Pima population. *Diabetes* 2003;**52**:187–93.

81 Casteels K, Ong K, Phillips D, Bendall H, Pembrey M. Mitochondrial 16189 variant, thinness at birth, and type-2 diabetes. ALSPAC study team. Avon Longitudinal Study of Pregnancy and Childhood. *Lancet* 1999;**353**:1499–500.

82 Vagero D, Leon D. Ischaemic heart disease and low birthweight: a test of the fetal-origins hypothesis from the Swedish Twin Registry. *Lancet* 1994;**343**:260–3.

83 Christensen K, Vaupel JW, Holm NV, Yashin AI. Mortality among twins after age 6: fetal origins hypothesis versus twin method. *Br Med J* 1995;**310**:432–6.

84 Christensen K, Wienke A, Skytthe A, Holm NV, Vaupel JW, Yashin AI. Cardiovascular mortality in twins and the fetal origins hypothesis. *Twin Res* 2001;**4**:344–9.

85 Williams S, Poulton R. Twins and maternal smoking: ordeals for the fetal origins hypothesis? A cohort study. *Br Med J* 1999;**318**:897–900.

86 De Geus EJ, Posthuma D, IJzerman RG, Boomsma DI. Comparing blood pressure of twins and their singleton siblings: being a twin does not affect adult blood pressure. *Twin Res* 2001; **4**:385–91.

87 Phillips DI, Davies MJ, Robinson JS. Fetal growth and the fetal origins hypothesis in twins—problems and perspectives. *Twin Res* 2001;**4**:327–331.

88 Leveno KJ, Santos-Ramos R, Duenhoelter JH, Reisch JS, Whalley PJ. Sonar cephalometry in twins: a table of biparietal diameters for normal twin fetuses and a comparison with singletons. *Am J Obstet Gynecol* 1979;**135**:727–30.

89 Taylor GM, Owen P, Mires GJ. Foetal growth velocities in twin pregnancies. *Twin Res* 1998;**1**: 9–14.

90 Phillips DI. Twin studies in medical research: can they tell us whether diseases are genetically determined? *Lancet* 1993;**341**:1008–9.

91 Hubinette A, Cnattingius S, Ekbom A, De Faire U, Kramer M, Lichtenstein P. Birthweight, early environment, and genetics: a study of twins discordant for acute myocardial infarction. *Lancet* 2001;**357**:1997–2001.

92 Hubinette A, Cnattingius S, Johasson ALV, Henriksson C, Lichtenstein P. Birthweight and risk of angina pectoris: analysis in Swedish twins. *Eur J Epidemiol* 2003;**18**:539–44.

93 Davey Smith G, Hart C, Ferrell C, Upton M, Hole D, Hawthorne V *et al.* Birthweight of offspring and mortality in the Renfrew and Paisley study: prospective observational study. *Br Med J* 1997;**315**:1189–93.

94 Davey Smith G, Whitley E, Gissler M, Hemminki E. Birth dimensions of offspring, premature birth, and the mortality of mothers. *Lancet* 2000;**356**:2066–7.

95 Davey Smith G, Harding S, Rosato M. Relation between infants' birthweight and mothers' mortality: prospective observational study. *Br Med J* 2000;**320**:839–40.

96 Lawlor DA, Davey Smith G, Whincup P, Wannamethee G, Papacosta O, Dhanjil S *et al.* The association between offspring birthweight and atherosclerosis in middle aged men and women: British Regional Heart Study. *J Epidemiol Commun Health* 2003;**57**:462–3.

97 Rasmussen F, Sterne J, Davey Smith G, Tynelius P, Leon DA. Fetal growth is associated with parents' cardiovascular mortality. *Am J Epidemiol* 2001;**153**(suppl):S98.

98 Smith GC, Pell JP, Walsh D. Pregnancy complications and maternal risk of ischaemic heart disease: a retrospective cohort study of 129,290 births. *Lancet* 2001;**357**:2002–6.

99 Klebanoff MA, Schulsinger C, Mednick BR, Secher NJ. Preterm and small-for-gestational-age birth across generations. *Am J Obstet Gynecol* 1997;**176**:521–6.

100 Ramakrishnan U, Martorell R, Schroeder DG, Flores R. Role of intergenerational effects on linear growth. *J Nutr* 1999;**129**(suppl 2S):544S–549S.

101 Magnus P, Gjessing HK, Skrondal A, Skjaerven R. Paternal contribution to birthweight. *J Epidemiol Commun Health* 2001;**55**:873–7.

102 Hypponen E, Davey Smith G, Power C. Parental diabetes and offspring birthweight in an intergenerational cohort study. *Br Med J* 2003;**326**:19–20.

103 Lawlor DA, Davey Smith G, Ebrahim S. Birthweight of offspring and insulin resistance in late adulthood: cross sectional survey using data from the British Women's Heart and Health Study. *Br Med J* 2002;**325**:359–62.

104 Rasmussen F, Davey Smith G, Sterne J, Tynelius P, Leon DA. Birth characteristics of offspring and parental diabetes. *Am J Epidemiol* 2001;**153**(suppl):S47.

105 Wannamethee SG, Lawlor DA, Whincup PH, Walker M, Ebrahim S, Davey Smith G. Birthweight of offspring and paternal insulin resistance and diabetes in late adulthood: cross-sectional survey. *Diabetologia* 2003 (in press).

106 Davey Smith G. Genetic risk factors in mothers and offspring. *Lancet* 2001;**358**:1268.

107 Tanner JM. Catch-up growth in man. *Br Med Bull* 1981;**37**:233–8.

108 Fitzhardinge PM, Steven EM. The small-for-date infant. I. Later growth patterns. *Pediat* 1972;**49**:671–81.

109 Karlberg J, Albertsson-Wikland K. Growth in full-term small-for-gestational-age infants: from birth to final height. *Pediat Res* 1995;**38**:733–9.

110 Pelletier DL, Frongillo EA, Jr., Habicht JP. Epidemiologic evidence for a potentiating effect of malnutrition on child mortality. *Am J Pub Health* 1993;**83**:1130–3.

111 Eriksson JG, Forsen T, Tuomilehto J, Osmond C, Barker DJ. Early growth and coronary heart disease in later life: longitudinal study. *Br Med J* 2001;**322**:949–53.

112 Singhal A, Fewtrell M, Cole TJ, Lucas A. Low nutrient intake and early growth for later insulin resistance in adolescents born preterm. *Lancet* 2003;**361**:1089–97.

113 Osborn GR. Stages in development of coronary disease observed from 1,500 young subjects. Relationship of hypotension and infant feeding to aetiology. *Coll Int Centre National Rech Scient* 1967;**169**:93–139.

114 Burr ML, Beasley WH, Fisher CB. Breast feeding, maternal smoking and early atheroma. *Eur Heart J* 1984;**5**:588–91.

115 Cowen DD. Myocardial infarction and infant feeding. *Practitioner* 1973;**210**:661–3.

116 Wingard DL, Criqui MH, Edelstein SL, Tucker J, Tomlinson-Keasey C, Schwartz JC *et al.* Is breast-feeding in infancy associated with adult longevity? *Am J Pub Health* 1994;**84**:1458–62.

117 Plancoulaine S, Charles MA, Lafay L *et al.* Infant-feeding patterns are related to blood cholesterol concentration in prepubertal children aged 5–11 y: the Fleurbaix-Laventie Ville Sante study. *Eur J Clin Nutr* 2000;**54**:114–9.

118 Ravelli AC, van der Meulen JH, Osmond C, Barker DJ, Bleker OP. Infant feeding and adult glucose tolerance, lipid profile, blood pressure, and obesity. *Arch Dis Child* 2000;**82**:248–52.

119 Parsons TJ, Power C, Logan S, Summerbell CD. Childhood predictors of adult obesity: a systematic review. *Int J Obesity* 1999;**23**:S1-S107.

120 Singhal A, Cole TJ, Lucas A. Early nutrition in preterm infants and later blood pressure: two cohorts after randomised trials. *Lancet* 2001;**357**:413–9.

121 Leeson CP, Kattenhorn M, Deanfield JE, Lucas A. Duration of breast feeding and arterial distensibility in early adult life: population based study. *Br Med J* 2001;**322**:643–7.

122 Ebrahim S, Davey Smith G. Lowering blood pressure: a systematic review of sustained effects of non-pharmacological interventions. *J Pub Health Med* 1998;**20**:441–8.

123 Geleijnse JM, Hofman A, Witteman JC, Hazebroek AA, Valkenburg HA, Grobbee DE. Long-term effects of neonatal sodium restriction on blood pressure. *Hypertension* 1997;**29**:913–7.

124 Koletzko B, Agostoni C, Carlson SE, Koletzko B, Agostoni C, Carlson SE *et al.* Long chain polyunsaturated fatty acids (LC-PUFA) and perinatal development. *Acta Paediat* 2001;**90**:460–4.

125 Forsyth JS, Willatts P, Agostoni C, Bissenden J, Casaer P, Boehm G. Long chain polyunsaturated fatty acid supplementation in infant formula and blood pressure in later childhood: follow up of a randomised controlled trial. *Br Med J* 2003;**326**:953.

126 McGill HCJ, Greer JC, Strong JP. Natural history of human atherosclerotic lessions. In Standler M, Bourne GH, eds. *Atherosclerosis and its origin.* New York: Academic Press, 1963.

127 Berenson GS, Srinivasan SR, Freedman DS, Radhakrishnamurthy B, Dalferes ERJ. Atherosclerosis and its evolution in childhood. *Am J Med Sci* 1987;**294**:429–40.

128 Enos MWF, Holmes LCRH, Beyer CJ. Coronary disease among United States soldiers killed in action in Korea. *J Am Med Assoc* 1953;**152**:1090–3.

129 Tracy RE, Newman WP III, Wattigney WA, Berenson GS. Risk factors and atherosclerosis in youth autopsy findings of the Bogalusa Heart Study. *Am J Med Sci* 1995;**310**(suppl 1):S37–S41.

130 Lauer RM, Connor WE, Leaverton PE, Reiter MA, Clarke WR. Coronary heart disease risk factors in school children: the Muscatine study. *J Pediat* 1975;**86**:697–706.

131 Lauer RM, Lee J, Clarke WR. Factors affecting the relationship between childhood and adult cholesterol levels: The Muscatine Study. *Pediatrics* 1988;**82**:309–18.

132 Eggen DA, Strong JP, McGill HC Jr. Coronary calcification. Relationship to clinically significant coronary lesions and race, sex, and topographic distribution. *Circulation* 1965;**32**:948–55.

133 Mahoney LT, Burns TL, Stanford W *et al.* Coronary risk factors measured in childhood and young adult life are associated with coronary artery calcification in young adults: the Muscatine Study. *J Am Coll Cardiol* 1996;**27**:277–84.

134 Berenson GS, McMahan CA, Voors AW *et al. Cardiovascular risk factors in children. The early natural history of atherosclerosis and essential hypertension.* New York: Oxford University Press, 1980.

135 Wattigney WA, Webber LS, Srinivasan SR, Berenson GS. The emergence of clinically abnormal levels of cardiovascular disease risk factor variables among young adults: the Bogalusa Heart Study. *Prev Med* 1995;**24**:617–26.

136 Myers L, Coughlin SS, Webber LS, Sriivasan SR, Berenson GS. Prediction of adult cardiovascular multifactorial risk status from childhood risk factor levels: the Bogalusa Heart Study. *Am J Epidemiol* 1995;**142**:918–24.

137 Bao W, Srinivasan SR, Wattigney WA, Berenson GS. Persistence of multiple cardiovascular risk clustering related to syndrome X from childhood to young adulthood. The Bogalusa Heart Study. *Arch Intern Med* 1994;**154**:1842–7.

138 McCarron P, Hart CL, Hole D, Davey Smith G. The relation between adult height and haemorrhagic and ischaemic stroke in the Renfrew/Paisley study. *J Epidemiol Commun Health* 2001; **55**:404–5.

139 Palmer JR, Rosenberg L, Shapiro S. Stature and the risk of myocardial infarction in women. *Am J Epidemiol* 1990;**132**:27–32.

140 Rich-Edwards JW, Manson JE, Stampfer MJ, Colditz GA, Willett WC, Rosner B *et al.* Height and the risk of cardiovascular disease in women. *Am J Epidemiol* 1995;**142**:909–17.

141 Leon DA, Davey Smith G, Shipley M, Strachan D. Adult height and mortality in London: early life, socioeconomic confounding, or shrinkage? *J Epidemiol Commun Health* 1995;**49**:5–9.

*142 Gunnell D. Commentary: Can adult anthropometry be used as a 'biomarker' for prenatal and childhood exposures? *Int J Epidemiol* 2002;**31**:390–4.

143 Gerver WJM, Bruin RD. Relationship between height, sitting height and subischial leg length in Dutch children: presentation of normal values. *Acta Paediat* 1995;**84**:532–5.

144 Tanner JM, Hayashi T, Preece MA, Cameron N. Increase in length of leg relative to trunk in Japanese children and adults from 1957 to 1977: comparison with British and with Japanese Americans. *Ann Hum Biol* 1982;**9**:411–23.

145 Davey Smith G, Greenwood R, Gunnell D, Sweetnam P, Yarnell J, Elwood P. Leg length, insulin resistance, and coronary heart disease risk: the Caerphilly Study. *J Epidemiol Commun Health* 2001;**55**:867–72.

146 Gunnell DJ, Davey Smith G, Frankel S *et al.* Childhood leg length and adult mortality: follow up of the Carnegie (Boyd Orr) Survey of Diet and Health in Pre-war Britain. *J Epidemiol Commun Health* 1998;**52**:142–52.

147 Lawlor DA, Ebrahim S, Davey Smith G. The association between components of adult height and type II diabetes and insulin resistance: British Women's Heart and Health Study. *Diabetologia* 2002;**45**:1097–106.

148 **Lawlor DA, Taylor M, Davey Smith G, Gunnell D, Ebrahim S.** The associations of components of adult height with coronary heart disease in postmenopausal women: the British Women's Heart and Health Study. *Heart* 2003 (in press).

149 **Gunnell D, Whitley E, Upton MN, McConnachie A, Davey Smith G, Watt GCM.** Associations of height, leg length and lung function with cardiovascular disease risk factors in the Midspan Family Study. *J Epidemiol Commun Health* 2003;**57**:141–6.

150 **Gunnell DJ, Davey Smith G, Frankel SJ, Kemp M, Peters TJ.** Socioeconomic and dietary influences on leg length and trunk length in childhood: a reanalysis of the Carnegie (Boyd Orr) survey of diet and health in prewar Britain (1937–39). *Paediat Perinat Epidemiol* 1998; **12(suppl 1)**:96–113.

151 **Martin R, Gunnell D, Mangtani P, Frankel S, Davey Smith G.** Association between breast feeding and growth in childhood through to adulthood: the Boyd Orr cohort study. *J Epidemiol Commun Health* 2000;**54**:784.

*152 **Wadsworth MEJ, Hardy RJ, Paul AA, Marshall SF, Cole TJ.** Leg and trunk length at 43 years in relation to childhood health, diet and family circumstances; evidence from the 1946 national birth cohort. *Int J Epidemiol* 2002;**31**:383–90.

153 **Elwood PC, Sweetnam PM, Gray OP, Davies DP, Wood PDP.** Growth of children from 0–5 years: with special reference to mother's smoking in pregnancy. *Ann Hum Biol* 1987;**14**:543–57.

154 **Goldstein H.** Factors influencing the height of seven year old children—results from the national child development study. *Hum Biol* 1971;**43**:92–111.

155 **Wingerd J, Schoen EJ.** Factors influencing length at birth and height at five years. *Pediatrics* 1974;**53**:737–41.

156 **Lawlor DA, Ebrahim S, Davey Smith G.** Is there a sex difference in the association between birthweight and systolic blood pressure in later life? Findings from a meta-regression analysis. *Am J Epidemiol* 2002;**156**:1100–4.

157 **Nieto FJ.** Infections and atherosclerosis: new clues from an old hypothesis? *Am J Epidemiol* 1998;**148**:937–48.

158 **Mattila KJ.** Viral and bacterial infections in patients with acute myocardial infarction. *J Intern Med* 1989;**225**:293–6.

159 **Thom DH, Grayston JT, Siscovick DS, Wang SP, Weiss NS, Daling JR.** Association of prior infection with *Chlamydia pneumoniae* and angiographically demonstrated coronary artery disease. *J Am Med Assoc* 1992;**268**:68–72.

160 **Saikku P, Leinonen M, Tenkanen L et al.** Chronic *Chlamydia pneumoniae* infection as a risk factor for coronary heart disease in the Helsinki Heart Study. *Ann Intern Med* 1992;**116**:273–8.

161 **Patel P, Mendall MA, Carrington D et al.** Association of *Helicobacter pylori* and *Chlamydia pneumoniae* infections with coronary heart disease and cardiovascular risk factors. *Br Med J* 1995;**311**:711–4.

162 **Murray LJ, Bamford KB, O'Reilly DP, McCrum EE, Evans AE.** *Helicobacter pylori* infection: relation with cardiovascular risk factors, ischaemic heart disease, and social class. *Br Heart J* 1995;**74**:497–501.

163 **Mendall MA, Carrington D, Strachan D et al.** *Chlamydia pneumoniae*: risk factors for seropositivity and association with coronary heart disease. *J Infect* 1995;**30**:121–8.

164 **Martin-de-Argila C, Boixeda D, Canton R, Gisbert JP, Fuertes A.** High seroprevalence of *Helicobacter pylori* infection in coronary heart disease. *Lancet* 1995;**346**:310.

165 **Whincup PH, Mendall MA, Perry IJ, Strachan DP, Walker M.** Prospective relations between *Helicobacter pylori* infection, coronary heart disease, and stroke in middle aged men. *Heart* 1996;**75**:568–72.

166 **Whincup P, Danesh J, Walker M** *et al.* Prospective study of potentially virulent strains of *Helicobacter pylori* and coronary heart disease in middle-aged men. *Circulation* 2000; **101**:1647–52.

167 **Danesh J, Whincup P, Lewington S** *et al.* *Chlamydia pneumoniae* IgA titres and coronary heart disease; prospective study and meta-analysis. *Eur Heart J* 2002;**23**:371–5.

168 **Mendall MA, Goggin PM, Molineaux N** *et al.* Childhood living conditions and *Helicobacter pylori* seropositivity in adult life. *Lancet* 1992;**339**:896–7.

169 **McCallion WA, Murray LJ, Bailie AG, Dalzell AM, O'Reilly DP, Bamford KB.** *Helicobacter pylori* infection in children: relation with current household living conditions. *Gut* 1996;**39**:18–21.

170 **Buck C, Simpson H.** Infant diarrhoea and subsequent mortality from heart disease and cancer. *J Epidemiol Commun Health* 1982;**36**:27–30.

171 **Mendall MA, Patel P, Ballam L, Strachan D, Northfield TC.** C reactive protein and its relation to cardiovascular risk factors: a population based cross sectional study. *Br Med J* 1996;**312**:1061–5.

172 **Danesh J, Whincup P, Walker M** *et al.* Low grade inflammation and coronary heart disease: prospective study and updated meta-analyses. *Br Med J* 2000;**321**:199–204.

173 **Danesh J.** Is there a link between chronic *Helicobacter pylori* infection and coronary heart disease? *Euro J Surg* 1998;**582**:27–31.

174 **Patel P, Mendall MA, Khulusi S, Northfield TC, Strachan DP.** *Helicobacter pylori* infection in childhood: risk factors and effect on growth. *Br Med J* 1994;**309**:1119–23.

175 **Yajnik CS.** Commentary: fetal origins of cardiovascular risk-nutritional and non-nutritional. *Int J Epidemiol* 2001;**30**:57–9.

176 **Victora CG, Barros FC.** Commentary: The catch-up dilemma—relevance of Leitch's 'low-high' pig to child growth in developing countries. *Int J Epidemiol* 2001;**30**:217–20.

177 **Yajnik CS.** The lifecycle effects of nutrition and body size on adult adiposity, diabetes and cardiovascular disease. *Obesity Rev* 2002;**3**:217–24.

178 **Aboderin I, Kalache A, Ben-Shlomo Y, Lynch JW, Yajnik CS, Kuh D** *et al.* *Life course perspectives on coronary heart disease, stroke and diabetes: key issues and implications for policy and research.* Geneva: World Health Organization, 2002.

179 **Leon DA, Koupilova I, Lithell HO** *et al.* Failure to realise growth potential *in utero* and adult obesity in relation to blood pressure in 50-year old Swedish men. *Br Med J* 1996;**312**:401–6.

180 **Lithell HO, McKeigue PM, Berglund L** *et al.* Relation of size at birth to non-insulin dependent diabetes and insulin concentrations in men aged 50–60 years. *Br Med J* 1996;**312**:406–10.

Chapter 4

Life course approaches to socioeconomic differentials in health

George Davey Smith and John Lynch

A strong case can be made for the contribution of socioeconomic conditions at different stages of the life course to health in adulthood. The particular weightings of the contributions of early and later life socioeconomic conditions may differ according to the outcome (for example, stronger early life contributions for cardiovascular disease (CVD) than unintentional injury). They will also vary according to how risk factors for a particular outcome are linked to socioeconomic circumstances over the life course (for example, different socioeconomic patterns of growth). These links between socioeconomic conditions and particular risk factors may differ across place (for example, different countries may have different socioeconomic configurations of risk factors such as diet) and time (for example, different birth cohorts may experience these risk factors differently) and may differentially affect population subgroups (for example, socioeconomic by gender interactions in the uptake and maintenance of smoking). Socioeconomic differentials in CVD are best understood through consideration of how a variety of exposures that increase CVD risk are influenced by social circumstances across the life course and how this social dependence can lead to them clustering across time. The accumulation of—and interaction between—these influences acting at different stages of life helps determine socioeconomic patterns of CVD within and between populations.

4.1 Introduction

Differences in life expectancy between social groups have been demonstrated since the early days of industrialization.[1] In 1845, Frederick Engels presented a multilevel examination of how both area-based and individual indicators of socioeconomic position (SEP) affected mortality (Fig. 4.1).[2] Engels described the wretched housing conditions of the working people, the soul- and body-destroying work, the poor sanitary state of the city environment and their inadequate diet. The direct contribution of such factors to poor health seemed obvious to Engels, as it would to any reader of his book today.

As Fig.4.2 shows, Engels was writing at a time when the mortality experience of the inhabitants of some of the great cities was worsening[3,4] and the decline in overall

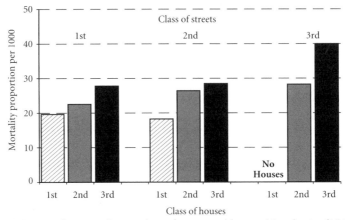

Fig. 4.1 Mortality according to class of street and house, Manchester (1844).

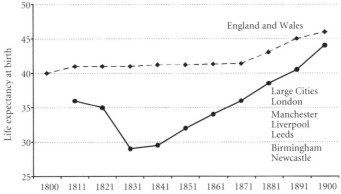

Fig. 4.2 Life Expectancy at birth, England and Wales (1800–1900).

population mortality rates that had been occurring in the UK had ceased.[5] From the 1860s on, however, life expectancy increased, first for children and young adults and then for older adults[6] (see Chapter 2). Infant mortality rates, interestingly, failed to fall until after the turn of the century, when subsequent generations of women born into these better circumstances began to have their own children.[7]

Over the twentieth century there have been at least three noteworthy features of population health in more developed nations.[8] One is the improvement in overall levels of population health, as indicated by increased life expectancy and reduced all-cause mortality. The components of this improvement have involved enormous increases in the survival of infants and children, substantial declines in haemorrhagic stroke and some cancers (stomach, lip and scrotum)[9] that have continued unabated since the beginning of the century, and dramatic reductions in coronary heart disease (CHD) and ischaemic stroke since the peak of the epidemics in the 1960s and 1970s. The second is spectacular deviations from such general trends as evidenced in the mortality crisis in post-Soviet countries.[10] The third major feature of population health in developed countries has been that socioeconomic differentials have persisted and in some cases increased against this background of general improvements. The topic of this chapter is to consider how influences acting at different stages of the life course contribute to the social distribution of risk factors that help determine socioeconomic differentials in health.

4.1.1 Socioeconomic health differentials: the need to understand heterogeneity across outcomes, place, and time

In the UK, from around the 1921 census onwards, routine statistics on social class mortality differences have been produced. Figure 4.3 shows that for men, from the 1921 to the 1991 census, dramatic declines in mortality have occurred for social classes I and II, while for social classes IV and V, smaller and less consistent decreases in mortality are seen. Increases in both the relative and absolute differentials in mortality between the social class groups have occurred since the early 1950s[11,12] and continued through the 1990s.[13]

In considering socioeconomic differentials we need to understand both relative and absolute components. Absolute differentials are arithmetic differences between the rates, percentages, or means (depending on the outcome—for example, mortality rate, percentage smokers, or mean blood pressure) between two socially defined groups (for example, rich versus poor, black versus white). Relative socioeconomic differentials are

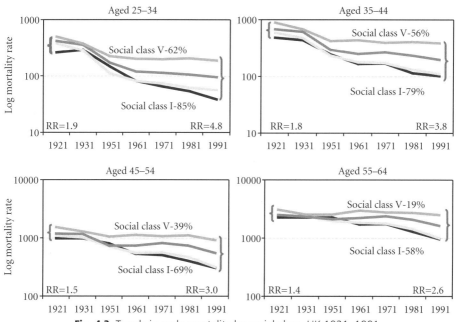

Fig. 4.3 Trends in male mortality by social class, UK 1921–1991.

based on a ratio of the rates, percentages, or means in the two groups being compared. We need both kinds of information when comparing the magnitude of socioeconomic differentials between causes or whether they have changed magnitude over time because declines in absolute inequality can be accompanied by increases in relative inequality. For example, suppose that at one point in time the disease rate per 100 000 was 100 in social group A but 40 in Group B. This means the relative differential in the rates would be would 2.5 (100/40) and the absolute differential 60 (100–40). Suppose that rates then declined over time so that they reduced to 40 in Group A (a reduction of 60%) and 10 in B (a reduction of 75%). The absolute differential would thus have halved from 60 to 30 but the relative difference would have increased four fold. Did inequality increase or decrease? Such situations are commonplace in population health and show why our current reliance on relative inequality statistics presents only part of the picture.

Time trends in relative and absolute socioeconomic health differentials are not necessarily the same in all countries. While the available time series are shorter for other countries, there is evidence that in Canada from 1971 to 1996, both absolute and relative socioeconomic mortality differences actually declined for some outcomes, such as infant, ischaemic heart disease (IHD), uterine cancer, and liver cirrhosis mortality among women, while absolute and relative inequality increased for female suicide.[14] In Sweden, absolute differences declined but relative gaps between the classes remained stable or even slightly increased for some outcomes,[15,16] while in the USA relative but not absolute income differences widened.[17] It is clear that time trends in the extent of socioeconomic inequalities in different types of health outcomes vary between countries, suggesting that the magnitude and composition of socioeconomic health differentials are sensitive to context and thus dynamic within and between countries.

One of the most commonly cited examples of this dynamism is the supposed social class crossover in heart disease mortality that occurred in the earlier part of the twentieth century. While we are advocates for the utility of considering the heterogeneity of socioeconomic differentials in health, this may not be one of the best examples. It has been widely considered that CVD used to affect the rich more than the poor. This generalization is, in fact, only true if the category of IHD is considered alone. In the analysis of social class differences in mortality around the 1911 census,[18] non manual social class men did have high mortality attributed to 'angina pectoris and arteriosclerosis', but for overall circulatory disease mortality this was not the case. Differences in the classification of causes of death between social classes could have generated spurious gradients for some causes of death, like CHD, that were becoming increasingly recognized.

Table 4.1 summarizes the results of UK or US studies with defined samples, initial recruitment up until 1960, and standardized measures of disease prevalence or incidence among men. The overall picture is one of no association or an inverse association between social position and CHD prevalence and incidence. A full rendering of the evidence on the socioeconomic crossover of CHD was provided in the first edition of this book.[19] Thus, the evidence for a marked positive social gradient in CHD disease earlier this century is considerably weaker than is generally supposed. There is certainly no strong support for the notion that such an association ever existed among women.

Table 4.1 Associations between socioeconomic position and coronary heart disease in US and UK studies with defined samples and standardized measures of disease prevalence or incidence among men, with initial recruitment up until 1960.[19]

Study name	Period of study entry	Country	Socioeconomic indicator	CHD measure	Association between socioeconomic position and CHD
Bell Telephone	1935	USA	Education	30-year CHD mortality prevalence in survivors in 1962	mortality = − prevalence = −
Framingham	1949	USA	Education	6-year CHD incidence	−
Chapman	1949	USA	Occupation	5-year CHD mortality	0
Lee	Early 1950s	USA	Occupation	5-year cumulative prevalence CHD	−
Commission on Chronic Illness	1953–55	USA	Income	prevalence CHD	−
Albany	1953–54	USA	Income, education	6-year CHD incidence	−
Stamler	1954–57	USA	Occupation, education, income	prevalent CHD; 4-year CHD incidence	0
Thomas	1954–58	UK	Social class	prevalent CHD	0
Brown	1956	UK	Social class	prevalent CHD; 1-year CHD incidence	all forms = 0 myocardial infarction = + other forms of CHD = −
Du Pont	1956	USA	Occupation, income group	1- and 6-year CHD incidence	1 year = − 6 years = −
Western Electric	1957	USA	Occupation	4.5-year CHD incidence	0
Evans County	1960	USA	Social status, based on income, education, and occupation	prevalence CHD; 2-year CHD incidence	prevalence = +* incidence = 0

CHD, coronary heart disease; 0, no consistent association; −, inverse socioeconomic gradient; +, positive socioeconomic gradient.

*Statistically significant; otherwise not significant or not reported.

This does not detract from the general principle that socioeconomic health differentials are dynamic across cause, place, and time. Perhaps the most dramatic example comes from the historical record, where available evidence suggests that before the 1700s social advantage was actually associated with lower life expectancy—some rural peasants lived longer than the aristocracy and their urban dwelling counterparts. Johannson has argued that '… what matters most to explaining pre-transition mortality is location not income'.[20(p4)] Location was crucial because of geographical proximity to sources of infection. Kunitz explained that '… until the turn of the eighteenth century, the dominant pattern of mortality was largely independent of wages, the price of food, and nutritional status. When an association did become evident, it was because certain infectious diseases had declined, most likely because human intervention and social organization had become effective …'.[21(p280)]

The particular pattern of how socioeconomic health differentials are expressed in a population, that is, their magnitude, their cause-specific composition and their trends over time, is sensitive to interdependencies between the extant disease environment, broadly defined social (political, economic, behavioural, cultural, and educational) differences between countries and changing social conditions within countries. This makes the task of linking particular distributions of risk factors from both early and later life to particular socioeconomic distributions of adult disease complex. It may, however, inform the general explanations about what determines socioeconomic health differences with more historically contextualized understandings of how risk factors for specific outcomes were socially distributed.[22] Life course processes are likely to be important in understanding the social distributions of risk factors over time.

There is ample evidence for heterogeneity of socioeconomic mortality differentials in the major CVDs. Figure 4.4 shows relative manual versus non manual differences in

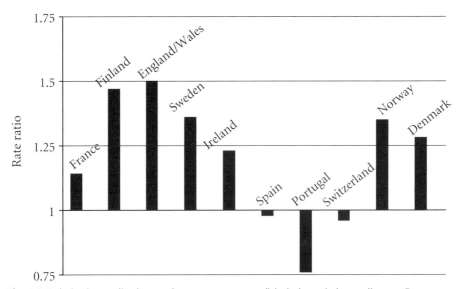

Fig. 4.4 Relative inequality (manual versus non manual) in ischaemic heart disease, Europe (circa 1980s), men aged 45–59.[23]

CHD mortality for selected European countries.[23] For CHD there are relatively large socioeconomic differentials favouring non manual workers in Finland, England, and Wales, small or no differences in Spain and Switzerland, and differences favouring manual workers in Portugal. However, data for stroke show manual workers have higher rates in all countries, but the magnitude of the association differs.[23] This heterogeneity in the magnitude and direction of absolute and relative socioeconomic differentials in CHD and stroke implies between-country differences in the socioeconomic distribution of CHD risk factors and within-country differences in the prevalence and socioeconomic distribution of risk factors for stroke.

The departure point for a more complete understanding of socioeconomic health differentials should be from a life course perspective that incorporates the heterogeneity of associations across outcomes, place, and time. This focus on specificity of associations[24] facilitates greater flexibility in considering how a particular indicator of SEP, from a particular point in the life course, might be linked via different risk factors to different outcomes in different places at different times.

4.2 What is the evidence for the contribution of socioeconomic factors over the life course to poorer adult health?

Despite the fact that the role of early life exposures has experienced a recent scientific renaissance, the notion that unfavourable social environments in early life could adversely affect health in adulthood has long been held (see Chapter 2).[25] Writing on the state of health in poor areas of the UK during the depression of the 1930s, Wal Hannington, leader of the National Unemployed Workers Movement, considered that 'unemployment has existed for so long in the Distressed Areas that many of the youths who are to-day leaving school were probably handicapped from the moment of their birth as the result of under-nourishment of the mothers during pregnancy'.[26(p78)] Vernon wrote that with '... the provision of adequate nourishment at all stages of human existence, we should find a further diminution of infant mortality, ... and ... we should find considerable improvement in the health and physique of the children. Such improvement would certainly lead to a healthier adult life'.[27(p9)] Similar views were expressed in the USA[28] and even in the mid 1960s, when the focus on adult lifestyle had gained prominence, René Dubos—invoking Milton in *Paradise Regained*—wrote 'From all points of view, the child is father of the man, and for this reason we need to develop an experimental science that might be called biological Freudianism. Socially and individually the response of human beings to the conditions of the present is always conditioned by the biological remembrance of things past.'[29(p789)]

In 1992, Elo and Preston[30] reviewed the effects of childhood exposures on adult mortality. While they focused mainly on the role of childhood infections on adult chronic disease, in reference to studies on early socioeconomic conditions, they commented, 'We have found surprisingly few studies that investigate the relationship between features of one's home, including parental characteristics and adult mortality' (p. 201). They mentioned only three studies that examined childhood socioeconomic conditions in relation to adult disease.[31–33] More than a decade later, there are now many studies that have examined the influence of childhood socioeconomic conditions on a range of health-related outcomes in adulthood. Such investigations have focused on the role of childhood socioeconomic conditions—usually indicated by the occupation and/or education of parents—in relation to biological risk factors such as blood pressure, lipid levels, body mass index, and fibrinogen,[34–48] health behaviours such as smoking, physical activity, and alcohol consumption,[49–51] psychosocial characteristics such as hostility, hopelessness, and depression,[52,53] psychiatric outcomes,[54–58] and perceptions of health.[59–64] In addition, there are now many studies of early life exposures and outcomes that are often socioeconomically patterned, such as birth anthropometry,[64,65] child neglect and abuse,[66] IQ,[67] pollutants,[68,69] and allergic exposures.[70] While these studies have not specifically investigated early life SEP, they are indicative of the potential for exposures that are differentially distributed across socioeconomic groups *in utero*, in infancy, and in childhood to have important effects on adult health.

4.2.1 Early life socioeconomic factors and coronary heart disease

Early studies of links between childhood SEP and CHD investigated 'social incongruity'—the stress of moving from a disadvantaged background into the hypothesized stressful environment of the professional and managerial world.[71] Investigation of socioeconomic deprivation in early life on later health was made prominent by the work of Forsdahl who demonstrated that areas with high infant mortality rates earlier this century had currently high CHD rates.[42,43,72] Forsdahl interpreted this as demonstrating that deprivation in early life, followed by later affluence, worked together to increase coronary risk, in part mediated by elevation of blood cholesterol.[43] This work was influential in Barker's early studies.[73] Forsdahl's interpretation is qualitatively similar to one of the recent thrusts of Barker's programming hypothesis whereby *in utero* nutritional disadvantage (resulting in sub-optimal growth) may be followed by nutritional advantage and rapid growth in childhood.[95]

Table 4.2 details 24 studies that have investigated associations between childhood socioeconomic circumstances and adult CHD.[31,32,65,74–94] Table 4.2 is arranged according to type of study—case–control (7 studies), prospective (15 studies), and cross-sectional/cumulative prevalence (2 studies). Of the 24 studies, 14 collected information on childhood socioeconomic circumstances in adulthood and 10 collected data either in childhood or early life—before age 20. Presumably, data collected in early life should be more reliable than that recalled in adulthood. These studies show stronger effects of childhood SEP on CHD than studies that collected data in adulthood. Moreover, all these studies with SEP data collected in early life used objectively defined CHD outcomes and controlled for indicators of adulthood SEP. There is one exception however. In the 1924–1933 Finnish cohort that has been used to investigate the *in utero* programming hypothesis, childhood social class was unrelated to CHD in women or stroke in men.[95,96] This is perhaps due to insufficient variation in the childhood SEP measure with 85% of fathers being classified as labourers.

4.2.2 Early life socioeconomic factors and stroke

Stroke risk has generally been found to be higher in those with less favourable socioeconomic circumstances in childhood, perhaps even more strongly than CHD,[97] but not in all studies.[98] There may also be important differences between stroke sub-types

Table 4.2 Review of studies examining childhood socioeconomic conditions and adult mortality and morbidity

Study	Number of cases (male and female)	Childhood measures	When childhood social position recorded	Design	Disease outcome	Odds ratio or relative risk—unadjusted or age adjusted	Multivariable odds ratio or relative risk	Comments
Case–control studies								
Hasle (1990)[74]	154 M	Father's occupational class; father unemployed; economic problems	Adulthood, around 58	Nested case–control	Non-fatal CHD	Father unskilled: 1.13 (0.80–1.58) Father unemployed: 1.04 (0.69–1.57) Economic problems: 1.16 (0.83–1.62)	Not reported	'Cases were participants self-reporting that they had had a heart attack
Bobák (2000)[75]	282 M and 80 F	Mother's and father's occupations	Adulthood, middle-age	Case–control	Hospital and out-patient MI cases	Adjusted for age, sex, and district *Mother's occupation* Industrial worker: 1.0 Agricultural worker: 1.02 (0.72–1.45) Non-manual: 1.55 (0.96–2.50) Professional: 1.00 (0.63–1.61) Not working: 1.44 (1.02–2.03) *Father's occupation* Industrial worker:1.0 Agricultural worker: 0.92 (0.66–1.29)	Adjusted for age, sex, district, education, car ownership, crowding, height, mother's education, and father's education *Mother's occupation* Industrial worker:1.0 Agricultural worker: 1.05 (0.69–1.59) Non manual: 1.77 (1.07–2.93) Professional: 0.84 (0.44–1.63)	Findings with respect to mother's and father's education also reported. If anything, a positive association of increasing risk with higher educational achievement of the mother, seen

Table 4.2 (*Cont.*)

Study	Number of cases (male and female)	Childhood measures	When childhood social position recorded	Design	Disease outcome	Odds ratio or relative risk—unadjusted or age adjusted	Multivariable odds ratio or relative risk	Comments
						Non manual: 1.07 (0.74–1.55) Professional: 0.76 (0.51–1.14) Not working: 1.62 (0.50–5.32)	Not working: 1.55 (1.07–2.24) *Father's occupation* Industrial worker: 1.0 Agricultural worker: 0.95 (0.63–1.43) Non manual: 1.04 (0.69–1.56) Professional: 0.87 (0.51–1.48) Not working: 1.63 (0.48–5.50)	
Coggon (1990)[76]	74 M and 25 F	Father's social class	Adulthood, middle-age	Case–control	Hospital admissions for MI	Adjusted for age and sex Non manual: 1.0 III manual: 2.0 (0.6–6.7) IV or V: 2.1 (0.6–7.5) Armed forces: 4.7 (1.0–22.7)	Adjusted for age, sex, smoking, and current social class Non manual: 1.0 III manual: 1.9 (0.5–7.6) IV or V: 2.0 (0.5–7.6) Armed forces: 3.9 (0.8–19.2)	

Study	N	Exposure	Period	Design	Outcome	Results	Adjustment	Comments
Donnan et al.[77] (1994)	358 M and 174 F	Father's occupation; mother worked; overcrowding; sibling died before 5; ever-inadequate food intake, meat included in the daily diet	Adulthood	Case–control, hospital control participants	Hospitalized acute MI	*Males* Father's social class Blue collar: 0.86 (0.61–1.28) Mother worked—yes: 1.79 (1.30–2.46) Crowding >3 per room: 1.0 (0.61–1.64) Inadequate food often: 2.51 (1.51–4.18) *Females* Father's social Class: 0.98 (0.56–1.71) Mother worked—yes: 1.98 (1.13–3.46) Crowding >3 per room: 0.69 (0.45–1.07) Inadequate food often: 1.58 (0.78–3.21)	Not reported	
Brasche et al.[78] (2001)	129 M	Housing conditions	Adulthood	Case–control	Non-fatal CHD	From best to worst housing conditions—best 1.00 (baseline), intermediate 2.07 (1.11–3.87), worst 8.99 (3.22–25.13)	Adjusted for cigarette smoking and other questionnaire-based social risk factors from best housing in childhood—best 1.00 (baseline), intermediate 2.03 (1.00–4.11), worst 5.14 (1.46–18.09)	Control participants were trauma cases

Table 4.2 (Cont.)

Study	Number of cases (male and female)	Childhood measures	When childhood social position recorded	Design	Disease outcome	Odds ratio or relative risk— unadjusted or age adjusted	Multivariable odds ratio or relative risk	Comments
Kaplan et al.[32] (1990)	940 M	Score based on father's education, mother's and father's occupational prestige, whether lived on farm, size of farm, and whether family perceived as wealthy	Adulthood, middle-age	Cross-sectional prevalence survey	Electro-cardiogram ischaemia or angina on exercise, or maximal heart rate <130 beats/min during exercise	High 1.0 medium: 1.35 (1.12–1.64) Low: 1.44 (1.17–1.78)	*Age and adult socioeconomic status* High: 1.0 Medium: 1.20 (0.98–1.45) Low: 1.21 (0.97–1.51)	Definition of CHD included failure to obtain a heart rate of 130 beats/min or more during exercise, which is a non-standard definition. This study population also provided the baseline data for a prospective mortality follow-up, which found little evidence of childhood socioeconomic effects (see prospective studies section of table)

Study	N	Measure	Life stage	Study design	Outcome	Results	Comments
Burr and Sweetnam (1980)	297 M	Father's social class; father unemployed for more than 1 year during childhood or father died during childhood (mainly unemployed, referred to as 'unemployed' in results section); family size	Adulthood, middle-age	Case-control, with hospital control participants	Hospitalized MI	*Social class* I/II: 1.0 III: 1.04 (0.59–1.86) (0.61–1.79) IV/V: 1.0 (0.51–1.95) (0.54–1.87) P for trend = 0.94 Father unemployed: 1.45 (1.03–2.05) (our calculations) 1.48 (1.03–2.13) Cases had more siblings ($P<0.05$)	Not given; father unemployed related to MI after adjustment for current social class ($P<0.05$); number of siblings related to MI after adjustment for current social class ($P<0.05$)

Prospective studies

Study	N	Measure	Life stage	Study design	Outcome	Results	Comments
Beebe-Dimmer et al,[80] (in press)	580	Father's occupation and education	Adulthood	Prospective	CVD (ICD-9 codes, 410–414) and cerebrovascular disease (ICD-9 codes, 430–438)	Father manual: 1.34 (1.13–1.58)	Father manual: 1.29 (1.09–1.54) Adjusted for respondent's own education, occupation and household income, smoking, physical activity, and body mass index—all as time-dependent covariates	Father's occupation more strongly associated with CVD than all-cause mortality. Even more strongly associated with premature (<age 70) CVD mortality (heart rate = 1.77; 95% confidence interval = 0.94–3.32)

Table 4.2 (Cont.)

Study	Number of cases (male and female)	Childhood measures	When childhood social position recorded	Design	Disease outcome	Odds ratio or relative risk— unadjusted or age adjusted	Multivariable odds ratio or relative risk	Comments
Pensola and Valkonen[81] (2002)	187 M	Father's social class	During childhood (1970 census for men born 1956–1960)	Whole-country cohort	CVD mortality (ICD-9 codes, 390–459)	Adjusted for own social class and education Upper non manual: 1.0 Lower non manual: 1.11 (0.5–2.4) Skilled manual: 1.50 (0.8–3.0) Unskilled manual: 2.76 (1.3–5.8) Farmer: 2.26 (1.0–5.0) Small farmer: 1.97 (0.9–4.3) Self-employed: 2.81 (1.3–6.0) Other: 3.93 (1.5–10)	Adjusted for own social class and education Upper non manual: 1.0 Lower non manual: 0.90 (0.4–2.0) Skilled manual: 1.04 (0.5–2.1) Unskilled manual: 1.75 (0.8–3.8) Farmer: 1.54 (0.7–3.5) Small farmer: 1.28 (0.6–2.9) Self-employed: 2.09 (1.0–4.6) Other: 2.55 (1.0–6.7)	
Davey Smith et al.[82] (2001)	339 M	Father's social class	Adolescence/ early adulthood	Prospective	Cardiovascular mortality	*Father's social class* I: 1.0 II: 1.51 (1.08–2.11) III: 1.63 (1.17–2.27) IV:1.85 (1.12–3.07) V: 2.36 (1.11–4.99) *P* for trend = 0.002	Adjusted for age, systolic blood pressure, and smoking *Father's social class* I: 1.0 II: 1.46 (1.05–2.05) III: 1.66 (1.19–2.32) IV: 1.91 (1.15–3.17) V: 2.31 (1.09–4.89) *P* for trend = 0.001	

Study	N	Exposure	Life stage	Design	Outcome	Results	Adjustments
Davey Smith et al.[83] (1998)	618 M	Father's social class	Adulthood, middle-age	Prospective	Cardiovascular mortality	Age-adjusted odds ratio manual:non manual father: 1.52 (1.24–1.87) I and II: 1.0 III non manual: 0.96 (0.65–1.40) III manual: 1.47 (1.13–1.92) IV and V: 1.53 (1.16–2.01) P for trend = 0.0003	Relative risk manual: non manual father adjusted for age, adult social class, deprivation category, car ownership, smoking, diastolic blood pressure, cholesterol, body mass index, and forced expiratory volume in 1 s: 1.26 (1.01–1.58)
Heslop et al.[84] (2001)	128 F	Father's social class	Adulthood, middle-age	Prospective	Cardiovascular mortality	Age-adjusted odds ratio manual:non manual father 1.56 (0.76–3.20)	Adjusted for age, diastolic blood pressure, cholesterol, body mass index, forced expiratory volume in 1 s, smoking, exercise, and alcohol. Manual:non manual father 1.57 (0.76–3.23)
Oslo mortality study[85] (2003)	201 M and 54 F	Housing conditions	Childhood	Prospective	Cardiovascular mortality	Age-adjusted relative index of inequality Men: 2.79 (1.71–4.55) Women: 3.96 (1.52–10.3)	Adjusted for age and income in adulthood, relative index of inequality Men: 2.68 (1.64–4.38) Women: 3.80 (1.45–9.96)

Table 4.2 (*Cont.*)

Study	Number of cases (male and female)	Childhood measures	When childhood social position recorded	Design	Disease outcome	Odds ratio or relative risk—unadjusted vs age adjusted	Multivariable odds ratio or relative risk	Comments
Gliksman[86] (1995)	607 F non fatal MI and 233 F fatal CHD	Father's social class (manual versus non manual)	Adulthood, 30–55	Prospective	Non-fatal MI and fatal CHD from physician record review and death registration	*Manual/ vs non manual fathers* Total CHD: 1.19 (1.03–1.37) Non-fatal MI: 1.25 (1.06–1.47) Fatal CHD: 1.07 (0.82–1.39) 0.94 (0.72–1.25)	Adjusted for age, smoking, BMI, parental CHD, alcohol, exercise, diet, medications, and post-medical history Manual vs non manual 1.12 (0.98–1.29) 1.18 (1.01–1.39)	In sub-sample with data on birthweight and breastfeeding, additional adjustment did not alter findings
Vågerö and Leon[87] (1994)	153 M	Father's social class	Childhood (1960 Swedish census)	Nested case–control; all IHD deaths compared to 4% sample of total population	CHD death (ICD-8 codes 410–414)	Non manual: 1.00 Manual: 2.29 (1.51–3.46) Not employed: 2.23(1.08–4.59)	Adjusted for adulthood social class Non manual: 1.00 Manual: 1.99 (1.30–3.05) Not employed: 1.82 (0.88–3.77)	Father's social class more strongly related to CHD mortality than all-cause mortality
Frankel et al.[88] (1999)	189 M and F	Father's occupational social class	Childhood, 0–14	Prospective	CHD mortality (ICD-9 codes 410–415)	I/II: 0.41 III: 1.0 IV: 0.88 V: 1.14 Unemployed: 1.04 P for trend = – 0.12	Adjustment for Townsend deprivation score in adulthood I/II: 0.43 (0.19–0.98) III: 1.0 IV: 0.89 (0.56–1.42) V: 1.12 (0.71–1.76) Unemployed: 1.04 (0.68–1.59) P for trend = – 0.15	Father's social class related to household food expenditure. Same study as Dedman (see below)

Study	N and sex	Exposure measure	Life stage	Study design	Outcome	Results	Adjusted	Other
Dedman et al.[89] (2001)	222 M and F	Overcrowding; water supply	Childhood, 0–14	Prospective	CHD mortality (ICD-9 codes 410–414)	Overcrowding index from least overcrowded to most overcrowded: 0.72, 1.0, 1.12, 1.11 (P for trend = 1.11); indoor private tapped water supply—no versus yes: 1.57 (1.03–2.41)	Adjusted for income, food expenditure and social class in childhood, and adult Townsend deprivation score— Overcrowding index: 0.74, 1.0, 1.13, 1.17 (P for trend = 0.15); indoor tapped water supply—no versus yes: 1.73 (1.13–2.64)	Other not directly socioeconomic measures, including cleanliness in the house and adequacy of ventilation, showed inconsistent relationships to CHD
Lynch et al.[90] (1994)	85 M	[see entry for Kaplan and Salonen]	Adulthood, middle-age	Prospective	CVD mortality (ICD-9 codes 390–459)	*Father low SEP respondent* Low: 2.02 (0.90–4.54) High: 0.99 (0.39–2.51) *Father mid-SEP respondent* Low: 2.26 (1.02–4.99) High: 0.78 (0.32–1.92) *Father high SEP respondent* Low: 1.59 (0.52–4.88) High: 1.0	Stratified by adult income	No effect of father's low SEP within strata of adult income
Forsen et al.[95] (1999) (note: 1924–1933 birth cohort)	279 W	Father's occupational social class	Childhood	Prospective	Hospital	No association admission or death from CHD	Effect size not reported	

Table 4.2 (Cont.)

Study	Number of cases (male and female)	Childhood measures	When childhood social position recorded	Design	Disease outcome	Odds ratio or relative risk— unadjusted or age adjusted	Multivariable odds ratio or relative risk	Comments
Barker et al.[65] (2001) (note: 1934–1944 birth cohort)	270 M	Father's occupational social class	Childhood	Prospective	Hospital admission or death from CHD	Upper middle class: 1.00 Lower middle class: 1.44 (0.86–2.43) Labourer: 2.10 (1.27–3.18) P for trend = 0.0006	Influence of father's social class remains significant (P = 0.0005) after adjustment for weight at 1	
Gillum et al.[92] (1978)	166 M	Father's social class	University entry, 15–29	Prospective	CHD death or reported history of doctor-diagnosed MI	Manual father: 1.75 (P<0.03)	Adjusted for multivariate confounder score containing age, smoking, blood pressure, height, ponderal index, and exercise, amongst others Manual: 1.53 (0.94–2.48)	Angina not associated with father's social class (odds ratio = 0.91), based on 48 cases

Study	N/Sex	Exposure	Source	Study type	Outcome	Results	Adjustment	Comments
Notkola[91] (1985)	198 M	Combination of father's occupation and land ownership (the landless taken as the lowest socioeconomic category)	From parish registers and other records during the childhood and early adulthood of the cohort members	Prospective	Fatal CHD	Landless: 1.39 Small farmers: 1.29 Major farmers: 1.00 (baseline) Confidence interval not reported but findings said to be non-significant Larger differences seen in the more deprived East Finland than West Finland.	Adjustment for SEP in adulthood had relatively small effect on the findings; adjustment for smoking, cholesterol, and body height attenuated the relative risk in East Finland by about 50%	Similar findings reported for non-fatal IHD and combined MI and combined endpoints. Some differences in numerical results between the two reports

Cumulative prevalence studies

Study	N/Sex	Exposure	Source	Study type	Outcome	Results	Adjustment	Comments
Wannamethee et al.[93] (1996)	434 M	Father's social class	Adulthood, 52–73 years at 1992 follow-up of original 1978–80 survey	Cumulative prevalence	Either reported doctor-diagnosed MI at baseline (1978–1980) or MI in doctor's records between baseline and 1992 follow-up	Manual father: 1.5 (1.1–1.8)	Adjusted for age, adult social class, smoking, systolic blood pressure, total cholesterol, body mass index and height Manual: 1.3 (1.0–1.7)	Similar findings with a broader definition of CHD

Table 4.2 (*Cont.*)

Study	Number of cases (male and female)	Childhood measures	When childhood social position recorded	Design	Disease outcome	Odds ratio or relative risk—unadjusted or age adjusted	Multivariable odds ratio or relative risk	Comments
Marmot et al.[94] (2001)	277 M and 51 F	Father's social class	Adulthood, middle-age	Nested case–control	Self-reported CHD symptoms or doctor diagnosis of CHD at phase 2 or phase 3 (those dying of CHD or not responding at phases 2 and 3 not included)	Father's social class *Men* I or II: 1.0 III non manual: 0.79 III manual: 1.05 IV or V: 0.86 *P* for trend = 0.93 *Women* I or II: 1.0 III non manual: 1.17 III manual 1.28 IV or V:1.32 *P* for trend = 0.20	Adjusted for current employment grade (father's social class) *Men* I or II: 1.0 III non manual: 0.77 (0.5–1.1) III manual: 1.02 (0.8–1.4) IV or V: 0.83 (0.5–1.3) *P* for trend = 0.77 *Women* I or II: 1.0 III non manual: 1.13 (0.6–2.0) III manual: 1.19 (0.8–1.8) IV or V: 1.20 (0.7–2.1) *P* for trend = 0.20	Self-reported CHD. Higher incidence of this outcome in women than in men

CHD, coronary heart disease; MI, myocardial infarction; CVD, cardiovascular disease; ICD, International Classification of Disease; IHD, ischaemic heart disease; SEP, socioeconomic position.
The following study was excluded, because high blood pressure was included in definition of CVD: Blackwell DL, Hayward MD, Crimmins EM. Does childhood health affect chronic morbidity in later life? *Soc Sci Med* 2001;**52**:1269–84.

in this regard. Haemorrhagic stroke has declined across the twentieth century in the UK, as social conditions improved, while ischaemic stroke increased and then decreased in parallel to changes in CHD.[99] Several indicators of early life socioeconomic disadvantage—low birthweight, short stature, large family size, and low paternal social class—have been shown to have much stronger links with haemorrhagic than with ischaemic stroke.[100] This heterogeneity in the strength of association suggests specificity of the aetiological links between socioeconomically patterned exposures early in life and adult disease outcomes. If some exposure in childhood—possibly infectious—is associated with poorer socioeconomic conditions and is correlated with birthweight, then it may suggest that the decline in haemorrhagic stroke over the last century is partly due to improved early life environments, as indexed by congruent secular trends in improving infant mortality over the century.

The dependence of haemorrhagic stroke on early life deprivation may also contribute to the considerable excess risk from this cause seen among African-Americans in the USA.[101,102] In both the USA and the UK, men of African origin have a considerable and unexplained elevation in stroke risk compared to white men, but they are relatively protected against CHD once conventional adult risk factors have been taken into account.[101,103]

4.2.3 Socioeconomic mobility and cardiovascular disease

There is little evidence that upward mobility from poor childhood background to advantaged adult social position increases the risk of CVD through generating the stress of status incongruity. In fact, some evidence would suggest the opposite—that upward social mobility is protective relative to the socioeconomic group of origin[90]—although those who are upwardly mobile seem not to attain the same levels of health as those who were advantaged over the whole life course.[104] Downward intergenerational social mobility—from a non manual occupational background of father to a manual occupation in middle-age—has rarely been directly studied in the context of adult CVD. Data from Finland showed that intergenerationally downwardly mobile men had the highest CVD risk of any social group.[90] Without detailed information on the precise timing of downward mobility, however, it is hard to know which particular life course processes might be implicated in generating the adult health differences. Early life critical period exposures, followed by later effect modifiers and accumulation models are both possible explanations for the downward mobility effects on adult health.[105,106]

These issues are also of interest with respect to health-related social selection models of the genesis of health inequalities. The social selection argument suggests that people destined to be unhealthy in adulthood have characteristics in earlier life that influence both later SEP and health and that this generates the social distribution of CVD risk in adulthood. These characteristics can either be childhood illnesses (which could influence both later SEP and health), height, obesity, or behavioural factors such as smoking or drug use. However, in one study of social mobility, the main determinant of CVD was the cumulative influence of social position across the life course, rather than CVD being a product of social mobility.[104] The only exception to this general pattern was related to the small percentage of the population who moved from non manual jobs at labour market entry to manual jobs in middle-age, who experienced a high rate of heart disease mortality. For this small group, it is possible that health status had an influence on future occupational trajectory. Nevertheless, the evidence suggests that these mechanisms make a small contribution to socioeconomic differentials in adult health.[107]

4.3 Early life socioeconomic factors and cardiovascular disease risk factors

Studies examining socioeconomic circumstances in early life and later affluence provide little support for the component of the Forsdahl hypothesis relating to an interaction between childhood deprivation and affluence in adult life.[42] The suggestion that the effects of early life deprivation are mediated through high blood cholesterol concentrations in adulthood has also received little support,[31] although in a Finnish cohort, there were residual effects of lower SEP on low-density lipoprotein (LDL) cholesterol, even among those who had attained high SEP as adults.[48,108] In the West of Scotland cohort who were born between 1916 and 1938, CVD risk factors were analysed in relation to childhood and adult social class.[37] Men with manual social class fathers had lower, rather than higher, total serum cholesterol concentrations compared to men with non manual fathers. Behavioural risk factors—such as smoking and exercise—were more dependent on adult than parental social class. This supports the notion that in some circumstances, behaviours like smoking are powerfully affected by the social environment experienced during adult life and that modifying such behaviours is dependent upon the presence of the social circumstances required for maintaining favourable health-related behaviours. Blood pressure and lung function were associated with both current and parental social class, but more strongly with the former. This suggests that smoking and occupational exposures for lung function or alcohol and other dietary factors for blood pressure are, in this male cohort, more dependent upon adult than childhood social circumstances. However, body mass index and triglyceride levels were dependent on childhood social class rather than current social class. Men with manual fathers had higher body mass indices and higher triglyceride levels than men with non manual fathers and once the father's social class was taken into account there was no association of current social class with body mass index and a reverse association for triglycerides. High body mass index and elevated triglycerides are components of the insulin resistance syndrome. This is compatible with evidence that the concomitants of adverse childhood socioeconomic circumstances are associated with an elevated risk of diabetes and impaired glucose tolerance in adulthood.[47,109] The components of insulin resistance syndrome (see Chapter 7) cluster in childhood[110,111] and this clustering tracks into adulthood[112] suggesting that a common factor, already active in young childhood, may underlie the risk of insulin resistance syndrome.

A Finnish study also failed to find an association between poor childhood socioeconomic circumstances and total cholesterol levels in adulthood.[31] In this study there was no consistent influence of childhood SEP on smoking behaviour or blood pressure, as is true of a Norwegian study.[43] In both the 1946 and 1958 UK birth cohort studies, obesity and high body mass index in adulthood were more prevalent among participants with fathers in manual social class occupations[38,64,113] as was found in the

Netherlands.[49] Evidence from Finland shows very little overall socioeconomic variation in blood pressure and triglyceride levels among men aged 42–64 in 1989[48] but there were childhood socioeconomic differences in waist-to-hip ratio and LDL cholesterol.[108] It was only those men with the most disadvantaged lifetime SEP who had significantly higher blood pressure. In the same data, levels of fibrinogen showed strong patterning by income but no effects of the father's occupation.[114] For fibrinogen—a general acute phase inflammatory reactant—it might be expected that it would be most sensitive to contemporaneous SEP and underlying adult disease, however in the Whitehall study, fibrinogen was found to reflect both early and later life socioeconomic factors.[34]

Thus, the relatively few studies that have examined the influence of early and later life socioeconomic factors on CVD risk factors have consistently found associations, but the patterning of links between socioeconomic factors in early life and particular CVD risk factors is somewhat inconsistent across studies. This is complicated by the fact that the studies are in different countries with cohorts of different ages and the relationships between SEP at different life course stages and CVD risk factors will not necessarily show the same patterns in different contexts. Life course socioeconomic patterning of behaviours like smoking, diet, and exercise may show period and cohort effects that are reflected in their biological sequelae and thus be specific to particular cohorts, countries, regions, and subgroups of the population.

For example, in the UK there is evidence that early life social circumstances have a stronger influence on smoking among women than among men,[115,116] although this is not necessarily the case in other countries or in other time periods. These potential gender-by-cohort interactions are evident in the educational patterning of smoking initiation in Switzerland, where higher education was a risk factor for early smoking initiation but over time eventually became protective and this effect was lagged by 20 years in women compared to men.[117] In the USA there are different education by sex by race/ethnic group patterns for smoking uptake by different birth cohorts.[118] These studies show how socioeconomic factors leave very different imprints on patterns of smoking initiation and cessation according to gender, race/ethnicity, and birth cohort, which in turn correspond to the timing of subgroup specific experiences of the overall trends in smoking or other risk factors in the population.

An example of the potential complexity of lifetime socioeconomic patterning of CVD risk factors can be seen in Table 4.3, which shows data from the Alameda County Study, on smoking and overweight according to father's occupation and respondent's average income in the period 1965–1994. Table 4.3 shows risk factor patterns at two points in time—first at the baseline exam in 1965 and then 29 years later among those cohort members who had not died or been lost to follow-up. These data show positive income gradients in smoking in 1965 but by 1994 those income gradients had reversed so that greater smoking was associated with lower income. This mirrors the secular pattern for smoking in the latter half of the twentieth century. Thus, even though the adult socioeconomic pattern of smoking changed from being more common among the well-off to being more common among lower socioeconomic groups, at every level of adult income, those from poorer backgrounds had higher smoking exposures. Thus, within the high income group in 1965, those from manual

Table 4.3 Father's occupation, adult income in 1965–1974, and age-adjusted mean level of smoking and odds ratios (95% confidence interval) for overweight for women and men in the Alameda County study at baseline in 1965 (n = 5707) and in 1994 (n = 2381)

Father's occupation	Mean adult income (1965–1974)	At baseline interview in 1965, median age = 35		At follow-up interview in 1994, median age = 64	
		Smoking (pack-years)	Overweight (high 25% body mass index)	Smoking (pack-years)	Overweight (high 25% body mass index)
Non manual	High 25% (n = 467)	12.0	Reference	12.9	Reference
	Middle 50% (n = 400)	11.0	1.22 (1.0–1.50)	16.2*	1.16 (0.84–1.61)
	Low 25% (n = 304)	8.8*	1.36 (1.1–1.67)	14.8	1.53 (1.09–2.15)
Manual	High 25% (n = 313)	13.9*	1.66 (1.35–2.4)	16.5*	1.59 (1.11–2.26)
	Middle 50% (n = 368)	12.5	1.6 (1.31–1.95)	16.9*	1.53 (1.12–2.10)
	Low 25% (n = 443)	9.9*	1.85 (1.52–2.25)	19.3*	2.81 (2.06–3.85)

*Significantly different from reference category (non manual + high income) in pair-wise comparison ($P < 0.05$).

backgrounds had higher pack-years of smoking exposure compared to those from non manual backgrounds. The same is true in 1994, except by that time the adult socioeconomic patterning of smoking had completely reversed so that it was then more common among lower socioeconomic groups. Contrast this with patterns of overweight where the early and later life socioeconomic distributions of the risk factors for being overweight were apparently maintained over time so that those most cumulatively disadvantaged had the highest risk of being overweight in both 1965 and 1994.

Such patterns could not be revealed without socioeconomic data from across the life course and may provide useful information on heterogeneity of risk among adult socioeconomic groups, even under social conditions where powerful period changes occur in the link between adult SEP and a risk factor such as smoking. Those from poorer childhood backgrounds were at increased risk of smoking even under conditions where the adult socioeconomic patterning of smoking had completely reversed. Similar period by socioeconomic group interactions may also be present for other life course CVD risk factors such as the period rise (in the early twentieth century) and social distribution of high-fat diets in the USA, followed by the socially patterned shifts to greater consumption of fruit and vegetables. Tastes for certain foods may be 'programmed' early in life but are also then subject to later modification based on adult socioeconomic influences.[48]

4.4 Explanations for socioeconomic differentials in cardiovascular disease: towards an integration of knowledge of exposures from across the life course

The long incubation period for CVD has been recognized for many years[119] and a life course approach to its aetiology and socioeconomic distribution is a natural extension of this view. In this discussion we have concentrated on studies for which the main focus is the social patterning of CVD risk. Table 4.4 summarizes factors which are putative CVD risk factors or are of particular interest from a life course perspective, according to their period of influence. Indeed, most of these important CVD risk factors are socially patterned. It is clear that CVD can be considered the archetype of diseases that have potential determinants across the entire life course—from conditions existing before conception, during intrauterine development, through nutrition, growth, and health in childhood, to social conditions, occupation, diet, physical activity, and smoking throughout adult life.

Nevertheless, for CHD and probably ischaemic stroke, current evidence suggests that levels of biologically and temporally proximal factors such as blood pressure, smoking, cholesterol, and insulin resistance can account for the major part of these diseases. It is helpful to separate the epidemic from the background portion of these diseases. The bulk of the epidemic portion of CHD and stroke can probably be accounted for by these risk factors.[120–122] Thus, life course influences could be important for two reasons. First, it seems clear that these major proximal risk factors can be influenced by biological, social, economic, and behavioural life course processes. Second, if we can account for the major part of the epidemic of CVD with these established risk factors, then there may be other aetiological pathways involved in determining the background

Table 4.4 Life course risk factors for coronary heart disease

Maternal health, development, and diet before and during pregnancy

Parental history of coronary heart disease

Intrauterine growth retardation

Socioeconomic deprivation from childhood onward

Stress from childhood onward

Poor growth in childhood

Short leg length in childhood

Obesity in childhood

Certain infections acquired in childhood

Diet from childhood onwards

Blood pressure in late adolescence

Serum cholesterol in late adolescence

Smoking from late adolescence onwards

Little physical activity from late adolescence onwards

Blood pressure in adulthood

Serum cholesterol in adulthood

Obesity in adulthood

Job insecurity and unemployment in adulthood

Short stature in adulthood

Binge alcohol drinking in adulthood

Diabetes and components of syndrome X in adulthood

Elevated fibrinogen and other acute phase reactants in adulthood

Certain infections acquired in adulthood

rates of CHD and ischaemic stroke in populations. These may include less well understood processes involving homocysteine, infection, inflammation, or even psycho-neuroendocrine pathways to ischaemic disease and it is likely that life course socioeconomic conditions would also contribute to these mechanisms either through behavioural or cumulative biological pathways.

4.4.1 Explanations for socioeconomic differentials based on adult risk factors

There have been several investigations into the contribution of adult physiological and behavioural factors in generating socioeconomic mortality differentials. In the first Whitehall study, considerable differences in all-cause mortality risk according to two socioeconomic measures—employment grade in the civil service and car ownership—could not be explained by smoking.[123,124] Cholesterol levels were also greater among high- rather than low-grade civil servants in the late 1960s, when this study was established.[125] Differences in cholesterol levels could not, therefore, account for the higher rates of CHD among the lower-grade employees. Indeed, simultaneous consideration of a range of risk factors—including smoking, blood pressure, cholesterol levels, and prevalent cardiorespiratory disease—failed to account for the grade differences in cardiovascular and non-cardiovascular mortality.

A prospective study of a third of a million men screened for the Multiple Risk Factor Intervention Trial between 1970 and 1973, with 16 years of mortality follow-up, found a strong inverse association between the income level of the area of residence and mortality risk from CHD and stroke.[102,103] While adjustment for smoking, cholesterol levels, blood pressure, and diabetes somewhat attenuated these associations, it did not remove them. Prospective studies from Sweden, Finland, Denmark, and the USA, using a variety of indices of social position have reached essentially the same conclusions.[126–132] This includes one with women participants,[132] which yielded the same results as the studies involving only men.

It is important to understand the role of measurement error in contributing to the residual associations seen between social class and health. Single measurements of risk factors may be poor proxies of lifetime exposure.[133] Whilst measurement imprecision in these factors renders the exploration of causes of differentials problematic,[134,135] it is also the case that the use of adult socioeconomic indicators alone may lead to an underestimation of the strength of the relationship between SEP and mortality.[83]

Nevertheless, these apparent residual effects have motivated an extensive research agenda aimed at identifying novel risk factors that can help completely explain socioeconomic health differentials.[136] The Whitehall II study was initiated in 1985 to particularly explore psychosocial factors. Baseline examinations demonstrated that higher-grade civil servants had lower prevalence of cardiorespiratory disease, among both sexes.[137] Average cholesterol levels were similar in each grade, but concentrations of serum apolipoprotein AI, the main structural protein of high-density lipoprotein (HDL) cholesterol, showed an association with grade[138] and suggested that characteristic disturbances of lipid metabolism associated with lower occupational status were potentially identifiable. Several of the components of the insulin resistance syndrome—waist–hip ratio, glucose 2 h after an oral load, insulin 2 h after an oral load, triglyceride levels, and (inversely) HDL cholesterol levels—clustered amongst civil servants in low employment grades.[36]

An influential finding that has emerged from Whitehall II[139] is that adult job stress—associated with a low degree of job control—is a major contributor to socioeconomic differentials in CVD. Indeed, statistical adjustment for self-reported job control essentially abolished the socioeconomic gradient in self-reported angina, severe chest pain, and self-reports of doctor-diagnosed CHD.[139] These associations were unaffected by adjustment for childhood social class, although height remained important suggesting additional influence of unmeasured early life factors.[139]

In some circumstances, low control over work can be virtually synonymous with other indicators of low SEP. In the case of civil servants in Whitehall, the links between job control and employment grade may be particularly close. The formal job descriptions that underlie 'employment grade' classifications are inherently based on organizational concepts concerning the degree of autonomy over work and the span of managerial control over the work of others. In populations comprising more than one employer and more diverse occupational classifications, the links between the degree of job control and other markers of SEP may not be as close. For instance, it is unlikely that levels of job control reveal as much about the socioeconomic conditions of farmers, those working in the home, or the unemployed as they do about particular job hierarchies within one work place.[140] This may help explain recent negative findings from other studies with regard to the role of job stress on CVD.[141,142]

A study of Finnish men constitutes the most detailed prospective investigation of risk factors measured in adulthood that contribute to socioeconomic gradients in CVD.[143] The risk of CVD mortality and incident acute myocardial infarction (AMI) across extreme quintiles of adult income showed three-fold (CVD) to four-fold (AMI) differences. It was possible to adjust for 22 biological, behavioural and psychosocial risk factors. On adjustment for all these factors the association between income and CVD mortality was essentially removed, while the associations between income and AMI was attenuated to 2.83. However, in analyses updated to 1998 conducted for this chapter, with a total of 205 events from 6 additional years of follow-up, the age-adjusted relative hazard (RH) for incident AMI comparing the low- to high-income quintile was 1.98 (1.26–3.12). This is considerably but not surprisingly reduced from the previous analysis[143] involving only 88 incident events. After adjustment for the same 22 risk factors the RH was 1.31 (0.79–2.17). Thus, with longer follow-up, this same set of risk factors eliminated the income gradient in AMI. Interpretation of these findings remains difficult as some of the adjustment factors (leukocytes, fibrinogen, and cardiorespiratory fitness) may be consequences of disease. Nevertheless, it would appear from these analyses that some finite set of risk factors measured in adulthood can at least statistically account for the bulk of the association between SEP in adulthood and objectively defined CVD endpoints. These risk factors may, however, have roots early in life.

4.4.2 Explanations for socioeconomic differentials based on childhood risk factors

As discussed above, the apparent difficulty of uncovering socially patterned biological and behavioural influences in the adult environment that adequately account for the social distribution of CVD led Barker[144] to postulate that the environment during fetal and infant life biologically 'programmes' people for later elevated CVD risk. Referring to the demonstration that infant mortality earlier this century correlated with later CVD mortality,[145] Barker considered that in a similar way early life factors could influence the social distribution of these (and other) diseases. He concluded that the origins of inequalities in health are being sown today through adverse influences that impair the growth, nutrition and health of mothers and their infants.

The centrepiece of this potential early life explanation for socioeconomic health differentials is poor growth *in utero*. As the direct effect of early life exposures such as birthweight or ponderal index on adult health outcomes may be relatively small in absolute terms,[146,147] it seems unlikely that early life exposures in and of themselves could play a large direct part in explaining adult socioeconomic distributions of CVD. In this regard it is interesting that research on *in utero* growth has increasingly examined interactions with later life exposures such as postnatal and childhood growth, which can also be socioeconomically patterned. This body of work has also suggested intergenerational components, so that the risks associated with less optimal birth outcomes (low birthweight, thinness, and so on) were modified both by intergenerational factors such as mother's anthropometry and by patterns of later growth during infancy and childhood.[95] Many of these intergenerational and intragenerational modifying forces are likely to be socioeconomically patterned. This means that socioeconomic health differences accumulated over the mother's life course can be transmitted across generations and further interact with socially patterned exposures in childhood such as diet and lack of exercise, to help generate adult socioeconomic health differences in the next generation. However compelling this is in theory, it will be difficult to capture its sequential complexity in the relatively crude statistical models we are forced to employ as caricatures of these life course processes.

Additionally, there may be sex differences, so that covariation of intergenerational factors, early life growth, and socioeconomic influences may be differently configured to produce increased CVD risk for men and women. For men, risk is increased with thinness at birth and catch-up growth in weight, especially in men whose mothers were shorter with higher body mass index.[148] For women, it is apparently shortness at birth and catch-up growth in height combined with having a tall mother that increases CHD risk.[95] For men, these *in utero* and postnatal growth parameters and intergenerational influences seem consistent with what is known about their socioeconomic distribution and appear consistent with observed adult socioeconomic distributions of CVD, but this is not so easily reconciled for the socioeconomic distribution of CVD in women.

These modifying factors have been extended beyond intergenerational and intragenerational anthropometric influences to include socioeconomic circumstances in both childhood[149] and adulthood.[150] In fact, Barker and colleagues have written 'Men who were not thin at birth were largely resilient to the later effects of poor living standards' (p. 3)[150] effectively suggesting that the negative health effects of adult socioeconomic disadvantage are obliterated by favourable *in utero* and postnatal growth.

This claim has not been widely investigated in other sources of data, so the idea that adult CVD differentials can be explained by early life growth is rather speculative. In fact, Barker's own data show suggestive evidence that the apparently protective effects of better *in utero* growth for CVD among socioeconomically disadvantaged adults may be specific to men, limited to one of the Finnish cohorts under study (1924–1933 cohort), not consistent across all CVD-related outcomes, and sensitive to how adult SEP is measured. For instance, for women in the 1924–1933 cohort, the combination of short birth length and greater height at age 7 was associated with higher CHD risk when the mother was tall.[95] As taller women are likely to have higher SEP this would be inconsistent with the finding for men in the same birth cohort. In the 1933–1944 birth cohort there was no overall effect (and therefore unlikely to be a reliable modifying effect) of adult SEP on hypertension.[149] Instead this study showed a modifying effect of low childhood SEP on growth and hypertension risk. Finally, the protective effects of better *in utero* growth were observed when adult social class was used as the measure of SEP but not income.[150] Thus the finding that the health effects of low SEP in adulthood can be explained by *in utero* growth requires more investigation. Nevertheless, such potentially modifying effects of early and later exposures are of particular interest to life course investigations[105,106] and should be encouraged, despite difficulties of interpretation.

There is limited evidence on the role of early life exposures in directly explaining adult socioeconomic differentials in CVD, though it is clear from the studies outlined in Table 4.3 that early life socioeconomic factors play a role. As in other areas of life course epidemiology, it is not clear how assessments of the contribution of early life exposures should be judged with regard to proper adjustments for factors that may lie on the causal pathway between early life and later exposures and CVD. Nevertheless, it is clear that social, biological, and behavioural factors operating early in life can influence the major risk factor pathways to CVD and thus socioeconomic differentials in CVD. There is more evidence that the time courses of changes in CVD differentials are more congruent with increasing socioeconomic differences in cigarette smoking and consumption of micronutrients than with trends in socioeconomic differentials in infant mortality or height[19,151,152]—understood as potential markers of early life growth. Thus, with regard to life course influences, this would seem to favour the development and maintenance of health behaviours and their cumulative biological sequelae as the main life course processes linking SEP to CVD—at least to epidemics of CVD.

4.5 Conceptualizing socioeconomic differentials within a life course perspective

The evidence presented here suggests that a strong case can be made for the contribution of socioeconomic conditions at different stages of the life course to health differentials in adulthood. However, the specific weights of the contribution of early and later life socioeconomic conditions will differ according to the outcome. For CVDs, poor socioeconomic conditions in early life appear to make a significant contribution to disease risk in adulthood especially when early life influences on the developmental trajectories of important adult risk factors are considered. Furthermore, there is growing evidence that the effect of early life socioeconomic conditions may depend on interactions with other risk factors in later life.

The interaction of socially patterned exposures at different periods of the life course to health status in adulthood renders the explanation of trends in both overall health status and in socioeconomic differentials in health potentially complex. For instance, the socially patterned exposure of low birthweight appears to interact with a socially patterned adulthood factor, obesity, to produce elevated risk of high blood pressure and CHD mortality.[153] Countervailing trends at different times would lead to different expectations regarding present-day disease risk and socioeconomic differentials. For example, reductions in infant mortality and improvements in birthweight happening around the time a cohort was born would be expected to reduce CVD risk for this cohort in adult life. If there is an increasing trend in obesity, however, this would be expected to increase the risk and trends in an opposite direction. As exposures acting across the life course, together with interactions between exposures acting at different times, contribute to disease risk, studies that only have data concerning one period of the life course are inadequate for further advancing our understanding of disease aetiology and socioeconomic differentials in health.

The specificity of associations between exposure measures and various health outcomes provides clues to aetiology. For example, height is inversely associated with CHD, stroke, respiratory disease, and stomach cancer risk, all known to be related to early life exposures. Height is not related to lung cancer risk—even though the latter is strongly related to adult socioeconomic circumstances, mainly through a strongly socially patterned risk factor, smoking, which itself may have been influenced by conditions earlier in life. There is also evidence for heterogeneity in links between height and CVD risk. Recent studies in Korea and Japan suggest that height is not associated with increased CVD risk,[154] suggesting an intriguing possibility that the effect of height and early growth may be partly dependent on dietary factors. Is height associated with CVD risk in societies with higher-fat diets but not in countries with historically lower levels of dietary fat?

The life course approach to chronic disease in adulthood—and therefore the life course approach to socioeconomic differentials in CVD—uses the tools of individual risk factor epidemiology but attempts to move on from an epidemiology that concentrates on risk factors acting in a supposedly independent and atemporal manner. This search for independent contributors to risk is in part an outcome of the underlying model of disease causation, captured in the well-known metaphor of the 'web of causation'.[155] While the idea of a complex web of causal components is certainly useful, it obscures the fact that what we observe at any one point in time as an array of adult risk factors may be the result of interlacing chains of social and biological influences that have coevolved over time.[156,157]

A life course approach embeds individual life trajectories in their historical, geographical, and cultural contexts. Indeed the long-term and sometimes irreversible outcomes of social circumstances at different stages of life are seen as becoming literally embodied.[158] Human bodies and minds in different social locations become crystallized reflections of the social experiences within which they have developed. The socially patterned nutritional, health, and environmental experiences of parents and self, influence, for example, birthweight, height, weight, and lung function. These biological and psychological aspects of bodies should be viewed as frozen 'snapshots' of social relations, rather than as asocial explanations of health inequalities, which, once accepted, exclude the social from consideration.[158]

The life course approach to socioeconomic health differentials views the physical and the social as being mutually constitutive, because aspects of bodily form can influence social trajectory in the same way as social experiences become embodied. Low birthweight, growth in childhood (and final adult height), persistent infections acquired in early life or the failure to acquire certain infections (leading to immunological programming increasing the risk of atopy), lung function, degree of adiposity, a habitus that embraces particular dispositional characteristics (including attitudes, health-related behaviours, and mood), modes of self-presentation, and ways of dealing with misfortune, may seem to fall within different categories, but they are all components of socially patterned life course trajectories that influence the social distribution of health in populations.[159]

Acknowledgements

John Lynch and George Davey Smith are supported by a Robert Wood Johnson, Investigators Award in Health Policy Research. John Lynch was also supported by grants from the US National Institutes of Health (RO1 HD35120-01A2; P50 HD38986-01). This work has also been facilitated by the European Science Foundation Programme on Health Variations, of which John Lynch and George Davey Smith are members.

References

Those marked with an asterisk are especially recommended for further reading.

1 **Woods R, Williams N.** Must the gap widen before it can be narrowed? Long-term trends in social class mortality differentials. *Continuity Change* 1995;**10**:105–37.

*2 **Engels F.** *The condition of the working class in England.* Harmondsworth: Penguin, 1987.

3 **Williams R.** Medical, economic and population factors in areas of high mortality: the case of Glasgow. *Sociol Health Illness* 1994;**16**:143–81.

4 **Szreter S.** The population health approach in historical perspective. *Am J Pub Health* 2002;**93**:421–31.

5 **Wrigley EA, Scholfield RS.** *The population history of England, 1541–1871.* Cambridge, Massachusetts: Harvard University Press, 1981.

6 **Kuh D, Davey Smith G.** When is mortality risk determined? Historical insights into a current debate. *Soc Hist Med* 1993;**6**:101–23.

7 **Kermack WO, McKendrick AG, McKinlay PL.** Death-rates in Great Britain and Sweden. Some general regularities and their significance. *Lancet* 1934;**31**:698–703. Reprinted in *Int J Epidemiol* 2001;**30**:678–83.

8 **Leon DA.** Common threads. In Leon DA, Walt G, eds. *Poverty, inequality and health.* Oxford: Oxford University Press, 2001:58–87.

9 **Swerdlow A, Dos Santos S, Doll R.** *Cancer incidence and mortality in England and Wales: Trends and risk factors.* Oxford: Oxford University Press, 2001.

10 **Shkolnikov V, McKee M, Leon DA.** Changes in life expectancy in Russia in the mid-1990s. *Lancet* 2001;**357**:917–21.

11 **Blane D, Bartley M, Davey Smith G.** Disease aetiology and materialist explanations of socio-economic mortality differentials. *Eur J Pub Health*1998;**8**:259–60.

12 **Najman JM.** Health and poverty: past, present and prospects for the future. *Soc Sci Med* 1993;**36**:157–66.

13 **Harding S.** Social class differences in mortality of men: recent evidence from the OPCS Longitudinal Study. *Pop Trends* 1995;**80**:31–7.

14 **Wilkins R, Ng E, Berthelot J-M.** Trends in mortality by income in urban Canada from 1971 to 1996. *Statistics Canada Health Reports* 2002;**13**:45–72 (supplement).

15 **Persson G, Bostrom G, Diderichsen F, *et al.*** Health in Sweden. The National Public Health Report, 2001. *Scand J Public Health* 2001;**29(suppl 58)**:199–218.

16 **Lundberg O, Diderichsen F, Aberg Yngwe M.** Changing health inequalities in a changing society? Sweden in the mid-1980s and mid-1990s. *Scand J Public Health* 2001;**29(suppl 55)**:31–40.

17 **Schalik LM, Hadden WC, Pamuk E, Navarro V, Pappas G.** The widening gap in death rates among income groups in the United States from 1967 to 1986. *Int J Health Serv* 2000;**30**:13–26.

18 **Stevenson THC.** The social distribution of mortality from different causes in England and Wales, 1910–12. *Biometrika* 1923;**15**:382–40.

19 **Davey Smith G.** Socioeconomic differentials. In Kuh D, Ben Shlomo Y, eds. *A life course approach to chronic disease epidemiology.* Oxford: Oxford University Press, 1997: 242–76.

20 **Johansson SR.** *Death and the doctors: medicine and eilite mortality in Britain from 1500 to 1800.* Cambridge: Cambridge Group for the History of Population and Social Structure, Working Paper Series No. 7, 1999.

21 **Kunitz S.** Making a long story short: A note on men's height and mortality in England from the first through the nineteenth centuries. *Med Hist* 1987;**31**:269–80.

22 **Davey Smith G, Egger M.** Commentary: understanding it all—health, meta-theories, and mortality trends. *Br Med J* 1996;**313**:1584–5.

*23 **Kunst AE, Groenhof F, Mackenbach JP, EU Working Group on Socioeconomic Inequalities in Health.** Occupational class and cause specific mortality in middle aged men in 11 European countries: comparison of population based studies. *Br Med J* 1998;**316**:1636–42.

24 **Weiss NS.** Can the 'specificity' of an association be rehabilitated as a basis for supporting a causal hypothesis? *Epidemiology* 2002;**13**:6–8.

25 **Davey Smith G, Kuh D.** Does early nutrition affect later health: Views from the 1930s and 1980s. In Smith D, ed. *The history of nutrition in Britain in the twentieth century: Science, scientists and politics.* London: Routledge, 1996:214–237.

26 **Hannington W.** *The problem of the distressed areas.* Golancz, London: Left Book Club Publications, 1937.

27 **Vernon HM.** *Health in relation to occupation.* London: Oxford University Press, 1939.

28 **Ciocco A, Klein H, Palmer CE.** Child health and the selective service physical standards. *Pub Health Rep* 1941;**56**:2365–75.

29 **Dubos R.** Biological Freudianism. Lasting effects of early environmental influences. *Pediatrics* 1966;**38**:789–800.

30 **Elo IT, Preston SH.** Effects of early-life conditions on adult mortality: a review. *Pop Ind* 1992;**58**:186–212.

31 **Notkola V, Punsar S, Karvonen MJ, Haapakoski J.** Socioeconomic conditions in childhood and mortality and morbidity caused by coronary heart disease in adulthood in rural Finland. *Soc Sci Med* 1985;**21**:517–23.

32 **Kaplan GA, Salonen JT.** Socioeconomic conditions in childhood and ischaemic heart disease during middle age. *Br Med J* 1990;**301**:1121–3.

33 **Mare RD.** Socio-economic careers and differential mortality among older men in the United States. In Vallin J, D'Souza S, Palloni A, eds. *Measurement and analysis of mortality.* Oxford: Clarendon Press, 1990:362–87.

34 **Brunner E, Davey Smith G, Marmot M, Canner R, Beksinska M, O'Brien J.** Childhood social circumstances and psychosocial and behavioural factors as determinants of plasma fibrinogen. *Lancet* 1996;**347**:1008–13.

35 **Parsons TJ, Power C, Logan S, Summerbell CD.** Childhood predictors of adult obesity: a systematic review. *Int J Obes Relat Metab Disord* 1999;**23**(**suppl 8**):S1–107.

*36 **Brunner E, Shipley MJ, Blane D, Davey Smith G, Marmot MG.** When does cardiovascular risk start? Past and present socioeconomic circumstances and risk factors in adulthood. *J Epidemiol Commun Health* 1999;**53**:757–64.

37 **Blane D, Hart CL, Davey Smith G, Gillis CR, Hole DJ, Hawthorne VM.** Association of cardiovascular disease risk factors with socioeconomic position during childhood and during adulthood. *Br Med J* 1996;**313**:1434–8.

*38 **Power C, Matthews S.** Origins of health inequalities in a national population sample. *Lancet* 1997;**350**:1584–9.

39 **Davey Smith G, Hart C.** Insulin resistance syndrome and childhood social conditions. *Lancet* 1997;**349**:284–5.

40 **Davey Smith G, Hart C.** Lifecourse socioeconomic and behavioural influences on cardiovascular disease mortality: the Collaborative study. *Am J Pub Health* 2002;**92**:1295–8.

41 **Wadsworth MEJ, Cripps HA, Midwinter RE, Colley JRT.** Blood pressure in a national birth cohort at the age of 36 related to social and familial factors, smoking, and body mass. *Br Med J* 1985;**291**:1534–8.

42 **Forsdahl A.** Are poor living conditions in childhood and adolescence an important risk factor for arteriosclerotic heart disease? *Br J Prev Soc Med* 1977;**31**:91–5.

*43 **Forsdahl A.** Living conditions in childhood and subsequent development of risk factors for arteriosclerotic heart disease. The cardiovascular survey in Finnmark 1974–75. *J Epidemiol Commun Health* 1978;**32**:34–7.

44 **Arnesen E, Forsdahl A.** The Tromso heart study: coronary risk factors and their association with living conditions during childhood. *J Epidemiol Commun Health* 1985;**39**:210–14.

45 **McKeigue PM.** Diabetes and insulin action. In Kuh D, Ben-Shlomo Y, eds. *A life course approach to chronic disease epidemiology.* Oxford: Oxford University Press, 1997:78–100.

46 **Laitinen J, Power C, Jarvelin MR.** Family social class, maternal body mass index, childhood body mass index, and age at menarche as predictors of adult obesity. *Am J Clin Nutr* 2001;**74**:287–94.

*47 **Lawlor DA, Ebrahim S, Davey Smith G.** Socioeconomic position in childhood and adulthood and insulin resistance: cross sectional survey using data from British women's heart and health study. *Br Med J* 2002;**325**:805–9.

*48 **Lynch JW, Kaplan GA, Salonen JT.** Why do poor people behave poorly? Variation in adult health behaviours and psychosocial characteristics by stages of the socioeconomic lifecourse. *Soc Sci Med* 1997;**44**:809–19.

49 **van de Mheen H, Stronks K, Looman CWN, Mackenbach JP.** Does childhood socioeconomic status influence adult health through behavioural factors? *Int J Epidemiol* 1998;**27**:431–7.

50 **van de Mheen H, Stronks K, Van Den Bos J, Mackenbach JP.** The contribution of childhood environment to the explanation of socio-economic inequalities in health in adult life: a retrospective study. *Soc Sci Med* 1997;**44**:13–24.

51 **Harper S, Lynch J, Hsu W-L, Everson SA, Hillemeier MM, Raghunathan TE, *et al*.** Life course socioeconomic conditions and adult psychosocial functioning. *Int J Epidemiol* 2002;**31**:395–403.

52 **Gilman SE, Kawachi I, Fitzmaurice GM, Buka SL.** Socioeconomic status in childhood and the lifetime risk of major depression. *Int J Epidemiol* 2002;**31**:359–67.

53 **Jones P.** The early origins of schizophrenia. *Br Med Bull* 1997;**53**:135–55.

54 **Power C, Manor O.** Explaining social class differences in phychological health among young adults: a longitudinal perspective. *Soc Psychiatry Psychiat Epidemiol* 1992;**27**:284–91.

55 **Fan AP, Eaton WW.** Longitudinal study assessing the joint effects of socio-economic status and birth risks on adult emotional and nervous conditions. *Br J Psychiat* 2001;**40**:S78–83.

56 **Eaton WW, Muntaner C, Bovasso G, Smith C.** Socioeconomic status and depressive syndrome: the role of inter- and intra-generational mobility, government assistance, and work environment. *J Health Soc Behav* 2001;**42**:227–94.

57 **Ritsher JE, Warner V, Johnson JG, Dohrenwend BP.** Inter-generational longitudinal study of social class and depression: a test of social causation and social selection models. *Br J Psychiat* 2001;**40**:S84–90.

58 **Power C, Matthews S, Manor O.** Inequalities in self-rated health: explanations from different stages of life. *Lancet* 1998;**351**:1009–14.

59 **Power C, Li L, Manor O.** A prospective study of limiting longstanding illness in early adulthood. *Int J Epidemiol* 2000;**29**:131–9.

60 **Power C, Matthews S, Manor O.** Inequalities in self rated health in the 1958 birth cohort: lifetime social circumstances or social mobility? *Br Med J* 1996;**313**:449–53.

61 Power C, Manor O, Matthews S. The duration and timing of exposure: effects of socioeconomic environment on adult health. *Am J Pub Health* 1999;**89**:1059–65.

62 Hertzman C, Power C, Matthews S, Manor O. Using an interactive framework of society and lifecourse to explain self-rated health in early adulthood. *Soc Sci Med* 2001;**53**:1575–85.

63 Wagstaff A, Paci P, Joshi H. Inequalities in health: who you are? Where you live? Or who your parents are? Evidence from a cohort of British 33-year olds. Presentation at International Health Economics Association Conference, York, July 17–21, http://econ.worldbank.org/files/3003_wps2713.pdf, 2001.

64 Kuh D, Hardy R, Chaturvedi N, Wadsworth ME. Birth weight, childhood growth and abdominal obesity in adult life. *Int J Obes Relat Metab Disord* 2002;**26**:40–7.

65 Barker DJP, Forsén T, Uutela A, Osmond C, Eriksson JG. Size at birth and resilience to effects of poor living conditions in adult life: longitudinal study. *Br Med J* 2001;**323**:1–5.

66 Bremne JD, Vermetten E. Stress and development: behavioral and biological consequences. *Dev Psychopathol* 2001;**13**:473–89.

67 Whalley LJ, Deary IJ. Longitudinal cohort study of childhood IQ and survival up to age 76. *Br Med J* 2001;**322**:819–823.

68 Tong S, Baghurst P, McMichael A, Sawyer M, Mudge J. Lifetime exposure to environmental lead and children's intelligence at 11–13 years: the Port Pirie cohort study. *Br Med J* 1996;**312**:1569–75.

69 Tong S, Baghurst PA, Sawyer MG, Burns J, McMichael AJ. Declining blood lead levels and changes in cognitive function during childhood: the Port Pirie Cohort Study. *J Am Med Assoc* 1998;**280**:1915–9.

70 von Mutius E, Illi S, Nicolai T, Martinez FD. Relation of indoor heating with asthma, allergic sensitisation, and bronchial responsiveness: survey of children in south Bavaria. *Br Med J* 1996;**312**:1448–50.

71 Marks RU. Social stress and cardiovascular disease. Factors involving social and demographic characteristics. A review of empirical findings. *Milbank Memorial Fund Q* 1967;**45**:S51–108.

72 Forsdahl A. Observations throwing light on the high mortality in the county of Finnmark: Is the high mortality today a late effect of very poor living conditions in childhood and adolescence? *Int J Epidemiol* 2002;**31**:302–8.

73 Barker DJP, Osmond C. Diet and coronary heart disease in England and Wales during and after the second world war. *J Epidemiol Commun Health* 1986;**40**:37–44.

74 Hasle H. Association between living conditions in childhood and myocardial infarction. *Br Med J* 1990;**300**:512–13.

75 Bobák M, Hertzman C, Skodová Z, Marmot M. Own education, current conditions, parental material circumstances, and risk of myocardial infarction in a former communist country. *J Epidemiol Commun Health* 2000;**54**:91–6.

76 Coggon D, Margetts B, Barker DJ, Carson PH, Mann JS, Oldroyd KG *et al.* Childhood risk factors for ischaemic heart disease and stroke. *Paediatr Perinat Epidemiol* 1990;**4**:464–9.

77 Donnan SPB, Ho SC, Woo J, Wong SL, Woo KS, Tse CY *et al.* Risk factors for acute myocardial infarction in a Southern Chinese population. *Ann Epidemiol* 1994;**4**:46–58.

78 Brasche S, Galbas C, Störl B. Kindheit und Herzinfarkt: sozioökonmische und psychosoziale Kindheitseinflüsse auf das Herzinfarktrisiko. *Sozial Und Präventivmedizin* 2001;**46**:311–19.

79 Burr ML, Sweetnam PM. Family size and paternal unemployment in relation to myocardial infarction. *J Epidemiol Commun Health* 1980;**34**:93–5.

*80 Beebe-Dimmer J, Lynch JW, Turell G, Lustgarten S, Raghunathan T, Kaplan GA. Childhood and adult socioeconomic conditions and 31-year mortality risk in women. *Am J Epidemiol* (in press).

81 Pensola TH, Valkonen T. Effect of parental social class, own education and social class on mortality among young men. *Eur J Pub Health* 2002;**12**:29–36.

82 Davey Smith G, McCarron P, Okasha M, McEwen J. Social circumstances in childhood and cardiovascular disease mortality: prospective observational study of Glasgow university students. *J Epidemiol Commun Health* 2001;**55**:340–1.

*83 Davey Smith G, Hart C, Blane D, Hole D. Adverse socioeconomic conditions in childhood and cause specific adult mortality: prospective observational study. *Br Med J* 1998;**316**:1631–5.

84 Heslop P, Davey Smith G, Macleod J, Hart C. The socioeconomic position of employed women, risk factors and mortality. *Soc Sci Med* 2001;**53**:477–85.

85 Claussen B, Davey Smith G, Thelle D. Impact of childhood and adulthood socioeconomic position on cause specific mortality: the Oslo Mortality Study. *J Epidemiol Commun Health* 2003;**57**:40–45.

86 Gliksman MD, Kawachi I, Hunter D, Colditz GA, Manson JE, Stampfer MJ *et al*. Childhood socioeconomic status and risk of cardiovascular disease in middle aged US women: a prospective study. *J Epidemiol Commun Health* 1995;**49**:10–15.

87 Vågerö D, Leon D. Effect of social class in childhood and adulthood on adult mortality. *Lancet* 1994;**343**:1224–5.

88 Frankel S, Davey Smith G, Gunnell D. Childhood socioeconomic position and adult cardiovascular mortality: the Boyd Orr cohort. *Am J Epidemiol* 1999;**150**:1081–4.

89 Dedman DJ, Gunnell D, Davey Smith G, Frankel S. Childhood housing conditions and later mortality in the Boyd Orr cohort. *J Epidemiol Commun Health* 2001;**55**:10–15.

90 Lynch JW, Kaplan GA, Cohen RD, Kauhanen J, Wilson TW, Smith NL *et al*. Childhood and adult socioeconomic status as predictors of mortality in Finland. *Lancet* 1994;**343**:524–7.

91 Notkola V. Living conditions in childhood and coronary heart disease in adulthood. *Commentationes Scientiarum Socialium* 1985;**29**:15–119.

92 Gillum RF, Paffenbarger RS. Chronic disease in former college students. *Am J Epidemiol* 1978;**108**:289–98.

93 Wannamethee SG, Whincup PH, Shaper G, Walker M. Influence of fathers' social class on cardiovascular disease in middle-aged men. *Lancet* 1996;**348**:1259–63.

94 Marmot M, Shipley M, Brunner E, Hemingway H. Relative contribution of early life and adult socioeconomic factors to adult morbidity in the Whitehall II study. *J Epidemiol Commun Health* 2001;**55**:301–7.

95 Forsen T, Eriksson JG, Tuomilehto J, Osmond C, Barker DJ. Growth *in utero* and during childhood among women who develop coronary heart disease: longitudinal study. *Br Med J* 1999;**319**:1403–7.

96 Eriksson JG, Forsén T, Tuomilehto J, Osmond C, Barker DJP. Early growth, adult income, and risk of stroke. *Stroke* 2000;**31**:869–74.

97 Hart CL, Hole DJ, Davey Smith G. Influence of socioeconomic circumstances in early and later life on stroke risk among men in a Scottish cohort study. *Stroke* 2000;**31**:2093–7.

98 Eriksson JG, Forsen T, Tuomilehto J, Osmond C, Barker DJP. Early growth, adult income, and risk of stroke. *Stroke* 2000;**31**:869–74.

99 Lawlor DA, Davey Smith G, Leon D, Sterne J, Ebrahim S. Secular trends in mortality by stroke subtype over the twentieth century: resolution of the stroke-coronary heart disease paradox? *Lancet* 2002;**360**:1818–23.

100 Hart CL, Davey Smith G. Relation between number of siblings and adult mortality and stroke risk: 25 year follow up of men in the Collaborative study. *J Epidemiol Commun Health* 2003;**57**:464–5.

101 Davey Smith G, Neaton JD, Wentworth D, Stamler R, Stamler J. Mortality differences between black and white men in the USA: contribution of income and other risk factors among men screened for the MRFIT. *Lancet* 1998;**351**:934–9.

102 Davey Smith G, Wentworth D, Neaton JD, Stamler R, Stamler J. Socioeconomic differentials in mortality risk among men screened for the Multiple Risk Factor Intervention Trial: Part II— results for 20,224 Black men. *Am J Pub Health* 1996;**86**:497–504.

103 Davey Smith G, Neaton JD, Wentworth D, Stamler R, Stamler J. Socioeconomic differentials in mortality risk among men screened for the Multiple Risk Factor Intervention Trial: Part I— results for 300,685 White men. *Am J Pub Health* 1996;**86**:486–96.

104 Hart CL, Davey Smith G, Blane D. Social mobility and 21 year mortality in a cohort of Scottish men. *Soc Sci Med* 1998;**47**:1121–30.

105 Kuh D, Ben Shlomo Y, Lynch J, Hallqvist J, Power C. A glossary for life course epidemiology. *J Epidemiol Commun Health* 2003;**57**:778–83.

106 Hallqvist J, Lynch JW, Blane D, Bartley M, Lange T. Critical period, accumulation and social trajectory: Can we empirically distinguish lifecourse processes? *Soc Sci Med* (in press).

107 Blane D, Davey Smith G, Bartley M. Social selection: what does it contribute to social class differences in health? *Sociol Health Illness* 1993;**15**:1–15.

108 Davey Smith G, Ben-Shlomo Y, Lynch JW. Lifecourse approaches to inequalities in coronary heart disease risk. In Stansfield S, Marmot M, eds. *Stress and the heart: psychosocial pathways to coronary heart disease.* London: British Medical Journal Books, 2002:20–49.

109 Alvarsson M, Efendic S, Grill VE. Insulin responses to glucose in healthy males are associated with adult height but not with birth weight. *J Intern Med* 1994;**236**:275–9.

110 Bao W, Srinivasan SR, Wattigney WA, Berenson GS. Persistence of multiple cardiovascular risk clustering related to syndrome X from childhood to young adulthood. *Arch Intern Med* 1994;**154**:1842–7.

111 Raitakari OT, Porkka KV, Rasanen L, Ronnemaa T, Viikari JS. Clustering and six year cluster-tracking of serum total cholesterol, HDL-cholesterol and diastolic blood pressure in children and young adults. *J Clin Epidemiol* 1994;**47**:1085–93.

112 Berenson GS, Srinivasan SR, Bao W, Newman WP, Tracy RE, Wattigney WA. Association between multiple cardiovascular risk factors and atherosclerosis in children and young adults. *New Engl J Med* 1998;**338**:1650–6.

113 Hardy R, Wadsworth M, Kuh D. The influence of childhood weight and socioeconomic status on change in adult body mass index in a British national birth cohort. *Int J Obes Relat Metab Disord* 2000;**24**:725–34.

114 Wilson TW, Kaplan GA, Kauhanen J, Cohen RD, Wu M, Salonen R *et al.* Association between plasma fibrinogen concentration and five socioeconomic indices in the Kuopio Ischemic Heart Disease Risk Factor Study. *Am J Epidemiol* 1993;**137**:292–300.

115 Graham H, Hunt K. Socio-economic influences on women's smoking status in adulthood: insights from the West of Scotland Twenty-07 study. *Health Bull* 1998;**56**:757–65.

116 Graham H, Der G. Influences on women's smoking status. The contribution of socioeconomic status in adolescence and adulthood. *Eur J Pub Health* 1999;**9**:137–41.

117 Curtin F, Morabia A, Bernstein M. Smoking behavior in a Swiss urban population: the role of gender and education. *Prev Med* 1997;**26**:658–63.

118 Escobedo L, Peddicord J. Smoking prevalence in US birth cohorts: the influence of gender and education. *Am J Pub Health* 1996;**86**:231–6.

119 Rose G. Incubation period of coronary heart disease. *Br Med J Clin Res Ed* 1982;**284**:1600–1.

120 **Magnus P, Beaglehole R, Rodgers A, Bennett S.** The real contribution of the major risk factors to the coronary epidemics—time to end the 'only-50%' myth. *Arch Intern Med* 2001;**161**:2657–60.

121 **Yusuf S, Reddy S, Ounpuu S, Anand S.** Global burden of cardiovascular diseases: part 1: general considerations, the epidemiologic transition, risk factors, and impact of urbanization. *Circulation* 2001;**104**:2746–53.

122 **Yusuf S, Reddy S, Ounpuu S, Anand S.** Global burden of cardiovascular diseases: part 2: variations in cardiovascular disease by specific ethnic groups and geographic regions and prevention strategies. *Circulation* 2001;**104**:2855–64.

123 **Davey Smith G, Shipley MJ.** Confounding of occupation and smoking: its magnitude and consequences. *Soc Sci Med* 1991;**32**:1297–300.

124 **Davey Smith G, Blane D, Bartley M.** Explanations for socioeconomic differentials in mortality: evidence from Britain and elsewhere. *Eur J Pub Health* 1994;**4**:131–44.

125 **Marmot MG, Rose G, Shipley M, Hamilton PJ.** Employment grade and coronary heart disease in British civil servants. *J Epidemiol CommunHealth* 1978;**32**:244–9.

126 **Salonen J.** Socioeconomic status and risk of cancer, cerebral stroke, and death due to coronary heart disease and any disease: a longitudinal study in eastern Finland. *J Epidemiol Commun Health* 1982;**36**:294–7.

127 **Holme I, Helgeland A, Hjermann I, Leren P, Lund-Larsen PG.** Physical activity at work and at leisure in relation to coronary risk factors and social class. A 4-year mortality follow-up. The Oslo study. *Acta Med Scand* 1981;**209**:277–83.

128 **Buring JE, Evans DA, Fiore M, Rosner B, Hennekens CH.** Occupation and risk of death from coronary heart disease. *J Am Med Assoc* 1987;**258**:791–2.

129 **Hein HO, Suadicani P, Gyntelberg F.** Ischaemic heart disease incidence by social class and form of smoking: the Copenhagen Male Study—17 years' follow-up. *J Intern Med* 1992;**231**:477–83.

130 **Pekkanen J, Tuomilehto J, Uutela A, Vartiainen E, Nissinen A.** Social class, health behaviour, and mortality among men and women in eastern Finland. *Br Med J* 1995;**311**:589–93.

131 **Rosengren A, Wedel H, Wilhelmsen L.** Coronary heart disease and mortality in middle aged men from different occupational classes in Sweden. *Br Med J* 1988;**297**:1497–500.

132 **Eaker ED, Pinsky J, Castelli WP.** Myocardial infarction and coronary death among women: psychosocial predictors from a 20-year follow-up of women in the Framingham Study. *Am J Epidemiol* 1992;**135**:854–64.

133 **Pocock SJ, Shaper AG, Cook DG, Phillips AN, Walker M.** Social class differences in ischaemic heart disease in British men. *Lancet* 1987;**2**:197–201.

134 **Davey Smith G, Phillips A.** Declaring independence: why we should be cautious. *J Epidemiol Commun Health* 1990;**44**:257–8 (erratum appears in *J Epidemiol Commun Health* 1991;**45**:88).

135 **Phillips AN, Davey Smith G.** How independent are 'independent' effects? Relative risk estimation when correlated exposures are measured imprecisely. *J Clin Epidemiol* 1991;**44**:1223–31.

136 **Adler NE, Boyce T, Chesney MA, Cohen S, Folkman S, Kahn RL** *et al.* Socioeconomic status and health. The challenge of the gradient. *Am Psychol* 1994;**49**:15–24.

137 **Marmot MG, Davey Smith G, Stansfeld S, Patel C, North F, Head J** *et al.* Health inequalities among British civil servants: the Whitehall II study. *Lancet* 1991;**337**:1387–93.

138 **Brunner EJ, Marmot MG, White IR, O'Brien JR, Etherington MD, Slavin BM** *et al.* Gender and employment grade differences in blood cholesterol, apolipoproteins and haemostatic factors in the Whitehall II study. *Atherosclerosis* 1993;**102**:195–207.

139 Marmot MG, Bosma H, Hemingway H, Brunner E, Stansfeld S. Contribution of job control and other risk factors to social variations in coronary heart disease incidence. *Lancet* 1997;**350**:235–9.

140 Davey Smith G, Harding S. Is control at work the key to socio-economic gradients in mortality? *Lancet* 1997;**350**:1369–70.

141 Lee S, Colditz G, Berkman L, Kawachi I. A propospective study of job strain and coronary heart disease in US women. *Int J Epidemiol* 2003;**31**:1147–53.

142 Rosvall M, Ostergren P-O, Hedblad B, Isacsson S-O, Janzon L, Berglund G. Work-related psychosocial factors and carotid atherosclerosis. *Int J Epidemiol* 2003;**31**:1169–78.

143 Lynch JW, Kaplan GA, Cohen RD, Tuomilehto J, Salonen JT. Do cardiovascular risk factors explain the relation between socioeconomic status, risk of all-cause mortality, cardiovascular mortality, and acute myocardial infarction? *Am J Epidemiol* 1996;**144**:934–42.

144 Barker DJ. The foetal and infant origins of inequalities in health in Britain. *J Pub Health Med* 1991;**13**:64–8.

145 Barker DJP, Osmond C. Infant mortality, childhood nutrition, and ischaemic heart disease in England and Wales. *Lancet* 1986;**1**:1077–81.

146 Huxley R, Neil A, Collins R. Unravelling the fetal origins hypothesis: is there really an inverse association between birthweight and subsequent blood pressure? *Lancet* 2002;**360**:659–65.

147 Joseph KS, Kramer MS. Review of the evidence on fetal and early childhood antecedents of adult chronic disease. *Epidemiol Rev* 1996;**18**:158–74.

148 Forsén T, Eriksson JG, Tuomilehto J, Teramo K, Osmond C, Barker DJP. Mother's weight in pregnancy and coronary heart disease in a cohort in Finnish men: follow up study. *Br Med J* 1997;**315**:837–40.

149 Barker DJ, Forsen T, Eriksson JG, Osmond C. Growth and living conditions in childhood and hypertension in adult life: a longitudinal study. *J Hypertens* 2002;**20**:1951–6.

150 Barker DJP, Forsen T, Uutela A, Osmond C, Eriksson JG. Size at birth and resilience to effects of poor living conditions in adult life: longitudinal study. *Br Med J* 2001;**323**:1273.

151 Watterson PA. Infant mortality by father's occupation from the 1911 census of England and Wales. *Demography* 1988;**25**:289–306.

152 Kuh DL, Power C, Rodgers B. Secular trends in social class and sex differences in adult height. *Int J Epidemiol* 1991;**20**:1001–9.

153 Frankel S, Elwood P, Sweetnam P, Yarnell J, Davey Smith G. Birthweight, body-mass index in middle age, and incident coronary heart disease. *Lancet* 1996;**348**:1478–80.

154 Song Y-M, Davey Smith G, Sung J. Adult height and cause-specific mortality: evidence on early-life origins of adult disease from a large prospective study of Korean men. *Am J Epidemiol* 2003;**158**:479–85.

155 MacMahon B, Pugh TF. *Epidemiology. Principles and methods.* Boston: Little, Brown and Company, 1970.

156 Davey Smith G. Income inequality and mortality: why are they related? *Br Med J* 1996;**312**:987–8.

157 Krieger N. Epidemiology and the web of causation: has anyone seen the spider? *Soc Sci Med* 1994;**39**:887–903.

158 Najman JM, Davey Smith G. The embodiment of class-related and health inequalities: Australian policies. *Aust NZ J Pub Health* 2000;**24**:3–4.

159 Davey Smith G. *Health inequalities: Lifecourse approaches.* Bristol: Policy Press, 2003.

Chapter 5

Ischaemic heart disease and cerebrovascular disease mortality trends with special reference to England and Wales: are there cohort effects?

Clive Osmond and Rebecca Hardy

Trends in ischaemic heart disease (IHD) death rates in many western industrialized countries have risen to a peak around the 1960s or 1970s and then declined. In these same countries there has generally been a continuous decline in rates subsequently. An important role for early life factors would produce cohort effects. Detailed statistical modelling of death rates for IHD and cerebrovascular disease (CVD) in England and Wales from 1951–1955 to 1996–2000 provides evidence of a cohort effect for IHD, as well as stronger period effects. A cohort-related peak in death rates affected those born during the early 1920s. The fact that the trends in CVD exhibit no turning points means that it is difficult to distinguish cohort from period effects. Improving trends in adult coronary heart disease (CHD) risk factors have probably played a major role in the mortality trends observed, as have declining case fatality rates. The increasing rates of smoking in women in some countries and in obesity remain a public health concern, as do the increasing mortality rates in eastern Europe. Birthweight, although associated with later risk of IHD and CVD in many individual-level studies, does not explain the cohort effects in IHD. Increasing growth tempo and attained height may explain some of the recent decline in both diseases, but not the peak observed in IHD. Given the growing evidence that the risk associated with birth characteristics is modified by subsequent growth and development, it is perhaps unreasonable to expect any cohort effect simply to be matched by a trend in mean birthweight. The further study of time trends in CVD would benefit from the separation of stroke subtype, as haemorrhagic and thrombotic stroke have different trends over time.

5.1 Introduction

Popular belief is that trends in IHD death rates in many countries have risen to a synchronized peak at every age and then fallen. This has been taken as evidence that the factors responsible for the rise and fall in rates—whether harmful or beneficial changes in lifestyle, beneficial interventions, or improvements in treatment—have acted in adult life.[1] It has also been taken as evidence against an important influence of early life factors on the incidence of the disease, as would be suggested by the 'fetal origins' hypothesis.[2] The argument is that early life factors would produce 'cohort' effects, that is, changes in the rates that were synchronized according to year of birth (cohort, generation), rather than year of death. The purpose of this chapter is to take a closer look at trends in IHD death rates in England and Wales to assess whether this popular belief is true. We also analyse the CVD death rates in England and Wales. CVD has also been related to early growth and development and so might also be expected to have death rates that depend on year of birth.

It is necessary to be modest about what may be achieved through time trend analyses. The 'ecological fallacy' (Chapter 6), in which we assume that observations made on populations will also apply to individuals within those populations, could apply to studies of time trend. Time trend analyses may be viewed as only a supplement to studies of individuals. For example, the 'fetal origins' hypothesis is being tested through studies of cohorts of individuals whose early growth had been characterized in detail, through mechanistic studies in individuals, and through animal models. However, one test of the importance of early life factors in terms of public health might be whether they can help to explain variations across populations in time and place.[3]

There are many difficulties in time trend analysis of death rates. Ideally we would study incidence rates rather than death rates. The survival processes that stand between incidence and death are likely to have shown important variation over age, year, and generation—some due to changes in treatment. But extensive incidence data are not available in England and Wales. Further, we depend on death certification of the underlying cause of death. This is vulnerable to fashion, rule change, and revision of the disease classification. In this chapter we use codes recommended by the Office for National Statistics (ONS). Another problem is that cohort effects can be created quite accidentally. For example, it has been argued[4] that the successive application of improved diagnostic tools to older age groups, and hence greater ascertainment of the disease, has created an artefactual cohort effect in multiple myeloma death rates.

5.2 Trends in ischaemic heart disease and cerebrovascular disease in England and Wales

5.2.1 Definition of ischaemic heart disease and cerebrovascular disease

In Table 5.1 we specify the International Classification of Disease codes that we have used to define both IHD and CVD. These codes are recommended in the ONS review article,[5] which includes a comprehensive discussion about comparability and use of codes throughout the twentieth century. There have been fewer problems since 1951. It is difficult to distinguish subtypes of stroke. The combination used is broad to enable a long time series.

Table 5.1 International Classification of Disease (ICD) codes used to define cause of death as either ischaemic heart disease or cerebrovascular disease

ICD revision in use Cause of death	1951–1957, 1958–1967 ICD6, ICD7 Codes used		1968–1978 ICD8 Codes used		1979–2000 ICD9 Codes used	
			Year of death			
Ischaemic heart disease	420	Arteriosclerotic heart disease, including coronary disease	410	Acute myocardial infarction	410	Acute myocardial infarction
	422	Other myocardial degeneration—fatty degeneration	411	Other acute and subacute forms of ischaemic heart disease	411	Other acute and subacute forms of ischaemic heart disease
			412	Chronic myocardial infarction	412	Chronic myocardial infarction
			413	Angina pectoris	413	Angina pectoris
			414	Asymptomatic ischaemic heart disease	414	Other form of chronic ischaemic heart disease
Cerebrovascular disease	330	Subarachnoid haemorrhage	430–438	Cerebrovascular disease	430–438	Cerebrovascular disease
	331	Cerebral haemorrhage	293.0	Psychosis with cerebral arteriosclerosis	290.4	Arteriosclerotic dementia
	332	Cerebral embolism and thrombosis	293.1	Psychosis with other cerebrovascular disturbances	342	Hemiplegia
	333	Spasm of cerebral arteries	344	Other cerebral paralysis	344	Other paralytic syndromes
	334	Other and ill-defined vascular lesions affecting central nervous system				
	352	Other cerebral paralysis				

5.2.2 Basic data and initial description

The numbers of deaths from IHD in men and corresponding death rates are given in Table 5.2 for 10 five-year periods of time from 1951–1955 through to 1996–2000 and for 13 five-year age groups from age 25–29 years through to ages 80–84 and 85 and over. Corresponding data follow for IHD in women (Table 5.3), CVD in men (Table 5.4), and CVD in women (Table 5.5). Too few deaths occur below age 25 to warrant analysis. Death certification is likely to be more reliable at ages under 70 years. The death rates are derived from the ONS annual estimates of population.

The death rates in Tables 5.2–5.5 are plotted against year of death in Figs 5.1–5.4 respectively. Rates are plotted on a log-scale with points corresponding to the same age group connected by a line. For each disease the death rates increase with age so that the lines do not overlap. Using a log-scale enables all the rates to be distinguishable on one graph, but disguises the fact that so many of the deaths occur at older ages. Lines at different age groups are parallel when there has been the same proportional change in death rates.

In men, at ages below 40 years, IHD rates rose to a peak in 1961–1965 and have subsequently fallen (Table 5.2, Fig. 5.1). Between ages 40 and 54 years the peak was delayed until 1971–1975. The peak between ages 55 and 64 was delayed a further 5 years until 1976–1980. Between ages 65 and 74 there was less of a distinct rise to a peak, but rates have clearly fallen since 1976–1980. At ages above 75, rates have fallen continuously. The pattern in women was similar to that seen in men, though the rates were lower (Table 5.3, Fig. 5.2). The rises to peaks were shallower, but the subsequent falls have been just as pronounced. Below age 40 years, the rates peaked before 1970, between 40 and 49 they peaked in 1971–1975, and between 50 and 64 they peaked in 1976–1980. At age 70 and above the rates have fallen throughout the period, particularly at the beginning and end.

Between ages 45 and 79, where most of the deaths occur, CVD rates have fallen progressively in men in each 5-year period (Table 5.4, Fig. 5.3). At younger and older ages there have also been steady declines, but these have been slower to start and shallower. The pattern of rates for women is very similar to that for men (Table 5.5, Fig. 5.4).

Figure 5.5 shows the same data as Fig. 5.1, but the rates are now plotted against year of birth, not year of death. This arrangement emphasizes changes in rates that are indexed by cohort and suggests a wave in the death rates with higher rates for men born around the 1920s. A similar impression is obtained from the IHD death rates in women. The CVD graphs are less affected by this presentation, though the stable rates at the very highest ages in the early part of the period are more distinct.

5.2.3 Age standardization

Calculation of an age-standardized index condenses information from several age groups into one summary figure. For example, we may pool the age groups from ages 35 to 64 by using the European standard population to generate a directly standardized index. This has been done for each of the 50 years from 1951 to 2000 and the results are presented in Figs 5.6 (IHD) and 5.7 (CVD). For IHD in men, the standardized rates rise from 2190 deaths per million in 1953 to exceed 3000 between 1968 and 1981, before falling continuously and steeply to be 1178 in the year 2000 (36% of the peak in 1972). However, it would be wrong to infer that this pattern has been repeated at each component age. The index reflects the trend at age 60–64, where many of the deaths occurred. The approach

Table 5.2 Numbers of deaths and death rates from ischaemic heart disease in men in England and Wales during 1951–2000 according to age at death and year of death

Year of death	Age at death (years)												
	25–29	30–34	35–39	40–44	45–49	50–54	55–59	60–64	65–69	70–74	75–79	80–84	85+
(a) Numbers of deaths from ischaemic heart disease in men													
1951–1955	190	571	1472	3914	8793	16239	23074	34193	47234	59694	65192	51396	34896
1956–1960	205	704	2169	4558	10452	19869	30689	38148	48803	58956	61056	50452	35795
1961–1965	215	780	2783	6481	11965	23105	37468	51206	55795	61673	59806	48322	37805
1966–1970	234	784	2528	7078	14602	23060	39760	56204	66910	63258	56170	41168	32119
1971–1975	238	813	2457	6814	15386	27574	37766	58703	76152	76322	59518	41655	30857
1976–1980	217	799	2355	5975	13086	25665	41286	54260	76436	85292	70978	43529	31442
1981–1985	197	721	2169	4991	10941	20825	36151	54891	67078	85670	78669	52204	33301
1986–1990	151	574	1865	4643	8860	16314	28519	46456	65852	73306	79850	58927	40003
1991–1995	179	477	1468	3605	7576	12405	21134	35157	53876	70343	69464	62288	48970
1996–2000	133	412	1236	2902	5932	11009	16483	25676	39254	55120	64083	52763	51796
(b) Death rates per million from ischaemic heart disease in men													
1951–1955	25	70	195	475	1100	2318	4093	7165	12071	20079	34186	57298	100855
1956–1960	28	91	269	610	1292	2585	4685	7535	12198	19738	31263	51168	81724
1961–1965	29	105	359	801	1618	2961	5165	8596	13163	20129	30152	47310	79107
1966–1970	31	107	345	926	1850	3246	5402	8603	13467	19667	27726	37341	63152
1971–1975	26	108	341	947	2059	3627	5644	8807	13773	20126	27867	37295	53674
1976–1980	24	89	318	843	1857	3557	5758	8931	13420	19864	27946	37179	51451
1981–1985	23	83	246	685	1579	3046	5279	8371	12764	18957	26550	36105	50175
1986–1990	15	66	214	529	1237	2417	4366	7348	11454	17333	24833	33523	47572
1991–1995	17	47	167	415	874	1770	3254	5770	9599	14867	22401	31400	44960
1996–2000	13	38	120	330	686	1289	2426	4191	7137	11688	17934	26729	38621

Table 5.3 Numbers of deaths and death rates from ischaemic heart disease in women in England and Wales during 1951–2000 according to age at death and year of death

Year of death	Age at death (years)												
	25–29	30–34	35–39	40–44	45–49	50–54	55–59	60–64	65–69	70–74	75–79	80–84	85+
(a) Numbers of deaths from ischaemic heart disease in women													
1951–1955	83	146	305	773	1901	4019	8125	16603	31072	51129	69008	68145	67477
1956–1960	45	145	297	737	1792	3914	8403	16813	30125	49096	66781	68954	70632
1961–1965	61	149	390	1000	1959	4291	9479	18920	32513	50846	66948	70932	78045
1966–1970	51	140	405	1091	2227	4356	9506	19541	33362	48754	60254	61015	67937
1971–1975	51	143	372	1077	2500	5211	9585	20142	35019	52179	62669	61539	69517
1976–1980	68	171	360	996	2211	5024	10483	18807	34716	53729	66771	65351	73187
1981–1985	42	141	351	757	1724	4236	9549	19128	30769	52607	69058	69985	80687
1986–1990	32	117	319	699	1401	3219	7607	16926	30641	45668	66383	74164	93342
1991–1995	37	130	256	650	1329	2525	5495	12254	24389	41863	56209	72837	106588
1996–2000	38	96	260	569	1205	2233	4207	8520	16571	30380	47689	56875	100534
(b) Death rates per million from ischaemic heart disease in women													
1951–1955	11	18	39	91	230	524	1180	2700	5822	11899	23504	44598	87861
1956–1960	6	19	36	95	215	484	1136	2578	5381	10778	20435	37455	74664
1961–1965	9	21	50	122	255	524	1209	2691	5461	10562	18807	34174	66894
1966–1970	7	20	56	142	275	583	1199	2620	5145	9439	15972	25401	48781
1971–1975	6	20	53	151	331	658	1327	2673	5088	9181	15339	24082	40433
1976–1980	8	20	50	144	315	681	1368	2734	4988	8887	14698	23490	38079
1981–1985	5	16	40	106	252	614	1337	2620	4832	8528	13955	21699	36311
1986–1990	3	14	37	80	197	478	1134	2476	4504	8041	12972	20369	34274
1991–1995	4	13	30	75	154	360	837	1904	3818	6856	11799	19075	32062
1996–2000	4	9	26	65	140	260	611	1343	2731	5267	9237	15855	26992

Table 5.4 Numbers of deaths and death rates from cerebrovascular disease in men in England and Wales during 1951–2000 according to age at death and year of death

Year of death	Age at death (years)												
	25–29	30–34	35–39	40–44	45–49	50–54	55–59	60–64	65–69	70–74	75–79	80–84	85+
(a) Numbers of deaths from cerebrovascular disease in men													
1951–1955	220	390	602	1243	2644	5039	7854	13633	20968	28592	32213	23170	12655
1956–1960	211	357	667	1176	2531	5000	8914	13540	20371	27949	32173	26404	16159
1961–1965	221	363	617	1249	2213	4585	8866	14759	20520	27273	30714	26414	19632
1966–1970	204	354	630	1182	2351	4119	8193	14553	22155	26867	29579	25619	21797
1971–1975	248	328	564	1044	2185	4035	6727	13124	22155	29015	28628	25281	22060
1976–1980	220	306	525	892	1787	3446	6180	10197	19373	27974	29833	22339	19710
1981–1985	203	284	566	769	1451	2671	4988	9114	14965	25693	31089	25346	19849
1986–1990	173	293	439	776	1231	2037	3839	7446	13386	20730	30118	28733	23250
1991–1995	167	276	419	721	1264	1810	3083	5695	10485	18043	23873	27804	26691
1996–2000	154	257	409	703	1169	1938	2729	4684	8322	14788	21878	22906	28782
(b) Death rates per million from cerebrovascular disease in men													
1951–1955	28	48	80	151	331	719	1393	2857	5359	9617	16892	25831	36575
1956–1960	29	46	83	157	313	651	1361	2674	5091	9357	16474	26779	36893
1961–1965	30	49	80	154	299	588	1222	2478	4841	8901	15485	25861	41080
1966–1970	27	48	86	155	298	580	1113	2228	4459	8353	14600	23237	42857
1971–1975	27	43	78	145	292	531	1005	1969	4007	7651	13404	22635	38372
1976–1980	25	34	71	126	254	478	862	1678	3401	6515	11746	19080	32253
1981–1985	23	33	64	105	209	391	728	1390	2848	5685	10492	17530	29907
1986–1990	17	33	50	88	172	302	588	1178	2328	4902	9367	16346	27649
1991–1995	16	27	48	83	146	258	475	935	1868	3813	7698	14016	24505
1996–2000	15	23	40	80	135	227	402	764	1513	3136	6123	11604	21461

Table 5.5 Numbers of deaths and death rates from cerebrovascular disease in women in England and Wales during 1951–2000 according to age at death and year of death

Year of death	Age at death (years)												
	25–29	30–34	35–39	40–44	45–49	50–54	55–59	60–64	65–69	70–74	75–79	80–84	85+
(a) Numbers of deaths from cerebrovascular disease in women													
1951–1955	202	388	636	1432	3196	6106	9288	14930	24508	36871	44197	36301	26710
1956–1960	164	344	727	1288	2765	5363	8612	14127	23169	36764	48401	44736	35646
1961–1965	161	331	596	1253	2369	4584	7610	13270	21870	35868	48236	49938	46668
1966–1970	190	313	621	1173	2411	3899	6719	12276	20913	34264	47849	52373	58095
1971–1975	224	321	564	1048	2045	3707	5444	10559	19408	33668	47423	54536	68193
1976–1980	221	304	521	925	1655	2998	5024	8386	16613	30184	44953	51543	67870
1981–1985	195	305	475	764	1309	2157	3963	7476	12885	26355	42915	52989	72304
1986–1990	165	260	431	751	1039	1562	2869	5753	11520	21030	38812	53736	82332
1991–1995	138	247	401	692	1047	1427	2187	4292	8726	17827	29918	48097	86675
1996–2000	153	215	388	643	1035	1578	2104	3473	6567	13994	26409	38423	87403
(b) Death rates per million from cerebrovascular disease in women													
1951–1955	26	47	81	169	386	796	1349	2428	4592	8581	15053	23757	34779
1956–1960	23	44	88	166	332	663	1165	2166	4139	8071	14811	24300	37681
1961–1965	23	46	77	153	309	560	971	1887	3673	7451	13550	24060	40000
1966–1970	25	44	86	153	298	522	848	1646	3225	6634	12684	21803	41714
1971–1975	25	44	81	147	271	468	754	1401	2820	5924	11607	21341	39663
1976–1980	25	35	72	134	236	407	656	1219	2387	4992	9895	18527	35312
1981–1985	23	35	54	107	191	313	555	1024	2023	4273	8672	16429	32539
1986–1990	17	30	50	86	146	232	428	842	1693	3703	7584	14758	30231
1991–1995	13	25	46	80	121	203	333	667	1366	2920	6280	12596	26072
1996–2000	16	21	39	74	120	184	305	547	1082	2426	5115	10711	23466

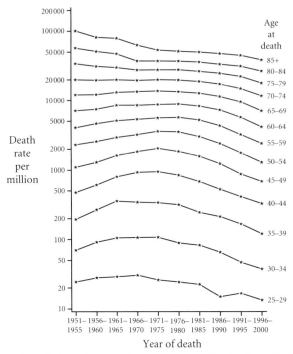

Fig. 5.1 Death rates from ischaemic heart disease in men in England and Wales during 1951–2000 according to age at death and year of death.

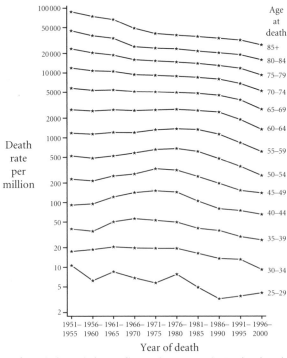

Fig. 5.2 Death rates from ischaemic heart disease in women in England and Wales during 1951–2000 according to age at death and year of death.

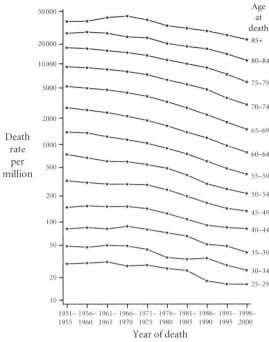

Fig. 5.3 Death rates from cerebrovascular disease in men in England and Wales during 1951–2000 according to age at death and year of death.

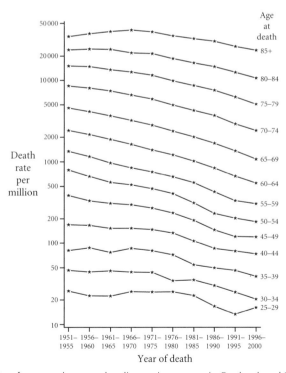

Fig. 5.4 Death rates from cerebrovascular disease in women in England and Wales during 1951–2000 according to age at death and year of death.

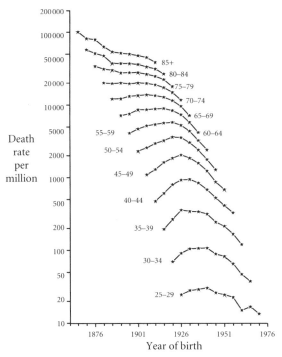

Fig. 5.5 Death rates from ischaemic heart disease in men in England and Wales during 1951–2000 according to age at death and year of birth.

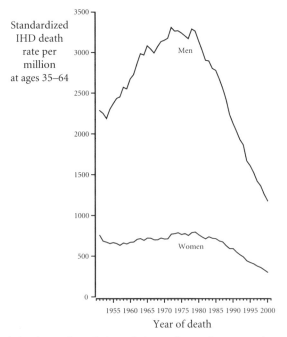

Fig. 5.6 Age-standardized death rate from ischaemic heart disease in men and women aged 35–64 in England and Wales during 1951–2000 according to year of death. Directly standardized according to the European standard population.

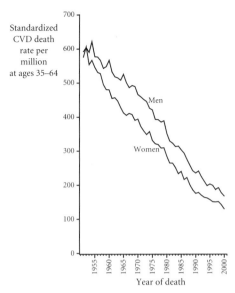

Fig. 5.7 Age-standardized death rate from cerebrovascular disease in men and women aged 35–64 in England and Wales during 1951–2000 according to year of death. Directly standardized according to the European standard population.

ignores the possibility of trends in the rates that are determined by year of birth. For IHD in women the age-standardized rate rose less steeply than for men, climbing from 634 per million in 1957 to 794 in 1979. Thereafter the rate fell year on year to reach 302 per million in 2000 (38% of the peak). For CVD in men, the age-standardized rate fell more or less continuously from a peak of 621 in 1954 to reach 168 in 2000 (27% of maximum). The pattern was almost identical for women, for whom the rates were slightly lower. The equivalent figures were 606 in 1952 dropping to 130 in 2000 (21% of maximum).

5.2.4 **Modelling rates**

5.2.4.1 Strategy

More satisfactory summaries of the rates may be obtained by statistical modelling. We first describe six models that we have used and then summarize the results of their application to IHD and CVD death rates. We analyse deaths separately by gender in the 13 five-year age groups and 10 five-year periods of time used in Tables 5.2–5.5. Each combination of age group and period of death can be linked to one of 22 overlapping periods of birth, referred to as cohorts. For example, those dying at ages 60–64 in 1971–1975 were born in the 1906–1915 cohort. In tables of rates, such as Tables 5.2–5.5, the rates from the same cohort fall on one diagonal.

In age group i and period of death j, let the cohort be k, the number of deaths be $d_{ij(k)}$, and the number of person-years of exposure be $y_{ij(k)}$. From these we derive the age- and period-specific death rate as $r_{ij(k)} = d_{ij(k)}/y_{ij(k)}$. We assume that the number of deaths is a random variable that follows a Poisson distribution[6] and seek simple models in terms of age, period, and cohort effects for the logarithm of the expected number of deaths, $\log(E(d_{ij(k)}))$, that will provide a useful summary of the trends in rates.[7] Models 1, 3, and 4 are standard log-linear models and can therefore be fitted in many standard software packages, while models 2, 5, and 6 are not and so require specific programming.

The goodness of fit of the model is determined by how closely the estimates match the observed rates. The deviances from such models measure goodness of fit, but because large numbers of deaths from IHD and CVD occur in each 5-year age group and period of time, there is a lot of power to detect small, possibly unimportant, departures from the models we use. As an additional diagnostic we measure the amount of 'extra Poisson variation' (φ) that needs to be introduced in order to reduce the χ^2 goodness-of-fit measure to its expected value under pure Poisson variation.[8] If the expected (fitted) number of deaths in a cell of the table is $f_{ij(k)}$, then we estimate the value of φ by setting.

$$\frac{\left(d_{ij(k)} - f_{ij(k)}\right)^2}{f_{ij(k)} \cdot \left(1 + \varphi \cdot f_{ij(k)}\right)}$$

to the number of degrees of freedom (cells minus fitted parameters). As an example to illustrate the impact of 'extra Poisson variation', if φ takes the value 0.001 (cf. IHD in men below), then the standard error associated with a fitted value of 10 000 deaths is inflated from 100 (Poisson error) to 332. Breslow[8] suggests estimating φ for a complicated model and using its value to assess simpler nested models. The less 'extra Poisson variation' and therefore the lower the value of φ, the better the fit of the model. Residuals (observed minus expected rate for each cell of the table) can also be used to assess the model fit. Examination of residuals allows us to distinguish for which specific rates a given model fits poorly.

Model 1: Age–period model

The simplest model we consider is the age–period model, in which

$$\log\left(E\left(d_{ij(k)}\right)\right) = \log\left(y_{ij(k)}\right) + \alpha_i + \beta_j \tag{1}$$

The log $(y_{ij(k)})$ term is declared as an offset. For a unique solution we may fix the sum of the β_j terms to be zero. Their anti-logs, $\exp(\beta_j)$, may be thought of as relative risks for that period of death. The anti-logs of the α_i terms, $\exp(\alpha_i)$, are then analogous to age-specific death rates. Our estimate of the age- and period-specific death rate is the product of $\exp(\alpha_i)$ and $\exp(\beta_j)$.

Informally, each cell of a table of rates (for example, Table 5.2) is approximated by multiplying a number for the column from which it comes (effectively an age-specific rate) with a number for the row from which it comes (effectively a relative risk). The modelling makes the best possible choice of column and row numbers.

Model 2: Lee–Carter model

The age–period model assumes that the same period trend is observed at each age group. This may not be the case, even without allowing for cohort effects. For example, the period effect may be attenuated at older ages. Actuaries have developed a model[9] that specifically allows for this possibility:

$$\log\left(E\left(d_{ij(k)}\right)\right) = \log\left(y_{ij(k)}\right) + \alpha_i + \delta_i \cdot \beta_j \qquad [2]$$

The term δ_i allows the period effect to have different strengths at different ages. There is no unique solution to this model, as we would obtain the same model fit if we replace β_j by $p \cdot \beta_j + q$, α_i by $\alpha_i - q \cdot \delta_i/p$, and δ_i by δ_i/p, for any constants p and q. We do obtain a unique solution by fixing the mean of the β terms to be zero and the mean of the δ terms to be unity. The $\exp(\alpha)$ terms are then of the same magnitude as age-specific rates. The $\exp(\beta)$ terms are the logarithm of relative risks pooled across age groups and the δ terms modify the relative risks that apply to each period.

Informally, there is an age-specific rate for each age group and there is a pattern of relative risks across all 5-year periods of time. Again, their product is used to estimate the rates. The difference from the age–period model is that the extent to which the pattern of relative risks is expressed is allowed to vary according to age group. For example, in young age groups, the relative risks could be 1.1, 1.3, 1.0, 0.7, 0.9, whereas in old age groups the relative risks could be 1.05, 1.15, 1.00, 0.85, 0.95—a weaker expression of the same pattern.

Model 3: Age–cohort model

The simplest model that makes explicit allowance for cohort effects is the age–cohort model:

$$\log\left(E\left(d_{ij(k)}\right)\right) = \log\left(y_{ij(k)}\right) + \alpha_i + \gamma_k \qquad [3]$$

The parameterization, fitting procedure, and interpretation are just as for the age–period model, but cohort effects (γ_k) replace period effects.

Informally, this uses the same idea as the age–period model. The difference is that each rate in the table is estimated as the product of its column (age-specific rate) and diagonal (relative risk for birth cohort).

Model 4: Age–period–cohort model

The classical age–period–cohort model[7] is a natural extension of the age–period model and age–cohort model, allowing both sets of parameters. Thus,

$$\log\left(E\left(d_{ij(k)}\right)\right) = \log\left(y_{ij(k)}\right) + \alpha_i + \beta_j + \gamma_k \qquad [4]$$

We fix the sets of β and γ parameters so that both have zero mean. However, this is not sufficient to define a unique solution. The ambiguity arises through the linear relation, 'time at birth plus age at death equals time at death'. The same fitted rates may be obtained in many ways. A simple example of this is provided by the analysis of a set of rates in which each successive rate is the same fixed percentage of its predecessor at each age group.

Informally, each rate in the table is approximated by multiplying together three terms; one for the column (age-specific rate), one for the row (relative risk for period of death), and one for the diagonal (relative risk for cohort). It turns out that the same best approximation can be achieved with different sets of terms. Interpretation of the estimates is therefore a problem, but interpretation of goodness of fit is not. Hence, comparing the goodness of fit of this model with the simpler models provides evidence of whether both a period and a cohort effect exist.

Model 5: Mixed model

A related model introduced to describe IHD trends in England and Wales for an earlier period[10] is

$$\log\left(E\left(d_{ij(k)}\right)\right) = \log\left(y_{ij(k)}\right) + \alpha_i \cdot \left(\beta_j + \gamma_k\right) \tag{5}$$

By fixing the sets of β and γ parameters so that both have mean 0.5, the $\exp(\alpha)$ terms have the same pattern as age-specific rates. There is no uniqueness problem with this model (cf. Age–period–cohort model above).

Informally, this is a mixture of age–period and age–cohort models. The logarithm of each rate is approximated by multiplying two terms: one representing the age group, the other a sum of terms representing period and cohort.

Model 6: Lee–Carter with cohort

An extension to the Lee–Carter model to allow for the possibility of cohort effects is

$$\log\left(E\left(d_{ij(k)}\right)\right) = \log\left(y_{ij(k)}\right) + \alpha_i + \delta_i \cdot \beta_j + \gamma_k \tag{6}$$

We fix the mean of the γ parameters to be zero, so that the $\exp(\gamma)$ terms are equivalent to relative risks for the cohort. As for the Lee–Carter model we set the mean of the β terms to be zero and the mean of the δ terms to be unity. If all the δ terms were equal to unity, then this model would correspond to the age–period–cohort model and would not have a unique solution.

Informally, this is a simple extension of the Lee–Carter model in which an extra term is allowed to describe variation due to cohort effects.

5.2.4.2 Results

Table 5.6 gives the goodness-of-fit statistics for each of the six models when applied to IHD and CVD death rates in men and women. The smaller the deviance and the smaller the value of φ, the better the model fit.

Ischaemic heart disease in men

The three simpler models all fit poorly. Period of death (model 1) explains more varia-tion than cohort (model 3). There is little gain over either of these models from using the Lee–Carter model. Allowing for variation in both period and cohort variables simultaneously improves the fit. This is especially true if the mixed model is used. The residuals indicate that the age–period–cohort model seriously overestimates the numbers of deaths observed below age 50 in 1951–1955, whilst the mixed model underestimates

Table 5.6 Deviances and measures of extra-Poisson variation for six models for the trend applied to ischaemic heart disease and cerebrovascular disease in men and women

Model for $\log\left(E\left(r_{ij(k)}\right)\right)$		n parameters, degrees of freedom	Ischaemic heart disease				Cerebrovascular disease			
			Men		Women		Men		Women	
			Deviance	φ	Deviance	φ	Deviance	φ	Deviance	φ
1 Age–period	$\alpha_i + \beta_j$	22/108	46454	0.0265	36755	0.0396	8122	0.0084	25467	0.0198
2 Lee–Carter	$\alpha_i + \delta_i\beta_j$	34/96	41628	0.0213	18241	0.0375	1382	0.0018	4119	0.0044
3 Age–cohort	$\alpha_i + \gamma_k$	34/96	61178	0.0463	20708	0.0389	3740	0.0157	2990	0.0163
4 Age–period–cohort	$\alpha_i + \beta_j + \gamma_k$	42/88	9546	0.0103	5445	0.0181	2036	0.0096	2568	0.0199
5 Mixed	$\alpha_i(\beta_j + \gamma_k)$	43/87	3064	0.0118	3466	0.0172	1241	0.0057	1241	0.0045
6 Lee–Carter–cohort	$\alpha_i + \delta_i\beta_j + \gamma_k$	55/75	1064	0.0010	992	0.0031	544	0.0011	507	0.0017

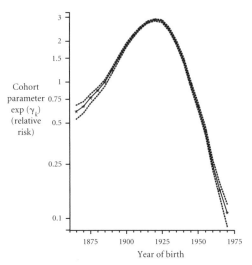

Fig. 5.8 Cohort parameters (γ_k) from the Lee–Carter model with cohort (model 6) applied to death rates from ischaemic heart disease in men in England and Wales during 1951–2000. Dotted lines represent 95% profile likelihood based confidence limits (which do not account for 'extra-Poisson variation').

the reduction in death rates at the two youngest age groups. The Lee–Carter with cohort model (model 6) fits most adequately of all six models. The β and δ parameters are both almost linear across time and age respectively, so their combination generates a linear-by-linear interaction. In the earliest periods this produces the higher fitted values at older ages and smaller ones at younger ages that are seen in Fig. 5.1. Strong cohort effects that rise to a peak between 1916 and 1925 and fall sharply are described by the γ parameters (Fig. 5.8).

Ischaemic heart disease in women

As for men, the three simpler models fit poorly. The best is the Lee–Carter model, suggesting that, again, period models describe the trends more adequately than cohort models. Simultaneous use of period and cohort effects improves the fits. The mixed model again fits better than the age–period–cohort model, but underestimates the reduction in death rates seen in the youngest age groups. There is further improvement in the Lee–Carter with cohort model. The β and δ terms fulfil the same function as in men. The cohort effect differs from that in men initially, in that it first decreases to a minimum at 1885, but then rises to a peak at 1925, similar to the timing in men, before falling sharply (Fig. 5.9). The early cohort parameters are flatter because there is a less distinct rise in rates in the earliest years studied for women than there is for men.

Cerebrovascular disease in men

The Lee–Carter model provides a simple summary of the CVD trends in men and is superior to the age–period and age–cohort models. The β terms that represent the logarithm of relative risks, pooled across age groups, decrease across the period 1951–2000

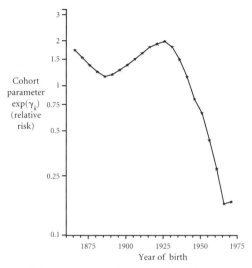

Fig. 5.9 Cohort parameters (γ_k) from the Lee–Carter model with cohort (model 6) applied to death rates from ischaemic heart disease in women in England and Wales during 1951–2000.

(Fig. 5.10(a)). The δ terms, which modify the relative risks that apply to each period (Fig. 5.10(b)), show the largest value at ages 60 to 64 and the smallest values at the youngest and oldest ages. The β terms and four illustrative δ terms are combined and anti-logged in Fig. 5.10(c) to produce age- and period-specific relative risks. The downward trend is much stronger at ages 60 to 64 (high δ) than at ages 35–39 or 75–79 (low δ) confirming that the rates have decreased throughout the period, but least in the youngest and oldest age groups. The largest residuals in this model occur in the 85 plus age group, where the model overestimates the rates during 1951–1960, but underestimates them during 1966–1970 (see also Fig. 5.3). The age–period–cohort model and mixed models have inferior fits. The Lee–Carter with cohort model fits slightly better than the simple Lee–Carter model, because the early cohort parameters can account for the low rates amongst the elderly at the beginning of the period.

Cerebrovascular disease in women

Among the age, period, and cohort models, the age–cohort model fits most adequately. It shows a pattern of reduced risk from the 1880 birth cohort onwards. The Lee–Carter model produces the same pattern of parameters as seen for CVD in men (Fig. 5.10), though the peak δ value occurs earlier at ages 55 to 59, but fits less well than in men. The mixed model shows a better fit. It has almost linear rising period (β) parameters and almost linear falling cohort (δ) parameters (Fig. 5.11). The residuals from this model show that it underestimates the decrease in rates in the youngest two age groups, but overestimates the decrease in rates in the next two age groups. The Lee–Carter model with cohort fits well and shows a pattern similar to that for IHD in men (Fig. 5.8). However, the cohort peak is timed later at 1940 and the rise is steeper than the fall.

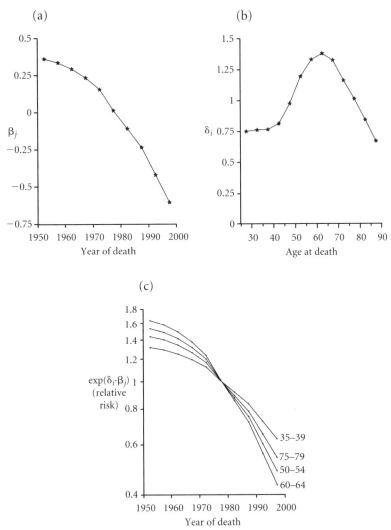

Fig. 5.10 Parameter estimates from the Lee–Carter model (model 2) applied to death rates from cardiovascular disease in men in England and Wales during 1951–2000: (a) shows the β parameter estimates; (b) shows the δ parameter estimates; (c) shows their combination for selected age groups. The combination gives estimates of period-specific relative risk for the given age groups.

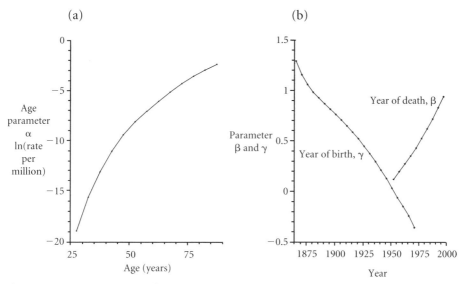

Fig. 5.11 Parameter estimates from the mixed model (model 5) applied to death rates from cardiovascular disease in women in England and Wales during 1951–2000: (a) shows the α parameter estimates; (b) shows the β and γ parameter estimates.

5.3 Trends in ischaemic heart disease and cerebrovascular disease and adult risk factors

5.3.1 Ischaemic heart disease

A clear rise and fall in IHD death rates have occurred among men in England and Wales at each age group during the 50-year study period, with the peak occurring in the 1970s. The rise to a peak was shallower in women than in men, but the subsequent fall has been just as marked in women. Similar patterns have been found in many other western industrialized nations.[1,11] The decline in rates occurred earlier in the USA, Canada, and possibly Switzerland and later in Germany, Ireland, the Netherlands, Northern Ireland, Spain, and Sweden. Countries in eastern Europe were the only ones out of the 27 considered in one study to show an increase in rates during the 1970s and 1980s.[11] In general, rates in these countries increased over the whole time period studied; that is, from around 1960. Among women, the decline in rates generally began earlier than in men and again increases were only seen in the countries of eastern Europe. One important conclusion from these secular trends is that a disease such as IHD, which shows such epidemic behaviour, must have a strong environmental rather than genetic trigger.

Much of the research attempting to explain these trends has been focused either on changes in case fatality due to improvements in the treatment and secondary prevention or on the impact on incidence of the classic adult CHD risk factors such as high blood pressure and high cholesterol levels, which are partly determined through diet, physical inactivity and body weight, and cigarette smoking. In England and Wales, the increasing mortality rates from the 1920s onwards probably reflected increasing incidence of disease rather than increasing case fatality.[5] The World Health Organization (WHO) MONICA (MONItoring trends and determinants of CArdiovascular disease) project found that in countries that experienced the largest increases or decreases in mortality rates during the 1980s, trends in coronary event rates and case fatality rates were both in the same direction.[12] In populations in countries such as England and Wales with declining mortality rates since the 1970s, the study suggests that contributions are partitioned so that two-thirds of the decline is due to falling incidence rates whilst the other third relates to a reduction in case fatality. Studies from the USA have, however, suggested that declines in mortality have been considerably greater than the declines in incidence.[13,14] The WHO MONICA project also estimated the contribution of changes in the adult CHD risk factors, serum cholesterol, blood pressure, cigarette smoking, and relative body weight to the mortality trends in CHD over 10 years from the mid-1980s to mid-1990s and found that around 15% of the CHD variability in women and 40% in men could be attributed to trends in these factors.[15] In general the risk factor trends were downwards in most populations, although increasing cigarette smoking in women in many populations and increasing body mass index do not match the declining mortality trends and present current and future public health concerns.[16] Decreasing cholesterol levels have the largest influence on the decreasing trends.[15] Decreases in intake of animal fat and saturated fat in the UK, USA, and some other industrialized nations[17,18] are likely to have played a role. This decreasing fat intake may also mark other beneficial dietary changes such as increases in fruit and vegetable consumption. In an analysis of the US Framingham Heart Study, the adult risk factors accounted for approximately 50% of the decline in rates between cohorts of 50–59 year olds in 1950 and 1970.[13] Although a considerable amount of any remaining variation in trends may be due to measurement error in the risk factors and the time delay between risk factor change and changes in incidence, as well as medical intervention, these findings suggest that there may be other risk factors that have contributed to the secular decline in mortality rates. The time lag between changes in risk-factor levels and changes in mortality rates is an important and challenging issue. A time lag hypothesis has, for example, been proposed as an explanation of why IHD mortality in France is low, although the major risk factors are very similar to those in the UK—the so-called 'French paradox'.[18] The MONICA study supports the existence of a time lag, but lack of knowledge regarding the distribution of the time lag across individuals in time and the fact that the time lag will vary between risk factors means that modelling the association between risk factor and mortality trends may not properly account for this.

5.3.2 Cerebrovascular disease

Death rates from CVD in men and women, unlike those in IHD, have decreased progressively throughout the 50-year period considered. In an analysis of trends in mortality from stroke between 1968 and 1994 for 51 countries, large variations in mortality rates and mortality trends were observed.[19] Throughout this period the steepest declines were observed in Japan, Australia, France, Switzerland, and the USA (for men and women) and Israel (for women). Among men, only a few countries in eastern Europe showed an increasing trend, such as Poland, Bulgaria, Romania, and the former

Yugoslavia. Mauritius and Mexico also showed increasing rates among the older age groups. Among women, only Poland and Mauritius exhibited increasing trends. As in IHD, separating changes in incidence from changes in case mortality is an issue for CVD. Some studies have failed to show any significant decline in the incidence of stroke.[20,21] An ONS review presents evidence that the decline in death rates in England and Wales is caused both by reductions in incidence and improvements in case fatality.[5]

The 'conundrum of time trends in stroke'[22]—that CVD and IHD trends are so different, despite some common risk factors and pathogenesis—has recently been addressed by Lawlor and colleagues.[23] They attempt to disentangle CVD trends into the component parts: thrombotic and haemorrhagic. They suggest that thrombotic stroke has a similar time trend to IHD and that haemorrhagic stroke, exhibiting a different time trend, must have a different aetiology. However, studies that have attempted to explain the trends in mortality rates in stroke have so far not been able to separate the subtypes. The WHO MONICA project, in an analysis similar to that reported earlier for CHD, estimated that the trend in stroke rates could only partially be explained by the traditional cardiovascular risk factors and, in contrast to CHD, the associations were much stronger in women than men.[24] Decreasing systolic blood pressure, having taken account of a 3–4-year time lag explained most variation (38%) in women. Although some of the declining stroke mortality during the 1970s and 1980s in many countries may be due to anti-hypertensive treatment, it cannot be the full explanation.[25] There is evidence that changes in environmental factors, most probably diet, have contributed more to the control of hypertension.[25,26] Such changes would shift the entire blood pressure distribution of a population rather then simply targeting the group at highest risk. Decreasing salt intake has been suggested as a likely candidate. In Japan, for example, there has been a sharp decrease in dietary salt intake and a corresponding decline in stroke mortality.[27] It has also been suggested that salt might have a direct effect on stroke risk, independent of blood pressure.[28,29] The widening gaps observed in trends between the nations of western and eastern Europe also point to differences in trends for risk factors such as smoking, alcohol consumption, and diet probably playing a primary role. The dramatic economic and political changes in eastern Europe and the former Soviet Union and the apparent immediate impact on life expectancy[30,31] also resulted in a focus of study on current risk factors. Although a life course approach should accommodate the influence of such acute events on health, little attention in the study of east–west differences has so far been given to the possibility that differences in circumstances and conditions in the past may explain some of the differences now observed.[32]

5.4 Are there cohort effects in ischaemic heart disease and cerebrovascular disease?

5.4.1 Ischaemic heart disease

The possibility of an early life effect having influenced mortality trends over time is supported by the fact that in the data from England and Wales the peak has not always been reached at the same time at each age group. The modelling approaches also suggest that, although year of death accounts for the majority of the time trend, there are also important variations associated with year of birth. There was a cohort-related increase in death rates affecting those born around 1920. There are similarly timed cohort effects, with a peak in 1925, but a shallower rise to the peak in women. Similar analysis using data from Norway also indicates a cohort effect as well as a period effect in men, but not women, with the peak occurring in cohorts born just after 1900.[33]

A cohort effect does not necessarily implicate an early life factor as the cohort effect due to cigarette smoking seen in lung cancer indicates (Chapter 12). Lung cancer rates peaked with the 1900 cohort in men, so it seems unlikely that cigarette smoking is the cause of the cohort peak in IHD. The peak in women does coincide with that in lung cancer, though the discordant timing in men makes it unlikely that cigarette smoking is responsible. Recent analysis of data from the USA shows that for both men and women, for cohorts born in the last third of the nineteenth century, as mortality due to influenza and pneumonia associated with the influenza pandemic in 1918–1919 increased so did CHD mortality from 1920 to1985 in the survivors from these cohorts.[34] The authors speculated that this association, together with a negative correlation between excess influenza and pneumonia mortality after 1930 and an early decline in CHD mortality across geographic regions of the USA, provide evidence of an infectious–inflammatory component to the peak in CHD. Such findings need to be reproduced in other populations.

5.4.2 Cerebrovascular disease

According to our analyses, the clearest decline in CVD mortality has been at the central ages studied. At younger and older ages the decreases have been shallower. The central ages, say 45–70, are the ages of greatest numbers of deaths with greatest diagnostic certainty. The observed rates in this age range have fallen by a comparable percentage in each 5-year group at each age group. This is the situation, described in the introduction to the age–period–cohort model, in which it is notoriously difficult to distinguish period and cohort effects as the trends have no turning points. In women, it may be that the preference of some of the models to assign variation to cohort rather than period is accounted for by the rise in rates that can be attributed to the cohorts from 1865 to 1880. This is rather insecure, because these rates were measured in those over age 70 years and their diagnostic accuracy is likely to be lower. Wolfe and Burney,[35] using age–period–cohort modelling of mortality data from 1931 to 1985 from England and Wales, suggested that there was a small, but significant, cohort effect as well as a stronger decreasing period effect. They describe a deceleration away from the previous trend in mortality rates in cohorts born between 1870 and 1910, followed by an acceleration in the trend of mortality rates in cohorts born after 1910, so far until age 65 years. The cohort effect was attributed to increasing survival rates of those with diabetes and CHD, increasing heavy alcohol consumption, and higher numbers of immigrants (who have higher cerebrovascular incidence rates) in these later cohorts and it was suggested that the cohort effect might eventually slow down the overall trends in the decline in stroke mortality. Data from other countries such as the USA[36] and Spain,[37] although without the use of formal statistical modelling, have also raised the possibility of a cohort as well as period effects in the recent decline in stroke mortality. Given the difficulty of distinguishing a cohort from a period effect where rates have fallen continuously over the period of study, these findings should be viewed with some caution.

5.4.3 Can the cohort effects be explained by early life factors?

The 'fetal origins' hypothesis proposes an individual susceptibility related to early growth and development. Birthweight is often the most conveniently available measure of fetal growth, though it is only a crude summary. Low birthweight has been associated with increased risk of both IHD and stroke in prospective observational studies (Chapter 3). A lack of any consistent trend in birthweight in England and Wales[38] suggests that poor fetal growth has had little impact on the mortality trends observed in either IHD or CVD. More recent evidence is accumulating to suggest that the risk associated with such birth characteristics is modified by subsequent growth and development (Chapter 3). This early life susceptibility may be tested in later life when an individual is exposed to 'affluence'. It would therefore be wrong to expect a cohort effect that is characterized simply by the mean birthweight of that generation, as account must also be made of the extent and timing of the later exposure to affluence. Our best prediction may be that rates of IHD will rise as susceptible generations encounter affluence, but then fall as the consequent improvements in growth and development reduce susceptibility. There will be a worst affected generation, but its timing will be determined by a trade-off between the introduction of affluence and the removal of susceptibility. A good example of this might be the high rates of IHD seen in immigrants to the UK from the Indian subcontinent who have been born in relative adversity, but have been exposed to affluent western lifestyle later in life. Further general tests of this idea come from comparisons of trends in social groups or geographical areas that introduce 'affluence' or remove susceptibility at different times. There is evidence that rates of IHD first rose in the socially advantaged, but have now transposed,[5] although this may be, at least to some extent, an artefact of differential classification of cause of death between the social classes over time (Chapter 4). Further the north–south divide in IHD mortality in England may be becoming greater.[39] The 'fetal origins' model for stroke appears to be simpler, although there is less research on this outcome at present (Chapter 3). It does not depend on an 'affluence' exposure, but only on an individual susceptibility acquired early in life.[2] There may still be interactions between early and later life risk factors.

Tall stature has been related to lower risk of both IHD and CVD in many studies (Chapter 3). Tall adult height may reflect early life influences on growth as Cole[40] suggested that the secular increase in adult height reflected secular increases in height in the first 2 years of life. In contrast to birthweight, there have been secular increases in adult height throughout the twentieth century in Europe, North America, and Australia, although most available data are from male conscripts.[38] Adult height showed a consistent increasing trend and does not reflect the increase and subsequent decrease in IHD mortality observed. The UK cohorts of 1870–1910, with a possible decelerating risk of stroke mortality in the analysis by Wolfe and Burney,[35] did show generational increases in growth tempo and final height and striking decreases in child mortality.[38] This may suggest a role for an as yet unidentified early life factor such as improved nutrition and reduced infection.[22] However, height contributed nothing to the explanation of the time trends in the MONICA study.[15]

Early evidence on the childhood origins of adult disease came from ecological studies that correlated infant mortality rates at the time of birth with CHD mortality over 50 years later in the survivors. Areas with high infant mortality showed high rates of later CHD, but the interpretation of such findings varied.[41,42] Infant mortality rates might either represent maternal health, and therefore fetal nutrition, or socioeconomic deprivation. Maheswaran and colleagues[43] identified a cohort effect on stroke mortality within England, which they identified by cross-over in the mortality rates of the two populations (Greater London and the surrounding South-East region) being compared taking place in the same year for all age bands. They concluded, however, that the effect was not explained by past maternal or neonatal mortality rates in the two populations as the same cross-over in trends was not observed. Olalla and colleagues[37] concluded that the cohort effect seen in Spain was not due to early life conditions as the later generations who were born and brought up in better economic conditions did not show sharper decreases than previous cohorts. The decline in infectious diseases over the course of the twentieth century in England and Wales does parallel the decline in stroke mortality,[22] even if we cannot distinguish cohort effects in stroke. Although trends in IHD mortality exhibit more obvious cohort effects than stroke mortality, other ecological evidence suggests that adverse conditions in early life are more important to stroke than to CHD. A study correlating infant mortality at the time of birth and at the time of death with various causes of adult mortality in those aged 65–74 years in 1991–1993 for 27 different countries observed that stroke exhibited strong correlations with both early and later mortality rates, while CHD showed the weakest correlation of any of the diseases considered with infant mortality at birth.[44] The authors also concluded that, given the similar associations seen with stomach cancer, risk of stroke may be influenced by an as yet undetermined infection in childhood that may be similar in epidemiological characteristics to *Helicobacter pylori*. It is possible that early life risk factors are more important for cerebral haemorrhage, which has a different time trend to IHD,[23] than cerebral infarct. Observational studies found stronger associations between birthweight, adult height, and number of siblings, which can indicate material resources in childhood, and cerebral haemorrhage than with cerebral infarct.[45–47]

5.5 **Conclusion**

There is evidence for cohort effects in the mortality trends for IHD in England and Wales. These are weaker than the trends associated with period of death. In relation to CVD, the continuous fall in rates throughout the years studied makes it more difficult to assign variation unambiguously to either period or cohort. Although birthweight is associated with later risk of CHD and CVD in individual-level studies, it does not appear to be a likely candidate for the decreasing trends in both of these diseases seen in recent decades. Increasing growth tempo and attained height may be responsible for some of the decline in both diseases, although it cannot explain the peak observed in IHD. Given that there are many risk factors that influence both IHD and CVD mortality risk and the recent evidence to suggest that the risk associated with birth characteristics is modified by subsequent growth and development, it is perhaps unreasonable to expect any cohort effect simply to be matched by a trend in mean birthweight. In order to assess the impact of multiple risk factors from across the life course and their interactions on time trends requires more complex modelling and the availability of the relevant data.[3] It may be that any cohort effects in CVD have been obscured due to the combination of thrombotic and haemorrhagic stroke and further work on stroke trends will benefit from a separation of these subtypes.

References

Those marked with an asterisk are especially recommended for further reading.

*1 **Beaglehole R.** International trends in coronary heart disease mortality and incidence rates. *J Cardiovasc Risk* 1999;**6**:63–8.

2 **Barker DJP.** *Mothers, babies and health in later life.* Edinburgh: Churchill Livingstone, 1998.

3 **Kuh D, Hardy R.** A life course approach to women's health: linking the past, present, and future. In Kuh D, Hardy R, eds. *A life course approach to women's health.* Oxford: Oxford University Press, 2002:397–412.

4 **Cuzick J, Velez R, Doll R.** International variations and temporal trends in mortality from multiple myeloma. *Int J Cancer* 1983;**32**:13–19.

5 **Charlton J, Murphy M, Khaw K-T, Ebrahim S, Davey Smith G.** Cardiovascular diseases. In Charlton J, Murphy M, eds. *The health of adult Britain: 1841–1994.* London: The Stationery Office, 1997:60–81.

6 **Brillinger DR.** The natural variability of vital rates and associated statistics. *Biometrics* 1986;**42**:693–734.

*7 **Clayton D, Schifflers E.** Models for temporal variation in cancer rates. I Age–period and age–cohort models. II Age–period–cohort models. *Stat Med* 1987;**6**:449–81.

8 **Breslow NE.** Extra-Poisson variation in log-linear models. *Appl Stat* 1984;**33**:38–44.

9 **Lee RD, Carter L.** Modelling and forecasting the time series of U.S. mortality. *J Am Stat Assoc* 1992;**87**:659–71.

*10 **Osmond C.** Coronary heart disease mortality trends in England and Wales, 1952–1991. *J Pub Health Med* 1995;**17**:404–10.

*11 **Thom TJ, Epstein FH.** Heart disease, cancer, and stroke mortality trends and their interrelations. An international perspective. *Circulation* 1994;**90**:574–82.

12 **Tunstall-Pedoe H, Kuulasmaa K, Mahonen M, Tolonen H, Ruokokoski E, Amouyel P.** Contribution of trends in survival and coronary-event rates to changes in coronary heart disease mortality: 10-year results from 37 WHO MONICA Project populations. *Lancet* 1999;**353**:1547–57.

13 **Sytkowski A, D'Agostino RB, Belanger A, Kannel WB.** Sex and time trends in cardiovascular disease incidence and mortality: the Framingham Heart Study, 1950–1989. *Am J Epidemiol* 1996;**143**:338–50.

14 **McGovern PG, Pankow JS, Shahar E, Doliszny KM, Folsom AR, Blackburn H** *et al.* Recent trends in acute coronary heat disease. Mortality, morbidity, medical care, and risk factors. *N Engl J Med* 1996;**334**:884–90.

*15 **Kuulasmaa K, Tunstall-Pedoe H, Dobson A, Fortmann S, Sans S, Tolonen H** *et al.* Estimation of contribution of changes in classic risk factors to trends in coronary-event rates across the WHO MONICA Project populations. *Lancet* 2000;**355**:675–87.

16 **Evans A, Tolonen H, Hense HW, Ferrario M, Sans S, Kuulasmaa K.** Trends in coronary risk factors in the WHO MONICA project. *Int J Epidemiol* 2001;**30**:S35–S40.

17 **Lynch WD, Glass GV, Tran ZV.** Diet, tobacco, alcohol and stress as causes of coronary artery heart disease: an ecological trend analysis of national data. *Yale J Biol Med* 1988;**61**:413–26.

18 **Law M, Wald N.** Why heart disease mortality is low in France: the time lag explanation. *Br Med J* 1999;**318**:1471–80.

*19 **Sarti C, Rastenyte D, Cepaitis Z, Tuomilehto J.** International trends in mortality from stroke, 1968 to 1994. *Stroke* 2000;**31**:1588–601.

20 **Bonita R, Broad JB, Beaglehole R.** Changes in stroke incidence and case fatality in Auckland, New Zealand, 1981–91. *Lancet* 1993;**342**:1470–3.

21 Harmsen P, Tsipogianni A, Wilkelmsen L. Stroke incidence rates were unchanged, while fatality rates declined, during 1971–1987 in Gotenburg, Sweden. *Stroke* 1992;**23**:1410–15.

*22 Gale CR, Martyn CN. The conundrum of time trends in stroke. *J R Soc Med* 1997;**90**:138–43.

23 Lawlor DA, Davey Smith G, Leon DA, Sterne JAC, Ebrahim S. Secular trends in mortality by stroke subtype in the 20th century: a retrospective analysis. *Lancet* 2002;**360**:1818–23.

*24 Tolonen H, Mahonen M, Asplund K, Rastenyte D, Kuulasmaa K, Vanuzzo D *et al.* Do trends in population levels of blood pressure and other cardiovascular risk factors explain trends in stroke event rates? Comparisons of 15 populations in 9 countries within the WHO MONICA stroke project. *Stroke* 2002;**33**:2367–75.

25 Bonita R, Beaglehole R. Increased treatment of hypertension does not explain the decline in stroke mortality in the United States, 1970–1980. *Hypertension* 1989;**13**(**suppl 1**):I169–I173.

26 Kesteloot H, Sasaki S, Xie J, Joossens JV. Secular trends in cerebrovascular mortality. *J Hum Hypertens* 1994;**8**:401–7.

27 Elliott P, Stamler J, Nichols R, Dyer AR, Stamler R, Kesteloot H *et al.* Intersalt revisited: further analyses of 24 hour sodium excretion and blood pressure within and across populations. *Br Med J* 1996;**312**:1249–53.

28 Perry IJ, Beeves DG. Salt intake and stroke, a possible direct effect. *J Hum Hypertens* 1992;**6**:23–5.

29 Antonios TFT, MacGregor GA. Salt—more adverse effects? *Lancet* 1996;**348**:250–1.

30 Chenet L, McKee M, Fulop N, Bojan F, Brand H, Hort A *et al.* Changing life expectancy in Central Europe: is there a single reason? *J Pub Health Med* 1996;**18**:329–36.

31 Leon DA, Chenet L, Shkolmikov VM, Zakharov S, Shapiro J, Vassin S *et al.* Huge variation in Russian mortality rates 1984–1994: artefact or alcohol or what? *Lancet* 1997;**350**:383–8.

32 Leon DA. Common threads: underlying components of inequalities in mortality between and within countries. In Leon DA, Walt G, eds. *Poverty, inequality and health: an international perspective.* Oxford: Oxford University Press, 2001:58–87.

33 Sverre JM. Secular trends in coronary heart disease mortality in Norway, 1966–1986. *Am J Epidemiol* 1993;**137**:301–9.

34 Azambuja MIR, Duncan BB. Similarities in mortality patterns from influenza in the first half of the 20th century and the rise and fall of ischemic heart disease in the United States: a new hypothesis concerning the coronary heart disease epidemic. *Cad Saude Publica, Rio de Janerio* 2002;**18**:557–77.

35 Wolfe CA, Burney PGJ. Is stroke mortality on the decline in England? *Am J Epidemiol* 1992;**136**:558–65.

36 Feinleib M, Ingster L, Rosenberg H, Maurer J, Singh G, Kochanek K. Time trends, cohort effects and geographic patterns in stroke mortality—United States. *AEP* 1993;**3**:458–65.

37 Olalla T, Medrano J, Sierra J, Almazan J. Time trends, cohort effect and spatial distribution of cerebrovascular disease. *Eur J Epidemiol* 1999;**15**:331–9.

*38 Kuh D, dos Santos Silva I, Barrett-Connor E. Disease trends in women living in established market economies: evidence of cohort effects during the epidemiological transition. In Kuh D, Hardy R, eds. *A life course approach to women's health.* Oxford: Oxford University Press, 2002:347–73.

39 Osmond C, Barker DJP. Ischaemic heart disease in England and Wales around the year 2000. *J Epidemiol Commun Health* 1991;**45**:71–2.

40 Cole TJ. Secular trends in growth. *Proc Nutr Soc* 2000;**59**:317–24.

41 Forsdahl A. Are poor living conditions in childhood and adolescence an important risk factor for arteriosclerotic heart disease? *Br J Prev Soc Med* 1977;**31**:91–5.

42 **Barker DJP, Osmond C.** Infant mortality, childhood nutrition, and ischaemic heart disease in England and Wales. *Lancet* 1986;**I**:1077–81.

43 **Maheswaran D, Strachan DP, Elliott P, Shipley MJ.** Trends in stroke mortality in Greater London and south east England—evidence for a cohort effect? *J Epidemiol Commun Health* 1997;**51**:121–6.

44 **Leon DA, Davey Smith G.** Infant mortality, stomach cancer, stroke, and coronary heart disease: ecological analysis. *Br Med J* 2000;**320**:1705–6.

45 **Hypponen E, Leon DA, Kenward MG, Lithell H.** Prenatal growth and risk of occlusive and haemorrhagic stroke in Swedish men and women born 1915–29. *Br Med J* 2001;**323**:1033–4.

46 **Eriksson JG, Forsen T, Tuomilehto J, Osmond C, Barker DJ.** Early growth, adult income, and risk of stroke. *Stroke* 2000;**31**:869–74.

47 **McCarron P, Hart CL, Hole D, Davey Smith G.** The relation between adult height and haemorrhagic and ischaemic stroke in the Renfrew/Paisley study. *J Epidemiol Commun Health* 2001;**55**:404–5.

Chapter 6

Geography and migration with special reference to cardiovascular disease

Jonathan Elford and Yoav Ben-Shlomo

Geographic variations in the risk of coronary heart disease (CHD) have been widely reported. Such variations may be genetic in origin, influenced by factors acting early in life, later in life, or a combination acting throughout the life course. Two epidemiological approaches to investigating geographic variations in disease are considered here—ecological studies and migrant studies. Ecological studies within countries have shown strong associations between past measures of early life conditions as well as current measures of deprivation and cardiovascular disease. Other conventional risk factors showed weak effects or no associations. Current birthweight distribution was also not associated with cardiovascular disease. At an international level, both early life and adult risk factors showed moderate associations, although these were greater for cerebrovascular disease rather than ischaemic heart disease (IHD).

Migrant studies conducted in the Pacific region, Israel, Kenya, and China showed that people moving from a low to high blood pressure community experienced a rise in blood pressure not seen in those who remained behind. This appeared to occur soon after moving and could not be explained by selective migration. For example, Tokelau Islanders (in the Pacific), who migrated to New Zealand experienced a faster annual rise in blood pressure during follow-up than non-migrants, the differential being 1 mm Hg/year for men and 0.4 mm Hg/year for women. Factors acting after migration were clearly of aetiological importance for blood pressure. Studies of mortality among migrants were more evenly divided than blood pressure studies however. While some clearly demonstrated the importance of factors acting later in life, others highlighted the long-term effect of genetic and other early life influences.

Ecological and migrant studies confirm that factors acting throughout the life course, and not simply at one stage, influence the geographic distribution of CHD and its risk factors.

6.1 Introduction

International comparisons of cardiovascular disease death rates reveal striking variations between countries. In 1989, among men aged 35 to 74 years, there was a six-fold difference in age-adjusted CHD mortality between Japan and Scotland. The differentials for women were even greater. While international comparisons of mortality may be hampered by varying practices of death certification, surveys using uniform clinical procedures have confirmed that vital statistics do reflect genuine differences in the risk of CHD between countries. Geographic differences in the risk of CHD may be genetic in origin, influenced by factors acting early in life, later in life, or through an accumulation model acting throughout the life course. This chapter considers two epidemiological approaches to investigating geographic variations in disease—ecological studies and migrant studies.

6.2 Ecological studies

Ecological studies examine the correlation between a potential explanatory variable and disease frequency both within and between countries. The distinction between this and other epidemiological study designs is that the unit of analysis is a group rather than an individual, for example, factories, cities, counties, or nations.[1]

6.2.1 Strengths and weaknesses of ecological studies

In general, ecological studies are regarded as providing fairly weak evidence for the following reasons: (i) explanatory variables are often taken from routinely collected data and may be proxy measures; (ii) the direction of causality between exposure and disease may not be clear; and (iii) interpreting any association between exposure and disease is complicated by the 'ecological fallacy' in that what is observed at a group level may not actually occur at an individual level. For example, areas with greater death rates from cardiovascular disease may also have a greater proportion of smokers. However it may actually be the non-smokers who are dying ('aggregation bias'). In addition exposure at a group level may be confounded by other risk factors ('specification bias').[2] The sum of these two components of bias is called 'cross-level bias' which can make ecological associations appear stronger or weaker than observed at an individual level.[2]

These limitations have led most epidemiologists to restrict ecological analyses to simple exploratory studies indicating '... the presence of effects worthy of further investigation' (p. 74).[1]

The importance of factors that determine disease at an individual level may be different from those at a population level.[3] There are two reasons for this. First, within populations the variation in an exposure may be far less than between populations. This can be illustrated by the weak relationships between sodium intake and blood pressure at an individual level, which are far stronger at a group level.[4] Second, at an individual level the relationship between exposure and outcome may be weaker due to the multi-factorial nature of disease causation. However, between groups these other factors may be more homogeneous and hence the relative importance of a key variable may be accentuated. In addition, some variables may be better characterized at an area level, for example, environmental exposures such as air pollution.[6,7] Similarly there may be cross-level interactions between individual- and area-level variables.[7–9] The advent of new techniques, such as multi-level modelling, has enabled these to be explicitly quantified. As Diez-Roux has highlighted, whilst we are all familiar with the ecological fallacy, we frequently fail to consider the psychologistic and sociologistic fallacies. The former occurs when individual-level data are used to infer causality at an individual level without group-level data. For example, immigrants may report greater levels of depression than non-migrants overall, but this may only be seen in communities where immigrants are the minority. Without appreciating this contextual modification, one may wrongly assume the immigration itself is always associated with depression or this reflects an underlying genetic characteristic.[8] The sociologistic fallacy occurs when group-level inferences are made without taking into account the distribution of individual-level exposures. In this case, areas with a high level of temporary residents are associated with higher levels of suicide. One might argue that this is the result of increased social disorganisation and worse social support structures in areas with a greater proportion of temporary residents. Yet it may be that temporary residents simply have a greater risk of suicide than permanent residents and this is seen equally across all areas regardless of the degree of social disorganisation.[8] These new technical developments in multi-level modelling 'challenge epidemiologists to develop models of disease causation that integrate macro- and micro-level determinants' (p.221).[8]

The failure to confirm an ecological association at the individual level may reflect the limitations of ecological analyses. However the failure to replicate an individual-based study at an ecological level does not negate the causal importance of that variable. Assuming this is not merely a measurement error problem, this either suggests other variables are more important in explaining ecological variations, or that there may be important interactions between different risk factors, which may be more marked at the ecological rather than individual level. For example, a correlation between prevalence of smoking and heart disease mortality would highlight Japan as an outlier as it has a very low rate of heart disease despite having a high rate of smoking.[10] However smoking is still a risk factor for heart disease amongst Japanese people as seen within individual-based studies.[11]

6.2.2 Variations in cardiovascular disease within countries

Geographical variations in disease rates have been noted in England and Wales since the mid-nineteenth century. William Farr reported that life expectancy for boys in Liverpool, inner London, and Surrey were 25, 35, and 44 years respectively (cited in Reference 12). Early attempts at ecological correlations often focused on environmental factors, such as air pollution, water hardness, and elevation above sea level.[13] Studies noted increasing mortality rates for degenerative disease, such as arteriosclerosis, with ecological measures of social deprivation (cited in Reference 14). These studies were to be replicated several decades later using similar but more sophisticated methods.[15–17]

6.2.2.1 Markers of early life influences

Forsdahl postulated that poverty in adolescence followed by later affluence might result in increased mortality from IHD. He noted strong correlations (men 0.79, women 0.61) between infant mortality between 1896 and 1925 and adult mortality from heart disease between 1964 and 1967 for the 19 counties in Norway.[18] This work was replicated for counties in England and Wales by Williams and colleagues, who noted however that correlations with both past and present infant mortality rates were strong, as poor areas in the past remain poorer today.[19] These studies grouped all infant deaths together.

Subsequent work from the Medical Research Council (MRC) unit in Southampton differentiated between neonatal (within first month) and postneonatal (after first month but within first year) mortality. Their results showed that stroke deaths were more strongly correlated with neonatal mortality, that bronchitis, stomach cancer, and rheumatic heart disease were more strongly correlated with postneonatal mortality, and that IHD was strongly correlated with both.[20] An earlier birth cohort analysis from the USA also suggested that infant mortality from diarrhoea and enteritis was a strong predictor of IHD.[21] Subsequent ecological analyses highlighted the relationships between maternal mortality and both stroke and IHD,[22] as well as infant mortality from bronchitis and pneumonia with subsequent adult mortality from chronic obstructive airways disease.[23] Despite the greater specificity of these findings, the authors did not try to control for any other confounding factors.

A later study, which did adjust for contemporary measures of deprivation, revealed that associations between infant mortality and adult mortality were greatly attenuated and most were no longer statistically significant except for bronchitis, emphysema, and asthma.[24] The authors concluded that geographical patterns in mortality could be explained by 'continued deprivation throughout life leading to an accumulation of detrimental health effects' (p.533).[24]

The results of these studies, despite using similar methods and exposures, were interpreted in very different ways. Some favoured an accumulation or interactive model whereby adverse early exposure, as indicated by infant mortality, increased disease risk in combination with social circumstances in later life. Forsdahl speculated on the possible role of 'programming' as he stated 'some form of permanent damage caused by a nutritional deficit may be involved' (p.95).[18] However he also believed that adverse disease outcome was dependent on later life affluence: '... our present way of life, with its high fat consumption, tends to increase serum cholesterol more in persons who have grown up in poor families than in those who have not experienced poverty' (p.95).[18] However, the concept of 'programming' was developed to a much greater extent by the MRC Southampton group.

An international analysis of past (1921–1923) and current (1991–1993) infant mortality with a variety of causes of adult mortality for 27 countries provides further informative clues as to the potential timing and importance of life course exposures.[25] Strong correlations were observed with past infant mortality and all-cause mortality, respiratory tuberculosis, stomach cancer, and stroke. Weak associations were apparent for IHD. Adjustment for current infant mortality attenuated the association with all-cause mortality but hardly altered the association with respiratory tuberculosis or stomach cancer. The association with stroke was more modestly attenuated. As respiratory tuberculosis and probably stomach cancer are due to an exposure with an infection in childhood, by analogy, this suggests that some of the risk for stroke is determined in early life, possibly with an undetermined infective agent.[25] A similar approach has also been used to examine the ecological association between cause-specific mortality and a measure of overcrowding, though the latter exposure was measured from contemporary rather than historical data as it should have been.[26] As one might have expected, overcrowding was positively associated with both acute respiratory infections and stomach cancer. In addition, mortality from IHD was also associated with overcrowding, suggesting a possible role of chronic infection.

6.2.2.2 Height: an indicator of childhood conditions?

Height is a measure that indicates both genetic and environmental factors acting from the perinatal period into early adulthood. Using data from the three UK birth cohorts, it is possible to rank counties in England and Wales into five groups based on the mean heights of their inhabitants. A clear trend is seen for both men and women, with taller counties having lower mortality rates from IHD, stroke, and bronchitis, but higher rates of cancers of the breast, ovary, and prostate.[27] Similarly an analysis based on the 1970 and 1946 birth cohorts related measures on maternal and child factors to geographical variations in adult cardiovascular disease.[28] Both maternal and child height showed strong inverse relationships with mortality, whilst mean birthweight showed no consistent pattern. This suggested that postnatal rather than prenatal factors may be more relevant in explaining the geographical variations. The geographic relationship between height and mortality may, however, be confounded by social class. 'Tall' counties, which tend to be in the south of England, may contain proportionately more people in high socioeconomic groups with lower mortality than 'short' counties, which tend to be in the north.

More direct evidence on the importance of height and hence childhood growth, independent of birthweight, comes from the Ten Towns study. Children from high-mortality towns were shorter, had a higher ponderal index, and higher blood pressure, although no differences were noted in cholesterol or post-load glucose measurements.[29] These differences persisted after adjustment for birthweight.

6.2.2.3 Urban and rural differences

Differences in mortality rates between urban and rural areas have been noted in several different countries (reviewed in Reference 30). Standardized mortality ratios for CHD in England (1950–1952)[31] showed lower mortality rates for rural districts than either county boroughs or urban districts, unrelated to the proportion of men in social classes I and II. This rural advantage has been seen in more contemporary data as well. Conventional risk factors appear inadequate to explain these observations as modelling differences in smoking, blood pressure, and cholesterol fail to account for the lower mortality rates.[32] The detrimental effects of urbanization have been proposed but this evidence is based on communities undergoing a transitional phase rather than on stable communities.[33] One possible explanation is that rural areas provide more favourable conditions for early life. Infant mortality rates in 1925 for England show a linear decline from 87 per 1000 births for county boroughs to 72 per 1000 births for other urban districts and 64 per 1000 births for rural districts. Similarly, standardized height ratios measured on school children between 1908 and 1910 show the opposite gradient with rural children being taller than their urban counterparts (manufacturing towns 97.9, urban county councils 100.5, rural county councils 102.4).[34] A recent report demonstrated that differences in birthweight and child height still persist today and appear to be independent of socioeconomic status.[35] Temporal data from the USA[36] and Norway[37] demonstrate that the rural advantage for IHD is rapidly disappearing. It is unclear whether these observations are more consistent with alterations in adult rather than early life factors.

6.2.2.4 Adult risk factors and early life measures

Data from the 1993 *Health Survey for England*[38] enables one to examine the geographical relationship across regional health authorities in England between the more important

Table 6.1 The relationship between cardiovascular risk factors and prevalent ischaemic heart disease or stroke in 14 English Regional Health Authorities

	Male ischaemic heart disease or stroke	Female ischaemic heart disease or stroke
Smoking 20+ cigarettes per day*	0.55†	0.28
Mean body mass index	0.23	0.13
High blood pressure	0.12	0.03
Fibrinogen*	0.02	0.28
Mean cholesterol	−0.03	0.41
Birthweight in 1986	−0.26	−0.01
Infant mortality rate (1925)	0.78†	0.53†
Townsend deprivation score	0.65†	0.51

Data taken from 1993 Health Survey for England, 1981 Census, Registrar's General Statistical Review of England and Wales 1925, and unpublished birth statistics (VS2) 1985, kindly provided by the Office of National Statistics.

*indicates a standardized ratio measure was used.

†$P<0.05$.

adult cardiovascular risk factors, two proxy measures of early life influences (infant mortality in 1925 and birthweight for 1985), current socioeconomic deprivation (Townsend Index), and prevalent IHD or stroke (see Table 6.1). Ideally data on birthweight from an earlier period would be used but is not available.

Infant mortality in 1925 showed the strongest relationships with both male and female IHD or stroke, closely followed by current socioeconomic deprivation. These results reflect the relative importance of factors acting both in early and later life. Conventional risk factors such as smoking and body mass index (BMI) showed moderate to weak associations, with cholesterol and fibrinogen showing no association or an inverse association in men and weak to moderate associations for women. The poor ability of cholesterol to predict geographical variations in IHD mortality has been noted in the British Regional Heart Study.[39] Birthweight, measured in 1986, surprisingly had a negative correlation and did not show the same pattern as infant mortality rates (see Fig. 6.1), similar to a previous birth cohort analysis.[28] This may either reflect a problem with using mean birthweight, unadjusted for gestational age, or because current birthweight should be compared with future regional mortality rather than current rates. Alternatively, low birthweight today may reflect different factors than those operating at the beginning of the century, which resulted in high rates of infant mortality. If this is the case, then the low birthweight–IHD relationship may well differ over time for future cohorts.

6.2.3 Variations in cardiovascular disease between countries

The Seven Countries study was one of the earliest international studies that demonstrated a strong correlation (0.84) between percentage of dietary energy from saturated fatty acids and mortality from CHD.[40] The ratio of monounsaturates to saturated dietary fat, age, BMI, systolic blood pressure, serum cholesterol, and cigarette

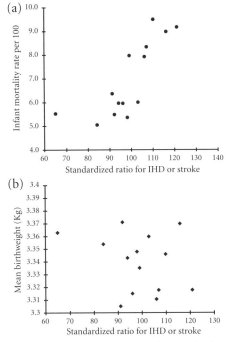

Fig. 6.1 Scatterplot showing the association between the standardized prevalence ratio for IHD or stroke and (a) infant mortality rates in 1925 and (b) mean birthweight for English Regional Health Authorities.

consumption explained 96% of the variance between countries.[41] Estimates of the strength of the relationship between cholesterol and IHD mortality suggest that a difference of 0.6 mmol/l (about 10% of the average value in Western countries) is associated with an average difference of 37% in IHD mortality in 55–64 year olds.[42] A more detailed analysis based on 27 countries and examining lipid sub-fractions noted correlations of 0.67, −0.57, and 0.74 for serum cholesterol, HDL cholesterol, and serum cholesterol:HDL cholesterol ratio respectively.[43] Analyses have failed to demonstrate an independent effect of alcohol, fish, fibre, and antioxidant vitamin intake after adjustment for saturated fatty acids.[44]

The large international MONICA (MONItoring trends and determinants of CArdiovascular disease) study obtained standardized data on 39 centres from 26 countries.[45] Using cross-sectional data on risk factors and routine mortality, it found much weaker associations between conventional risk factors and IHD with only 25% of the variance explained by smoking, blood pressure, and total cholesterol. However these studies fail to include a temporal perspective so that there is no time lag between measurement of exposure and disease outcome.

We have undertaken a further analysis using the MONICA data but also including data on infant mortality rates (1932) for selected countries, which is shown in Table 6.2. Because China is an extreme outlier, results have been presented both including and excluding it. Smoking shows no significant association with IHD but a strong

Table 6.2 The relationship between all-cause and cardiovascular disease by several risk factors for 19 countries involved in the MONICA World Health Organization project

	Males			Females		
	Cardiovascular disease	Ischaemic heart disease	Stroke	Cardiovascular disease	Ischaemic heart disease	Stroke
Smoking (%)	0.21	−0.05	0.62*	−0.06	−0.01	−0.10
	0.39†	0.10	0.61*	−0.05	−0.03	−0.06
Hypertension (%)	0.44	0.19	0.59*	0.56*	0.40	0.47*
	0.44	0.19	0.61*	0.60*	0.39	0.53*
Raised cholesterol (%)	0.08	0.14	−0.25	−0.19	0.10	−0.32
	−0.10	−0.03	−0.18	−0.10	0.05	−0.18
Infant mortality rate, 1932 (15 countries)	0.17	−0.10	0.66*	0.40	0.15	0.38
	0.32	0.01	0.60*	0.31	0.17	0.27

MONICA, MONItoring trends and determinants of CArdiovascular disease.

*P<0.05.

†Second row shows correlation coefficients excluding China.

association with stroke for men. Raised cholesterol, as noted in the previous MONICA publication, surprisingly shows no significant associations.[45] Another analysis using 18 countries from the MONICA project found that smoking and elevated blood pressure explained 21% of the variation in stroke incidence in men and 42% in women, leaving the authors to conclude that other unmeasured variables were also of considerable importance.[46] Infant mortality shows moderately strong correlations with cardiovascular disease, similar in magnitude to hypertension. However these associations mask a strongly positive correlation with stroke mortality and a weak or negative correlation with IHD, in marked contrast to the pattern seen within countries. This suggests that any perinatal influences may play a greater role for cerebrovascular disease rather than IHD. Individual-level analyses from the WHO MONICA project examining trends in risk factors with trends in coronary events show only modest associations, with smoking (0.22) and BMI (−0.23) having the strongest associations.[47]

6.2.4 Going beyond cross-sectional associations

Most ecological studies report associations between present and past exposure with disease outcome. Because many of these area-level exposures will be confounded with other variables, it is hard to determine causal associations despite multi-variable analysis. One approach that may disentangle such confounding is to examine temporal trends either within or between countries where there are marked period or cohort effects that may or may not be consistent with temporal changes in risk factors (see Chapters 5 and 12). This approach has been most elegantly demonstrated with the marked period effect for changes in life expectancy seen in Russia between 1994 and 1998 where declines in life expectancy dramatically reversed.[48] Cause-specific analyses strongly suggested the importance of changes in alcohol consumption.

Whilst IHD and stroke mortality rates show very high correlations across local authority districts in England and Wales ($r=0.72$ for men, $r=0.94$ for women),[49] their descriptive epidemiology suggest some marked differences. Age-standardized IHD mortality rates rose from the 1920s peaking around the 1970s and then declined whilst stroke rates showed a slow progressive decline from the beginning of the twentieth century (see Reference 49 for a detailed review). In addition, there are marked differences in the sex ratios for these two diseases over time. Ischaemic heart disease showed a marked period effect with the ratio of male to female mortality dramatically increasing in the immediate post-war period from a previous ratio of 1.5 to a peak of 3.5 in 1972. In contrast stroke ratios remained around unity over the same time period.[50]

A recent speculative hypothesis has been that the rise and fall of the IHD epidemic was the result of the influenza infection.[51] Most deaths from the influenza pandemic were thought to be due not to the viral infection *per se* but rather the immune inflammatory response. It is possible that exposed survivors were therefore 'primed' to be predisposed for future IHD. Birth cohort plots of death rates from influenza and pneumonia (1918–1919) and standardized IHD mortality rates show marked similarity, though the rise in IHD rates preceded the influenza epidemic. Within the USA, the decline in IHD mortality rates showed a marked correlation ($r=-0.68$, $P=0.04$) with the persistence of excess influenza and pneumonia mortality after 1930. This correlation could also be explained by variations in area deprivation, which the authors failed to examine.

Whilst concordance of risk factors with disease trends is appealing, it is less convincing than discordance. An analysis of time trends for IHD mortality in Poland showed a turning point in rates with marked dramatic declines (26%) in IHD rates around 1994 despite constant rates for influenza and lung cancer.[52] Patterns of risk factors also remained relatively constant except for an acute switch between animal and vegetable fats and a doubling of citrus fruit consumption. Such an acute effect could not be mediated directly through atherosclerosis but may reflect changes in coagulability. No data were presented on early life factors such as maternal or infant mortality from the corresponding historical time period as was undertaken by Maheswaran and colleagues.[53] They compared period and cohort plots of stroke mortality for Greater London and South East England between 1951 and 1991. Whilst both areas showed marked declines, the rates of decline varied so that south-east England, which had previously higher rates in the earlier time period, had lower rates in the later period. These patterns were not consistent with a period effect but a marked cohort effect with the cross-over point emerging for birth cohorts around 1916–1921. This was not consistent with either patterns of maternal or neonatal mortality. Childhood influences however cannot be excluded as data on height patterns between these two areas may be consistent with this apparent cross-over.[54]

Further ecological studies that exploit natural experiments or discordance in patterns across time and place provide a more robust test of the role of early and later life influences. It is important that such studies do not solely focus on an either/or model but consider the accumulative or interactive influences of factors across the life course.

6.3 Migrant studies

Migration provides a naturally occurring experiment, which may establish the aetiological importance of factors acting at different points in the life course. If the risk of

CHD among people migrating from a low incidence to a high incidence country increases with time it is highly probable that factors acting later in life, following migration, are of aetiological importance. On the other hand, if migrants retain the risk of their country of origin, then it is likely that genetic characteristics or factors operating early in life exert a greater influence than exposures later on.

Migration also provides the opportunity to test Forsdahl's hypothesis that poverty in early life followed by later affluence increases the risk of CHD.[18] According to this hypothesis, migrants who encounter prosperity in adult life, having experienced relative deprivation during childhood, should face an even *greater* risk of CHD than long-term residents of the country they migrate to.

One of the major methodological challenges presented by these studies is that migration may be selective. Migrants may differ from non-migrants and so may not be representative of the population they left.

For the first edition of this book, the most comprehensive migrant studies available for review were those that examined changes in *blood pressure* on migration rather than CHD incidence or mortality. Blood pressure studies among migrants from the Tokelau Islands or Ethiopia and among the Yi in China or Luo in Kenya were particularly important. These studies remain in the second edition. However, since the publication of the first edition, a number of studies have emerged examining *mortality* among migrants. These are now included in the chapter

6.4 Migration and blood pressure

6.4.1 Tokelau Island Migrant Study

Tokelau, a former New Zealand dependency, comprises three small atolls in the south Pacific. Following a hurricane in 1966, many Tokelauauns migrated to New Zealand. The migration of Tokelauauns from their traditional life on the atoll to urban life in New Zealand provided the opportunity to study the effects of migration on their health.

The strength of the Tokelau Island Migrant Study lay in its ability to collect detailed information on Tokelauans prior to, as well as after, migration enabling the authors to investigate any selection effects among migrants.[55,56] A number of papers examined changes in blood pressure associated with migration.[57–61] Some were longitudinal in nature, initially examining people in Tokelau and then re-examining them several years later either in New Zealand (migrants) or in Tokelau (non-migrants).[57–59] Other studies were cross-sectional in nature, comparing Tokelauans who had migrated with those who had not at the same point in time.[60,61]

6.4.1.1 Longitudinal studies—children

In 1971, of all 518 children aged 5 to14 years resident in Tokelau, 502 (97%) were examined. Follow-up examinations of 456 (91%) of these children were conducted 5 years later in New Zealand (121 migrants) and Tokelau (335 non-migrants). At baseline, in 1971, there were no significant differences between non-migrants and migrants in mean systolic or diastolic blood pressure, weight, height, or BMI.

At follow-up examination, mean systolic and diastolic blood pressures were higher in male migrants than in non-migrants, significantly so at ages 5–9 years. Adjusted for age at follow-up, the difference between migrants and non-migrants aged 5–9 years was

6.4 mm Hg for systolic and 10.0 mm Hg for diastolic blood pressure ($P<0.01$). For girls, younger migrants (5–9 years) had higher mean blood pressure than non-migrants although this difference was only significant for diastolic pressure (62.4 versus 54.0, adjusted for age, $P<0.01$). For the older girls, however, the situation was reversed, with non-migrants having a higher mean blood pressure than migrants although this difference was significant only for systolic pressure.[57] The authors suggested that psychosocial factors may have contributed to the different blood pressure patterns among male and female migrants. In particular, anthropologists had observed that the behaviour of non-migrant girls (but not boys) living in Tokelau was particularly constrained by family and social pressures.

6.4.1.2 Longitudinal studies—adults

Of 1018 adults aged 15–69 years who were examined in Tokelau between 1968 and 1971, 812 were re-examined approximately 5 years later (1975–1977) in New Zealand (280 migrants) or Tokelau (532 non-migrants). At baseline, there were no systematic significant differences between migrants and non-migrants in blood pressure or BMI. On re-examination, blood pressures among male migrants had risen by an average of 10 mm Hg systolic and 7 mm Hg diastolic during follow-up. It was found that after adjusting for baseline age, BMI, blood pressure, and rate of change of BMI, the blood pressure of migrants had risen faster than that of non-migrants—by a factor of about 1 mm Hg a year for males ($P<0.001$) and 0.4 mm Hg/year for females (systolic $P=0.054$; diastolic $P=0.02$).[59] No information was available on corresponding increases in blood pressure among long-term New Zealand migrants.

The authors commented that the lack of systematic differences between migrants and non-migrants at the premigration survey ruled out measurable selection bias in these analyses.

6.4.1.3 Cross-sectional studies

In a study conducted in the mid-1970s, 856 Tokelauan children living in New Zealand had significantly higher mean systolic blood pressure than 571 children still living in Tokelau (non-migrants), even after adjusting for height and weight ($P<0.001$).[60] A mean difference in blood pressure of 6.0 mm Hg was recorded. Similarly, the prevalence of hypertension was higher among 1181 Tokelauan adults examined in New Zealand than among 807 still in Tokelau (non-migrants) (definite hypertension, males 9.4% versus 2.6%, females 10.3% versus 7.6% respectively).[61] It was thought unlikely that the findings of these cross-sectional studies, which were consistent with the longitudinal studies, were the result of non-response, biased assessment, or selection.

6.4.2 Yi Migrant Study—China

The Yi people are an ethnic minority who live principally in remote mountainous areas in south-west China. Isolated from the outside world they have preserved their own language and traditional lifestyle. Since the 1950s, Yi farmers have migrated to Xichang City and urban 'county seats' within the prefecture. The traditional residents of these urban areas are Han people, the majority ethnic group in China. A survey conducted in 1979–1980 (and only published in Chinese) found that among Yi people still living in mountain areas, blood pressure was low and did not increase with age during adult-hood and that hypertension, CHD, and stroke were extremely rare.[62] Two large-scale surveys have subsequently been conducted among Yi farmers (non-migrants), Yi migrants, and Han residents, the first in 1986–1988,[62] the second in 1989.[63] Both were cross-sectional in design. The main aims were to compare blood pressure patterns (1) among the same ethnic group living in different environments and (2) among different ethnic groups living in the same environment.

6.4.2.1 The 1986–1988 survey

Between 1986 and 1988 a survey was undertaken among more than 6000 men and women (overall response exceeded 80%), comparing 2327 Yi farmers living in high-mountain areas and 2631 Yi farmers living in mountainside areas (mean age of both groups 30 years) with 517 Yi migrants and 1143 Han residents in Puge county seat (mean age of both groups 34 years).

For men, mean systolic blood pressure was similar for Yi migrants and Han residents (107.3 and 108.3 mm Hg) but significantly lower ($P < 0.01$) among Yi farmers (101.8 and 100.8 for high-mountain and mountainside farmers respectively). A similar pat-tern was seen for diastolic pressure ($P < 0.001$). The differential was reduced, but nonetheless persisted after adjusting for age and BMI (Yi migrants and Han residents were older and had higher BMI than non-migrants). For women, after adjusting for age, BMI, and altitude, diastolic but not systolic blood pressure was lower among Yi farmers than in migrants and Han residents. The prevalence of hypertension was higher among Yi migrants and Han residents than among non-migrant farmers. Mean blood pressure rose very little with age after puberty among Yi farmers, but there was a trend of increasing blood pressure with age in Yi migrants and Han residents.[62]

6.4.2.2 The 1989 survey

Of 16 301 men and women aged 15–89 years eligible for the 1989 study, 14 505 (89%) were examined—8241 Yi farmers living in remote mountain villages (mean age 31 years), 2575 Yi migrants, and 3689 Han people living in urban county seats (mean age 34 and 35 years respectively). Median length of residence in the county seats by Yi migrants was 10 years.

Although blood pressure rose significantly with age in all three groups, the rate of increase was lowest in Yi farmers (systolic 0.13 mm Hg/year men, 0.06 women) and highest in Yi migrants (systolic 0.33 mm Hg/year men, 0.37 women) and Han people (systolic 0.36 mm Hg/year men, 0.56 women) ($P < 0.01$). After adjusting for BMI the differences remained significant except for diastolic pressure in women. The age-adjusted prevalence of definite hypertension (systolic ≥ 160 mm Hg and/or diastolic ≥ 95 mm Hg) in men was higher among Yi migrants and Han people (4–5%) than in Yi farmers (<1%). A similar pattern was seen in women. The differentials were slightly reduced after adjusting for age, BMI, heart rate, alcohol use, and smoking but still remained statistically significant ($P < 0.05$).[63,64] While blood pressure levels rose steadily with alcohol consumption in all three groups, Yi farmers consistently had lower blood pressure than Yi migrants and Han people at all daily alcohol intake levels.[65]

Although the ethnic background of Yi migrants was similar to that of the Yi farmers, their mean blood pressure levels, rate of increase of blood pressure with age, and prevalence of hypertension closely resembled the Han people. Differences between Yi migrants and farmers in blood pressure could only be partially explained by age, BMI, heart rate, smoking, and alcohol use. Compared with Yi farmers, however, Yi migrants ate more sodium, fat, and cholesterol and less potassium, calcium, and magnesium. In fact their diet was similar to that of the Han people. Thus dietary changes appear to have contributed to the development of raised blood pressure in Yi migrants.

6.4.3 Ethiopian migrants to Israel

Living in remote rural areas, only a relatively small number of Ethiopian Jews emigrated to Israel in the 1970s and 1980s. However, during a dramatic airlift in 1984–1985, known as Operation Moses, more than 6500 Ethiopian Jews were airlifted to Israel from Sudanese refugee camps having left Ethiopia during a drought.[66] The migration from rural villages in Ethiopia to urban areas in Israel provided the opportunity to examine changes in blood pressure among Ethiopians by duration of residence in Israel and to compare their blood pressure levels with those of long-term Israeli residents.[67–73]

6.4.3.1 Longitudinal studies

In 1984, blood pressure was measured in 483 Ethiopians aged 5 years and above a few weeks after their arrival in Israel (Operation Moses). One year later, blood pressure was measured again in 265 of these people. Mean blood pressure at baseline among those who were re-examined and those who were not was similar for all but one age group. Average diastolic blood pressure increased by about 4 mm Hg in those who were re-examined, a differential which remained after adjusting for age and weight change over the year. Systolic pressures, however, changed only slightly over the year.[67]

Of 87 Ethiopian immigrants in their early 20s who were examined within 3 months of their arrival in Israel, in a residential agricultural college, 53 were still living in the college 2 years later. Most of those lost to follow-up had been drafted for regular army service but they were not significantly different at baseline from those who were available for re-examination. Among the 53 immigrants, there was a significant rise in blood pressure over the 2-year period ($P < 0.01$). Mean systolic pressure increased from 118 to 129 mm Hg and diastolic from 62 to 71 mm Hg. Eleven of the 53 people (21%) were found to be hypertensive at 2 years; none were at baseline. Mean BMI did not change during follow-up. The authors thought it unlikely that alcohol consumption had increased during the 2 years, due to its lack of ready availability at the schools, but salt intake could have increased.[68]

6.4.3.2 Cross-sectional studies

Ethiopian immigrants who had recently arrived in Israel had lower mean blood pressure than those who had lived there for 2–3 years.[69–72] For example, mean blood pressure among new Ethiopian immigrants in their early 20s living in a residential college (n = 87) was 118.6 mm Hg compared with 125.7 mm Hg in immigrants (n = 63) who had been there at least 2 years.[72] Conversely, Ethiopians who had lived in Israel for 4 years had a blood pressure distribution similar to 'veteran' Israeli people of the same age.[73] This suggested to the authors that Ethiopian immigrants to Israel developed the blood pressure patterns of the society to which they migrated. The cross-sectional studies were not as methodologically robust as the longitudinal investigations. Nonetheless, all the studies reported an increase in blood pressure among Ethiopians associated with duration of residence in Israel.

6.4.4 Luo migrants—Kenya

The Luo tribe live in a rural area to the north of Lake Victoria in western Kenya. Seeking work, a number of Luo people have migrated to Nairobi. The migration of Luo people from a rural to an urban area provided the opportunity to examine blood pressure in migrants before and after they moved, by duration of residence in Nairobi and to compare their blood pressure with non-migrants who remained in the rural areas.[74–77]

6.4.4.1 Longitudinal studies

One-hundred Luo migrants to Nairobi (90 men, 10 women, mean age 21 years) were traced who had already been examined on average 10 months earlier, prior to migration. Among the 90 men, mean systolic blood pressure increased from 120.9 mm Hg before migration to 127.2 mm Hg after migration (diastolic 59.0–65.3) ($P < 0.01$). Mean body weight and mean sodium/potassium ratio also increased. Pre-migration mean blood pressures among the migrants, however, were almost identical to those seen in age-matched rural non-migrants who were examined at the same time. Mean body weights were also similar. The authors concluded that while selective migration was a theoretical and sometimes real cause for concern in the interpretation of migrant studies, it did not appear to play an important role in the Kenya Luo migrant study.[74]

Between 1981 and 1985 rural non-migrants and urban migrants aged 15–34 years were recruited for an investigation of changes in blood pressure over time. Migrants (n=63) were examined shortly after migration and then 3, 6, 12, 18, and 24 months later. Age–sex-matched non-migrants (n=143) were examined at the same time periods. Mean systolic blood pressure was significantly higher in migrants than in non-migrants throughout the study ($P < 0.02$). Mean diastolic pressures were also elevated among migrants, although not always significantly. The distributions of both systolic and diastolic blood pressures for migrants were shifted to the right of non-migrants. Selective migration was not a factor because blood pressure measurements in male migrants prior to migration were not significantly different from rural non-migrants. The authors concluded that differences in blood pressure between rural and urban groups were apparent, on average, 1 month after migration.[75]

6.4.4.2 Cross-sectional studies

In a 1980 study, the rate of increase of blood pressure with age was greater among 310 migrants aged 20 years and over living in Nairobi than among 861 rural non-migrants (men 0.56 mm Hg/year compared with 0.14 mm Hg/year, $P < 0.001$). Mean blood pressures were similar in migrant and non-migrants until the age of 35 years but above that age were consistently higher among migrants. After age adjustment, systolic, but not diastolic blood pressure was significantly correlated with duration of urban residence.[76]

6.4.5 Migrants within the UK

For the British Regional Heart Study, approximately 300 men aged 40–59 years were recruited between 1978 and 1980 from one general practice in each of 24 towns throughout England, Scotland, and Wales (7735 participants in all). Overall, mean blood pressure was higher in the north of England and Scotland than in the south. For example, systolic and diastolic blood pressures in Guildford (south of England) were 135.9 and 77.6 mm Hg respectively compared with 152.4 and 88.5 mm Hg in Dunfermline (Scotland).[77]

The men were divided into two groups: non-migrants who were born in the town where they were examined for the study (n = 3144) and migrants who were born elsewhere in the UK (n = 4147). Regardless of where they were born, men living in the south of England had lower mean blood pressures than men living in the north of England or Scotland. Furthermore, men born in the south who moved to Scotland had higher mean blood pressure levels than those who stayed in the south (systolic 156.7 compared with 141.7 mm Hg, diastolic 88.5 compared with 79.9 mm Hg). Equally, men born in Scotland who moved south had lower mean blood pressure than those who stayed put (systolic 143.1 compared with 147.7 mm Hg, diastolic 80.1 compared with 84.9 mm Hg).[78] Yet according to Forsdahl,[18] migrants from Scotland to the south of England should have experienced an increased risk of CHD (that is, raised blood pressure) because they had lived in a relatively deprived area as children and then moved to a relatively prosperous region later in life.

Clearly, geographic variations in blood pressure were strongly influenced by where the men had lived for most of their adult lives rather than by where they were born and brought up. It was thought unlikely that selective migration could account for these findings.[79] The authors concluded that regional differences in blood pressure in the UK were more closely linked to factors acting in adult life rather than those present early in life.

6.5 Migration and mortality

6.5.1 Migration within the UK

A study based on a 1% sample of residents living in England and Wales provided the opportunity of investigating whether geographic variations in mortality from IHD and stroke were influenced by factors acting early or later in life.[80] All participants were born before 1939 and were enumerated in the 1971 census. The authors compared the relative influence of area of residence in 1971 and 1939 on mortality from IHD (n = 18 221 deaths) and stroke (n = 9899 deaths). They found that the north–south gradient in mortality from IHD and stroke was related significantly ($P < 0.05$) to both the 1939 and 1971 area of residence. They concluded that geographic variations in mortality from cardiovascular disease in the UK may therefore be partly determined by genetic or early life factors, although the risk of fatal IHD or stroke appeared to change on migration between areas of high and low mortality. In other words, cardiovascular mortality was related equally to factors acting both early and later during the life course.

A study by Elford and colleagues[81] from the British Regional Heart Study tried to disentangle the independent effects on cardiovascular risk of place of birth and place of residence in middle-age. This study found that men born in the south of England who moved north experienced a greater risk of IHD than men who remained in the south (7.3 compared with 4.4 per 1000 per year). Similarly men born in the north who moved south experienced a lower risk than men who remained in the north (7.9 compared with 3.3 per 1000 per year). In a multi-variate logistic model the zone of examination was significantly associated with IHD risk (odds ratio 1.34, 95% confidence interval 1.11, 1.3, $P=-0.003$) whereas there was no significant association with zone of birth (odds ratio 0.93, 95% confidence interval 0.78, 1.13, $p=0.5$). This study suggested that geographic area of adult residence was of far greater importance in determining cardiovascular risk than place of birth. In other words, factors acting later in life exerted a greater influence than those earlier in the life course. A criticism of this study was that it was based on only 24 incident cases of IHD among migrants during 6 years of follow-up. However, the analysis of Elford and colleagues was repeated using data gathered over 22 years of follow-up (1978–2000).[82] During this period of time there were 1392 cases of incident CHD of which 114 events occurred in internal migrants from either the rest of the UK or the south. After adjusting for standard risk factors, zone of examination was, as in the original analysis, more strongly associated with both CHD incidence and mortality than zone of birth. After more than 20 years of follow-up, area of residence in adult life continued to exert a stronger influence on CHD risk than place of birth, confirming the findings from the earlier analysis of Elford and colleagues.

6.5.2 Migration into the UK

By way of comparison, the importance of genetic factors that are resistant to change was highlighted in a study of mortality among immigrants to England and Wales.[83] Compared with the population as a whole, mortality from cerebrovascular disease among immigrants from the Caribbean was elevated (standardized mortality ratios (SMRs) 1989–1992, males 168, females 157, $P<0.05$). SMRs for cerebrovascular disease were also raised among immigrants from West Africa (males 271, females 181, $P<0.05$). Mortality from hypertensive diseases showed a similar pattern as did the prevalence of hypertension. The authors wrote that 'as migrants from the Caribbean and from West Africa have not shared a common environment for the past 300 years, a genetic explanation for the susceptibility to hypertension in people of West African descent is likely' (p. 709).[83]

Excess mortality persisting after migration was also reported among the Irish. Studies among Irish people living in England and Wales have found that mortality among the second and third generation (that is, the descendants of migrants) remains elevated.[84,85] This excess could not be explained by socioeconomic disadvantage. An editorial in the *British Medical Journal* commented that 'the apparent persistence of excess mortality into the second generation for those of Irish parentage suggests that some important elements of being Irish persist long beyond the initial migration. … although what these (factors) are and the mechanisms by which they contribute to the relatively poor health of Irish people in England and Wales remains unclear' (p. 1374).[86]

Thus findings from mortality studies are more evenly divided than those from the blood pressure studies concerning the relative contribution of factors acting early and later in the life course. While some mortality studies clearly demonstrate the importance of factors acting later in life, others highlight the long-term effect on adults of genetic or other early life influences.

6.6 **Conclusions**

6.6.1 **Ecological studies**

Ecological studies have provided useful clues as to important risk factors for cardiovascular disease. Within England, both measures of past early life conditions and current deprivation show strong associations. Current measures of birthweight do not however show the same patterns suggesting that this is either an inadequate measure or that the biological relationships between poor fetal growth and cardiovascular disease are different today from those in the past. Internationally, current adult risk factors and past measures of early life influences show associations with cardiovascular disease. In both cases, these appear stronger for cerebrovascular disease and there appears to be no or a weak relationship between past infant mortality rates and current IHD. These results highlight the importance of a life course approach because focusing solely on adult or early life factors is unlikely to explain adequately geographic variations in disease.

6.6.2 **Migrant studies**

The migrant studies conducted among Tokelau islanders, Yi farmers, Ethiopian Jews, and the Luo people all provide compelling evidence that people moving from a low- to high-blood pressure community experience a rise in blood pressure not seen in those who remain behind. This was observed in both children and adults, appeared to occur fairly rapidly after moving, and could not be explained by selective migration. Nor could corresponding changes in weight fully account for the increase in blood pressure. Although the mechanism for the rise in blood pressure among migrants is not fully understood, the consistency of the findings in different migrant groups highlights the aetiological importance of factors acting *after* migration, in late childhood or adult life, on blood pressure levels. Interestingly, blood pressure studies among migrants provide no evidence to support Forsdahl's hypothesis that poverty early in life followed by later affluence raises the risk of CHD (and in this case blood pressure) to a level over and above that of long-term residents in the host population. While findings from some studies of migrant mortality reflected those from the blood pressure studies, other mortality studies highlighted the lasting effect of genetic or other early life influences.

To conclude, although genetic and early life factors may play a role in determining blood pressure levels and the risk of CHD, migrant studies reveal that factors acting at a later stage in the life cycle can exert an even greater influence. Looking to the future, migrant studies will continue to provide researchers with invaluable evidence for evaluating the impact of factors acting at different stages in the life course on cardiovascular risk.

References

Those marked with an asterisk are especially recommended for further reading.

1 Rothman KJ. *Modern epidemiology.* Boston/Toronto: Little, Brown and Company, 1986.

2 Morgenstern H. Uses of ecological analysis in epidemiological research. *Am J Pub Health* 1982;**72**:1336–44.

3 Rose G. Sick individuals and sick populations. *Int J Epidemiol* 1985;**14**:32–8.

4 **Intersalt Cooperative Research Group.** Intersalt: an international study of electrolyte excretion and blood pressure. Results for 24 hour urinary sodium and potassium excretion. *Br Med J* 1988;**297**:319–28.

5 **Schwartz S.** The fallacy of the ecological fallacy: the potential misuse of a concept and the consequences. *Am J Pub Health* 1994;**84**:819–23.

6 **Susser M.** The logic in ecological: I. The logic of analysis. *Am J Pub Health* 1994;**84**:825–9.

7 **Susser M.** The logic in ecological: II. The logic of design. *Am J Pub Health* 1994;**84**:830–5.

8 **Diez-Roux AV.** Bringing context back into epidemiology: variables and fallacies in multilevel analysis. *Am J Pub Health* 1998;**88**:216–22.

9 **Shouls S, Congdon P, Curtis S.** Modelling inequality in reported long term illness in the UK: combining individual and area characteristics. *J Epidemiol Commun Health* 1996;**50**:366–76.

10 **Marmot MG, Davey Smith G.** Why are the Japanese living longer? *Br Med J* 1989;**299**:1547–51.

11 **Szatrowski TP, Peterson AVJ, Shimizu Y, Prentice RL, Mason MW, Fukunaga Y** *et al.* Serum cholesterol, other risk factors, and cardiovascular disease in a Japanese cohort. *J Chron Dis* 1984;**37**:569–84.

12 **Charlton J.** Which areas are healthiest? *Pop Trends* 1996;**83**:17–24.

13 **Sauer HI.** Epidemiology of cardiovascular mortality—geographic and ethnic. *Am J Pub Health* 1962;**52**:94–105.

14 **Antonovsky A.** Social class and the major cardiovascular diseases. *J Chron Dis* 1968;**21**:65–106.

15 **Carstairs V, Morris R.** Deprivation: explaining differences in mortality between Scotland and England and Wales. *Br Med J* 1989;**299**:886–9.

16 **Townsend P, Phillimore P, Beattie A.** *Health and deprivation. Inequality and the North.* London: Croom Helm, 1988.

17 **Eames M, Ben-Shlomo Y, Marmot MG.** Social deprivation and premature mortality: regional comparison across England. *Br Med J* 1993;**307**:1097–102.

*18 **Forsdahl A.** Are poor living conditions in childhood and adolescence an important risk factor for arteriosclerotic heart disease? *Br J Prev Soc Med* 1977;**31**:91–5.

19 **Williams DRR, Roberts SJ, Davies TW.** Deaths from ischaemic heart disease and infant mortality in England and Wales. *J Epidemiol Commun Health* 1979;**33**:199–202.

*20 **Barker DJP, Osmond C.** Infant mortality, childhood nutrition, and ischaemic heart disease in England and Wales. *Lancet* 1986;**1**:1077–81.

21 **Buck C, Simpson H.** Infant diarrhoea and subsequent mortality from heart disease and cancer. *J Epidemiol Commun Health* 1982;**36**:27–30.

22 **Barker DJP, Osmond C.** Death rates from stroke in England and Wales predicted from past maternal mortality. *Br Med J* 1987;**295**:83–6.

23 **Barker DJP, Osmond C.** Childhood respiratory infection and adult chronic bronchitis in England and Wales. *Br Med J* 1986;**293**:1271–5.

*24 **Ben-Shlomo Y, Davey Smith G.** Deprivation in infancy or in adult life: which is more important for mortality risk? *Lancet* 1991;**337**:530–5.

25 **Leon D, Davey Smith G.** Infant mortality, stomach cancer, stroke, and coronary heart disease: ecological analysis. *Br Med J* 2000;**320**:1705–6.

26 **Wong YK, Dawkins KD, Ward ME.** The association between deaths from myocardial infarction and household size in England and Wales. *J Cardiovasc Risk* 2001;**8**:159–63.

27 **Barker DJP, Osmond C, Golding J.** Height and mortality in the counties of England and Wales. *Ann Hum Biol* 1990;**17**:1–6.

*28 **Barker DJP, Osmond C, Golding J, Kuh D, Wadsworth MEJ.** Growth *in utero*, blood pressure in childhood and adult life, and mortality from cardiovascular disease. *Br Med J* 1989;**298**:564–7.

*29 **Whincup PH, Cook DG, Adshead F, Taylor S, Papacosta O, Walker M** *et al.* Cardiovascular risk factors in British children from towns with widely differing adult cardiovascular mortality. *Br Med J* 1996;**313**:79–84.

30 **Marks RU.** A review of empirical findings. *Milbank Mem Fund Q* 1967;**45**:51–108.

31 **Martin WJ.** The distribution in England and Wales of mortality from coronary disease. *Br Med J* 1956;**June 30**:1523–5.

32 **Kleinman JC, DeGruttola VG, Cohen BB, Madans JH.** Regional and urban-suburban differentials in coronary heart disease mortality and risk factor prevalence. *J Chron Dis* 1981;**34**:11–9.

33 **Tyroler HA, Cassel J.** Health consequences on culture change—II. The effect of urbanization on coronary heart mortality in rural residents. *J Chronic Dis* 1964;**17**:67–77.

34 **Greenwood A.** *The health and physique of school children.* Westminster: King, 1913.

35 **Reading R, Raybould S, Jarvis S.** Deprivation, low birthweight, and children's height: a comparison between rural and urban areas. *Br Med J* 1993;**307**:1458–62.

36 **Barnett E, Strogatz D, Armstrong D, Wing S.** Urbanisation and coronary heart disease mortality among African Americans in the US South. *J Epidemiol Commun Health* 1996;**50**:252–7.

37 **Krüger O, Aase A, Westin S.** Ischaemic heart disease mortality among men in Norway: reversal of urban–rural difference between 1966 and 1989. *J Epidemiol Commun Health* 1995;**49**:271–6.

38 **Bennett N, Dodd T, Flately J, Freeth S, Bolling K.** *Health survey for England* (1st edn). London: Her Majesty's Stationery Office, 1993.

39 **Shaper AG, Elford J.** Regional variations in coronary heart disease in Great Britain: risk factors and changes in environment. In Marmot M, Elliot P, eds. *Coronary heart disease epidemiology: from aetiology to public health* (2nd edn). Oxford: Oxford University Press, 1995:127–39.

*40 **Keys A.** Seven countries: a multivariate analysis of death and coronary heart disease. Cambridge, Massachusetts: Harvard University Press, 1980.

41 **Keys A, Menotti A, Karvonen MJ, Aravanis C, Blackburn H, Buzina R** *et al.* The diet and 15-year death rate in the Seven Countries Study. *Am J Epidemiol* 1986;**124**:903–15.

42 **Law MR, Wald NJ.** An ecological study of serum cholesterol and ischaemic heart disease between 1950 and 1990. *EurJ Clin Nutr* 1994;**48**:305–25.

43 **Simons LA.** Interrelations of lipids and lipoproteins with coronary artery disease mortality in 19 countries. *Am J Cardiol* 1986;**57**:5–10G.

44 **Kromhout D, Bloemberg PM, Feskens EJM, Hertog MGL, Menotti A, Blackburn H.** Alcohol, fish, fibre and anti-oxidant vitamin intake do not explain population differences in coronary heart disease mortality. *Int J Epidemiol* 1996;**25**:753–9.

45 **The World Health Organization (WHO) MONICA project.** Ecological analysis of the association between mortality and major risk factors of cardiovascular disease. *Int J Epidemiol* 1994;**94**:705–16.

46 **WHO MONICA project.** Stroke incidence and mortality correlated to stroke risk factors in the WHO MONICA project: an ecological study of 18 populations. *Stroke* 1997;**28**:1367–74.

47 **Kuulasmaa K, Tunstall-Pedoe H, Dobson A, Fortmann S, Sans S, Tolonen H** *et al.* Estimation of contribution of changes in classic risk factors to trends in coronary-event rates across the WHO MONICA Project populations. *Lancet* 2000;**355**:675–87.

48 **Shkolnikov V, McKee M, Leon D.** Changes in life expectancy in Russia in the mid-1990s. *Lancet* 2001;**357**:917–21.

49 **Charlton J, Murphy M, Khaw KT, Ebrahim S, Davey Smith G.** Cardiovascular diseases. In Murphy M, Charlton J, eds. *Health of adult Britain 1841–1994, Volume 2.* London: Office of National Statistics, 1997:60–81.

50 Lawlor DA, Ebrahim S, Davey Smith G. Sex matters: secular and geographical trends in sex differences in coronary heart disease mortality. *Br Med J* 2001;**323**:541–5.

51 Azambuja MIR, Duncan BB. Similarities in mortality patterns from influenza in the first half of the 20th century and the rise and fall of ischaemic heart disease in the United States: a new hypothesis concerning the coronary heart disease epidemic. *Cad Saude Publica* 2002;**18**:557–67.

52 Zatonski WA, McMichael AJ, Powles JW. Ecological study of reasons for sharp decline in mortality from iscaemic heart disease in Poland since 1991. *Br Med J* 1998;**316**:1047–51.

53 Maheswaran R, Strachan DP, Elliott P, Shipley MJ. Trends in stroke mortality in Greater London and south east England—evidence for a cohort effect? *J Epidemiol Commun Health* 1997;**51**:121–6.

54 Davey Smith G, Ben-Shlomo Y. Geographical and social class differentials in stroke mortality—the influence of early life factors: comments on papers by Maheswaran and colleagues. *J Epidemiol Commun Health* 1997;**51**:134–7.

55 Prior IAM, Stanhope JM, Grimley Evans J, Salmond CE. The Tokelau Island Migrant Study. *Int J Epidemiol* 1974;**3**:225–32.

56 Stanhope JM, Prior IAM. The Tokelau Island migrant study: prevalence of various conditions before migration. *Int J Epidemiol* 1976;**5**:259–66.

57 Beaglehole R, Eyles E, Prior I. Blood pressure and migration in children. *Int J Epidemiol* 1979;**8**:5–10.

58 Ward RH, Chin PG, Prior IAM. Tokelau Island Migrant Study, effect of migration on the familial aggregation of blood pressure. *Hypertension* 1980;**2(suppl 1)**:I-43–54.

*59 Salmond CE, Joseph JG, Prior IAM, Stanley DG, Wessen AF. Longitudinal analysis of the relationship between blood pressure and migration: the Tokelau Island migrant study. *Am J Epidemiol* 1985;**122**:291–301.

60 Beaglehole R, Eyles E, Salmond C, Prior I. Blood pressure in Tokelauan children in two contrasting environments. *Am J Epidemiol* 1978;**108**:283–8.

61 Joseph JG, Prior IAM, Salmond CE, Stanley D. Elevation of systolic and diastolic blood pressure associated with migration: the Tokelau Island migrant study. *J Chron Dis* 1983;**36**:507–16.

62 He J, Tell GS, Tang YC, Mo PS, He GQ. Effect of migration on blood pressure: the Yi people study. *Epidemiology* 1991;**2**:88–97.

*63 He J, Klag MJ, Whelton PK, Chen JY, Mo JP, Qian MC *et al.* Migration, blood pressure pattern, and hypertension: the Yi migrant study. *Am J Epidemiol* 1991;**134**:1085–101.

64 He J, Klag MJ, Whelton PK, Chen JY, Qian MC, He GQ. Body mass and blood pressure in a lean population in southwestern China. *Am J Epidemiol* 1994;**139**:380–9.

65 Klag MJ, He J, Whelton PK, Chen JY, Qian MC, He GQ. Alcohol use and blood pressure in an acculturated society. *Hypertension* 1993;**22**:365–70.

66 Rosen H. Ethiopian Jews: an historical sketch. *Israel J Med Sci* 1991;**27**:242–3.

*67 Goldbourt U, Khoury M, Landau E, Reisin LH, Rubinstein A. Blood pressure in Ethiopian immigrants: relationship to age and anthropometric factors, and changes during their first year in Israel. *Israel J Med Sci* 1991;**27**:264–7.

68 Bursztyn M, Raz I. Blood pressure and insulin in Ethiopian immigrants: longitudinal study. *J Hum Hypertens* 1995;**9**:245–8.

69 Rosenthal T, Grossman E, Knecht A, Goldbourt U. Blood pressure in Ethiopian immigrants in Israel: comparison with resident Israelis. *J Hypertens* 1989;**7(suppl 1)**:S53–55.

70 Rosenthal T, Grossman E, Knecht A, Goldbourt U. Levels and correlates of blood pressure in recent and earlier Ethiopian immigrants to Israel. *J Hum Hypertens* 1990;**4**:425–30.

71 Goldbourt U, Rosenthal T, Rubinstein A. Trends in weight and blood pressure in Ethiopian immigrants during their first few years in Israel: epidemiological observations and implications for the future. *Israel J Med Sci* 1991;**27**:260–3.

72 Bursztyn M, Raz I. Blood pressure, glucose, insulin and lipids of young Ethiopian recent immigrants to Israel and in those resident for 2 years. *J Hypertens* 1993;**11**:455–9.

73 Green MS, Etzion T, Jucha E. Blood pressure and serum cholesterol among male Ethiopian immigrants compared to other Israelis. *J Epidemiol Commun Health* 1991;**45**:281–6.

74 Poulter NR, Khaw KT, Sever PS. Higher blood pressures of urban migrants from an African low-blood pressure population are not due to selective migration. *Am J Hypertens* 1988;**1**:143-5S.

*75 Poulter NR, Khaw KT, Hopwood BEC, Mugambi M, Peart WS, Rose G *et al.* The Kenyan Luo migration study: observations on the initiation of a rise in blood pressure. *Br Med J* 1990;**300**:967–72.

76 Poulter N, Khaw KT, Hopwood BEC, Mugambi M, Peart WS, Rose G *et al.* Blood pressure and its correlates in an African tribe in urban and rural environments. *J Epidemiol Commun Health* 1984;**38**:181–6.

77 Shaper AG, Ashby D, Pocock S. Blood pressure and hypertension in middle-aged British men. *J Hypertens* 1988;**6**:367–74.

78 Elford J, Phillips AN, Thomson AG, Shaper AG. Migration and geographic variations in blood pressure in Britain. *Br Med J* 1990;**300**:291–5.

79 Elford J, Whincup P, Shaper AG. Selective migration by birthweight. *J Epidemiol Commun Health* 1993;**47**:336.

80 Strachan DP, Leon DA, Dodgeon B. Mortality from cardiovascular disease among interregional migrants in England and Wales. *Br Med J* 1995;**310**:423–7.

81 Elford J, Phillips AN, Thomson AG, Shaper AG. Migration and geographic variations in ischaemic heart disease in Great Britain. *Lancet* 1989;**i**:343–6.

82 Wannamethee SG, Shaper AG, Whincup PH, Walker M. Migration within Great Britain and cardiovascular disease: early life and adult environmental factors. *Int J Epidemiol* 2002;**31**:1054–60.

83 Wild S, McKeigue P. Cross sectional analysis of mortality by country of birth in England and Wales, 1970–92. *Br Med J* 1997;**314**:705–10.

84 Harding S, Balarajan R. Patterns of mortality in second generation Irish living in England and Wales: longitudinal study. *Br Med J* 1996;**312**:1389–92.

85 Harding S, Balarajan R. Mortality of third generation Irish people living in England and Wales: longitudinal study. *Br Med J* 2001;**322**:466–7.

86 Haskey J. Mortality among second generation Irish in England and Wales. Poorer health is not fully explained by continuing socioeconomic disadvantage. *Br Med J* 1996;**312**:1373–4.

Chapter 7

A life course approach to diabetes

Nita Forouhi, Elizabeth Hall, and Paul McKeigue

This chapter reviews the evidence that the risk of type 2 diabetes mellitus (T2DM) in adult life may be set by factors operating early in the life course of an individual. An inverse association between birthweight and the prevalence of glucose intolerance in later life has been demonstrated in several populations around the world. Birthweight has also been reported to be inversely associated with future gestational diabetes (GDM) risk in women and with plasma glucose levels after oral glucose challenge in children and young adults. Known predictors of diabetes such as obesity do not account for these associations.

Impairment of insulin secretion, resistance to the action of insulin, or both could mediate the association between size at birth and diabetes. Epidemiological evidence demonstrates that low birthweight predicts insulin resistance, while the evidence for an association with impaired beta-cell function is weak and inconsistent.

A genetic explanation for this association is plausible, but there is more evidence at present that the association may be environmental in origin. However, genetic factors may be more important in explaining ethnic differences in the prevalence of T2DM.

Whatever the basis of the association between reduced size at birth and glucose intolerance, prevention and control of obesity is likely to be the most effective measure to reduce diabetes risk in those born small. Strategies aimed at reducing fetal exposure to maternal hyperglycaemia, which exposes both mother and offspring to future diabetes risk and is readily amenable to intervention, should be the focus of public health efforts.

7.1 Introduction

The prevalence of T2DM, previously known as non-insulin dependent diabetes mellitus, is rising worldwide—it is projected to double from a baseline of 124 million in 1995 to 221 million in 2010[1] and to 300 million by the year 2025. This represents an estimated 42% increase in developed countries and a 170% increase in developing countries.[2] As T2DM has a life course epidemiology and is associated with greatly increased morbidity and premature mortality, reduced quality of life, and huge health care and personal costs, the search is on to identify causative and risk factors to enable prevention strategies.

It is known that prevalence of T2DM increases with increasing age, physical inactivity, obesity, in particular central obesity,[3] and family history. It is also now known that T2DM is four to six times more prevalent in some non-European populations such as south Asians, where its onset also occurs earlier than in European-descent counterparts.[3] That the origins of T2DM may lie in fetal and early life stages was proposed in the early 1990s—a study in Hertfordshire, England, was the first to show that people with low birthweights had higher rates of glucose intolerance and T2DM later in life.[4] The past decade has seen, simultaneously, confirmation of such associations by independent investigators in different parts of the world, extensions of the hypothesis, challenges and alternatives to the hypothesis, and a search for the underlying mechanisms. This chapter reviews some of the important epidemiological associations and mechanisms acting across the life course that influence the development of T2DM.

7.1.1 Definitions

Type 2 diabetes occurs as a result of disturbances in glucose and insulin metabolism. Plasma glucose levels are regulated by the beta-cells of the pancreatic islets, which sense glucose levels in extracellular fluid and respond to raised levels by secreting insulin. Insulin lowers plasma glucose by stimulating uptake of glucose from blood (mainly by skeletal muscle) and by suppressing production of glucose by the liver. Failure to keep plasma glucose down to normal levels implies either that the secretion of insulin is inadequate, or that there is resistance to the action of insulin in lowering plasma glucose. The relationship between size at birth and T2DM could be mediated through insulin resistance, a defect in insulin secretion, or both. In addition there is evidence for a state of pre-diabetes, which may exist for a number of years before clinical diabetes becomes manifest. This has been called various names such as the insulin resistance syndrome, Reaven's syndrome, syndrome X, and the metabolic syndrome. This is defined as a cluster of related abnormalities, which include central obesity, resistance to insulin-mediated glucose uptake, glucose intolerance, hyperinsulinaemia, dyslipidaemia, and hypertension.[5] Insulin resistance may underpin the pathogenesis of both T2DM and coronary heart disease.[5]

7.2 Epidemiological evidence relating birth size to glucose and insulin metabolism—the fetal origins hypothesis

7.2.1 Studies in adult men and women

In the first UK study, 408 men born in Hertfordshire between 1920 and 1930 underwent glucose tolerance tests at a mean age of 64 years.[4] Glucose intolerance was defined by a 2 h glucose of 7.8 mmol/l or more. There was a linear inverse relationship between prevalence of glucose intolerance and birthweight, from 14% prevalence in the highest two birthweight categories to 36% in the lowest two birthweight categories. Adjustment for body mass index (BMI) strengthened the relationship: the adjusted odds ratios (ORs) for prevalence in the lowest birthweight category compared with the highest was 6.6. There was an equally strong relationship between glucose intolerance and weight at 1 year.

Further studies in the 1990s in England,[6] Sweden,[7] and the USA[8] confirmed the initial findings of an inverse association between birthweight and glucose intolerance or T2DM. Some studies showed that thinness at birth, defined by low ponderal index (weight divided by cubed length), had a stronger association with diabetes than did birthweight. In the Swedish study, prevalence of diabetes at age 60 years was three times higher in the lowest quintile of ponderal index at birth than in the other four quintiles. This association was independent of BMI.[7]

Somewhat different results have come from studies in populations at high risk of diabetes, including native Americans and south Asians. Pima native Americans were the first non-European group where birth size associations were examined: 1179 Pimas whose birthweights had been recorded between 1965 and 1972 were examined between ages 20 and 39 years.[9] There was a U-shaped relationship between birthweight and the prevalence of diabetes. Prevalence of diabetes was raised only in those with birthweight less than 2.5 kg or more than 4.5 kg. Although the OR for diabetes in those with low birthweight compared with those with normal birthweight was 3.8, the excess risk associated with low birthweight accounted for only 6% of all cases in the population. When maternal diabetes was included in the model, the excess prevalence in the high birthweight group was no longer significant. In the Mysore study, the prevalence of diabetes in south Asian adults was not related to birthweight.[10] When the association was adjusted for age, sex, and BMI, there was a non-significant positive association between birthweight and diabetes prevalence. A recent matched-pairs case–control study of the association between T2DM and birthweight among 3992 native Americans in Saskatchewan, Canada found a positive association:[11] a greater proportion of those with T2DM had high birthweight (>4000 g) than non-diabetic individuals (16.2% compared with 10.7%; $P<0.01$). In analyses unadjusted for maternal diabetes, there was a significant association between high birthweight and diabetes (OR, 1.63, 95% confidence interval (CI), 1.20, 2.24), which was stronger in women, but no such association was found with low birthweight (<2500 g).

The most likely explanation for these results is that in high-risk populations, the associations of GDM with increased size at birth and increased risk of diabetes in the offspring (during adult life) obscure any associations of reduced fetal growth with diabetes in adult life.

Some of the key studies to date relating size at birth to diabetes or impaired glucose tolerance in adult life are summarized in Table 7.1. The largest study (n = 69 526) of these associations is the Nurses' Health Study where self-reported birthweight was related prospectively to the incidence of self-reported T2DM.[12] This study showed an increased risk of diabetes associated with lower birthweight, but also an increased risk in those with birthweight greater than 4.5 kg. When adjusted for current BMI or maternal history of diabetes, the increased risk in the high birthweight group was eliminated revealing an inverse association between birthweight and T2DM across the range of birthweights.

7.2.2 Birth size and gestational diabetes

Women with GDM are at an increased risk of developing T2DM in later life, thus it has been of interest to examine the relationship between size at birth of female infants and the risk of GDM when these women become pregnant.

A case (n = 440)–control (n = 22 955) study of healthy New York women with first pregnancies found a U-shaped association between risk of medically recorded GDM and the women's own low (<2000 g) and high (>4000 g) birthweights (obtained from

Table 7.1 Studies relating diabetes or impaired glucose tolerance to size at birth

Population	n	Age (years)	Outcome	Measurement of size at birth	Form of relationship	Odds ratio highest/ lowest categories
Hertfordshire men[4]	468	64	IGT/new T2DM	Birthweight	Linear	6.6*
Preston adults[6]	266	46–54	IGT/new T2DM	Birthweight	Linear	6.4*
Pima-American adults[9]	1179	20–39	T2DM	Birthweight	U-shaped	3.8*
US male health professionals[8]	22 693	61	Diagnosed T2DM	Birthweight (recalled)	Non-linear	1.9
Uppsala men[7]	1093	60	T2DM	(1) birthweight	Step wise	1.9, 2.3*
				(2) ponderal index	Step wise	4.4
Helsinki adults[30]	7086	64–73	Treated T2DM	(1) birthweight	Linear	1.38 per kg decrease
				(2) birth length	Linear	1.07 per cm decrease
				(3) ponderal index	Linear	1.04 per unit decrease
US nurses[12]	69 526	46–71	T2DM	Birthweight (recalled)	Linear	1.87*
Dutch adults[44]	720	51–55	IGT	Birthweight	Linear	
Stockholm men[118]	2237	35–56	(1) T2DM	Birthweight (recalled)	Step wise	4.5*
			(2) IGT			1.9*
Icelandic adults[119]	4648	33–65	IGT/T2DM	Birthweight	Linear	1.1–1.2*
Indian adults[10]	506	39–60	T2DM	Birthweight	None	1.6
				Birth length	Linear	

IGT, impaired glucose tolerance; T2DM, type 2 diabetes mellitus.

*Adjusted for body mass index.

birth certificates).[13] Odds ratios for GDM with adjustment for gestational age were 2.2 and 1.5 respectively for low and high birthweight. Adjustment for prepregnancy BMI and maternal diabetes increased the OR for low birthweight to 4.2 (95% CI, 1.5–11.5), but eliminated the OR for high birthweight (OR, 0.92, 95% CI, 0.54–1.57), leaving a strong inverse dose–response relationship between birthweight and risk of GDM (*P*-value for trend <0.001). A population-based cohort study linked birth certificate data of 41 839 women from four ethnic groups in the USA with completed pregnancies between 1987 and 1995.[14] There was a significant (adjusted) association of low birthweight (<2000 g) with GDM risk (obtained from obstetric and neonatal records) in all ethnic groups (White, African-American, native American, and Hispanic) when compared with higher birthweight (3000–3999 g). In this study women of African-American origin were the only group with a significant association between high birthweight (>4000 g) and GDM.[14] A Norwegian study of 138 714 women with singleton pregnancies with birth size data from the birth registry found self-reported GDM risk to increase with lower birthweight.[15] The increased risk of GDM was 80%, 60%, and 40% in women whose birthweights were <2500 g, 2500–2999 g, and 3000–3499 g respectively compared with women in the 4000–4500 g group. Thus there is an accumulating body of consistent evidence, from epidemiologically rigorous studies in different parts of the world, that there is an inverse association between female birthweight and the future risk for GDM.

7.2.3 Studies in children and young adults

Studies in children and young adults are useful because measures of birth size are more readily available and they afford the opportunity to study the association between birth size and intermediate variables on the causal pathway to T2DM. Studies of children in Jamaica,[16] India,[17,18] England,[19] and South Africa[20] have reported inverse associations of birthweight or ponderal index with glucose levels (Table 7.2). However, not all studies have consistently found such an inverse association. For example, one UK study of 10–11-year-old children found no consistent association between either birthweight or ponderal index and either fasting or 30-min post-load glucose levels.[21] In analyses adjusted for current body size, in Pima American children the relationship between 2 h glucose and birthweight was U-shaped.[22] A recent study from Taiwan also reported a U-shaped relationship between birthweight and T2DM in children aged 6–18 years.[23] In this study both low (<2500 g) and high (>4000 g) birthweight were associated with an increased risk for T2DM and the higher risk among the high birthweight children persisted after adjustment for GDM.[23] It is important to note that the nature of the association between birth size and future glucose intolerance is complex and may be affected by the growth pattern in infancy and childhood, as discussed in Section 7.3.1.

7.2.4 Summary

In summary, the findings of the epidemiological associations between birth size and glucose tolerance suggest that in populations of European descent, where prevalence of diabetes is low in young adults and GDM is uncommon, there is a consistent association of reduced size at birth with raised glucose levels in children or glucose intolerance in adults. In populations at high risk for diabetes, such as native North Americans or

Table 7.2 Studies relating glucose levels in children and young adults to size at birth

Population	n	Age (years)	Outcome	Measurement	Relationship
Southampton men[120]	40	21	30-min glucose	Birthweight	Inverse association*
Mexican-American adults[36]	564	31	Fasting glucose	Birthweight	Higher mean level of glucose in bottom tertile of birthweight compared to top tertile
Salisbury children[19]	250	7	30-min glucose	Ponderal index	Inverse association*
Pune children[17,18]	379	4	30-min glucose	Birthweight	Higher mean glucose in low birthweight group*
		8	30-min glucose	Birthweight	Inverse association*
French adults[121]	517	20	30-min glucose	Birthweight	Higher mean glucose in those born small for gestational age*
South African children[20]	152	7	30-min glucose	Birthweight	Inverse association
Pima native Americans[22]	3061	10–29	2-h glucose	Birthweight	U-shaped association*

*Adjusted for body mass index.

Mexican-Americans, the inverse relationship between glucose intolerance and size at birth is less clear and the relationship may be U-shaped or flat. A possible explanation for this reversal of the direction of association is that in high-risk populations the prevalence of glucose intolerance in pregnancy is high. A recent systematic review has examined the association of birthweight with glucose and insulin metabolism after 1 year of age.[24] Based on 48 papers included in the review, the authors provide useful summary tabulations of studies that confirm the inverse associations of birthweight and adverse later glucose and insulin metabolism as well as those studies that show positive, U-shaped, or no associations.[24]

7.3 Pathways of the fetal origins of diabetes

7.3.1 Accelerated postnatal growth

The effects of impaired fetal growth are modified by subsequent growth: the highest risks of T2DM or glucose intolerance are in those who are small at birth but become overweight adults. This led to the second part of the hypothesis proposed by Barker and Hales: the idea of a 'thrifty phenotype', where undernutrition in fetal and infant life, followed by relative overnutrition later, predisposes to high risk for T2DM.[25] Supportive evidence exists that the most unfavourable growth pattern for insulin resistance and T2DM risk is smallness or thinness at birth followed by acceleration of growth through childhood and beyond, so-called 'catch up growth' or 'accelerated postnatal growth'.[20,26–30]

There is much debate on the importance of the timing of the weight and height gain in relation to risk for T2DM. In a study of 8760 Helsinki people, Eriksson and colleagues[26] recently reported that an early adiposity rebound (lowest BMI of childhood at or before 5 years of age) was associated with a significantly higher incidence of T2DM than if the adiposity rebound was later (at greater than 7 years of age). Early adiposity rebound was also associated with low weight gain between birth and age one year in their study. However, the clinical and public health implications of early adiposity rebound and of the importance of the timing and determinants of postnatal growth patterns are not yet clear and need to be addressed in further research studies.

7.3.2 Insulin resistance or insulin secretion?

Hales and colleagues initially suggested that inadequate fetal nutrition might impair the development of the endocrine pancreas,[4] leading to defects of insulin secretion. According to this hypothesis the pathways of association between low birthweight and T2DM would be as in Fig. 7.1. The Southampton–Cambridge group subsequently suggested that the association may be mediated through an effect of malnutrition in fetal life leading to thinness at birth and insulin resistance in adult life.[31,32] The pathways by which this would give rise to T2DM are shown in Fig. 7.2. This is in line with other evidence that insulin resistance has a primary role in the pathogenesis of T2DM.[33]

A summary of some of the key studies that have examined the role of insulin resistance and insulin secretion with birth size is given in Table 7.3. In various studies insulin resistance has been measured by euglycaemic clamp, intravenous glucose tolerance test,

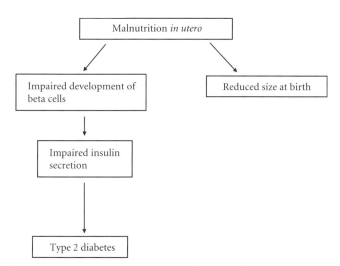

Fig. 7.1 How impaired beta-cell function could mediate an effect of malnutrition *in utero* on reduced size at birth and the risk of diabetes in adult life.

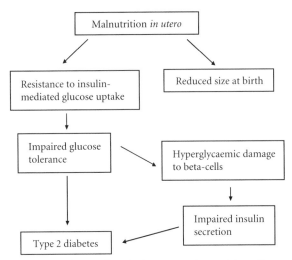

Fig. 7.2 How resistance to insulin-mediated glucose uptake could mediate an effect of malnutrition *in utero* on the risk of diabetes in adult life.

glucose–insulin product (homeostasis model assessment (HOMA)), or slope of (log) glucose decrease during an insulin tolerance test. Insulin secretion has been measured by insulin secretion during a hyperglycaemic clamp, insulin secretion during an intravenous glucose tolerance test, formula using fasting glucose and insulin (HOMA-beta cell function), and insulin increment during an oral glucose tolerance test. Few studies have used the gold standard method of the acute insulin response to intravenous glucose challenge as a direct measure of beta-cell function; those that have failed to demonstrate that reduced size at birth predicts impairment of the acute insulin response.[7,31] Associations of birth size with T2DM appear to be mediated mainly through insulin resistance,[24,34] rather than reduced insulin secretion.[24,31]

7.3.3 Small baby syndrome or insulin resistance syndrome?

Investigating associations with the metabolic syndrome,[5] Barker and colleagues have demonstrated that when glucose intolerance, hypertension, and lipid disturbances are combined to define a single binary trait, there is a strong inverse relationship between birthweight and the prevalence of this trait in middle-age, with an OR of 18 between the highest and the lowest categories.[35] They suggested that impaired fetal growth could account for the clustering of glucose intolerance, hypertension, and lipid disturbances in the population and that the insulin resistance syndrome should therefore be renamed 'small baby syndrome'.[35] In other studies that have examined the associations of size at birth with glucose intolerance, hypertension, and disturbances of plasma lipid levels separately, with diabetic individuals excluded,[7,36] reduced fetal growth has been found to predict hyperinsulinaemia, glucose intolerance, and hypertension but not to predict the lipid abnormalities characteristic of the insulin resistance syndrome—elevated triglyceride and low high-density lipoprotein (HDL) cholesterol levels—which are correlated with central obesity. In particular, HDL-cholesterol

Table 7.3 Studies relating insulin resistance or insulin levels to size at birth

Population	n	Age (years)	Outcome	Measurement	Relationship
Southampton men[120]	40	21	30-min insulin	Birthweight	Positive association
Mexican-Americans[36]	564	31	Fasting and 2-h insulin	Birthweight	Higher mean insulin level in bottom tertile of birthweight than in top
Preston adults[32]	103	47–55	Insulin tolerance test	Ponderal index	Inverse association*
Uppsala men[7]	1032	50	60-min insulin in IVGTT	Ponderal index	Inverse association*
Salisbury children[19]	250	7	Fasting insulin	Ponderal index	Inverse association
Pune children[17,18]	379	4	30-min insulin	Birthweight	Inverse association
		8	Fasting, 30-min and 2-h insulin	Birthweight	Inverse association with fasting and 30-min plasma insulin*. No association with 2-h insulin
UK women[122]	1394	60–79	HOMA score	Birthweight	Inverse association*
Indian adults[10]	506	39–60	Fasting and 30-min insulin*	Birthweight	Inverse association with fasting insulin*
US adolescents[123]	296	15	Fasting insulin, insulin sensitivity (euglycaemic clamp)	Birthweight	Inverse association of birthweight with fasting insulin, if adjusted for weight. No association of birthweight with insulin sensitivity
Chinese adults[124]	627	45	Fasting and 2-h insulin	Birthweight	Inverse association*
French adults[121]	517	20	Fasting, 30-min and 2-h insulin*	Birthweight	Higher mean levels in those born small for gestational age*
UK children[21]	1138	10–11	Fasting and 30-min insulin	Birthweight	Inverse association*
South African children[20]	152	7	Total insulin secretion in 30 min	Birthweight	Inverse association
Pima native Americans[22]	2272	5–29	Fasting and 2-h insulin	Birthweight	Inverse association*
Korean men[79]	22		Insulin sensitivity index (IVGTT)	Birthweight	Positive association
			Acute insulin response during FSIGT		No association

IVGTT, intravenous glucose tolerance test; HOMA, homeostasis model assessment; FSIGT, frequently sampled intravenous glucose tolerance test.
*Adjusted for body mass index.

concentrations are positively, and triglyceride concentrations inversely, related to birthweight in some[18,37] but not all studies.[7,38,39] It is thus possible to distinguish two patterns of clustering: a 'small baby syndrome' characterized by hypertension, insulin resistance, and glucose intolerance and a central obesity syndrome characterized by raised triglyceride levels, low HDL cholesterol, insulin resistance, and glucose intolerance.

7.4 Potential mechanisms

7.4.1 Does the association have a genetic or an environmental explanation?

Both genetic and environmental explanations have been forwarded to account for the association between low birthweight and T2DM. The 'thrifty phenotype' hypothesis[25] posits that inadequate nutrition in early life may lead to impairment of the ability to maintain glucose homeostasis in later life (discussed in Section 7.4.1.1). However, it is also known that insulin regulates fetal growth, so a primary genetic defect in insulin action would reduce growth *in utero* and also predispose to glucose intolerance in later life. The pathways by which this would produce an association between reduced size at birth and T2DM are shown in Fig. 7.3 and discussed in Section 7.4.1.2.

7.4.1.1 Does fetal malnutrition explain the association?

Although experimental models exist for undernutrition in early life causing impairment of beta-cell function,[40,41] there is no clear experimental support for undernutrition *in utero* causing insulin resistance.[40] Epidemiological evidence to support an environmental hypothesis in humans comes from a Danish study that compared birthweights of monozygotic and dizygotic twins discordant for T2DM.[42,43] Within twin pairs, the twin with T2DM was more likely to have lower birthweight than their non-diabetic twin, suggesting that the association is, at least in part, independent of genotype.

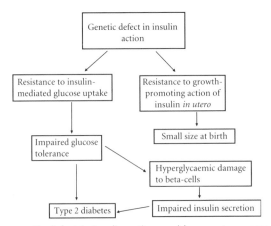

Fig. 7.3 How a primary genetic defect in insulin action could generate an association between birth size and diabetes in adult life.

Further support for an environmental cause is provided by a study of adults whose mothers were exposed to starvation while pregnant during the Dutch Hunger Winter of 1944–1945, which demonstrated an association between exposure to famine *in utero* and reduced glucose tolerance in middle-age.[44] However, the Leningrad study, which compared Russian adults exposed *in utero* to malnutrition during the 1941–1942 siege of Leningrad with controls born before the siege or outside Leningrad,[45,46] found no significant difference in fasting and 2 h glucose levels, insulin, blood pressure, and lipid concentrations between the group exposed to malnutrition *in utero* and control participants. It is possible that the dissimilar effects of exposure to the two famines may contribute to our understanding of the mechanisms of the thrifty phenotype and support the importance of accelerated postnatal growth—after the Dutch famine, conditions improved quite quickly in the Netherlands, whereas in Leningrad nourishment remained poor for a considerable time after the famine.

It is noteworthy that offspring who were exposed to the Dutch famine in early gestation had an increased risk of adult dyslipidaemia that was independent of size at birth and adult obesity,[47] while those exposed in late or mid-gestation had reduced glucose tolerance.[44] The long-term effects of intrauterine undernutrition seem to depend on its timing during gestation and on the tissues and systems undergoing critical periods of development at that time and maternal malnutrition may affect adult health without affecting the size of the baby at birth. Birthweight is a crude marker of the dynamic process of fetal growth and may not capture the effects of fetal undernutrition on body composition or the development of tissues. Thus the full impact of intrauterine undernutrition may not be known until there are studies with better tissue-level markers than birthweight.

7.4.1.2 Genetic influences on birthweight and on diabetes

One argument against genetic explanations for associations with size at birth has been that genetic effects on size at birth are weak in comparison to the effects of maternal environment.[48] However, such studies were based on heritability estimates derived from data on half siblings and twins. Alternative study designs with offspring of monozygotic and dizygotic twins[49,50] and grandchildren of twins[51] from the Norwegian twin panel have estimated that of the total variance in birthweight, 50–70% was accounted for by fetal genes.[49–51] Thus fetal genetic effects on birthweight are plausible.

Experimental manipulations that reduce insulin secretion *in utero* also reduce fetal growth.[52] It has also been demonstrated that diabetes caused by a genetic defect in insulin secretion (a rare mutation of the pancreatic glucose sensing gene, glucokinase), is associated with a 500 g birthweight reduction.[53] However, fetal genes that cause insulin resistance would be more consistent with the observation that insulin resistance, and not defects in insulin secretion, mediate the association between low birthweight and diabetes.

Hattersley and Tooke elaborated the 'fetal insulin hypothesis'[54] suggesting that genetically determined insulin resistance results in impaired insulin-mediated growth in the fetus as well as insulin resistance in adult life. Low birthweight, measures of insulin resistance in later life, and ultimately glucose intolerance, diabetes, and hypertension could all be phenotypes of the same insulin resistant genotype. That this is biologically plausible is shown by the fact that birthweight is reduced in a number of rare genetic syndromes causing insulin resistance.[55,56] A positive association between a polymorphism of the insulin variable number of tandem repeats (INS-VNTR) locus and birthweight, head circumference, and length at birth was found in a study of 758 term births.[57] It is difficult to reconcile the higher birthweight effect of this gene with the fetal origins hypothesis, but the same group also described an association between a variant mitochondrial DNA (transmitted maternally) and thinness at birth and the risk of T2DM or insulin resistance in men from the original UK studies of fetal origins.[58,59] Recently, a polymorphism of the promoter region of the insulin-like growth factor-1 gene has been associated with lower birthweight in a Dutch study of 463 adults.[60] However, this finding was not replicated in a UK case–control study of 640 people, where no association was found between birthweight and the polymorphism.[61] There is lack of consistency in the studies examining a genetic basis for low birthweight and the robustness of these associations remains to be tested in further studies.

An analysis of the British Women's Heart and Health Study has recently reported that birthweight of first offspring is inversely related to the mother's glucose–insulin product (HOMA insulin resistance score) in late adulthood, despite the association of glucose intolerance during pregnancy with heavier offspring at birth.[62] This has been interpreted as providing support for the fetal insulin hypothesis, but an alternative explanation could be that these women were lean during their first pregnancies, but gained weight in subsequent pregnancies and in later life. There is also emerging evidence that paternal diabetes but not maternal diabetes is associated with low birthweight, providing supportive evidence for genetic effects.[63,64] In contrast, a small but well-designed French study found that in 15 non-diabetic adult offspring of mothers with type 1 diabetes (exposed participants) and 16 offspring of type 1 diabetic fathers (control participants), there was a 33% higher prevalence of adult impaired glucose tolerance in the group with intrauterine exposure ($P=0.02$).[65] Early insulin secretion after an oral glucose tolerance test was lower in exposed participants than in control participants. This suggests a more powerful role for maternal environmental than fetal genetic factors. It is possible, however, that maternal genes may have conferred increased susceptibility to deficient insulin secretory response compared to paternal genes.

There is evidence that T2DM has a genetic basis: people with a family history of diabetes are at greater risk of the disease. Some of the genetic influence on diabetes is likely to be mediated through central obesity and this trait appears to be more closely under genetic control than obesity in general.[66,67] The insulin resistance atherosclerosis study group (IRAS) have recently reported in people of African-American and Hispanic origin, estimates of heritability as 0.08 for fasting insulin and HOMA (frequently sampled glucose tolerance test (GTT)), 0.28 for fasting glucose, and 0.54 for BMI. After adjustment for age, sex, and ethnicity, all heritability estimates were significantly greater than zero ($P<0.05$).[68] These results are consistent with the expectation that intermediate measures of insulin resistance and visceral adiposity are heritable. Further studies, including those of the human genome, will help elucidate further the role of genetic factors in T2DM risk.

7.4.1.3 Does the thrifty phenotype hypothesis or the thrifty genotype hypothesis explain ethnic differences in diabetes risk?

Neel proposed the 'thrifty genotype' hypothesis in 1962 to explain the emergence of T2DM in populations shifting from vigorous activity and subsistence nutrition to abundance and obesity of urban societies.[69] This hypothesis was challenged however, when a decline in T2DM and glucose intolerance prevalence was reported in Nauru, where there has been a recent transition from undernutrition to relative affluence.[70] This was seen by Hales and Barker as lending support to the 'thrifty phenotype' alternative.[25] Other evidence, however, points strongly to genetic influences underlying the high rates of diabetes in such populations. One line of evidence comes from migrant studies. Prevalence of diabetes is uniformly high (around 20% in those aged over 35 years) in Indian populations overseas whose migration occurred during the mid-nineteenth century.[71] While it is plausible that an effect of maternal environment could persist over one or two generations after migration, it is unlikely that such an effect would persist five or six generations after migration as an exposure specific to Indians. In Singapore, for instance, a rapid transition to affluence has been shared by all three of the main ethnic groups (Chinese, Malay, and Indian people) but the prevalence of diabetes is much higher in Indian than in Chinese people.[72] In several of the populations at high risk of diabetes, it has been reported that prevalence of diabetes is lower in those of mixed descent than in those without admixture from other populations at lower risk. In Nauru, for instance, prevalence of diabetes in those who had genetic markers of non-Nauruan admixture was found to be less than one-quarter of the prevalence in those without evidence of admixture.[73] Admixture in this population resulted mainly from unions between Nauruan women and European sailors: thus admixture introduced European genes but not European maternal environment. Similar relationships between diabetes and admixture have been reported for Pima-Americans.[74] It is of course possible that ethnic differences in the risk of diabetes could be a consequence of ethnic differences in fetal growth that have a genetic basis: average ponderal index at birth has been reported to be lower in the infants of Indian than European mothers in England. Such an explanation, however would still assign a primary role to genetic influences.

7.4.1.4 Summary

In summary, environmental and genetic factors are both likely to be important in determining the association between birth size and adult diabetes. It is more likely, however, that within-population diabetes risk is determined by a larger element of environmental factors, while between-population risk (ethnic difference in risk) is determined by a larger genetic element.

7.4.2 Alterations to the fetal hypothalamic–pituitary–adrenal axis

It has been suggested that changes to the hypothalamic–pituitary–adrenal (HPA) axis in the fetus leading to increased adrenal glucocorticoid secretion may be the physiological basis of insulin resistance in those who were small at birth. A study in three populations including Australian people and people from the Preston and Hertfordshire UK historical cohort studies, found that low birthweight was associated with raised fasting plasma cortisol concentrations in all three populations. A combined analysis that allowed for differences in the gender composition, age, and BMI between the studies showed that cortisol concentrations fell by 23.9 nmol/l per kg increase in birthweight (95% CI, 9.6–38.2, $P < 0.001$).[75] However, these associations are complex as shown by a Finnish birth cohort study of 421 people, where the relationship between size at birth and cortisol concentrations in adult life was different in people born at different gestational ages: both hyper- and hypocortisolism may arise as a consequence of fetal programming of the HPA axis during intrauterine life.[76] In this study there was no association of birthweight with fasting cortisol, but a positive association with ponderal index in both genders, and an inverse association with birth length in women.[76]

In experimental models, rats exposed to high glucocorticoid levels *in utero* are of low birthweight and insulin resistant.[77] However, this has not been replicated in humans. A study in Finland tested whether maternal consumption of glycyrrhizin (an inhibitor of the placental enzyme, which protects the fetus from maternal cortisol) in licorice affects birthweight in humans. Although glycyrrhizin consumption was associated with reduced gestational age, it was not significantly associated with a reduction in birthweight independent of gestational age.[78] In addition, raised cortisol levels would be expected to lead to central obesity in addition to glucose intolerance. There is no convincing evidence that the association between low birthweight and insulin resistance is paralleled by an association between low birthweight and central obesity or dyslipidaemia.[38,79] There is evidence however that the density of glucocorticoid receptors on muscle is associated with insulin resistance, indicating that changes in cortisol sensitivity rather than cortisol levels may be more relevant.[80]

7.4.3 Potential effects of confounding

It has been argued that the observed associations of the fetal origins hypothesis may be the result of confounding.[81,82] Body mass index is strongly related to prevalence of diabetes and also has a weak positive correlation ($r = 0.1$) with birthweight.[7] To address the issue that birthweight may be correlated with later size, it has been suggested that relationships between early life and later outcome should be presented according to a standard set of regression equations.[83] These equations take the outcome (a measure of glucose tolerance) and assess its relationship with (1) size at birth only (*early model*), (2) with a *combined model* of birth size and current size together, (3) the *interaction model*, which includes the combined model and interaction of size at birth and current size, and (4) the *late model* where current size alone is related to outcome, to interpret the relative importance of early and late size separately and together.[83] Few studies have used this thorough statistical approach.

Moreover, most studies have used BMI as the measure of obesity, which has limitations because of uncertainties about what underlying physiological variables are adjusted for: these are components of fat mass, lean tissue mass, and skeletal proportions. Adiposity probably underlies the association of glucose intolerance with raised BMI, whereas it is possible that lean tissue mass underlies the correlation of adult BMI with birthweight. Adjusting for BMI could produce an association between T2DM and low birthweight simply because of confounding by adiposity. Measures of adiposity other than BMI, such as skinfold thickness and percentage body fat would provide useful alternatives. The issue of the potential role of socioeconomic status in the fetal origins hypothesis[82] is addressed below (Section 7.6).

7.4.4 Could selective survival explain the association?

It has been suggested that the inverse association between fetal growth and diabetes could be accounted for by an inverse association between genetic susceptibility to diabetes and mortality among low birthweight infants.[9] In other words, low birthweight infants are more likely to survive if they are genetically predisposed to diabetes—the 'surviving small baby hypothesis'.[9] The results from the Uppsala study are not consistent with this explanation.[7] When the men in this cohort were born in 1920–1924, the infant mortality rate in Uppsala County was around 60 per 1000 live births, similar to the national rate for Sweden. Even if all these deaths had occurred in the lowest quintile of ponderal index among infants who were not susceptible to diabetes, such selection at birth could account only for a prevalence ratio for diabetes in adults of 1.3 in the lowest quintile compared to the other four quintiles. This contrasts with the observed prevalence ratio of 3.0.

7.5 Life course epidemiology of diabetes beyond fetal origins

7.5.1 The role of obesity in childhood and beyond

Evidence is emerging that insulin resistance in childhood is associated more strongly with obesity than with low birthweight. The Early Bird Study from Plymouth, England reported recently that the insulin–glucose product (HOMA insulin resistance) in 300 contemporary 5-year olds was a function of excess current weight rather than of low birthweight (no association) or change in weight (weaker association and merely correlated with current weight).[84] In a school-based survey of 1148 UK children aged 10–11 years, Whincup and colleagues found that current childhood obesity was a stronger determinant of insulin level and insulin resistance than size at birth:[21] (1) fasting and 30-min glucose was not consistently related with either birthweight or birth ponderal index; (2) after adjustment for childhood height and ponderal index, both fasting and 30-min insulin levels fell with increasing birthweight; and (3) the proportional change in insulin level for a one standard deviation increase in childhood ponderal index was much greater than that for birthweight (27.2% and –8.8% respectively for fasting insulin).[21] In a population-based study of 428 people in Finland, Vanhala and colleagues[85] found no association between birthweight and adult metabolic syndrome defined as a cluster of hypertension, dyslipidaemia, and insulin resistance. Among obese children at the age of 7 (BMI in the highest quartile), the OR for the metabolic syndrome in adulthood was 4.4 (95% CI, 2.1–9.5) as compared to the other children (the three other quartiles combined).[85] In a further study the same group reported that associations between adult obesity and the metabolic syndrome were stronger when obesity had been present in childhood (age 7).[86]

Cross-sectional surveys over the last few decades show that the prevalence of obesity has increased steadily in all age groups, including children as young as 3–4 years old (see Chapter 8).[87,88] This is likely to be one factor contributing to the emergence of T2DM in children.[89–92]

In adults as well the association with insulin resistance and T2DM is stronger for obesity than for birth size.[7,93] It is likely that a life course approach, which focuses on exposures and outcomes separated by many years, may be less relevant for obesity than an approach using a shorter time frame that focuses on the balance between energy intake and expenditure. Falling physical activity levels with sedentary lifestyles and energy-intense diets in all age groups,[94,95] rather than factors operating in early life, likely exert a stronger influence on obesity and T2DM risk. However, further research with carefully designed studies is necessary to disentangle the relative contribution of early life factors and of lifestyle factors to the risk for insulin resistance and T2DM.

7.5.2 Gestational diabetes

Offspring of mothers with GDM are at increased risk of developing T2DM. Experimental and epidemiologic data suggest that maternal hyperglycaemia itself affects glucose homeostasis. Induction of hyperglycaemia in female rats leads to glucose intolerance, insulin resistance, and impaired beta-cell function in the adult offspring,[96,97] an effect which is transmissible from one generation to the next.[98] This has now been shown in studies of Pima-Americans.[99] Dabelea and colleagues found that 70% of people exposed prenatally to a diabetic environment were diabetic at 25–34 years of age.[100] The risk of diabetes is much higher in the offspring of mothers who are diabetic during pregnancy than in the offspring of mothers who develop diabetes subsequently.[101,102]

The detrimental effects of GDM can be escalated through the potential for its intergenerational effects. Although the mechanisms are not understood, it is likely that a cycle is set in motion whereby women who were low-birthweight babies develop GDM in their own pregnancies and in turn have offspring that are exposed *in utero* to increased diabetes risk in later life. The importance of GDM as a factor in the worldwide epidemic of T2DM is not known and there are few recent data of GDM prevalence or incidence. However, GDM prevalence is high among women of non-European ancestry who have migrated to the West. In London, UK, 6% of south Asian mothers and 3% of Afro-Caribbean mothers developed GDM compared with 1% of white women, while in Melbourne, Australia, the prevalence was 15%, 14%, and 10% in Asian, Chinese, and African origin women respectively, compared with 5% among white women.[103] The intergenerational effects may be particularly important among such populations worldwide.

7.6 Influence of lifetime socioeconomic factors on diabetes risk

Social gradients in risk for both obesity and risk for T2DM have been observed. The direction of the association with both childhood and adulthood socioeconomic status is generally noted to be inverse in developed countries (lower socioeconomic status and higher obesity prevalence[104–106] and higher diabetes prevalence[107,108]). The converse is true for developing countries where this association is positive: higher socioeconomic status is associated with greater obesity prevalence[104,109,110] and with higher diabetes prevalence.[107,111] Few studies have examined the association between socioeconomic status and insulin resistance.[112–114]

The social gradients in risk for insulin resistance or T2DM are likely to be explained by the social gradients in obesity risk, but most studies have not controlled for the confounding effect of obesity on the association.[112–114] For example, the Whitehall II study reported an inverse social gradient in the prevalence of the metabolic syndrome (central obesity, post-load glucose, and triglycerides).[112] While statistical adjustment was made for lifestyle factors such as smoking, alcohol, and exercise level, which contributed little to the observed association between socioeconomic status and prevalence of the metabolic syndrome, notably the analyses were not adjusted for obesity.[112] In a recent study of 4286 UK women aged 60–79 years, those in manual social classes in childhood and adulthood had increased prevalence of insulin resistance (measured by the insulin–glucose product or HOMA), dyslipidaemia (reduced HDL cholesterol and increased triglycerides), and general obesity (higher BMI).[113] While those in manual social classes, compared with non manual classes, were 2.4 times more likely to be obese, the authors did not adjust for the potential confounding effects of obesity on the social class and insulin resistance association. Thus it is not clear whether the observed association with insulin resistance is independent of the effect of obesity.

Adult leg length is regarded as a more a sensitive indicator of early social environment, in particular of infant nutrition, than is height or trunk length.[115–117] Davey Smith and colleagues reported an independent inverse association between leg length and glucose–insulin product (HOMA) in Caerphilly men[116] and leg length and HOMA insulin resistance and T2DM in women of the British Women's Heart and Health Study.[117] It is hard to interpret whether there was an independent inverse association of insulin resistance with leg length: in the Caerphilly study there was no adjustment for men's current obesity for the HOMA-insulin resistance association and in the women's study the fully adjusted models included weight and waist hip ratio, but a more direct measure of obesity such as percentage fat, skinfold thickness, or waist circumference was not included.

In summary, the pathways underlying the associations between socioeconomic factors and birthweight, obesity, insulin resistance, insulin resistance syndrome, and T2DM are complex, operate at different times of the life course of individuals, and are not yet fully understood. While the observed associations between social deprivation and insulin resistance or T2DM cannot be ignored, a major challenge is to understand and ameliorate socioeconomic differences in obesity that may underlie these associations.

7.7 Public health implications

There is compelling evidence that T2DM may be a deferred consequence of successful adaptation *in utero* and hence primary prevention would lie in protecting fetal development. The public health implications of this for developing countries such as India are even greater than in the developed nations, owing to widespread prevalence of fetal malnutrition and low birthweight. An additional factor may be intergenerational effects of GDM, occurring in mothers who grew poorly in early life and become obese as adults. There is a case for more rigorous efforts in screening for and intensively managing GDM, particularly in women who were of low birthweight themselves.

Public health implications lie also in curbing the rise of childhood and adult obesity and physical inactivity and in promoting healthier lifestyles given the global epidemic of diabetes.[2] There is a public health need for healthy public policy interventions that include government actions directed at entire populations, including health promotion, over and above curative interventions that are individual focused.

7.8 Conclusions

There is a consistent body of evidence linking small size at birth and T2DM in later life. This association appears to be mediated through insulin resistance and to be at least partly explained by the effects of environmental exposures *in utero*. However this 'small baby syndrome' is unlikely to be the main explanation for ethnic differences in rates of diabetes and insulin resistance, where genetic factors are more important. The effects of reduced fetal growth on risk of diabetes are modest in comparison with the effects of other factors that may be amenable to intervention: exposure to maternal hyperglycaemia and obesity.

References

Those marked with an asterisk are especially recommended for further reading.

1 Amos AF, McCarty DJ, Zimmet P. The rising global burden of diabetes and its complications: estimates and projections to the year 2010. *Diabet Med* 1997;**14(suppl 5)**:S1–85.

2 King H, Aubert RE, Herman WH. Global burden of diabetes, 1995–2025: prevalence, numerical estimates, and projections. *Diabet Care* 1998;**21**:1414–31.

3 McKeigue PM, Pierpoint T, Ferrie JE, Marmot MG. Relationship of glucose intolerance and hyperinsulinaemia to body fat pattern in south Asians and Europeans. *Diabetologia* 1992;**35**:785–91.

*4 Hales CN, Barker DJ, Clark PM, Cox LJ, Fall C, Osmond C *et al.* Fetal and infant growth and impaired glucose tolerance at age 64. *Br Med J* 1991;**303**:1019–22.

5 Reaven GM. Banting lecture 1988. Role of insulin resistance in human disease. *Diabetes* 1988;**37**:1595–607.

*6 Phipps K, Barker DJ, Hales CN, Fall CH, Osmond C, Clark PM. Fetal growth and impaired glucose tolerance in men and women. *Diabetologia* 1993;**36**:225–8.

*7 Lithell HO, McKeigue PM, Berglund L, Mohsen R, Lithell UB, Leon DA. Relation of size at birth to non-insulin dependent diabetes and insulin concentrations in men aged 50–60 years. *Br Med J* 1996;**312**:406–10.

8 Curhan GC, Willett WC, Rimm EB, Spiegelman D, Ascherio AL, Stampfer MJ. Birth weight and adult hypertension, diabetes mellitus, and obesity in US men. *Circulation* 1996;**94**:3246–50.

*9 McCance DR, Pettitt DJ, Hanson RL, Jacobsson LT, Knowler WC, Bennett PH. Birth weight and non-insulin dependent diabetes: thrifty genotype, thrifty phenotype, or surviving small baby genotype? *Br Med J* 1994;**308**:942–5.

10 Fall CH, Stein CE, Kumaran K, Cox V, Osmond C, Barker DJ *et al.* Size at birth, maternal weight, and type 2 diabetes in South India. *Diabet Med* 1998;**15**:220–7.

11 Dyck RF, Klomp H, Tan L. From "thrifty genotype" to "hefty fetal phenotype": the relationship between high birth weight and diabetes in Saskatchewan Registered Indians. *Can J Pub Health* 2001;**92**:340–4.

12 Rich-Edwards JW, Colditz GA, Stampfer MJ, Willett WC, Gillman MW, Hennekens CH *et al.* Birth weight and the risk for type 2 diabetes mellitus in adult women. *Ann Intern Med* 1999;**130**:278–84.

13 Innes KE, Byers TE, Marshall JA, Baron A, Orleans M, Hamman RF. Association of a woman's own birth weight with subsequent risk for gestational diabetes. *J Am Med Assoc* 2002;**287**:2534–41.

14 Williams MA, Emanuel I, Kimpo C, Leisenring WM, Hale CB. A population-based cohort study of the relation between maternal birth weight and risk of gestational diabetes mellitus in four racial/ethnic groups. *Paediatr Perinat Epidemiol* 1999;**13**:452–65.

15 Egeland GM, Skjaerven R, Irgens LM. Birth characteristics of women who develop gestational diabetes: population based study. *Br Med J* 2000;**321**:546–7.

16 Forrester TE, Wilks RJ, Bennett FI, Simeon D, Osmond C, Allen M *et al.* Fetal growth and cardiovascular risk factors in Jamaican schoolchildren. *Br Med J* 1996;**312**:156–60.

17 Yajnik CS, Fall CH, Vaidya U, Pandit AN, Bavdekar A, Bhat DS *et al.* Fetal growth and glucose and insulin metabolism in four-year-old Indian children. *Diabet Med* 1995;**12**:330–6.

18 Bavdekar A, Yajnik CS, Fall CH, Bapat S, Pandit AN, Deshpande V *et al.* Insulin resistance syndrome in 8-year-old Indian children: small at birth, big at 8 years, or both? *Diabetes* 1999;**48**:2422–9.

19 Law CM, Gordon GS, Shiell AW, Barker DJ, Hales CN. Thinness at birth and glucose tolerance in seven-year-old children. *Diabet Med* 1995;**12**:24–9.

20 Crowther NJ, Cameron N, Trusler J, Gray IP. Association between poor glucose tolerance and rapid post natal weight gain in seven-year-old children. *Diabetologia* 1998;**41**:1163–7.

21 Whincup PH, Cook DG, Adshead F, Taylor SJ, Walker M, Papacosta O *et al.* Childhood size is more strongly related than size at birth to glucose and insulin levels in 10–11-year-old children. *Diabetologia* 1997;**40**:319–26.

22 Dabelea D, Pettitt DJ, Hanson RL, Imperatore G, Bennett PH, Knowler WC. Birth weight, type 2 diabetes, and insulin resistance in Pima Indian children and young adults. *Diabet Care* 1999;**22**:944–50.

23 Wei JN, Sung FC, Li CY, Chang CH, Lin RS, Lin CC *et al.* Low birth weight and high birth weight infants are both at an increased risk to have type 2 diabetes among schoolchildren in Taiwan. *Diabet Care* 2003;**26**:343–8.

*24 Newsome CA, Shiell AW, Fall CH, Phillips DI, Shier R, Law CM. Is birth weight related to later glucose and insulin metabolism?—a systematic review. *Diabet Med* 2003;**20**:339–48.

*25 Hales CN, Barker DJ. Type 2 (non-insulin-dependent) diabetes mellitus: the thrifty phenotype hypothesis. *Diabetologia* 1992;**35**:595–601.

*26 Eriksson JG, Forsen T, Tuomilehto J, Osmond C, Barker DJ. Early adiposity rebound in childhood and risk of Type 2 diabetes in adult life. *Diabetologia* 2003;**46**:190–4.

27 Eriksson JG, Forsen T, Tuomilehto J, Jaddoe VW, Osmond C, Barker DJ. Effects of size at birth and childhood growth on the insulin resistance syndrome in elderly individuals. *Diabetologia* 2002;**45**:342–8.

28 Ong KK, Ahmed ML, Emmett PM, Preece MA, Dunger DB. Association between postnatal catch-up growth and obesity in childhood: prospective cohort study. *Br Med J* 2000;**320**:967–71.

29 Cianfarani S, Germani D, Branca F. Low birth weight and adult insulin resistance: the "catch-up growth" hypothesis. *Arch Dis Child Fetal Neonatal Ed* 1999;**81**:F71–73.

30 Forsen T, Eriksson J, Tuomilehto J, Reunanen A, Osmond C, Barker D. The fetal and childhood growth of persons who develop type 2 diabetes. *Ann Intern Med* 2000;**133**:176–82.

31 Phillips DI, Hirst S, Clark PM, Hales CN, Osmond C. Fetal growth and insulin secretion in adult life. *Diabetologia* 1994;**37**:592–6.

32 **Phillips DI, Barker DJ, Hales CN, Hirst S, Osmond C.** Thinness at birth and insulin resistance in adult life. *Diabetologia* 1994;**37**:150–4.

33 **Yki-Jarvinen H.** Evidence for a primary role of insulin resistance in the pathogenesis of type 2 diabetes. *Ann Med* 1990;**22**:197–200.

34 **Phillips DI.** Insulin resistance as a programmed response to fetal undernutrition. *Diabetologia* 1996;**39**:1119–22.

35 **Barker DJ, Hales CN, Fall CH, Osmond C, Phipps K, Clark PM.** Type 2 (non-insulin-dependent) diabetes mellitus, hypertension and hyperlipidaemia (syndrome X): relation to reduced fetal growth. *Diabetologia* 1993;**36**:62–7.

36 **Valdez R, Athens MA, Thompson GH, Bradshaw BS, Stern MP.** Birth weight and adult health outcomes in a biethnic population in the USA. *Diabetologia* 1994;**37**:624–31.

37 **Fall CH, Osmond C, Barker DJ, Clark PM, Hales CN, Stirling Y** *et al.* Fetal and infant growth and cardiovascular risk factors in women. *Br Med J* 1995;**310**:428–32.

*38 **Byberg L, McKeigue PM, Zethelius B, Lithell HO.** Birth weight and the insulin resistance syndrome: association of low birth weight with truncal obesity and raised plasminogen activator inhibitor-1 but not with abdominal obesity or plasma lipid disturbances. *Diabetologia* 2000;**43**:54–60.

39 **Levitt NS, Lambert EV, Woods D, Hales CN, Andrew R, Seckl JR.** Impaired glucose tolerance and elevated blood pressure in low birth weight, nonobese, young south african adults: early programming of cortisol axis. *J Clin Endocrinol Metab* 2000;**85**:4611–8.

40 **Crace CJ, Swenne I, Milner RD.** Long-term effects on glucose tolerance and insulin secretory response to glucose following a limited period of severe protein or energy malnutrition in young rats. *Ups J Med Sci* 1991;**96**:177–83.

41 **Dahri S, Snoeck A, Reusens-Billen B, Remacle C, Hoet JJ.** Islet function in offspring of mothers on low-protein diet during gestation. *Diabetes* 1991;**40(suppl 2)**:115–20.

42 **Poulsen P, Vaag AA, Kyvik KO, Moller JD, Beck-Nielsen H.** Low birth weight is associated with NIDDM in discordant monozygotic and dizygotic twin pairs. *Diabetologia* 1997;**40**:439–46.

43 **Poulsen P, Vaag A.** Glucose and insulin metabolism in twins: influence of zygosity and birth weight. *Twin Res* 2001;**4**:350–5.

44 **Ravelli AC, van der Meulen JH, Michels RP, Osmond C, Barker DJ, Hales CN** *et al.* Glucose tolerance in adults after prenatal exposure to famine. *Lancet* 1998;**351**:173–7.

45 **Stanner SA, Bulmer K, Andres C, Lantseva OE, Borodina V, Poteen VV** *et al.* Does malnutrition *in utero* determine diabetes and coronary heart disease in adulthood? Results from the Leningrad siege study, a cross sectional study. *Br Med J* 1997;**315**:1342–8.

46 **Stanner SA, Yudkin JS.** Fetal programming and the Leningrad Siege study. *Twin Res* 2001;**4**:287–92.

47 **Roseboom TJ, van der Meulen JH, Osmond C, Barker DJ, Ravelli AC, Bleker OP.** Plasma lipid profiles in adults after prenatal exposure to the Dutch famine. *Am J Clin Nutr* 2000;**72**:1101–6.

48 **Morton NE.** The inheritance of human birth weight. *Ann Hum Genet* 1955;**20**:125–34.

49 **Magnus P, Berg K, Bjerkedal T, Nance WE.** Parental determinants of birth weight. *Clin Genet* 1984;**26**:397–405.

50 **Magnus P.** Causes of variation in birth weight: a study of offspring of twins. *Clin Genet* 1984;**25**:15–24.

51 **Magnus P.** Further evidence for a significant effect of fetal genes on variation in birth weight. *Clin Genet* 1984;**26**:289–96.

52 **Fowden AL.** The role of insulin in prenatal growth. *J Dev Physiol* 1989;**12**:173–82.

53 **Hattersley AT, Beards F, Ballantyne E, Appleton M, Harvey R, Ellard S.** Mutations in the glucokinase gene of the fetus result in reduced birth weight. *Nat Genet* 1998;**19**:268–70.

54 Hattersley AT, Tooke JE. The fetal insulin hypothesis: an alternative explanation of the association of low birth weight with diabetes and vascular disease. *Lancet* 1999;**353**:1789–92.

55 Frayling TM, Hattersley AT. The role of genetic susceptibility in the association of low birth weight with type 2 diabetes. *Br Med Bull* 2001;**60**:89–101.

56 Gluckman PD. The role of pituitary hormones, growth factors and insulin in the regulation of fetal growth. *Oxf Rev Reprod Biol* 1986;**8**:1–60.

57 Dunger DB, Ong KK, Huxtable SJ, Sherriff A, Woods KA, Ahmed ML *et al.* Association of the INS VNTR with size at birth. ALSPAC Study Team. Avon Longitudinal Study of Pregnancy and Childhood. *Nat Genet* 1998;**19**:98–100.

58 Ong KK, Phillips DI, Fall C, Poulton J, Bennett ST, Golding J *et al.* The insulin gene VNTR, type 2 diabetes and birth weight. *Nat Genet* 1999;**21**:262–3.

59 Casteels K, Ong K, Phillips D, Bendall H, Pembrey M. Mitochondrial 16189 variant, thinness at birth, and type-2 diabetes. ALSPAC study team. Avon Longitudinal Study of Pregnancy and Childhood. *Lancet* 1999;**353**:1499–500.

60 Vaessen N, Janssen JA, Heutink P, Hofman A, Lamberts SW, Oostra BA *et al.* Association between genetic variation in the gene for insulin-like growth factor-I and low birth weight. *Lancet* 2002;**359**:1036–7.

61 Frayling TM, Hattersley AT, McCarthy A, Holly J, Mitchell SM, Gloyn AL *et al.* A putative functional polymorphism in the IGF-I gene: association studies with type 2 diabetes, adult height, glucose tolerance, and fetal growth in U.K. populations. *Diabetes* 2002;**51**:2313–6.

62 Lawlor DA, Davey SG, Ebrahim S. Birth weight of offspring and insulin resistance in late adulthood: cross sectional survey. *Br Med J* 2002;**325**:359–62.

63 Lindsay RS, Dabelea D, Roumain J, Hanson RL, Bennett PH, Knowler WC. Type 2 diabetes and low birth weight: the role of paternal inheritance in the association of low birth weight and diabetes. *Diabetes* 2000;**49**:445–9.

64 Hypponen E, Smith GD, Power C. Parental diabetes and birth weight of offspring: intergenerational cohort study. *Br Med J* 2003;**326**:19–20.

65 Sobngwi E, Boudou P, Mauvais-Jarvis F, Leblanc H, Velho G, Vexiau P *et al.* Effect of a diabetic environment *in utero* on predisposition to type 2 diabetes. *Lancet* 2003;**361**:1861–5.

66 Perusse L, Despres JP, Lemieux S, Rice T, Rao DC, Bouchard C. Familial aggregation of abdominal visceral fat level: results from the Quebec family study. *Metabolism* 1996;**45**:378–82.

67 Hong Y, Rice T, Gagnon J, Despres JP, Nadeau A, Perusse L *et al.* Familial clustering of insulin and abdominal visceral fat: the HERITAGE Family Study. *J Clin Endocrinol Metab* 1998;**83**:4239–45.

68 Henkin L, Bergman RN, Bowden DW, Ellsworth DL, Haffner SM, Langefeld CD *et al.* Genetic epidemiology of insulin resistance and visceral adiposity. The IRAS Family Study design and methods. *Ann Epidemiol* 2003;**13**:211–17.

69 Neel JV. Diabetes mellitus: a 'thrifty' genotype rendered detrimental by 'progress'. *Am J Hum Genet* 1962;**14**:353–62.

70 Dowse GK, Zimmet PZ, Finch CF, Collins VR. Decline in incidence of epidemic glucose intolerance in Nauruans: implications for the "thrifty genotype". *Am J Epidemiol* 1991;**133**:1093–104.

71 McKeigue PM, Miller GJ, Marmot MG. Coronary heart disease in south Asians overseas: a review. *J Clin Epidemiol* 1989;**42**:597–609.

72 Hughes K, Yeo PP, Lun KC, Thai AC, Sothy SP, Wang KW *et al.* Cardiovascular diseases in Chinese, Malays, and Indians in Singapore. II. Differences in risk factor levels. *J Epidemiol Commun Health* 1990;**44**:29–35.

73 Serjeantson SW, Owerbach D, Zimmet P, Nerup J, Thoma K. Genetics of diabetes in Nauru: effects of foreign admixture, HLA antigens and the insulin-gene-linked polymorphism. *Diabetologia* 1983;**25**:13–17.

74 Knowler WC, Williams RC, Pettitt DJ, Steinberg AG. Gm3;5,13,14 and type 2 diabetes mellitus: an association in American Indians with genetic admixture. *Am J Hum Genet* 1988;**43**:520–6.

75 Phillips DI, Walker BR, Reynolds RM, Flanagan DE, Wood PJ, Osmond C *et al*. Low birth weight predicts elevated plasma cortisol concentrations in adults from 3 populations. *Hypertension* 2000;**35**:1301–6.

76 Kajantie E, Phillips DI, Andersson S, Barker DJ, Dunkel L, Forsen T *et al*. Size at birth, gestational age and cortisol secretion in adult life: foetal programming of both hyper- and hypocortisolism? *Clin Endocrinol (Oxf)* 2002;**57**:635–41.

77 Lindsay RS, Lindsay RM, Waddell BJ, Seckl JR. Prenatal glucocorticoid exposure leads to offspring hyperglycaemia in the rat: studies with the 11 beta-hydroxysteroid dehydrogenase inhibitor carbenoxolone. *Diabetologia* 1996;**39**:1299–305.

78 Strandberg TE, Jarvenpaa AL, Vanhanen H, McKeigue PM. Birth outcome in relation to licorice consumption during pregnancy. *Am J Epidemiol* 2001;**153**:1085–8.

79 Choi CS, Kim C, Lee WJ, Park JY, Hong SK, Lee MG *et al*. Association between birth weight and insulin sensitivity in healthy young men in Korea: role of visceral adiposity. *DiabetRes Clin Pract* 2000;**49**:53–9.

80 Reynolds RM, Chapman KE, Seckl JR, Walker BR, McKeigue PM, Lithell HO. Skeletal muscle glucocorticoid receptor density and insulin resistance. *J Am Med Assoc* 2002;**287**:2505–6.

81 Paneth N, Susser M. Early origin of coronary heart disease (the "Barker hypothesis"). *Br Med J* 1995;**310**:411–12.

82 Kramer MS, Joseph KS. Enigma of fetal/infant-origins hypothesis. *Lancet* 1996;**348**:1254–5.

*83 Lucas A, Fewtrell MS, Cole TJ. Fetal origins of adult disease—the hypothesis revisited. *Br Med J* 1999;**319**:245–9.

84 Wilkin TJ, Metcalf BS, Murphy MJ, Kirkby J, Jeffery AN, Voss LD. The relative contributions of birth weight, weight change, and current weight to insulin resistance in contemporary 5-year-olds: the Early Bird Study. *Diabetes* 2002;**51**:3468–72.

85 Vanhala MJ, Vanhala PT, Keinanen-Kiukaanniemi SM, Kumpusalo EA, Takala JK. Relative weight gain and obesity as a child predict metabolic syndrome as an adult. *Int J Obes Relat Metab Disord* 1999;**23**:656–9.

86 Vanhala M, Vanhala P, Kumpusalo E, Halonen P, Takala J. Relation between obesity from childhood to adulthood and the metabolic syndrome: population based study. *Br Med J* 1998;**317**:319.

87 Bundred P, Kitchiner D, Buchan I. Prevalence of overweight and obese children between 1989 and 1998: population based series of cross sectional studies. *Br Med J* 2001;**322**:326–8.

88 Ebbeling CB, Pawlak DB, Ludwig DS. Childhood obesity: public-health crisis, common sense cure. *Lancet* 2002;**360**:473–82.

89 Fagot-Campagna A. Emergence of type 2 diabetes mellitus in children: epidemiological evidence. *J Pediatr Endocrinol Metab* 2000;**13**(**suppl 6**):1395–402.

90 Ehtisham S, Barrett TG, Shaw NJ. Type 2 diabetes mellitus in UK children—an emerging problem. *Diabet Med* 2000;**17**:867–71.

91 Ludwig DS, Ebbeling CB. Type 2 diabetes mellitus in children: primary care and public health considerations. *J Am Med Assoc* 2001;**286**:1427–30.

92 Steinberger J, Daniels SR. Obesity, insulin resistance, diabetes, and cardiovascular risk in children: an American Heart Association scientific statement from the Atherosclerosis, Hypertension, and Obesity in the Young Committee (Council on Cardiovascular Disease in the Young) and the Diabetes Committee (Council on Nutrition, Physical Activity, and Metabolism). *Circulation* 2003;**107**:1448–53.

93 **Boyko EJ.** Proportion of type 2 diabetes cases resulting from impaired fetal growth. *Diabet Care* 2000;**23**:1260–4.

94 **World Health Organization (WHO).** *Obesity: preventing and managing the global epidemic.* Technical Report Series Number 894. Geneva: WHO, 2000.

95 **WHO.** Diet, nutrition and the prevention of chronic diseases. Report of a joint WHO/Food and Agriculture Organization expert consultation, Technical Report Series Number 916. Geneva: WHO, 2003

96 **Aerts L, Sodoyez-Goffaux F, Sodoyez JC, Malaisse WJ, Van Assche FA.** The diabetic intrauterine milieu has a long-lasting effect on insulin secretion by B cells and on insulin uptake by target tissues. *Am J Obstet Gynecol* 1988;**159**:1287–92.

97 **Grill V, Johansson B, Jalkanen P, Eriksson UJ.** Influence of severe diabetes mellitus early in pregnancy in the rat: effects on insulin sensitivity and insulin secretion in the offspring. *Diabetologia* 1991;**34**:373–8.

98 **Gauguier D, Bihoreau MT, Ktorza A, Berthault MF, Picon L.** Inheritance of diabetes mellitus as consequence of gestational hyperglycemia in rats. *Diabetes* 1990;**39**:734–9.

99 **Pettitt DJ, Bennett PH, Saad MF, Charles MA, Nelson RG, Knowler WC.** Abnormal glucose tolerance during pregnancy in Pima Indian women. Long-term effects on offspring. *Diabetes* 1991;**40**(**suppl 2**):126–30.

100 **Dabelea D, Knowler WC, Pettitt DJ.** Effect of diabetes in pregnancy on offspring: follow-up research in the Pima Indians. *J Maternal-Fetal Med* 2000;**9**:83–8.

101 **Pettitt DJ, Aleck KA, Baird HR, Carraher MJ, Bennett PH, Knowler WC.** Congenital susceptibility to NIDDM. Role of intrauterine environment. *Diabetes* 1988;**37**:622–8.

102 **Dabelea D, Hanson RL, Lindsay RS, Pettitt DJ, Imperatore G, Gabir MM *et al*.** Intrauterine exposure to diabetes conveys risks for type 2 diabetes and obesity: a study of discordant sibships. *Diabetes* 2000;**49**:2208–11.

103 **King H.** Epidemiology of glucose intolerance and gestational diabetes in women of childbearing age. *Diabet Care* 1998;**21**(**suppl 2**):B9–13.

104 **Wang Y.** Cross-national comparison of childhood obesity: the epidemic and the relationship between obesity and socioeconomic status. *Int J Epidemiol* 2001;**30**:1129–36.

105 **Power C, Moynihan C.** Social class and changes in weight-for-height between childhood and early adulthood. *Int J Obes* 1988;**12**:445–53.

106 **Hardy R, Wadsworth M, Kuh D.** The influence of childhood weight and socioeconomic status on change in adult body mass index in a British national birth cohort. *Int J Obes* 2000;**24**:1–10

*107 **Fall CH.** Non-industrialised countries and affluence. *Br Med Bull* 2001;**60**:33–50.

108 **Whitford DL, Griffin SJ, Prevost AT.** Influences on the variation in prevalence of type 2 diabetes between general practices: practice, patient or socioeconomic factors? *Br J Gen Pract* 2003;**53**:9–14.

109 **Ramachandran A, Snehalatha C, Vinitha R, Thayyil M, Kumar CK, Sheeba L *et al*.** Prevalence of overweight in urban Indian adolescent school children. *Diabetes Res Clin Pract* 2002;**57**:185–90.

110 **Shetty PS.** Obesity in children in developing societies: indicator of economic progress or a prelude to a health disaster? *Indian Pediatr* 1999;**36**:11–15.

111 **Abu SM, Ali L, Hussain MZ, Rumi MA, Banu A, Azad Khan AK.** Effect of socioeconomic risk factors on the difference in prevalence of diabetes between rural and urban populations in Bangladesh. *Diabet Care* 1997;**20**:551–5.

112 **Brunner EJ, Marmot MG, Nanchahal K, Shipley MJ, Stansfeld SA, Juneja M *et al*.** Social inequality in coronary risk: central obesity and the metabolic syndrome. Evidence from the Whitehall II study. *Diabetologia* 1997;**40**:1341–9.

113 **Lawlor DA, Ebrahim S, Davey SG.** British women's heart and health study. Socioeconomic position in childhood and adulthood and insulin resistance: cross sectional survey using data from British women's heart and health study. *Br Med J* 2002;**325**:805–9.

114 **Wamala SP, Lynch J, Horsten M, Mittleman MA, Schenck-Gustafsson K, Orth-Gomer K.** Education and the metabolic syndrome in women. *Diabet Care* 1999;**22**:1999–2003.

115 **Wadsworth ME, Hardy RJ, Paul AA, Marshall SF, Cole TJ.** Leg and trunk length at 43 years in relation to childhood health, diet and family circumstances; evidence from the 1946 national birth cohort. *Int J Epidemiol* 2002;**31**:383–90.

116 **Smith GD, Greenwood R, Gunnell D, Sweetnam P, Yarnell J, Elwood P.** Leg length, insulin resistance, and coronary heart disease risk: the Caerphilly Study. *J Epidemiol Commun Health* 2001;**55**:867–72.

117 **Lawlor DA, Ebrahim S, Davey SG.** The association between components of adult height and Type II diabetes and insulin resistance: British Women's Heart and Health Study. *Diabetologia* 2002;**45**:1097–106.

118 **Carlsson S, Persson PG, Alvarsson M, Efendic S, Norman A, Svanstrom L** *et al.* Low birth weight, family history of diabetes, and glucose intolerance in Swedish middle-aged men. *Diabet Care* 1999;**22**:1043–7.

119 **Birgisdottir BE, Gunnarsdottir I, Thorsdottir I, Gudnason V, Benediktsson R.** Size at birth and glucose intolerance in a relatively genetically homogeneous, high-birth weight population. *Am J Clin Nutr* 2002;**76**:399–403.

120 **Robinson S, Walton RJ, Clark PM, Barker DJ, Hales CN, Osmond C.** The relation of fetal growth to plasma glucose in young men. *Diabetologia* 1992;**35**:444–6.

121 **Leger J, Levy-Marchal C, Bloch J, Pinet A, Chevenne D, Porquet D** *et al.* Reduced final height and indications for insulin resistance in 20 year olds born small for gestational age: regional cohort study. *Br Med J* 1997;**315**:341–7.

122 **Lawlor DA, Davey SG, Ebrahim S.** Life course influences on insulin resistance: findings from the British Women's Heart and Health Study. *Diabet Care* 2003;**26**:97–103.

123 **Murtaugh MA, Jacobs DR Jr, Moran A, Steinberger J, Sinaiko AR.** Relation of birth weight to fasting insulin, insulin resistance, and body size in adolescence. *Diabet Care* 2003;**26**:187–92.

124 **Mi J, Law C, Zhang KL, Osmond C, Stein C, Barker D.** Effects of infant birth weight and maternal body mass index in pregnancy on components of the insulin resistance syndrome in China. *Ann Intern Med* 2000;**132**:253–60.

Chapter 8

A life course approach to obesity

Matthew W. Gillman

Obesity, a major risk factor for many chronic diseases, is rising in prevalence in the developing as well as the developed world. Early life prevention is important as treatment of established obesity is largely ineffectual. Evidence is growing that factors from the prenatal period through adolescence are important determinants of excess weight gain. These factors may span a wide spectrum from the societal level through lifestyle to biological factors. The current research agenda includes not only how to identify and quantify determinants at each life stage, but how to tackle the analytic challenges of figuring out how these determinants act in concert with each other and over time. Interventions that address multiple behaviours with tested behaviour change strategies may have the best chance of interrupting what appears to be a vicious cycle of increasing obesity and its complications over generations.

8.1 Introduction

The prevalence of obesity has risen dramatically—perhaps exponentially—in the developed world over the past four decades, in both children (Fig. 8.1) and adults (Fig. 8.2).[1–9] In the USA, the Surgeon General has estimated that obesity may soon surpass cigarette smoking as the leading cause of morbidity and mortality.[6] Adult obesity causes heart disease, stroke, gallbladder disease, infertility, respiratory disorders, some cancers, and most strikingly, type 2 diabetes (Fig. 8.3).[10,11] Emerging evidence shows that obesity in childhood and adolescence is also associated with both short- and long-term adverse outcomes.[12–17] The rise of obesity in the developed world could actually presage a recrudescence of ischaemic heart disease, which had been on the decline in the late twentieth century in most western countries.

Equally noteworthy, the developing world is beginning to witness the early stages of the obesity epidemic.[18] The tendency to urbanize and industrialize, featuring reductions in daily physical activity and increases in energy intake, is accompanied by increases in obesity and a transition from infections and undernutrition to chronic western illnesses (Fig. 8.4).[19] Indeed, Murray and Lopez[20] estimated that by 2020, cardiovascular diseases—well-known sequelae of obesity—will be the leading causes of death and disability worldwide.

Children who are overweight tend to become overweight adults, and once present, obesity is notoriously hard to treat.[21–24] Thus prevention, starting in early life, is

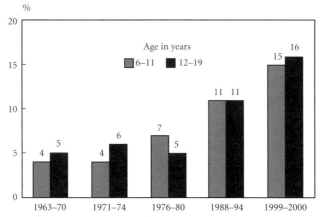

Fig. 8.1 Prevalence of overweight among children and adolescents aged 6–19 years. Data from US national surveys from 1960s to 1990s.[6,9] Overweight is body mass index exceeding the age- and sex-specific 95th percentile from US national reference data.[28]

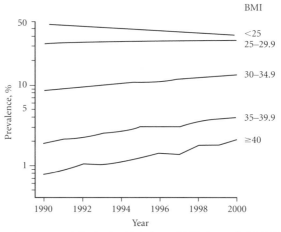

Fig. 8.2 Secular trends among adults in the USA from 1990 through 2000 in the prevalence of normal weight (body mass index (BMI) <25 kg/m^2), overweight (BMI 25–29.9), and classes 1, 2, and 3 obesity (BMI 30–34.9, 35–39.9, and ≥40).[8]

potentially crucial to stemming the rising tide of obesity. Prevention of obesity is particularly suited to a life course perspective. Its aetiology is multidimensional, including biological, behavioural, and social processes. In addition, its development likely encompasses both critical (or sensitive) periods and accumulation of risk over time.

A critical period involves the concept of biological programming, in which an environmental influence causes irreversible metabolic consequences that alter susceptibility to later adverse outcomes. As we outline in the section on fetal life, evidence exists that altered glucose–insulin metabolism *in utero* may lead to increased risk for obesity later in life. The term sensitive period is more often used for influences that can alter behaviour

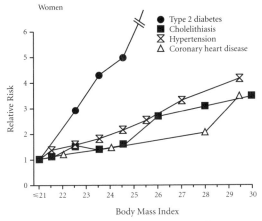

Fig. 8.3 Relationship between body mass index up to 30 kg/m² and the relative risk of type 2 diabetes, hypertension, coronary heart disease, and cholelithiasis. Data from participants in the US Nurses' Health Study, initially 30–55 years of age, who were followed for up to 18 years.[10]

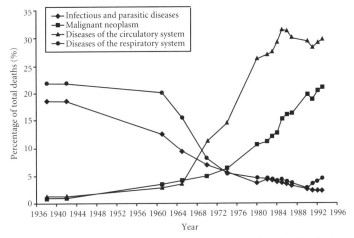

Fig. 8.4 Trends in cause of death in South Korea, 1938–1993, showing the 'epidemiologic transition' from respiratory and infectious diseases to cardiovascular diseases and cancer.[19]

or metabolism long-term, but are not as deterministic as critical periods. For example, long-term physical activity habits may be set during childhood or adolescence.[25] Another reason that early life prevention of obesity is vital is that with weight gain the organism may find a new metabolic 'set point,' in which efforts to lose weight are thwarted by the body's desire to return to recently acquired body weight status.[26] For all of these reasons, identification of modifiable early life determinants of obesity and effective strategies to alter them appear to be crucial steps in curbing the epidemic. Thus this chapter focuses on such non-genetic determinants from fetal life to adolescence.

8.2 Measurement of overweight and obesity

While fatness is the entity of interest, the inherent limitations of large epidemiologic studies often require use of proxies for adiposity. From early childhood to at least middle adulthood, body mass index (BMI; kg/m^2) is the best proxy. Height and weight are easily measured, even by self-report of children who are at least 10 years old.[27] However, BMI represents not only fat, but also lean tissue. Thus, for example, muscular adolescents can have relatively high BMI in the absence of excess adiposity. In addition, BMI changes with linear growth and sexual maturation, making it advisable to account for these covariates in analyses of children and adolescents. In smaller studies, it is feasible to use more direct measures of fatness, such as skinfold thicknesses or more extensive methods for assessing body composition, including dual x-ray absorptiometry, computed tomography, and magnetic resonance imaging.

In adulthood, one standard definition of obesity is BMI exceeding 30 kg/m^2; overweight is BMI between 25 and 30 kg/m^2. In childhood and adolescence, however, BMI rises with age even if adiposity is constant, so setting explicit numerical cut-points is impossible over a wide range of ages. Percentile cut-points are more useful, but even so, definitions vary for the dichotomous outcomes of obesity, overweight, and 'at risk for overweight'. The US Centers for Disease Control and Prevention defines overweight as BMI exceeding the 95th percentile for age and sex and 'at risk for overweight' as between the 85th and 95th percentiles.[28] They recommend against using the term obesity unless additional information about adiposity or comorbidities is available. But others do use BMI cut-points alone to define overweight and obesity, so readers should be careful to inspect the specific definitions used in each publication. For example, using combined growth data from six countries, Cole and colleagues[29] estimated BMI cut-points for overweight and for obesity from ages 2 to 17 years that correspond to 25 and 30 kg/m^2 at age 18 years.

In addition to overall adiposity, fat distribution is important. Centrally deposited fat is more metabolically active than peripheral fat. Compared with the peripheral pattern ('pear shape'), the central pattern ('apple shape') is more strongly associated with insulin resistance and its concomitants, glucose intolerance, hypertension, and dyslipidaemia.[30]

Most studies reviewed in this chapter use BMI as the primary measure of fatness. Where data are available we include more direct measures of adiposity as well as measures of central obesity in addition to overall obesity.

8.3 Critical or sensitive periods for obesity development

Dietz[31,32] has hypothesized three periods in early life that are particularly important for the development of obesity—the prenatal period, the period of adiposity rebound, and adolescence. Hypothesizing that environmental exposures may do more damage at these developmental stages than at other times, he called them critical periods, although he did not distinguish critical from sensitive periods in the way we have outlined above. While this hypothesis provides a convenient framework for exploring the life course approach to obesity, these three periods may not be the only ones that entrain the development of obesity. In particular recent data also suggest that infancy may be an important aetiologic period. The remainder of this chapter is devoted to

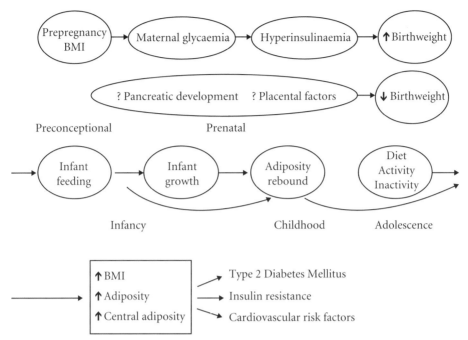

Fig. 8.5 Schematic of life course approach to obesity, showing selected determinants at various developmental stages and some hypothesized causal sequences among them.

discussing determinants of obesity during these four periods, as reflected in the examples depicted in Fig. 8.5.

8.4 The prenatal period

8.4.1 Higher birthweight is associated with later body mass index

More than a score of studies have addressed the association between birthweight and either childhood or, less commonly, adult BMI. Almost all of the studies have found that higher birthweight is associated with higher attained BMI.[33–49] Some of the smaller studies have found no association;[50–54] none has found an inverse association. The typical effect size ranges from 0.6 to 0.7 kg/m^2 for each 1 kg increment in birthweight.[49]

Limitations of most of these studies have included incomplete data on gestational age, birth length, socioeconomic factors, and parental adiposity. Parental adiposity is particularly important: one explanation for the birthweight–BMI findings is that a postnatal environment that includes adverse eating and activity habits shared by family members, and reflected in maternal obesity, is related to both higher birthweight and later adiposity. Another is that genes shared between parents and child entrain both birthweight and later obesity.

A few studies have attempted to control for parental obesity and other potentially confounding influences. In the US Growing Up Today Study, a cohort study of over

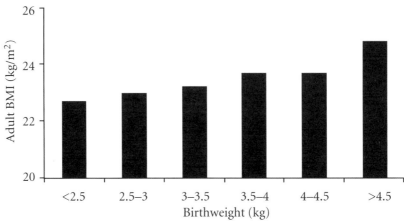

Fig. 8.6 Body mass index (BMI) at ages 18–26 years in Danish military conscripts by birthweight. Estimates are adjusted for gestational age, birth length, birth order, mother's marital status, age, and occupation. Adult BMI rises monotonically with birthweight.[49]

14 000 adolescents, a 1 kg increment in birthweight among full-term infants was associated with an approximately 50% increase in the risk of overweightness (BMI exceeding the age- and sex-specific 95th percentile) at ages 9–14 years. The effect declined to approximately 30% after adjustment for maternal BMI, with no further attenuation after control for additional social and economic factors.[55] In a study of Danish military conscripts, a monotonic increase of BMI with increasing birthweight was evident after adjustment for birth length and maternal factors (Fig. 8.6).[49] In contrast, Parsons and colleagues[56] published 33-year follow-up data from the 1958 British birth cohort showing that maternal BMI explained most or all of the association between birthweight and adult BMI. This study also had data on gestational age, paternal body size at one time point, social class, and maternal smoking.

Overall, the preponderance of evidence indicates that higher birthweight is associated with increased risk of adiposity in childhood and adulthood, as reflected by BMI. In most but not all of the few studies that have been able to control for confounding factors, the birthweight–obesity relationship remains, suggesting a persistent impact of the fetal environment.[57]

8.4.2 Possible mechanisms for an association between birthweight and later adiposity

Research into the fetal origins of adult diseases generally relies on the assumption of programming, the process by which a stimulus occurring at a critical period of development has lasting effect.[58] For fetal origins of obesity, most evidence to date comes from the special circumstance of diabetes during pregnancy. While maternal glucose freely crosses the placenta to the fetus, maternal insulin does not.[59] The developing fetal pancreas responds to a glucose load by producing additional insulin. As insulin acts as a fetal growth hormone, exposure to hyperglycaemia may produce fetal adiposity.[59,60]

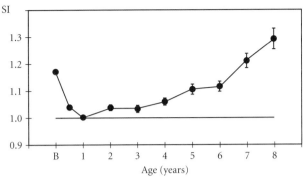

Fig. 8.7 Symmetry index (SI, mean ± SEM) in offspring of diabetic mothers from birth to 8 years of age. SI = (weight/National Center for Health Statistics median weight for age)/(height/National Center for Health Statistics median height for age).[195] Copyright American Diabetes Association © 1991.

Human studies have addressed this theory of 'fuel-mediated teratogenesis' by examining offspring of diabetic mothers. Silverman and colleagues found that between ages 14 and 17 years, offspring of mothers with gestational diabetes had a mean BMI of 26.0 kg/m^2, compared with 20.9 kg/m^2 in control participants.[53] Interestingly, the increased adiposity was apparent at birth and progressively after about the age of 4 years, but not at younger ages (Fig. 8.7). Also in that study, amniotic fluid insulin levels, which reflect fetal pancreatic insulin production, correlated with obesity during adolescence.

In a study from the Pima Indian community, Dabelea and colleagues[61] examined BMI among siblings aged 6–24 years whose fetal lives were discordant for the presence of maternal diabetes. From age 9 years onwards, offspring exposed to diabetes *in utero* had higher BMI than their unexposed siblings (Fig. 8.8). This study is important because it mitigates the roles of both shared genes and postnatal environment, likely similar within a sibling set, thus emphasizing the potential role of the fetal environment.

Other studies, perhaps because they took place in areas where diabetes is of lower prevalence than the studies cited above, have not shown clear associations of maternal gestational diabetes with offspring obesity.[55,62] This issue is critical to resolve, as programming of offspring adiposity by maternal glucose–insulin metabolism could lead to a vicious cycle of childhood obesity and gestational diabetes over generations.

To understand the mechanisms underlying a potential role of maternal diabetes in offspring obesity, Plagemann and colleagues have experimentally induced gestational diabetes among rats. In adulthood, the offspring of these rats demonstrate hyperphagia, hyperinsulinaemia, impaired glucose tolerance, and overweight.[63] These investigators have described several potential pathways, including increased levels of orexigenic (appetite-enhancing) neurotransmitters, increased sensitivity to orexigenic neurotransmitters, and decreased levels of satiety signals, potentially mediated through a hypothesized mechanism of induced hypothalamic insulin resistance.[64–67]

Animal findings cannot be directly translated to humans, as sensitive periods and mechanisms may differ between species. In addition, the animal studies noted above address just one possible set of mechanisms. Nevertheless these studies support

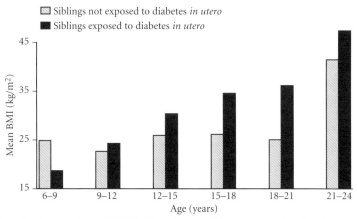

Fig. 8.8 Mean body mass index (BMI) in Pima Indian siblings exposed and not exposed to diabetic intrauterine environment, separated into 3-year age intervals. Siblings exposed have a higher BMI than those unexposed. Adapted from Reference 61.

epidemiologic observations that influences in fetal life, specifically nutrient excess and insulin exposure, can have long-term impact on gene expression and body weight regulation.

Scant epidemiologic evidence exists regarding the effects of maternal prenatal nutrition on offspring obesity. In one terrible 'natural experiment', pregnant women were exposed to severe malnutrition during the Nazi occupation of the Netherlands in the winter of 1944–1945. The effects of the severe energy restriction on birthweight were modest, but at age 18 years, male offspring of mothers exposed in the first trimester of pregnancy had higher rates of obesity than those exposed later in gestation.[68] In follow-up of males from this population at age 50 years, however, no BMI differences were apparent. At that age, females exposed in the first trimester appeared to have higher BMI than unexposed females.[69] Given that the malnutrition was balanced across nutrients and that the long-term findings are variable, the Dutch Hunger Winter experience teaches us that some aspects of prenatal maternal nutrition may be important in the genesis of obesity, but is non-specific as to which aspects and to timing of insults.

Food rationing also occurred during the siege of Leningrad between 1941 and 1945, with the worst energy deprivation during the winter of 1941–1942. Stanner and colleagues[70] followed up a group of approximately 450 survivors some 50 years later and compared outcomes among those whose mothers were exposed to famine prenatally, postnatally, and not at all. No differences were apparent among these groups in BMI, waist-to-hip ratio, or skinfold thicknesses. These data thus provide no corroborating evidence for long-lasting effects of maternal malnutrition during pregnancy, but in contrast to the Dutch Hunger Winter studies, trimester-specific data were not available.

8.4.3 Lower birthweight is associated with later central obesity

Several studies have addressed the association of birthweight with measures of central obesity in both childhood and adulthood,[34,71–74] as well as with measures of insulin resistance and the metabolic syndrome.[52,73,75–83] Although not evident in all populations studied, in general these studies show that, after adjustment for attained BMI, birthweight is *inversely* associated with these three outcomes. Thus, the lower the birthweight, the higher the risk of central obesity, insulin resistance, and the insulin resistance syndrome phenotype in later life. Rates of central obesity and insulin resistance are highest in those born small but who are overweight later.[34,35,84–86]

The mechanisms of these associations remain unknown. Inherited genetic factors such as alterations in insulin regulation may play a role.[87,88] It is also possible that intrauterine exposures lead to persistent metabolic changes, resulting in a 'thrifty phenotype'.[89] Indeed, long-term changes in the activation of the hypothalamic–pituitary–adrenal axis may mediate these associations.[90,91]

Whatever the mechanisms, it is becoming clear that after adjustment for attained BMI, lower birthweight is associated with increased later central adiposity and its metabolic consequences. Thus we are faced with the seeming paradox of increased adiposity at both ends of the birthweight spectrum—higher BMI with higher birthweight and increased central adiposity at lower birthweights.

8.4.4 Implications for public health

Further research is needed to disentangle these effects. For example, what are the relations of fat and lean among babies born at lower birthweights? Which determinants of birthweight underlie the BMI associations and which the central adiposity associations? Public health interventions to alter the fetal environment await these inquiries.

In the meantime, the data have clear implications for childhood interventions. Several studies now indicate that the highest risk for cardiovascular outcomes is associated with the phenotype of lower birthweight and higher BMI in childhood or adulthood. Examples include elevated incidence of coronary heart disease in Welsh men aged 45–59 years;[92] the highest systolic blood pressure among Swedish men at age 50;[93] highest risk ratios for coronary disease among Finnish men;[94] highest insulin resistance among 8-year-old Indian children,[35] and highest rates of central obesity among adolescent girls in England.[34] Moreover, the combination of lower birthweight and higher attained BMI is characteristic of developing world populations undergoing the transition to urban lifestyles as well as of groups of lower social class in the developed world.[95–97] The remainder of this chapter, therefore, addresses obesity determinants and prevention in childhood and adolescence.

8.5 Infancy

In the first year of life, a primary determinant of later obesity appears to be type and duration of infant feeding. Two decades ago, Kramer[98] published two linked case–control studies showing lower rates of obesity among Canadian adolescents who had been breastfed as infants and, to a lesser extent, duration of breastfeeding. In the interim, several other published studies produced variable results, but they had several limitations, including lack of data on duration of breastfeeding, inadequate sample sizes, lack of data on important confounding variables, and end-points measured at relatively young ages.[44,99–103] However, four studies have recently been published that have addressed these limitations, at least in part.

In 1999, von Kries and colleagues[104] investigated the relationship between breast-feeding and obesity among over 9000 German children given compulsory examinations for school entry. Two years later, the *Journal of the American Medical Association* published back-to-back articles addressing the same issue, one among over 15 000 US adolescents and the other among approximately 2700 young US children.[105,106] Within the following two years, three other similar articles appeared, one among over 2000 9–10-year German children,[107] another involving nearly 34 000 Czech children and adolescents,[108] and a third among 32 000 Scottish 3-year-olds.[109] Notwithstanding some differences in methodology, the six studies are quite consistent in showing a reduced risk of obesity among children and adolescents who had been breastfed as infants. Consistency of effect size was more evident with use of the more extreme BMI cut-points (90th or 97th percentile for the European studies, 95th for the US studies), which is more likely to represent true adiposity than the less extreme cut-points.[110,111] Using the more extreme cut-points, adjusted odds ratios for breast versus formula feeding ranged from 0.66 to 0.84 across the six studies. Three of the studies[104,105,107] also showed a 'dose–response' effect: the longer the duration of breastfeeding, the lower the risk of being overweight or obese later in childhood (Fig. 8.9).

If breastfeeding protects against later obesity, at least two mechanisms could be at play. Children naturally regulate their energy intake, but parents' behaviour may override the appetite signals. In cross-sectional studies, Birch and Fisher[112] have reported that pre-school children of parents who used a high degree of control over the quantity their children ate had lower self-regulation of energy intake. Among the girls but not the boys, there was also increased adiposity. During infancy, it is possible that, compared with parents who bottle feed, mothers who breastfeed may be more responsive to the infant's signals for frequency and volume of feedings. A second mechanism could be related to the metabolic influences of ingested breast milk. Lucas and colleagues[113,114] found lower concentrations of serum insulin in infants fed breast milk than those fed infant formula.

The key limitation of all such observational studies is the inability to control completely for the joint cultural determinants of both breastfeeding and later obesity. While all four of the highlighted studies made attempts to do so, residual confounding by these factors could still exist. This limitation highlights the need for new studies with information on these potentially confounding social and economic factors.[115]

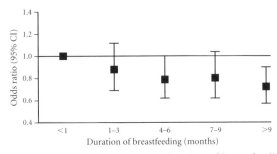

Fig. 8.9 Risk of being overweight in adolescence by duration of breastfeeding in infancy. Multivariate adjusted odds ratio and 95% confidence interval for each category compared with the reference group of never breastfed or breastfed less than 1 month.[105]

Nevertheless, the bulk of evidence to date indicates no adverse effects of breastfeeding on later obesity and a probable beneficial effect. Given the myriad reasons to promote breastfeeding in both the developed and developing world, it appears that adding the potential of obesity prevention to the list has few risks.

Two recent studies address the extent to which *infant growth* predicts later obesity. Among approximately 28 000 term infants born in the USA in the 1950s and 1960s, rapid weight gain in the first 4 months of life was associated with increased risk of overweight at age 7 years.[116] These findings were independent of birthweight and weight at 1 year. In a UK study, 848 full-term singleton babies were categorized as having 'catch-up growth' if they showed a gain of 0.67 standard deviations for weight between birth and 2 years. At age 5 years, these children had higher BMI as well as waist circumference, a measure of central adiposity, than other children.[117] Given their different metrics, the results of these two studies are difficult to compare directly. In addition, neither followed participants to older childhood or adolescence, when the long-term consequences of overweight are more clear. Nevertheless, they raise the possibility that growth in infancy may have a lasting impact on risk of later obesity. Another study showed that, after adjustment for adult BMI, both birthweight and relative weight at age 7 years were inversely associated with measures of central obesity at age 43 years.[74] In that study, however, the authors did not address the rapidity of growth between birth and age 7 years.

8.6 **The period of 'adiposity rebound'**

In general, individuals' BMIs increase rapidly in the first year of life, but then decrease to a nadir at 4–8 years before rising again into adulthood (Fig. 8.10). In the 1980s,

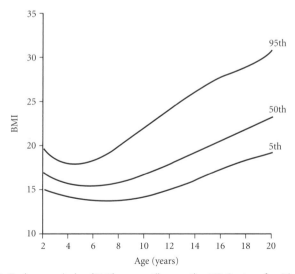

Fig. 8.10 Body mass index (BMI) percentiles on the US Centers for Disease and Prevention growth charts, showing the BMI nadir (adiposity rebound) at approximately ages 4–8 years. Earlier rebound occurs at higher BMI percentiles.[196]

Rolland-Cachera and colleagues[118] noted that in a small cohort of French children, those whose nadir came at younger ages had higher BMI in teenage years. Subsequently several studies have confirmed that younger age at 'adiposity rebound' is associated with higher BMI or risk of obesity one to two decades later.[118–124] However, several concerns may limit the usefulness of these findings.

The first limitation is that BMI is not a direct measure of adiposity, but incorporates both lean and fat mass. Whether a true adiposity nadir predicts increased risk of obesity is not known. One study[121] did show differences in adult subscapular skinfold thicknesses between early and late BMI rebounders, but no study has included skinfold thicknesses in childhood. Further, the curvilinear pattern of BMI over childhood years is a function of changing weight versus height^2 relationships with age, not necessarily an underlying biological phenomenon relating to fatness. For example, if (the square of) linear growth increases faster than weight at a certain point in childhood, BMI will go down, even if true fatness does not. Other adiposity indices do not show the same age pattern as BMI. Ponderal index (weight/height^3) decreases to about age 6 years and is flat thereafter; percentage of body fat follows a similar pattern; and in boys, triceps skinfold thickness shows two nadirs, one at 6–8 years and one at 15–17 years.[119]

These considerations have led investigators recently to question both the biological meaning and clinical application of the adiposity rebound. Freedman and colleagues[119] have shown that BMI at age 7–8 years is at least as good a predictor of young adult BMI as the age at minimum BMI. These findings extend the observations of Williams and colleagues,[124] who reported similar correlations between BMI at ages 18–21 years with both age at adiposity rebound and BMI at age 7 years. While Whitaker and colleagues[123] found associations of early versus late adiposity rebound with obesity at ages 21–29 years independent of childhood BMI, they used only three categories of childhood BMI at the time of the adiposity rebound rather than BMI at age 7–8 years.

While the influence of age at minimum BMI on later obesity is reproducible across studies, there is no current biological explanation for why this should be so. Rolland-Cachera and colleagues[118] hypothesized that early adiposity rebound is associated with increased number of fat cells, but no empirical data have supported this association. Another hypothesis is behavioural. The studies of Birch and Fisher[112] mentioned above, regarding self-regulation of energy intake among pre-school children, raise one possible explanation. It is possible that parents try harder to have children who are quickly losing 'baby fat' eat more, with no effect on timing of BMI minimum but an adverse influence on long-term overeating. However, these are speculations based on a small amount of cross-sectional research in selected populations and would need direct confirmation from careful longitudinal studies.

The clinical implications of early adiposity rebound are also not clear. In practice, one might want to 'prevent' early adiposity rebound, but identifying the age of minimum BMI for an individual child is by necessity retrospective. Also, prevention requires identification of determinants, but in a study of dietary and socioeconomic factors associated with early adiposity rebound among 889 UK children, the only consistent predictor was parental obesity, a known risk factor for offspring obesity itself.[125]

The final limitation is that children with early adiposity rebound actually have higher age-specific BMI than children with later rebound (see Fig. 8.10). As BMI is easier to ascertain and is equally predictive,[119] it is more useful clinically. In addition, given the shape of the BMI-for-age curve, pre-school children who are crossing BMI centiles in the upward direction will mathematically have earlier observed BMI rebound (Cole T, unpublished).

In conclusion, the observation that early age of minimum BMI is associated with later obesity is fascinating and may reveal biological insights, but may ultimately not be of much use in clinical medicine or public health. To a certain extent, the phenomenon seems to be a function of the fact that 'early rebounders' are really 'early weight gainers' and that the BMI nadir is an artefact of the limitations of the weight/height^2 measure that we accept as the most useful measure of adiposity. Currently it appears that the most useful childhood predictor of adult obesity is the child's own BMI, especially at older ages.[22] Parental obesity is also an important predictor in younger children, but becomes less important as the child grows.[22]

8.7 Older children and adolescents

While the pre-teen and teenage years may not constitute a truly critical period, they appear to be quite important in the life course development of obesity. Whitaker and colleagues[22] have shown that children who are obese between 10 and 17 years of age have about 20 times the odds of becoming obese in young adulthood compared with their non-obese counterparts. Adolescent obesity is associated both with short-term morbidity, including cardiovascular risk factors, orthopaedic conditions, lower self-esteem, poor social and economic outcomes in young adulthood,[12–15] and long-term adult morbidity and mortality.[16,17] Puberty is a time of rapid acceleration and deceleration of height growth; relative weight changes tend to be rapid as well. In girls, early menarche is associated with obesity.[126] In addition, post-pubertal fat deposition appears to favour the more adverse central pattern in both boys and girls.[127] While boys tend not to gain as much fat overall as girls during the teenage years, the tendency towards central deposition of fat may be more pronounced in boys.[31]

Fundamentally, excess weight gain and thus obesity are caused by a surplus of energy intake compared with energy expenditure over time, after accounting for energy intake needed for growth. Physical activity accounts for most variation in energy expenditure and what we eat provides energy intake. In this section we address physical activity and its relative, inactivity, as well as dietary factors in the context of older childhood and adolescence.

8.7.1 Physical activity

Over time, even a small daily increment of energy intake compared with energy expenditure leads to excess weight gain. This concept is particularly important in the adolescent years, during which time levels of physical activity decline, especially among girls.[128–131] For example, in the US National Growth and Health Study, a longitudinal study of black and white girls, the decline began at or before entry into the study at age 9–10 years. Particularly striking was the steep decline among black girls, to a median of 0 h/week in total activity by the age of 16 or 17 years.[131] Black girls also gained more weight than white girls over 10 years of follow-up in that study.[132] The combination of decreasing activity levels with age and an overall secular decrease with time[133] is particularly harmful. Counteracting these trends requires knowledge both of their modifiable determinants as well as effective behaviour change strategies.

Only recently have longitudinal data begun to emerge on the role of physical activity in the modulation of adiposity in older children and adolescents. Among 9–14-year-old girls in the US Growing Up Today Study each increment in 1 h/day of physical activity at baseline was associated with a relative BMI decrease of 0.03 kg/m^2 over a 1-year period.[134] More recent analyses from this cohort show that *changes* in physical activity level over a 1-year period were inversely associated with BMI change over the same year, especially among overweight girls and boys.[135] In addition, a study of young adults aged between 18 and 30 years at baseline, showed that increasing physical activity over a 10-year follow-up period was accompanied by decreasing body weight.[136]

Future interventions can benefit from increased knowledge of the determinants of physical activity level and change among adolescents. As physical activity among youth is a complex behaviour determined by multiple factors, most authors have divided variables into categories, such as personal (including biological, psychological, and behavioural), social/cultural, and physical environment.[137]

8.7.1.1 Personal variables

Some biological variables such as age, sex, and ethnicity[137–139] are not modifiable but can identify groups at risk of being inactive. Most studies that examined ethnicity as a correlate of physical activity found that non-Hispanic white people in the USA were more active than other ethnic groups.[140] In at least one study socioeconomic status was not closely related to physical activity in adolescents.[141]

A few psychological variables such as achievement orientation, perceived physical competence, and intention to be active are consistently correlated with physical activity in adolescents.[142,143] Some studies have found that perceived benefits, self-efficacy, and body image are positively related to the behaviour, whereas most studies have found general barriers, self-esteem, stress, and enjoyment of exercise are not associated with physical activity in adolescents.[142,144,145] However, most of these inferences derive from cross-sectional, not prospective, studies. Further, the ability to modify many of these factors is questionable. One exception is an analysis of a 1-year follow-up of participants in the National Longitudinal Study of Adolescent Health, a study of almost 10 000 US teenagers. In that cohort, depressed adolescents were twice as likely to develop obesity even after accounting for several potentially confounding variables.[146] Adolescent depression is a potentially treatable condition. Related lifestyle habits and other potential influences on maintenance of activity throughout the teenage years, such as type of activity, have not been well characterized.

Behavioural variables such as previous physical activity and participation in community sports appear to be positively related to physical activity in adolescents.[143,144,147] Previous studies looking at other behavioural variables such as cigarette and alcohol use, participation in school sports teams, healthy diet, and watching television have given variable results.[144,147,148] These inconsistent associations need to be explored in prospective studies that control for confounders.

8.7.1.2 Sociocultural variables

Social support from parents was strongly related to physical activity in most studies but parental physical activity level was inconsistently related.[144,145] More information is needed on parents' attitudes as well as behaviour. Sibling physical activity was consistently related to physical activity in adolescents.[149] Studies looking at perceived social support from peers and peer modelling found inconsistent associations.[145] Specific media influences may be predictive of activity level and change but few data exist.[144] One preliminary analysis from the US Growing Up Today Study suggests that the desire to emulate media role models is associated with increased physical activity.[150]

8.7.1.3 Physical environmental variables

Although some personal and social factors are potentially modifiable, effecting individual behaviour change is difficult and expensive. Thus recent interest has also focused on the possibility of modifying the child's environment, through which individual change is theoretically possible even without direct intervention on the child and family.[151] Potential determinants include access to programmes and settings where children can be active. Barriers to access could include geographical distance as well as lack of transportation, neighbourhood safety, and structured programmes. Previous studies of these factors have given variable results[144,145,148,152,153] due to several potential factors, including reliance only on self-report measures.[154] In addition, intervention studies to assess the effect of changing these factors are lacking.[155]

In summary, previous studies have identified some personal, social, and environmental factors that are related to level of physical activity in adolescents. However, almost all of the studies have been cross-sectional. Few longitudinal studies reported to date have adequate sample sizes or sufficient data on covariates. Many factors that could potentially be modified, for example, type of activity (a personal factor), media influences (a social factor), and proximity to playing areas (an environmental factor), are not well studied.

8.7.2 Inactivity

Inactivity is not just a lack of physical activity. Rather inactivity comprises activities that individuals do while they are sedentary, such as watching television. The notion that television watching causes obesity has existed for close to two decades.[156] It is an important issue, for the average child in the USA may spend as much as five of his or her waking years in front of the television set.[157] One possible mechanism is that children replace physical activity with sedentary television viewing, although correlations between activity and inactivity tend to be low. Another is that children who watch more television have higher energy intake, either because they eat while watching television or because they respond to food commercials.[158,159]

Most of the observational studies examining this issue have been cross-sectional.[156,159–167] Thus the temporal sequence is not clear; it is plausible that obesity could cause more television viewing. Prospective studies are few and possibly conflicting.[158] Fortunately intervention studies are now available, addressed in more detail below, which provide the strongest evidence that television watching causes obesity. Future studies of inactivity will benefit from taking into account newer activities, such as video and computer games and internet use.[148,159]

8.7.3 Diet

Recognizing that excess energy intake leads to obesity is easy. Much harder is identifying which dietary factors lead to excess energy intake. Surprisingly little is known about this topic in children and adolescents and not much more information is available among adults. For some time the role of dietary fat has been controversial. While some studies suggest a role of dietary fat in weight gain, others have criticized the data because studies are short term.[168,169] In addition, it is not clear from many of the existing intervention studies that reduction in dietary fat itself, as opposed to reduction in overall calories, causes weight reduction.[168] Despite the ambiguous role of total fat intake, it remains possible that reductions in saturated fat alone could have beneficial effects on obesity, especially if foods high in saturated fat are replaced by foods high in fibre, low in glycaemic index, or neutral in terms of other fatty acids.

Fibre and glycaemic index are two properties of foods that have garnered recent attention. One reason for the ineffectiveness of lowering dietary fat in reducing obesity rates may be that in many countries products marketed as low fat contain increased amounts of refined carbohydrate with very little fibre, resulting in a high glycaemic index. Glycaemic index is a property of carbohydrate-containing food that describes the rise of blood glucose after a meal. Foods that are rapidly digested and absorbed, such as refined grains and potatoes, have a high glycaemic index.[170,171] Physiologic responses to oral glucose suggest a mechanism linking glycaemic index to weight gain. Consumption of glucose—or high-glycaemic index foods—produces rapid elevations in blood glucose and insulin levels, followed in many individuals by a period of reactive hypoglycaemia with continued modest elevation of insulin levels. This situation results in hunger and increased food intake, possibly leading to cycles of hypoglycaemia and hyperphagia. The relative hyperinsulinaemia would also promote storage of fat.[172,173] In one feeding study among 12 obese teenage boys, voluntary energy intake after a high glycaemic index meal was 81% greater than after a low glycaemic index meal.[174] An observational study showing that consumption of sugar-sweetened drinks predicts increased BMI is consistent with the adverse role of high-glycaemic index foods.[175] Also consistent with this hypothesis, carbohydrate consumption has risen over time in the USA, from 46% of energy intake in 1965 to 55% in the mid-1990s.[176]

Fibre, one of several components of foods that lower their glycaemic index, may play a role itself in moderating weight gain. Dietary fibre can reduce insulin secretion by slowing post-prandial absorption of nutrients. Recent observational studies suggest that increased amounts of dietary fibre are associated with lower weight gain in young adults and with protection against development of ischaemic cardiovascular disease risk factors and end-points in adults.[177,178] Both reduced glycaemic index and increased dietary fibre may thus protect against development of obesity, but more and longer-term data in children and adolescents are needed.

In addition to effects of foods and nutrients, it is also of interest to examine the environments in which children and adolescents eat. For example, one study showed that children and adolescents who eat dinner with family members more often have diets of higher quality, as defined by a range of foods and nutrients.[179] But whether these measures of quality translate into appropriate weight gain over time is not known. No longitudinal studies address whether skipping breakfast predicts development of obesity. The extent and speed to which parental influence over adolescent diet wanes with age is also not known. Considerable scientific and lay interest exists in the ill effects of fast food, but published longitudinal data are not yet available on its role in promoting obesity.[180] Large portion size is one way in which fast food could contribute to excess weight gain,[18,181] but few data exist on the link between portion size and body weight in children.[182] The teenage years are ones of emerging independence, including obtaining and preparing food, so studies of these social and environmental influences over eating habits may help in designing strategies to prevent obesity.

8.7.4 Intervention studies to prevent obesity

This section contains a summary of selected population-based intervention studies to prevent obesity in older children and adolescents. We do not discuss treatment of established obesity.[183,184] The rationale for a population-based approach was articulated by Rose.[185] Although severely obese individuals are at the highest risk of morbidity and mortality, moderately overweight individuals are still at somewhat elevated risk. As many more people are moderately overweight than severely obese, the greatest burden of disease in the population rests mostly in the moderate range. Thus even a modest 'shift to the left' of the entire population distribution of adiposity should result in large decreases in its sequelae. Investigators have therefore designed intervention studies to increase physical activity, decrease inactivity, or improve diet by modest amounts among relatively unselected populations of children.

In addition, one can divide population approaches to disease prevention into two strategies: active and passive.[186] Active strategies require individual education to change behaviour, whereas passive strategies alter the environment to effect behaviour change. For example, to increase fibre intake, an active strategy might involve educating individuals about how to read nutrition labels on breakfast cereals and empowering them to choose high-fibre varieties; a passive strategy could involve manufacturers producing more high-fibre cereals and grocers placing them on the most accessible shelves. Obesity prevention interventions in children have incorporated both strategies.

In the past, active/educational obesity prevention interventions have relied primarily on changing knowledge and attitudes about diet and activity, without adequate attention to effective behaviour change strategies.[157] The moderate success of some recent studies is probably due, in part, to a focus of attention on strategies based on tested principles, such as social cognitive and social inoculation theories.[157] One such study involved multiple risk factor interventions among adolescents in California in the 1980s.[187] The investigators randomized four schools to a control or intervention, which consisted of 20 classroom lessons concerning physical activity, nutrition, smoking, stress reduction, and personal problem solving. In addition to knowledge, the intervention stressed cognitive and behavioural skills, including resisting social influences, as well as practising using the new skills. At the end of the 2-month intervention period, students in the intervention schools had increased aerobic exercise, increased low-fat/high-fibre food choices, and reduced BMI and skinfold thicknesses.[187]

While that small study appeared promising, the 1990s saw the failure of a very large multiple risk factor intervention trial to alter body weight. Conducted in 96 schools in four states of the USA, the Child and Adolescent Trial for Cardiovascular Health (CATCH) involved both active and passive strategies, including school curricula, school food service, physical education, and family-based components.[188] Some aspects of diet, such as fat intake, and physical activity, such as daily vigorous activity, did improve, but they were not effective in modifying body fat. One also suspects lack of complete fidelity to the intervention in such a widespread intervention.

Planet Health was a school-based randomized controlled intervention study among 10–12 year-olds. Its aims were to decrease television watching and high fat foods and to increase physical activity and intake of fruits and vegetables.[189] It was based on behavioural choice and social cognitive theories of behaviour change, with intervention material infused into school subject areas. Over a 2-year period, both boys and girls decreased their television viewing and among girls, BMI change was less in the intervention group. The BMI effect in girls appeared to be explained by the reduction in television viewing. There were also increases in fruit and vegetable consumption among the girls.

Another intervention study attempted to isolate the effects of reducing television viewing among 92 children of average age 9 years in a single school, with students in a neighbouring school serving as control participants.[190] The main intervention components comprised 18 classroom lessons to learn behaviour change skills, followed by a challenge to each child not to watch television or videos or play video games for 10 days, with a subsequent budget of 7 h/week. Absent were interventions to alter physical activity levels or dietary intake. Over a 7-month period, compared with control participants, children in the intervention group watched much less television and had modestly smaller increases in BMI (Fig. 8.11). Measures of moderate and vigorous physical activity and dietary intakes were only slightly changed. Although the BMI effect was relatively small, this is perhaps the most convincing evidence to date that television viewing causes obesity and it provides a prevention strategy to be tested in larger and more diverse settings.

Some elements seem to be common to successful interventions to reduce the development of obesity in children. One is adherence to a conceptual model of behaviour change that makes sense and has been empirically tested. Another is a focus on proximal

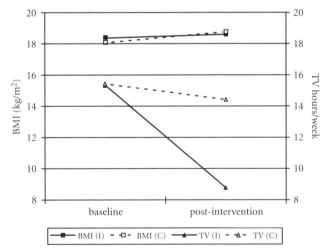

Fig. 8.11 Results from a school-based intervention trial to decrease television watching.[190] Compared with the control (C) group, the intervention (I) group had a reduction both in television viewing and in the expected age related increase in BMI.

factors that motivate children and adolescents, such as appearance, self-confidence, stress control, and autonomy, rather than remote health effects. The failure of CATCH also implies that intensive educational interventions may need to be mounted on relatively small scales to be effective. Current challenges are to test the efficacy of promising interventions in diverse populations and to translate them for optimal dissemination and evaluation in the 'real world'.

8.8 Analytical challenges

The life course approach to obesity posits that exposures that occur at different developmental stages interact with each other to produce excess weight gain. Analytical challenges include determining which exposures are independent of each other, how they interact with each other, and how to identify critical or sensitive periods. Which approaches are most useful is still a controversial area. An example from the study of early life origins of cardiovascular disease demonstrates this uncertainty. Analysing data from a cohort of 4630 Finnish men, Eriksson and colleagues[94(p949)] concluded that 'low weight gain during infancy is associated with increased risk of coronary heart disease'. Other investigators, however, using a different statistical approach, argued that these same data show that increased childhood growth after infancy constitutes a critical period for development of coronary disease.[191,192] Another approach uses a multilevel regression model of weight change over time, conditional on the previous period of growth, to account for the negative association in weight change between consecutive periods and regression to the mean.[193] How best to analyse highly correlated longitudinal data, such as individual relative weight over time, weight change between consecutive periods, dietary intake, and physical activity, to make causal inferences and to identify critical periods remains an important challenge.

In addition, the life course approach seeks to analyse not only the contribution of a factor over time, but also several levels of factors at any one time. For example, while this chapter has focused to a large extent on lifestyle and biological factors, 'upstream' social and economic factors are also clearly related to obesity. In the developed world, lower social class and other indicators of socioeconomic status in early life appear related to development of later obesity.[126,194] Exactly what it is about these social and economic factors that leads to the energy imbalance and results in excess weight gain is not yet known. Do they have direct biological influences or are they mediated through lifestyle choices? And what are the causes and sequelae of changes in socioeconomic status over time that are related to obesity? The answers to such questions will rely on robust longitudinal data sources and suitable data analysis techniques.

Acknowledgements

I thank Emily Oken and Nicolas Stettler for valuable comments on a draft of this chapter.

References

Those marked with an asterisk are especially recommended for further reading.

1 Mokdad AH, Serdula MK, Dietz WH, Bowman BA, Marks JS, Koplan JP. The spread of the obesity epidemic in the United States, 1991–1998. *J Am Med Assoc* 1999;**282**:1519–22.

2 Bundred P, Kitchiner D, Buchan I. Prevalence of overweight and obese children between 1989 and 1998: population-based series of cross sectional studies. *Br Med J* 2001;**322**:326–8.

3 Chinn S, Rona RJ. Prevalence and trends in overweight and obesity in three cross sectional studies of British children, 1974–94. *Br Med J* 2001;**322**:24–6.

4 Strauss RS, Pollack HA. Epidemic increase in childhood overweight, 1986–1998. *J Am Med Assoc* 2001;**286**:2845–8.

5 Mokdad AH, Serdula MK, Dietz WH, Bowman BA, Marks JS, Koplan JP. The continuing epidemic of obesity in the United States. *J Am Med Assoc* 2000;**284**:1650–1.

6 United States Department of Health and Human Services, Office of the Surgeon General. *The Surgeon General's call to action to prevent and decrease overweight and obesity.* Rockville: United States Department of Health and Human Services, 2001.

7 Flegal KM, Carroll MD, Ogden CL, Johnson CL. Prevalence and trends in obesity among US adults, 1999–2000. *J Am Med Assoc* 2002;**288**:1723–7.

8 Freedman DS, Khan LK, Serdula MK, Galuska DA, Dietz WH. Trends and correlates of class 3 obesity in the United States from 1990 through 2000. *J Am Med Assoc* 2002;**288**:1758–61.

9 Ogden CL, Flegal KM, Carroll MD, Johnson CL. Prevalence and trends in overweight among US children and adolescents, 1999–2000. *J Am Med Assoc* 2002;**288**:1728–32.

10 Willett WC, Dietz WH, Colditz GA. Guidelines for healthy weight. *N Engl J Med* 1999;**341**:427–34.

11 Jung RT. Obesity as a disease. *Br Med Bull* 1997;**53**:307–21.

12 Committee on Nutrition of the American Academy of Pediatrics. *Pediatric nutrition handbook* (4th edn). Elk Grove Village, Illinois: American Academy of Pediatrics, 1998.

13 Freedman DS, Dietz WH, Srinivasan SR, Berenson GS. The relation of overweight to cardiovascular risk factors among children and adolescents: the Bogalusa Heart Study. *Pediatrics* 1999;**103**:1175–82.

14 French SA, Story M, Perry CL. Self-esteem and obesity in children and adolescents: a literature review. *Obes Res* 1995;**3**:479–90.

15 Gortmaker SL, Must A, Perrin JM, Sobol AM, Dietz WH Jr. Social and economic consequences of overweight in adolescence and young adulthood. *N Engl J Med* 1993;**329**:1008–12.

16 Gunnell DJ, Frankel SJ, Nanchahal K, Davey Smith G. Childhood obesity and adult cardiovascular mortality: a 57- y follow-up study based on the Boyd Orr cohort. *J Clin Nutr* 1998;**67**:1111–18.

17 Must A, Jacques PF, Dallal GE, Bajema CJ, Dietz WH Jr. Long-term morbidity and mortality of overweight adolescents. A follow-up of the Harvard Growth Study of 1922 to 1935. *N Engl J Med* 1992;**327**:1350–5.

18 Ebbeling CB, Pawlak DB, Ludwig DS. Childhood obesity: public-health crisis, common sense cure. *Lancet* 2002;**360**:473–82.

19 Kim S, Popkin BM. The nutrition transition in South Korea. *Am J Clin Nutr* 2000;**71**:44–53.

20 Murray CJL, Lopez AD. Alternative projections of mortality and disability by cause 1990–2020: Global Burden of Disease Study. *Lancet* 1997;**349**:1498–504.

21 Serdula MK, Ivery D, Coates RJ, Friedman DS, Williamson DF, Byers T. Do obese children become obese adults? A review of the literature. *Prev Med* 1993;**22**:167–77.

*22 Whitaker RC, Wright JA, Pepe MS, Seidel KD, Dietz WH Jr. Predicting obesity in young adulthood from childhood and parental obesity. *N Engl J Med* 1997;**337**:869–73.

23 Douketis JD, Feightner JW, Attia J, Feldman WF. Periodic health examination, 1999 update: 1. Detection, prevention and treatment of obesity. *Can Med Assoc J* 1999;**160**:513–25.

24 Serdula MK, Mokdad AH, Williamson DF, Galuska DA, Mendlein JM, Heath GW. Prevalence of attempting weight loss and strategies for losing weight. *J Am Med Assoc* 1999;**282**:1353–8.

25 **Moore LL, Nguyen U, Rothman KJ, Cupples LA, Ellison RC.** Preschool physical activity level and change in body fatness. The Framingham Children's Study. *Am J Epidemiol* 1995;**142**:982–8.

26 **Keesey RE, Hirvonen MD.** Body weight set-points: determination and adjustment. *J Nutr* 1997;**127**:1875–83S.

27 **Goodman E, Hinden B, Khandelwal S.** Accuracy of teen and parental reports of obesity and body mass index. *Pediatrics* 2000;**106**:52–8.

28 **Centers for Disease Control and Prevention.** *CDC Growth Charts: United States 2000.* http://www.cdc.gov/nchs/about/major/nhanes/growthcharts/datafiles.htm.

29 **Cole TJ, Bellizzi MC, Flegal KM, Dietz WH.** Establishing a standard definition for child overweight and obesity worldwide: international survey. *Br Med J* 2000;**320**:1240–3.

30 **Meigs JB.** Insulin resistance syndrome? Syndrome X? Multiple metabolic syndrome? A syndrome at all? Factor analysis reveals patterns in the fabric of correlated metabolic risk factors. *Am J Epidemiol* 2000;**152**:908–10.

31 **Dietz WH.** Periods of risk in childhood for the development of adult obesity—what do we need to learn? *J Nutr* 1997;**127**:1884–6S.

32 **Dietz WH.** Critical periods in childhood for the development of obesity. *Am J Clin Nutr* 1994;**59**:955–9.

33 **Allison DB, Paultre F, Heymsfield SB, Pi-Sunyer F.** Is the intra-uterine period really a critical period for the development of adiposity? *Int J Obes Relat Metab Disord* 1995;**19**:397–402.

34 **Barker M, Robinson S, Osmond C, Barker D.** Birth weight and body fat distribution in adolescent girls. *Arch Dis Child* 1997;**77**:381–3.

35 **Bavdekar A, Yajnik CS, Fall CHD, Pandit AN, Bapat S, Deshpande V** *et al.* The insulin resistance syndrome in eight-year-old Indian children; small at birth, big at eight years or both? *Diabetes* 1999;**48**:2422–9.

36 **Braddon FEM, Rogers B, Wadsworth MEJ, Davies JMC.** Onset of obesity in a 36 year birth cohort study. *Br Med J* 1986;**293**:299–303.

37 **Charney E, Goodman HC, McBride M, Lyon B, Pratt R.** Childhood antecedents of adult obesity: do chubby infants become obese adults? *N Engl J Med* 1976;**295**:6–9.

38 **Curhan GC, Willett WC, Rimm EB, Spiegelman D, Ascherio AL, Stampfer MJ.** Birth weight and adult hypertension, diabetes mellitus and obesity in US men. *Circulation* 1996;**94**:3246–50.

39 **Fall CHD, Osmond C, Barker DJP, Clark PMS, Hales CN, Stirling Y** *et al.* Fetal and infant growth and cardiovascular risk factors in women. *Br Med J* 1995;**310**:428–32.

40 **Fall CHD, Stein CE, Kumaran K, Cox V, Osmond C, Barker DJP** *et al.* Size at birth, maternal weight, and type 2 diabetes in South India. *Diabet Med* 1998;**15**:220–7.

41 **Guillaume M, Lapidus L, Beckers F, Lambert A, Bjontorp P.** Familial trends of obesity through three generations: the Belgian–Luxembourg child study. *Int J Obes Relat Metab Disord* 1995;**19**:S5–9.

42 **Kramer MS, Barr RG, Leduc DG, Boisjoly C, Pless IB.** Infant determinants of childhood weight and adiposity. *J Pediatr* 1985;**107**:104–7.

43 **Maffeis C, Micciolo R, Must A, Zaffanello M, Pinelli L.** Parental and perinatal factors associated with childhood obesity in north-east Italy. *Int J Obes Relat Metab Disord* 1994;**18**:301–5.

44 **O'Callaghan MJ, Williams GM, Anderson MJ, Bor W, Najman JM.** Prediction of obesity in children at 5 years: a cohort study. *J Paediatr Child Health* 1997;**33**:311–16.

45 **Phillips DIW, Young JB.** Birth weight, climate at birth, and risk of obesity in adult life. *Int J Obes Relat Metab Disord* 2000;**24**:281–7.

46 **Rasmussen F, Johansson M.** The relation of weight, length and ponderal index at birth to body mass index and overweight among 18-year-old males in Sweden. *Eur J Epidemiol* 1998;**14**:373–80.

47 Seidman DS, Laor A, Gale R, Stevenson DK, Danon YL. A longitudinal study of birth weight and being overweight in late adolescence. *Am J Dis Child* 1991;**145**:782–5.

48 Shaheen SO, Sterne JAC, Montgomery SM, Azima H. Birth weight, body mass index and asthma in young adults. *Thorax* 1999;**54**:396–402.

49 Sorensen HT, Sabroe S, Rothman KJ, Gillman MW, Fischer P, Sorensen TIA. Relation between weight and length at birth and body mass index in young adulthood: cohort study. *Br Med J* 1997;**315**:1137.

50 Fomon SJ, Rogers RR, Ziegler EE, Nelson SE, Thomas LN. Indices of fatness and serum cholesterol at age eight years in relation to feeding and growth during early infancy. *Pediatr Res* 1984;**18**:1233–8.

51 Harland PSE, Watson MJ, Ashworth L. The effect of metabolic programming on atherosclerosis and obesity risk factors in UK adolescents living in poor socioeconomic areas. *Ann NY Acad Sci* 1997;**817**:361–4.

52 Hulman S, Kushner H, Katz S, Falkner B. Can cardiovascular risk be predicted by newborn, childhood, and adolescent body size? An examination of longitudinal data in urban African Americans. *J Pediatr* 1998;**132**:90–7.

53 Silverman BL, Cho NH, Rizzo TA, Metzger BE. Long-term effects of the intrauterine environment. *Diabet Care* 1998;**21**:B142–8.

54 Stettler N, Tershakovec AM, Zemel BS, Leonard MB, Boston RC, Katz SH *et al.* Early risk factors for increased adiposity: a cohort study of African American subjects followed from birth to young adulthood. *Am J Clin Nutr* 2000;**72**:378–83.

55 Gillman MW, Rifas-Shiman SL, Berkey CS, Field AE, Colditz GA. Maternal gestational diabetes, birth weight, and adolescent obesity. *Pediatrics* 2003;**111**:e221–6.

56 Parsons TJ, Power C, Manor O. Fetal and early life growth and body mass index from birth to early adulthood in 1958 British cohort: longitudinal study. *Br Med J* 2001;**323**:1331–5.

57 Oken E, Gillman MW. Fetal origins of obesity. *Obes Res* 2003;**11**:496–506.

58 Lucas A. Role of nutritional programming in determining adult morbidity. *Arch Dis Child* 1994;**71**:288–90.

59 Frienkel N. Of pregnancy and progeny. *Diabetes* 1980;**29**:1023–35.

60 Pederson J. Weight and length at birth of infants of diabetic mothers. *Acta Endocrinol* 1954;**16**:330–42.

*61 Dabelea D, Hanson RL, Lindsay RS, Pettitt DJ, Imperatore G, Gabir MM *et al.* Intrauterine exposure to diabetes conveys risks for type 2 diabetes and obesity: a study of discordant sibships. *Diabetes* 2000;**49**:2208–11.

62 Whitaker RC, Pepe MS, Seidel KD, Wright JA, Knopp RH. Gestational diabetes and the risk of offspring obesity. *Pediatrics* 1998;**101**:e9.

63 Plagemann A, Harder T, Melchior K, Rake A, Rohde W, Dorner G. Elevation of hypothalamic neuropeptide Y-neurons in adult offspring of diabetic mother rats. *NeuroReport* 1999;**10**:3211–16.

64 Heidel E, Plagemann A, Davidowa H. Increased response to NPY of hypothalamic VMN neurons in postnatal overfed juvenile rats. *NeuroReport* 1999;**10**:1827–31.

65 Plagemann A, Harder T, Rake A, Melchior K, Rittel F, Rohde W *et al.* Hypothalamic insulin and neuropeptide Y in the offspring of gestational diabetic mother rats. *NeuroReport* 1998;**9**:4069–73.

66 Plagemann A, Rake A, Harder T, Melchior K, Rohde W, Dorner G. Reduction of cholecystokinin-8S-neurons in the paraventricular hypothalamic nucleus of neonatally overfed weanling rats. *Neurosci Lett* 1998;**258**:13–16.

67 Plagemann A, Harder T, Rake A, Voits M, Fink H, Rohde W et al. Perinatal elevation of hypothalamic insulin, acquired malformation of hypothalamic galaninergic neurons, and syndrome X-like
alterations in adulthood of neonatally overfed rats. *Brain Res* 1999;**836**:146–55.

68 Ravelli G, Stein ZA, Susser MW. Obesity in young men after famine exposure *in utero* and early
infancy. *N Engl J Med* 1976;**295**:349–53.

69 Ravelli AC, vanDerMeulen JH, Osmond C, Barker DJ, Bleker OP. Obesity at the age of 50 y in
men and women exposed to famine prenatally. *Am J Clin Nutr* 1999;**70**:811–16.

70 Stanner SA, Bulmer K, Andres C, Lantseva OE, Borodina V, Poteen VV et al. Does malnutrition
in utero determine diabetes and coronary heart disease in adulthood? Results from the Leningrad
siege study, a cross sectional study. *Br Med J* 1997;**315**:1342–8.

71 Law CM, Barker DJP, Osmond C, Fall CHD, Simmonds SJ. Early growth and abdominal fatness
in adult life. *J Epidemiol Commun Health* 1992;**46**:184–6.

72 Okosun IS, Liao Y, Rotimi CN, Dever GEA, Cooper RS. Impact of birth weight on ethnic variations
in subcutaneous and central adiposity in American children aged 5–11 years. A study from the
Third National Health and Nutrition Examination Survey. *Int J Obes Relat Metab Disord*
2000;**24**:479–84.

73 Valdez R, Athens MA, Thompson GH, Bradshaw BS, Stern MP. Birthweight and adult health
outcomes in a biethnic population in the USA. *Diabetologia* 1994;**37**:624–31.

74 Kuh D, Hardy R, Chaturvedi N, Wadsworth MEJ. Birth weight, childhood growth and abdominal
obesity in adult life. *Int J Obes Relat Metab Disord* 2002;**26**:40–7.

75 Barker DJP, Hales CN, Fall CHD, Osmond C, Phipps K, Clark PMS. Type 2 (non-insulin dependent)
diabetes mellitus, hypertension and hyperlipidaemia (syndrome X); relation to reduced fetal
growth. *Diabetologia* 1993;**36**:62–7.

76 Choi CS, Kim C, Lee WJ, Park JY, Hong SK, Lee MG *et al.* Association between birth weight and
insulin sensitivity in healthy young men in Korea: role of visceral adiposity. *Diabet Res Clin Pract*
2000;**49**:53–9.

77 McCance DR, Pettitt DJ, Hanson RL, Jacobsson LT, Knowler WC, Bennett PH. Birth weight and
non-insulin dependent diabetes: thrifty genotype, thrifty phenotype, or surviving small baby
genotype? *Br Med J* 1994;**308**:942–5.

78 Mi J, Law C, Zhang KL, Osmond C, Stein C, Barker D. Effects of infant birthweight and maternal
body mass in pregnancy on components of the insulin resistance syndrome in China. *Ann Intern
Med* 2000;**132**:235–60.

79 Phillips DI. Birth weight and the future development of diabetes. A review of the evidence.
Diabet Care 1998;**21**:B150–5.

80 Phillips DIW, Barker DJP, Hales CN, Hirst S, Osmond C. Thinness at birth and insulin resistance
in adult life. *Diabetologia* 1994;**37**:150–4.

81 Reaven GM. Role of insulin resistance in human disease. *Diabetes* 1988;**37**:1595–607.

82 Robinson S, Walton RJCPM, Barker DJ, Hales CN, Osmond C. The relation of fetal growth to
plasma glucose in young men. *Diabetologia* 1992;**35**:444–6.

83 Vanhala MJ, Vanhala PT, Keinanen-Kiukaanniemi SM, Kumpusalo EA, Takala JK. Relative weight
gain and obesity as a child predict metabolic syndrome as an adult. *Int J Obes Relat Metab Disord*
1999;**23**:656–9.

84 Crowther NJ, Cameron N, Trusler J, Gray IP. Association between poor glucose tolerance and
rapid postnatal weight gain in seven-year-old children. *Diabetologia* 1998;**41**:1163–7.

85 McKeigue PM, Lithell HO, Leon DA. Glucose tolerance and resistance to insulin-
stimulated glucose uptake in men aged 70 years in relation to size at birth. *Diabetologia*
1998;**41**:1133–8.

86 Yarbrough DBS, Barrett-Connor E, Kirtz-Silverstein D, Wingard DL. Birth weight, adult weight, and girth predictors of the metabolic syndrome in postmenopausal women: the Rancho Bernando study. *Diabet Care* 1998;**21**:1652–8.

87 Hattersley AT, Beards F, Ballantyne E, Appleton M, Harvey R, Ellard S. Mutations in the glucokinase gene of the fetus result in reduced birth weight. *Nature Genet* 1998;**19**:268–70.

88 Terauchi Y, Kubota N, Tamemoto H, Sakura H, Nagai R, Akanuma Y *et al.* Insulin effect during embryogenesis determines fetal growth: a possible molecular link between birth weight and susceptibility to Type 2 diabetes. *Diabetes* 2000;**49**:82–6.

89 Hales CN, Barker DJP. Type 2 (non-insulin dependent) diabetes mellitus: the thrifty phenotype hypothesis. *Diabetologia* 1992;**35**:595–601.

90 Levitt NS, Lambert EV, Woods D, Hales CN, Andrew R, Seckl JR. Impaired glucose tolerance and elevated blood pressure in low birth weight, nonobese, young South African adults: early programming of cortisol axis. *J Clin Endocrinol Metab* 2000;**85**:4611–18.

91 Phillips DIW, Barker DJP, Fall CHD, Seckl JR, Whorwood CB, Wood PJ *et al.* Elevated plasma cortisol concentrations: a link between low birth weight and the insulin resistance syndrome? *J Clin Endocrinol Metab* 1998;**83**:757–60.

92 Frankel S, Elwood P, Sweetnam P, Yarnell J, Davey Smith G. Birthweight, body-mass index in middle age, and incident coronary heart disease. *Lancet* 1996;**348**:1478–80.

93 Leon DA, Koupilova I, Lithell HO, Berglund L, Mohsen R, Vagero D *et al.* Failure to realise growth potential *in utero* and adult obesity in relation to blood pressure in 50 year old Swedish men. *Br Med J* 1996;**312**:401–6.

94 Eriksson JG, Forsen T, Tuomilehto J, Osmond C, Barker DJP. Early growth and coronary heart disease in later life: longitudinal study. *Br Med J* 2001;**322**:949–53.

95 Chandalia M, Abate N, Garg A, Stray-Gunderson J, Grundy SM. Relationship between generalized and upper body obesity to insulin resistance in Asian Indian men. *J Clin Endocrinol Metab* 1999;**84**:2329–35.

96 Singh RB, Sharma JP, Rastogi V, Raghuvanshi RS, Moshiri M, Verma SP *et al.* Prevalence of coronary artery disease and coronary risk factors in rural and urban populations of north India. *Eur Heart J* 1997;**18**:1728–35.

97 Power C, Matthews S. Origins of health inequalities in a national population sample. *Lancet* 1997;**350**:1584–9.

98 Kramer MS. Do breast-feeding and delayed introduction of solid foods protect against subsequent obesity? *J Pediatr* 1981;**98**:883–7.

99 Agras WS, Kraemer HC, Berkowitz RI, Hammer LD. Influence of early feeding style on adiposity at 6 years of age. *J Pediatr* 1990;**116**:805–9.

100 Elliott KG, Kjolhede CL, Gournis E, Rasmussen KM. Duration of breastfeeding associated with obesity during adolescence. *Obes Res* 1997;**5**:538–41.

101 Strbak V, Skultetyova M, Hromadova M, Randuskova A, Macho L. Late effects of breast-feeding and early weaning: seven-year prospective study in children. *Endocr Regul* 1991;**25**:53–7.

102 Thorogood M, Clark R, Harker P, Mann JI. Infant feeding and overweight in two Oxfordshire towns. *J R Coll Gen Pract* 1979;**29**:427–30.

103 Zive MM, McKay H, Frank-Spohrer GC, Broyles SL, Nelson JA, Nader PR. Infant-feeding practices and adiposity in 4-y-old Anglo- and Mexican-Americans. *Am J Clin Nutr* 1992;**55**:1104–8.

104 von Kries R, Koletzko B, Sauerwald T, von Mutius E, Barnert D, Grunert V, *et al.* Breast feeding and obesity: cross sectional study. *Br Med J* 1999;**319**:147–50.

*105 Gillman MW, Rifas-Shiman SL, Camargo CA Jr, Berkey C, Frazier AL, Rockett HRH *et al.* Risk of overweight among adolescents who had been breast fed as infants. *J Am Med Assoc* 2001;**285**:2461–7.

106 Hediger ML, Overpeck MD, Kuczmarski RJ, Ruan WJ. Association between infant breastfeeding and overweight in young children. *J Am Med Assoc* 2001;**285**:2453–60.

107 Liese AD, Hirsch T, von Mutius E, Keil U, Leopold W, Weiland SK. Inverse association of overweight and breast feeding in 9 to 10-year-old children in Germany. *Int J Obes Relat Metab Disord* 2001;**25**:1644–50.

108 Toschke AM, Vignerova J, Lhotska L, Osancova K, Koletzko B, von Kries R. Overweight and obesity in 6- to 14-year-old Czech children in 1991: Protective effect of breastfeeding. *J Pediatr* 2002;**141**:764–9.

109 Armstrong J, Reilly JJ. Child Health Information Team. Breastfeeding and lowering the risk of childhood obesity. *Lancet* 2002;**359**:2003–4.

110 Ellis KJ, Abrams SA, Wong WW. Monitoring childhood obesity: Assessment of the weight/height^2 index. *Am J Epidemiol* 1999;**150**:939–46.

111 Himes JH, Dietz WH. Guidelines for overweight in adolescent preventive services: recommendations from an expert committee. *Am J Clin Nutr* 1994;**59**:307–16.

112 Birch LL, Fisher JO. Development of eating behaviors among children and adolescents. *Pediatrics* 1998;**101**:539–48.

113 Lucas A, Sarson DL, Blackburn AM, Adrian TE, Aynsley-Green A, Bloom SR. Breast vs. bottle: endocrine responses are different with formula feeding. *Lancet* 1980;**1**:1267–9.

114 Lucas A, Boyes S, Bloom SR, Aynsley-Green A. Metabolic and endocrine responses to milk fed in six-day-old term infants: differences between breast and cow's milk formula feeding. *Acta Paediatr Scand* 1981;**70**:195–200.

115 Gillman MW. Breast-feeding and obesity (editorial). *J Pediatr* 2002;**141**:749–50.

116 Stettler N, Zemel BS, Kumanyika SK, Stallings VA. Infant weight gain and childhood overweight status in a multicenter, cohort study. *Pediatrics* 2002;**109**:194–9.

117 Ong KKL, Ahmed ML, Emmett PM, Preece MA, Dunger DB (Avon Longitudinal Study of Pregnancy and Childhood Study Team). Association between postnatal catch-up growth and obesity in childhood: prospective cohort study. *Br Med J* 2000;**320**:967–71.

118 Rolland-Cachera M, Deheeger M, Bellisle F, Sempé M, Guilloud-Bataille M, Patois E. Adiposity rebound in children: a simple indicator for predicting obesity. *Am J Clin Nutr* 1984;**39**:129–35.

119 Freedman DS, Kettel Khan L, Serdula MK, Srinivasan SR, Berenson GS. BMI rebound, childhood height and obesity among adults: the Bogalusa Heart Study. *Int J Obes Relat Metab Disord* 2001;**25**:543–9.

120 Prokopee M, Bellisle F. Adiposity in Czech children followed from 1 month of age to adulthood: analysis of individual BMI patterns. *Ann Hum Biol* 1993;**20**:517–25.

121 Rolland-Cachera MF, Deheeger M, Guilloud-Bataille M, Avons P, Patois E, Sempé M. Tracking the development of adiposity from one month of age to adulthood. *Ann Hum Biol* 1987;**14**:219–29.

122 Siervogal RM, Roche AF, Guo SM, Mukhergee D, Chumlea WC. Patterns of change in weight/stature^2 from 2 to 18 y: findings from the long-term serial data for children in the Fels Longitudinal Growth Study. *Int J Obes Relat Metab Disord* 1991;**15**:479–85.

123 Whitaker RC, Pepe MS, Wright JA, Seidel KD, Dietz WH. Early adiposity rebound and the risk of adult obesity. *Pediatrics* 1998;**101**:e5.

124 Williams S, Davie G, Lam F. Predicting BMI in young adults from childhood data using two approaches to modelling adiposity rebound. *Int J Obes Relat Metab Disord* 1999;**23**:348–54.

125 Dorosty A, Emmett PM, Cowin IS, Reilly JJ. Factors associated with early adiposity rebound. *Pediatrics* 2000;**105**:1115–18.

126 Laitinen J, Power C, Jarvelin MR. Family social class, maternal body mass index, childhood body mass index, and age at menarche as predictors of adult obesity. *Am J Clin Nutr* 2001;**74**:287–94.

127 Hediger ML, Scholl TO, Schall JI, Cronk CE. One-year changes in weight and fatness in girls during late adolescence. *Pediatrics* 1995;**96**:253–8.

128 Andersen KL, lmarinen J, Rutenfranz J, Ottman W, Berndt I, Kylian H *et al.* Leisure time sport activities and maximal aerobic power during late adolescence. *Eur J Appl Occup Physiol* 1984;**52**:431–6.

129 Crocker PR, Bailey DA, Faulkner RA, Kowalski KC, McGrath R. Measuring general levels of physical activity: preliminary evidence for the Physical Activity Questionnaire for Older Children. *Med Sci Sports Exerc* 1997;**29**:1344–9.

130 Fuchs R, Powell KE, Semmer NK, Dwyer JH, Lippert P, Hoffmeister H. Patterns of physical activity among German adolescents: the Berlin–Bremen study. *Prev Med* 1988;**17**:746–63.

*131 Kimm SY, Glynn NW, Kriska AM, Barton BA, Kronsberg SS, Daniels SR *et al.* Decline in physical activity in black girls and white girls during adolescence. *N Engl J Med* 2002;**347**:709–15.

132 Kimm SY, Barton BA, Obarzanek E, McMahon RP, Sabry ZI, Waclawiw MA, *et al.* Racial divergence in adiposity during adolescence: the NHLBI Growth and Health Study. *Pediatrics* 2001;**107**:e34.

133 United States Department of Health and Human Services, Centers for Disease Control and Prevention, National Center for Chronic Disease Prevention and Health Promotion. *Physical activity and health: A report of the surgeon general.* Atlanta: United States Department of Health and Human Services, 1996.

134 Berkey CS, Rockett HRH, Field AE, Gillman MW, Frazier AL, Camargo CA Jr *et al.* Activity, dietary intake, and weight changes in a longitudinal study of preadolescent and adolescent boys and girls. *Pediatrics* 2000;**105**:e56.

135 Berkey CS, Rockett HRH, Gillman MW, Colditz G. One year changes in activity and in inactivity among 10 to 15 year old boys and girls: relationship to change in body mass index. *Pediatrics* (in press).

136 Schmitz KH, Jacobs DR, Leon AS, Schreiner PJ, Sternfeld B. Physical activity and body weight: assocations over 10 years in the CARDIA Study. *Int J Obes* 2000;**24**:1475–87.

137 Sallis JF, Prochaska JO, Taylor WC. A review of correlates of physical activity of children and adolescents. *Med Sci Sports Exerc* 2000;**32**:963–75.

138 Gordon-Larsen P, McMurray RG, Popkin BM. Adolescent physical activity and inactivity vary by ethnicity: The National Longitudinal Study of Adolescent Health. *J Pediatr* 1999;**135**:301–6.

139 Perusse L, Tremblay A, LeBlanc C, Bouchard C. Genetic and environmental influences on level of habitual physical activity and exercise participation. *Am J Epidemiol* 1989;**129**:1012–22.

140 Raitakari OT, Porkka KV, Taimela S, Telama R, Viikari J, Viikari JS. Effects of persistent physical activity and inactivity on coronary risk factors in children and young adults. The Cardiovascular Risk in Young Finns Study. *Am J Epidemiol* 1994;**140**:195–205.

141 Aaron DJ, Kriska AM, Dearwater SR, Anderson RL, Olsen TL, Cauley JA *et al.* The epidemiology of leisure time physical activity in an adolescent population. *Med Sci Sports Exerc* 1993;**25**:847–53.

142 Biddle S, Goudas M. Analysis of children's physical activity and its association with adult encouragement and social cognitive variables. *J Sch Health* 1996;**66**:75–8.

143 Reynolds KD, Killen JD, Bryson SW, Maron DJ, Taylor CB, Maccoby N *et al.* Psychosocial predictors of physical activity in adolescents. *Prev Med* 1990;**19**:541–51.

144 DiLorenzo TM, Stucky-Ropp RC, Vander Wal JS, Gotham HJ. Determinants of exercise among children. II. A longitudinal analysis. *Prev Med* 1998;**27**:470–7.

145 Zakarian JM, Hovell MF, Hofstetter CR, Sallis JF, Keating KJ. Correlates of vigorous exercise in a predominantly low SES and minority high school population. *Prev Med* 1994;**23**:314–21.

146 Goodman E, Whitaker RC. A prospective study of the role of depression in the development and persistence of adolescent obesity. *Pediatrics* 2002;**110**:497–504.

147 Terre L, Ghiselli W, Taloney L, DeSouza E. Demographics, affect, and adolescents' health behaviors. *Adolescence* 1992;**27**:12–24.

148 Trost SG, Pate RR, Saunders R, Ward DS, Dowda M, Felton G. A prospective study of the determinants of physical activity in rural fifth-grade children. *Prev Med* 1997;**26**:257–63.

149 Aarnto M, Winter T, Kujala UM, Kaprio J. Familial aggregation of leisure time physical activity: a three generation study. *Int J Sports Med* 1997;**18**:549–56.

150 Taveras EM, Rifas-Shiman SL, Field AE, Frazier AL, Colditz GA, Gillman MW. Association of adolescents wanting to look like figures in the media with physical activity levels. *J Adol Health* (in press).

151 Booth SL, Sallis JF, Ritenbaugh C, Hill JO, Birch LL, Frank LD *et al.* Environmental and societal factors affect food choice and physical activity: rationale, influences, and leverage points. *Nutr Rev* 2001;**59**:S21–39.

152 Dowda M, Ainsworth BE, Addy CL, Saunders R, Riner W. Environmental influences, physical activity, and weight status in 8 to 16 year olds. *Arch Pediatr Adolesc Med* 2001;**156**:711–17.

153 Gordon-Larsen P, McMurray RG, Popkin BM. Determinants of adolescent physical activity and inactivity patterns. *Pediatrics* 2000;**105**:1327–8.

154 Stettler N. Environmental factors in the etiology of obesity in adolescents. *Ethnicity Dis* 2002;**12**:41–5.

155 Williams Torres G, Pittman M, Hollander M, Kraft MK, Henry E. *Active living through community design.* Princeton: Robert Wood Johnson Foundation, 2001.

156 Dietz WH, Gortmaker SL. Do we fatten our children at the TV set? Television viewing and obesity in children and adolescents. *Pediatrics* 1985;**75**:807–12.

157 Robinson TN. Population-based obesity prevention for children and adolescents. In Johnston FE, Foster GD, eds. *Obesity and human growth.* London: Smith-Gordon, 2000.

158 Robinson TN. Does television cause childhood obesity? *J Am Med Assoc* 1998;**279**:959–60.

159 Gortmaker S, Must A, Sobol A, Peterson K, Colditz G, Dietz WH. Television viewing as a cause of increasing obesity among children in the United States, 1986–1990. *Arch Pediatr Adolesc Med* 1996;**150**:356–62.

160 DuRant RH, Baranowski T, Johnson M, Thompson WO. The relationship among television watching, physical activity, and body composition of young children. *Pediatrics* 1994;**94**:449–55.

161 Locard E, Mamelle N, Billette A, Miginiac M, Munoz F, Rey S. Risk factors of obesity in a five year old population: parental versus environmental factors. *Int J Obes Relat Metab Disord* 1992;**16**:721–9.

162 Obarzanek E, Schreiber GB, Crawford PB, Goldman SR, Frederick M, Lakatos E. Energy intake and physical activity in relation to indexes of body fat: the National Heart, Lung, and Blood Institute Growth and Health Study. *Am J Clin Nutr* 1994;**61**:15–22.

163 Pate RR, Ross JG, Dotson CO, Gilbert GG. The National Children and Youth Fitness Study: The new norms: a comparison with the 1980 AAHPERD norms. *J Phys Educ Recreat Dance* 1985;**56**:70–2.

164 Robinson TN, Hammer LD, Killen JD, Kraemer HC, Wilson DM, Taylor CB. Does television viewing increase obesity and reduce physical activity? Cross-sectional and longitudinal analyses among adolescent girls. *Pediatrics* 1993;**91**:273–80.

165 Robinson TN, Killen JD. Ethnic and gender differences in the relationships between television viewing and obesity, physical activity and dietary fat intake. *J Health Educ* 1995;**26**:S91–S98.

166 Shannon B, Peacock J, Brown MJ. Body fatness, television viewing and calorie intake of a sample of Pennsylvania sixth grade children. *J Nutr Educ* 1991;**23**:262–8.

167 Tucker LA. The relationship of television viewing to physical fitness and obesity. *Adolescence* 1986;**21**:797–806.

168 Willett WC. Dietary fat plays a major role in obesity: no. *Obes Rev* 2002;**3**:59–68.

169 Astrup A. The role of dietary fat in the prevention and treatment of obesity. Efficacy and safety of low-fat diets. *Int J Obes Relat Metab Disord* 2001;**25**:S46–50.

170 Wolever TMS, Jenkins DJ, Jenkins AL, Josse RJ. The glycemic index: methodology and clinical implications. *Am J Clin Nutr* 1991;**54**:846–54.

171 Foster-Powell K, Miller JB. International tables of glycemic index. *Am J Clin Nutr* 1995;**62**:871–93S.

172 Campfield L, Smith F, Rosenbaum M, Hirsch J. Human eating: evidence for physiological basis using a modified paradigm. *Neurosci Biobehav Rev* 1996;**20**:133–7.

173 Ludwig DS. The glycemic index: physiological mechanisms relating to obesity, diabetes, and cardiovascular disease. *J Am Med Assoc* 2002;**287**:2414–23.

174 Ludwig DS, Majzoub JA, Al-Zahrani A, Dallal GE, Blanco I, Roberts SB. High glycemic index foods, overeating, and obesity. *Pediatrics* 1999;**103**:e26.

175 Ludwig DS, Peterson KE, Gortmaker SL. Relation between consumption of sugar-sweetened drinks and childhood obesity: a prospective, observational analysis. *Lancet* 2001;**357**:505–8.

176 Cavadini C, Siega-Riz AM, Popkin BM. US adolescent food intake trends from 1965 to 1996. *Arch Dis Child* 2000;**83**:18–24.

177 Ludwig DS, Pereira MP, Kroenke CH, Hilner JE, VanHorn LV, Slattery ML *et al.* Dietary fiber, weight gain, and cardiovascular disease risk factors in young adults. *J Am Med Assoc* 1999;**282**:1539–46.

178 Pereira MA, Ludwig DS. Dietary fiber and body weight regulation: observations and mechanisms. *Ped Clin North Am* 2001;**48**:969–80.

179 Gillman MW, Rifas-Shiman SL, Frazier AL, Rockett HR, Camargo CA Jr, Field AE *et al.* Family dinner and diet quality among older children and adolescents. *Arch Fam Med* 2000;**9**:235–40.

180 Schlosser E. *Fast food nation*. Boston: Houghton Mifflin, 2001.

181 Nielsen SJ, Popkin BM. Patterns and trends in food portion sizes, 1977–1998. *J Am Med Assoc* 2003;**289**:450–3.

182 McConahy KL, Smiciklas-Wright H., Birch LL, Mitchell DC, Picciano MF. Food portions are positively related to energy intake and body weight in early childhood. *J Pediatr* 2002;**140**:340–7.

183 Epstein LH, Myers MD, Raynor HA, Saelens BE. Treatment of pediatric obesity. *Pediatrics* 1998;**101**:554–70.

184 Epstein LH, Paluch RA, Gordy CC, Dorn J. Decreasing sedentary behaviors in treating pediatric obesity. *Arch Pediatr Adolesc Med* 2000;**154**:220–6.

185 Rose G. *Strategy of preventive medicine*. London: Oxford University Press, 1993.

186 Gillman MW, Ellison RC. Childhood prevention of essential hypertension. *Ped Clin North Am* 1993;**40**:179–94.

187 Killen JD, Telch MJ, Robinson TN, Maccoby N, Taylor CB, Farquhar JW. Cardiovascular disease risk reduction for tenth graders. *J Am Med Assoc* 1988;**260**:1728–33.

188 Luepker RV, Perry CL, McKinlay SM, Nader PR, Parcel GS, Stone EJ *et al.* Outcomes of a field trial to improve children's dietary patterns and physical activity. The Child and Adolescent Trial for Cardiovascular Health (CATCH). *J Am Med Assoc* 1996;**275**:768–76.

189 Gortmaker SL, Peterson K, Wiecha J, Sobol AM, Dixit S, Fox MK *et al.* Reducing obesity via a school-based interdisciplinary intervention among youth: Planet Health. *Arch Pediatr Adolesc Med* 1999;**153**:409–18.

*190 **Robinson TN.** Reducing children's television viewing to prevent obesity: a randomized controlled trial. *J Am Med Assoc* 1999;**282**:1561–7.

191 **Cole TJ, Fewtrell MS, Lucas A.** Early growth and coronary heart disease in later life. Analysis was flawed. *Br Med J* 2001;**323**:572–3.

192 **Lucas A, Fewtrell MS, Cole TJ.** Fetal origins of adult disease—the hypothesis revisited. *Br Med J* 1999;**319**:245–9.

193 **Law CM, Shiell AW, Newsome CA, Syddall HE, Shinebourne EA, Fayers P** *et al.* Fetal, infant, and childhood growth and adult blood pressure: a longitudinal study from birth to 22 years of age. *Circulation* 2002;**105**:1088–92.

*194 **Parsons TJ, Power C, Logan S, Summerbell CD.** Childhood predictors of adult obesity: a systematic review. *Int J Obes Relat Metab Disord* 1999;**23**:S1–107.

195 **Silverman BL, Rizzo T, Cho NH, Winter RJ, Ogata ES, Richards GE** *et al.* Long-term prospective evaluation of offspring of diabetic mothers. *Diabetes* 1991;**40**:121–5.

196 **Dietz WH.** "Adiposity rebound": reality or epiphenomenon? *Lancet* 2000;**356**:2027–8.

Chapter 9

A life course approach to blood pressure

Peter H. Whincup, Derek G. Cook, and Johanna M. Geleijnse

Blood pressure is a major risk factor for cardiovascular disease. Though blood pressure in early adult life and in childhood may make small contributions to adult cardiovascular risk, blood pressure in middle and later life is the dominant factor. The emergence of adult blood pressure variation between individuals begins in early childhood and becomes stronger with age; adult differences between population groups probably emerge during later childhood or adolescence. Body mass is a strong influence on blood pressure differences at the individual and population level in adults and in children. Alcohol intake is an important influence on blood pressure level in adult life, with average exposure being particularly high in early adult life. High potassium intake is associated with lower mean blood pressure levels in adult life and with a lower rate of blood pressure rise with age in childhood, while high sodium intake is related to higher mean blood pressure levels in middle and later life and possibly also in infancy. The effects of all these factors are probably short-term and reversible, though it is conceivable that sodium intake in infancy could have longer-term effects on blood pressure. Fetal nutrition (of which birthweight is a marker) may also have a long-term influence on adult blood pressure. However, the influence of fetal factors on blood pressure is small, probably less important than that of factors acting in adult life (particularly obesity) and the underlying causes and mechanisms have yet to be defined.

9.1 Introduction

Blood pressure is a major risk factor for coronary heart disease (CHD) and stroke, diseases of middle and later life. The conventional view of high blood pressure in recent decades has been that it is, with specific exceptions, a condition of middle and later life (30 years plus).[1–3] The search for aetiological factors, reflecting this view, has concentrated on factors operating in adult life. Thus body build and alcohol intake, both strong determinants of blood pressure in middle-age,[4–7] have received particular attention.

Other factors that appear to have smaller effects on blood pressure in middle-age, including electrolyte intake,[4–6,8–10] physical activity,[11] and possibly psychosocial factors,[12] have also been studied. However, in recent years there has been increasing interest in the possibility that high blood pressure may have its origins in childhood[13] or even *in utero*.[14] It is therefore helpful to take a life course perspective on the development of blood pressure patterns, addressing three issues in particular. First, at what stages in the life course does blood pressure have an appreciable independent effect on adult cardiovascular risk? Second, at what stage in life do the patterns of blood pressure associated with cardiovascular risk actually develop? Third, what are the determinants of these blood pressure patterns and at which stages of the life course do they actually affect blood pressure level? To address this third question, it is necessary to consider whether the factors that affect blood pressure in middle-age also affect blood pressure earlier and whether their effects at earlier ages are reversible or not. It is also necessary to examine an alternative possibility, that environmental factors might influence blood pressure at very specific points of the life course in an irreversible manner, the implication of the 'programming hypothesis'.[14,15]

Blood pressure follows a continuous distribution in the population and its relationship with cardiovascular risk is also continuously graded. Definitions of 'high' blood pressure ('hypertension') are usually based on the levels of blood pressure at which intervention is likely to be beneficial.[3] Such definitions are somewhat arbitrary, depend on current evidence of treatment benefits, and are of very limited value for epidemiological purposes. In this overview, the focus will be on average blood pressure levels rather than on the prevalence of hypertension defined using arbitrary thresholds.

9.2 Blood pressure as a risk factor for cardiovascular disease: life course approach

At what stages in the life course is blood pressure actually a risk factor for adult cardiovascular risk? It has long been recognized that blood pressure levels in middle-age show a graded relationship to subsequent CHD and stroke events; because of the imprecision of blood pressure measurement, the strength of the association has frequently been underestimated.[16] Once imprecision in the measurement of blood pressure is taken into account, a 10 mm Hg increase in usual diastolic pressure at 60–69 years (equivalent to an 18 mm Hg increase in systolic pressure) is associated with a doubling in risk of stroke and with an increase of more than 50% in coronary risk.[17,18] The relative risks associated with a given degree of blood pressure elevation are particularly high in early middle-age (40–49 years), although the absolute risk of cardiovascular events is lower than at older ages.[18]

Comparisons of the reductions in cardiovascular risk that actually occurred in the major therapeutic trials of blood pressure reduction in middle-age with the reductions expected on the basis of observational data relating blood pressure to cardiovascular risk suggest that lowering blood pressure in middle-age reverses most if not all of the associated cardiovascular risk.[17,19] A therapeutic blood pressure reduction of 5–6 mm Hg in diastolic pressure (equivalent to a 10–14 mm Hg reduction in systolic pressure) for a 5-year period in adult life achieves all the expected reduction in stroke incidence and at least two-thirds of the expected reduction in CHD incidence in 5 years.[19]

These results suggest that the independent contributions of blood pressure level before middle-age to overall adult cardiovascular risk are very modest. Though several prospective studies have suggested that blood pressure in early adult life (18–20 years) is associated with subsequent cardiovascular risk,[20–23] the independent effect of blood pressure in early adult life on cardiovascular risk is difficult to assess precisely because these studies were unable to control for blood pressure nearer to the time of cardiovascular events. The same limitation applies to autopsy studies that have shown a relationship between blood pressure levels in childhood or adolescence and pathological evidence of coronary atherosclerosis in early adult life.[24,25]

9.3 Emergence of adult patterns of blood pressure

Blood pressure variation in adult life occurs at two levels, within populations and (especially on a geographic basis) between populations.[3] Though the factors responsible for variation in blood pressure level within and between populations overlap, there are important differences and the emergence of adult patterns needs to be considered separately. Within-population variation has an important genetic component, with estimates of heritability ranging from 30 to 60% depending on the degree of environmental homogeneity.[26] In contrast, the results of studies of migration, which have shown consistently that migrant people attain average blood pressure levels close to those of the host country within months, suggest that between-population variation in blood pressure has a strong environmental basis.[27,28]

9.3.1 Variation between individuals

The point at which the variations in blood pressure between individuals observed in middle-age emerge has been extensively studied in all periods between infancy and middle-age, although few studies have covered the whole period. Consistency of blood pressure ranking ('tracking') has been described during the first year of life[29] and at all stages in the life course thereafter.[30] However, the degree of consistency is weak. The tracking (correlation) coefficient for measurements of systolic pressure made at a 1-year interval rises from 0.1 or so in the first 2 years to about 0.4 between 3 and 4 years[31] and continues to rise during childhood. Although temporarily diminished during the period of rapid adolescent growth,[32] the coefficient rises to about 0.7 at the end of the second decade and remains reasonably stable thereafter.[30]

That blood pressure 'tracks' from an early age suggests that at least some degree of stability in the balance of genetic and environmental determinants of blood pressure is present from early in the life course. However, the proportion of variation not accounted for by previous blood pressure measurements is very high in childhood (more than 80%) and even in adulthood it remains substantial (50% or more). In childhood it is likely that intra-individual variations in weight gain and growth rate, which are strongly related to blood pressure change, play an important part in the marked intra-individual variability.[33,34] In adults, imprecision of blood pressure measurement and regression to the mean (the tendency for outlying measurements to be closer to the mean on repeated assessment) are probably of greater relative importance in explaining intra-individual variation.

9.3.2 Variation between populations

Although geographic variations in blood pressure between populations have been well described for many years,[35] the age at which adult differences in blood pressure between population groups emerge has had little systematic study. Many authors have assumed that variations in blood pressure between populations emerge during middle-age[2] and that mean blood pressures in childhood and early adult life (up to 30 years) do not differ between populations.[3] However, there have been few systematic attempts to study variation in the mean blood pressure levels of children and young adults from different populations or to relate them to average blood pressure levels in the same populations in middle-age. A standardized measurement study of 8- and 9-year-old children in 13 European countries[36] and a review of published studies on blood pressure in children[37] both suggested marked variation in average blood pressure levels between populations in childhood, but relationships with adult blood pressure or cardiovascular mortality were not explored. The Intersalt Study made standardized measurements of blood pressure in men and women aged between 20 and 59 years in 52 different populations from 32 countries. Examining published data from the study,[38] it is apparent that mean blood pressure levels at 20–29 years vary markedly between populations and are strongly related to levels at 50–59 years (Fig. 9.1), although level at 20 to 29 years is not strongly related to subsequent *change* in pressure.[39] This suggests that blood pressure differences of the middle-aged pattern are apparent at 20–29 years. The strong correlation between mean blood pressure levels and published stroke mortality data for 19 of the 32 countries in that study ($r=0.40$) makes between-centre observer bias an unlikely explanation for the finding. Strong associations are also observed between mean blood pressure levels at 15–19 years and those at 50–59 years in population-based studies of blood pressure that included participants in both these age groups (Table 9.1).[39] Comparable data for younger people are sparse. However, in the Tokelau Island Migrant Study, marked differences between the mean blood pressures of Tokelauan children (aged 2–14 years) on Tokelau

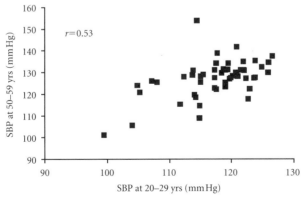

Fig. 9.1 Mean systolic blood pressure (males) at 20–29 years and 50–59 years in 52 populations based on published data from the Intersalt Study.[38]

Table 9.1 Relationship between blood pressure levels at 15–19 years and 50–59 years in population-based studies in different countries

	Number of centres	Slope	Standard error	*P*
Systolic				
Males	35	1.26	0.22	<0.0001
Females	28	1.55	0.35	0.0001
Diastolic				
Males	35	0.46	0.19	0.02
Females	28	0.51	0.22	0.03

Slopes refer to regression coefficients representing mean difference in population blood pressure at 50–59 years (mm Hg) associated with a 1 mm Hg difference in population blood pressure at age 15–19 years.[39]

and New Zealand were observed from 2 years upwards,[40] which paralleled adult differences and were not due to selection bias.[41] However, these striking findings in younger children may have been influenced by climatic factors and require further substantiation in other populations. In any event, it seems likely that geographic variations in blood pressure emerge before adult life, even if the precise point of emergence remains uncertain. The appearance of adult blood pressure differences between socioeconomic groups and ethnic groups, which are well-established by early adult life,[42] may also occur in childhood[43] though not all studies in children show a social class gradient.[42] The factors responsible for these differences between population groups are likely to include obesity, alcohol intake, and to a lesser extent other aspects of diet, including sodium and potassium intake. In the Intersalt Study,[38] between-population variations in blood pressure observed at 20–29 years are strongly correlated with variation in body mass index ($r=0.46$ in men) and to a lesser extent with alcohol intake ($r=0.20$ in men); sodium and potassium intake (more weakly correlated) appear less important. Fetal factors (q.v.) are an unlikely explanation for these population differences; populations with particularly low blood pressure have characteristics that suggest that average birthweights are likely to be low rather than high[44] and international associations between birthweight and blood pressure tend to be positive rather than inverse.[45] This is also borne out by ecological analyses of international differences in infant mortality rate to cardiovascular disease, which show little relationship to CHD mortality and no period-specific relationship to stroke[46] (see also Chapter 6).

There is no doubt that elevation of blood pressure level following movement from a 'low' blood pressure environment to a 'high' blood pressure environment occurs rapidly with changes beginning within a month of migration and complete by 6 months in widely differing age groups.[47–49] However, the degree to which these increases in blood pressure are reversible and the influence of age on reversibility remain uncertain. There have been few systematic migrations from 'high' to 'low' blood pressure areas for study. However, the results of two studies—one in Australian aborigines reverting from a Western lifestyle to a traditional lifestyle[50] and one in UK middle-aged men migrating from regions of UK with higher average blood pressure levels to those with lower levels[28]—suggest that blood pressure may fall on migration as well as rise, although this requires confirmation in other settings and the extent of reversibility at different ages needs to be studied.

9.4 Factors influencing blood pressure in middle-age: life course approach

Another potentially useful way to study the development of blood pressure during the life course is to consider the time course of exposures influencing blood pressure at different ages and the reversibility of their effects. The first way in which this can be done is by examining whether those exposure factors that influence blood pressure in middle-age are present earlier in life. The early presence of such exposures may be important either because they affect subsequent blood pressure directly (particularly if cumulative, irreversible effects were to occur) or because earlier exposure might influence the probability of exposure in middle-age. Thus, early exposures could be important either because they have direct long-term effects on blood pressure, particularly of a cumulative nature or because (particularly in the early setting of behavioural patterns) they make the continuation of exposure into adult life more likely. These possibilities are considered in the following subsections for several factors that have associations with blood pressure in middle-age that are likely to be causal—including adiposity, alcohol intake, dietary sodium and potassium intake, and physical activity levels. Dietary intakes of calcium and magnesium are not discussed here because their relationships with blood pressure in adults are inconsistent or weak.[51] The separate possibility that other exposures operating at specific points in the life course (particularly in early life) may have long-term effects on blood pressure—the phenomenon known as 'programming'[15]—is addressed separately in Section 9.5.

9.4.1 Adiposity

Body mass (weight for height or body mass index) has a strong relation to blood pressure in middle-age. However, this association is present at all stages of the life course; weight is positively related to blood pressure at birth[29] and the association persists through childhood and adolescence into adult life, although it becomes weaker in late middle-age.[13] Although the mechanisms of the association between obesity and blood pressure are not fully understood, the relationship is likely to be causal. Moreover, the distribution of fat may be important, with central obesity being particularly associated with raised blood pressure and hyperinsulinaemia both in adults[52] and in children.[53] Progressive weight gain in adult life, particularly on a diet high in saturated fat, is a consistent feature of populations at high risk of cardiovascular disease, particularly CHD.[54]

Although it has been shown that weight in childhood, adolescence, or early adult life predicts blood pressure in middle-age,[55] earlier weight does not appear to be an independent predictor of blood pressure once current weight is taken into account. Controlled studies of weight loss both in adults and in children have suggested that the effects of body mass on blood pressure are substantially reversible.[56] This finding is also supported by the results of longitudinal studies, showing that weight change is strongly related to changes in blood pressure, both in adults[55,57] and in children.[33,57] However, although the effects of body weight are theoretically reversible, the strong degree of tracking shown by body mass index from childhood through to adult life[58] suggests that becoming overweight in childhood increases the possibility of being overweight in adult life. Thus, though the effects of early obesity on blood pressure are theoretically reversible, they are not often reversed in practice. This is of particular concern in the context of the marked secular increases in obesity both in adults and children during the past 20 years.[59]

9.4.2 Alcohol intake

Alcohol intake has a strong and graded relation to blood pressure both in middle-age and in early adult life, when alcohol intake is often particularly high.[7,60,61] There is little information on the relationship of alcohol intake in early adult life with later blood pressure. However, the effects on blood pressure of reducing alcohol intake in middle-age[62] are consistent with the strength of associations in observational data,[60] suggesting that alcohol intake before middle-age probably has little if any sustained effect on later blood pressure. It is however possible that the establishment of alcohol intake patterns in adolescence and early adult life sets a pattern followed throughout adult life, though average intake tends to decline with increasing age.

9.4.3 Sodium intake

In adults there appears to be a positive association between sodium intake and blood pressure. However, the strength of the association and the scale of blood pressure reduction expected from reducing dietary sodium intake in middle-age are still debated. In observational studies based in general populations (and adjusted for regression dilution bias), a 100 mmol increase in daily sodium intake is associated with an increase of between 3 and 6 mm Hg in systolic pressure,[5,8,9] an association that tends to increase in strength with age between 20 and 59 years.[9,63] The most reliable evidence on the effects of reducing sodium intake comes from meta-analyses of the large number of mostly small randomized trials of reduced sodium intake carried out in adults. However, estimates of the effect on systolic pressure of a reduction in daily sodium intake of 100 mmol in normotensive people based on meta-analyses of these trials have varied markedly, depending on the inclusion criteria, between 1–2 mm Hg[64,65] and 10 mm Hg[10]; analyses restricted to longer-term trials correspond to a fall of about 4 mm Hg.[66] The results of the recent Dietary Approaches to Stop Hypertension (DASH) sodium trial were consistent with a large effect (8.7 mm Hg fall in systolic pressure for a 100 mmol daily sodium reduction on a normal diet)—though the results suggested that the effect of sodium reduction might depend on other aspects of dietary composition.[67] Taken together, these results suggest that the effect of dietary sodium intake on blood pressure in middle-age is reversible in middle-age, though the completeness of reversibility is uncertain.

Sodium intake in children in most affluent countries is high, about 100 mmol/day in early childhood[68] and increases further to early adult life.[38] However, it has been difficult to demonstrate associations between sodium intake and blood pressure in childhood. Although Cooper and colleagues[69] found a weak positive association between sodium excretion and blood pressure in 73 11–14-year-old boys (each producing seven repeat 24 h urine samples) the finding could not be replicated.[70] Similarly, no association was observed either in 887 8–9-year-old children with 24 h urine samples[36] or 3000 5–7-year-old children providing spot urine samples.[71] Moreover, in a small but detailed longitudinal study, Geleijnse and colleagues found no relationship between habitual sodium intake (based on annual 24 h urine assessments) and annual blood pressure change in 233 young people, studied from entry at 5 to 17 years for at least 7 years.[72] Though the absence of an association between sodium intake and blood pressure in children must be interpreted cautiously, because of the imprecision of assessment of habitual sodium intake, the limited range of sodium intake in many populations, and the possibility of dietary confounding, any association between dietary sodium intake and blood pressure in childhood appears to be small. This conclusion is also consistent with the results of both short-term and longer-term trials of sodium restriction in childhood, which showed no consistent effect on blood pressure follow-up either after 6 months[73] or after 3 years.[74]

Though sodium intake is not clearly related to blood pressure in childhood, the situation may be different in the immediate postnatal period. In a randomized controlled trial in 476 infants in Zoetermeer in the early 1980s (when sodium concentrations in commercially available formula milks were three times greater than those in human milk), it was reported that a 6-month period of sodium restriction in newborns produced a reduction in systolic pressure of 2.1 mm Hg at the end of the intervention period,[75] which was no longer detectable 6 months later.[76] The size of effect demonstrated in this trial (approximately 2.35 mm Hg in systolic pressure for a 10 mmol/day reduction in sodium intake), though imprecisely estimated, was stronger than the effect sizes observed in adults.[5,8,9] Though no replication of the Zoetermeer trial has been reported, the results of a small trial reducing the sodium composition of water used to dilute formula milk was associated with a marked short-term difference in blood pressure 8 weeks after birth (5.3/11.1 mm Hg), an effect which was attenuated 4 months later.[77]

These studies point to the possibility of a short-term effect of sodium intake on blood pressure in infancy. However, the results of a 15-year follow-up of the Zoetermeer trial[78] raised the possibility that sodium intake in infancy might have longer-term effects. Mean blood pressures at 15 years were markedly lower among the original low sodium group (3.6/2.2 mm Hg) than those of the control group; there was no marked difference in current sodium intake between the groups. However, this study was based on only 35% of the original participants and the differences in blood pressure between sodium groups were only statistically significant after adjustment for potential confounding factors, so the results should be treated cautiously. A trial of sodium restriction in premature neonates showed no long-term effect on blood pressure at 8 years.[79] Though longer-term follow-up of a subset of this study population in adolescence showed lower pressures in participants who had been breastfed, this difference was not related to sodium intake.[80] At present therefore the evidence to suggest that early sodium intake has long-term effects on blood pressure is not strong. However, it is well-recognized that sodium taste is acquired relatively early in life[81] and it is therefore possible that early sodium intake may indirectly affect sodium intake in adult life.

9.4.4 **Potassium intake**

An inverse relationship between potassium intake and blood pressure has been demonstrated in adults, both by observational studies[4,6] and by experimental studies.[82] The strength of association (an approximately 8–9 mm Hg fall in systolic pressure per 100 mmol/day increase in potassium intake) is similar in experimental and observational studies, suggesting that the hypotensive effect of potassium supplementation on blood pressure is substantially reversible.[82] Inverse associations between potassium intake and blood pressure have been described in children[71] and a high potassium intake also appears to be related to a smaller rate of rise in blood pressure with age in children and adolescents.[72] The relationship between potassium intake in infancy and later blood pressure has not been studied, though an intriguing report from an observational study suggests that high maternal potassium intake in pregnancy may be related to lower blood pressure levels in offspring.[83] At present, there is no convincing evidence that potassium intake before middle-age has longer-term influences on blood pressure, though further research is needed.

9.4.5 **Physical activity and fitness**

Observational studies have suggested that increased levels of physical activity are associated with lower levels of blood pressure, both in adults[11] and in children.[84,85] However, such studies need to be cautiously interpreted because of the possibility of confounding (for example, by social factors and alcohol intake), though this is less likely in childhood. There is no strong evidence that higher levels of physical activity have a long-term influence on blood pressure. In a longitudinal study of students followed up to middle-age, recent physical activity was much more strongly related to incidence of hypertension than physical activity in youth; the authors stated that only in the presence of high levels of recent activity did earlier activity have any effect.[86] Intervention studies, which have generally introduced vigorous activity, have been associated with sustained blood pressure reduction in some but not all cases, though the effects are only sustained as long as the activity levels are maintained.[87] Moreover, short-term changes in physical activity and fitness levels have been related to changes in blood pressure, both in adults and in children[11] again suggesting that the duration of effects of physical activity are limited. Overall there is little evidence that physical activity or fitness before adult life has sustained effects on later blood pressure; current physical activity and fitness level is the dominant influence on blood pressure. However, level of physical activity tends to 'track' strongly between childhood and adult life, so that physical activity behaviour in childhood may influence physical activity level in adult life.[88]

9.5 **Factors that may act at specific points in the life course with long-term effects on blood pressure**

There has been growing interest in the possibility that factors operating at very specific points in the life course are related to blood pressure. The recognition of 'programming' has increased the biological plausibility of such exposures.[15] The relationship between birthweight and blood pressure has been a particular focus of attention, but the possibility that infant feeding or postnatal growth, particularly early postnatal growth, may influence later blood pressure has also been considered.

9.5.1 Fetal factors and blood pressure

The observation that low birthweight is related to later blood pressure has been a central part of the 'fetal origins hypothesis' linking fetal nutrition and adult cardio-vascular disease.[14] By 2000, more than 40 studies had been published reporting the relationship, particularly for systolic pressure.[89] Most of those studies were in developed countries, though a few were from developing populations. The association has been described in adults, in children, and (despite early reports suggesting that the associa-tion might not be present in adolescents)[14] in adolescents.[90,91] It was initially suggested that the association between birthweight and blood pressure might be confounded, particularly by social class and its correlates,[92] but analyses in individual studies have suggested that the association is independent of alcohol intake, social class,[93,94] mater-nal age,[95,96] and birth rank.[95,96] Though it was suggested that maternal blood pressure might be an important potential confounder,[97] the relationship between maternal blood pressure and offspring birthweight is not graded across the population and adjustment for maternal blood pressure does not appear to confound the association.[98] Neither is this association confounded by maternal smoking, which is associated with lower mean birthweight.[99] Whether current body size can be regarded as a confounder of the birthweight–blood pressure relationship and whether adjustment for it is appropriate has been discussed in detail.[100,101] In adults, the justifi-cation for such adjustment is not clear and the unadjusted association (inverse but weak)[91] is likely to provide the best indicator of the overall strength of effect. In children, in whom the inverse association between birthweight and blood pressure is only observed after adjustment for current body size,[95,96,102,103] the situation is more complex. Throughout childhood, birthweight is related both to subsequent height and weight-for-height, which are themselves strong determinants of blood pressure. However, in this age group adjustment for current size, particularly for height, may be appropriate. Height, though a strong determinant of blood pressure in childhood, ceases to be an important determinant in adulthood. Childhood height may therefore be regarded as a temporary confounder of the birthweight–blood pressure association. Adjustment for current adiposity would be misleading if adiposity were a mechanism by which birthweight exerted its effects on blood pressure. Though a few studies have suggested that fetal undernutrition may be related to an increased degree of general obesity,[104] a very large number of studies (reviewed in detail in Chapter 8) have reported positive associations between birthweight and later body mass index, with lower birthweight associated with lower subsequent body mass index. However, several studies (reviewed in Chapter 8) have suggested that low birthweight is associated with greater degrees of central obesity in adult life—though this association is generally only apparent after adjustment for body mass index, which is itself closely correlated with central obesity measures.

How strong and how important is the influence of birthweight on blood pressure and what causal pathway does it represent? For the reasons discussed earlier, the importance of the birthweight–blood pressure association depends on its strength in adult life. A recent meta-analysis providing estimates of the strength of the birthweight–blood pressure association suggested that while the reported association in all studies was of the order of −1.5 mm Hg/kg, the association was related to size of study and was very much weaker (of the order of −0.6 mm Hg/kg) in very large studies (3000 plus participants).[91] These observations are difficult to interpret because of the possibility of greater error in exposure ascertainment in the largest studies, based on routine data collection. However, even the larger estimate of the strength of the association (−1.5 mm Hg/kg) represents a change in blood pressure of less than 0.2 standard deviations (SDs) for a very substantial (2 SDs) change in birthweight. Moreover, the associations become weaker (of the order of −0.4 mm Hg/kg) once examined without adjustment for current body size.[91] The weakness of the birthweight–blood pressure association is further emphasized if the strength of the associations between birthweight and blood pressure and current adiposity and blood pressure are compared; the potential influence of birthweight on blood pressure tends to be much less marked than the equivalent influence of current adiposity.[105] This is also the case for associations between birthweight and other risk markers, including blood cholesterol and insulin resistance.[106,107]

However, before concluding that fetal factors are of limited importance in the control of blood pressure, it is important to consider the possibility that the strength of the relevant association has been underestimated. There are three particular reasons why this might be the case. First, the relevant exposure may have been imprecisely measured—particularly if a maternal rather than a fetal exposure were important (q.v.). Second, the association may be concentrated among a particular section of the population. Third, the strength of the association that is most relevant for contemporary public health purposes is that which will apply in contemporary infants and children when they reach adulthood. If the association were to become stronger with increasing age with successive generations, the association in contemporary children could be important.

Though birthweight itself has been accurately assessed in most studies, either from maternal recall[106] or in many cases directly from birth records, it is possible that birthweight is acting as a proxy for other, possibly more complex measures of size at birth—perhaps relating to disturbance of growth at a specific period of pregnancy. Studies in adults have suggested that fetal growth rate (rather than birthweight *per se*) is the important factor.[93,94] However, the relationships between birthweight and blood pressure in children are similar in term and preterm offspring and adjusting birthweight for gestational age does not strengthen the association.[99,108,109] Two more specific markers, thinness at birth (that is, a low weight/height^3) and shortness at birth (that is, a low length/head circumference), were reported to be associated with particularly high adult levels of blood pressure in the Preston study.[110] However, neither of these markers, thought to be linked to fetal undernutrition in the second and third trimesters respectively, has been substantiated in later studies in adults[94,111] nor in studies of children.[112] In the Preston study, increasing placental weight and a high placental weight-to-birth weight ratio were both linked to particularly high mean blood pressure levels,[93] suggesting that fetal undernutrition might underlie the association between placental size and blood pressure.[14] However, these findings were strongly dependent on the results in a small subgroup of individuals with particularly low birthweight and high placental weight. Moreover, the association between placental size and blood pressure, although supported by some studies,[103,113] has not been replicated in several others, either in adults[94,111] or in children.[108,114] At present therefore, no more specific marker of size at birth has been consistently found to relate more closely to blood pressure than birthweight. It has also been hypothesized that it is not low birthweight but rapid early postnatal growth that is responsible for the association between birthweight and blood pressure. However, several studies have now shown that early postnatal weight gain has no longer-term influence on blood pressure once current body size is taken into account, either in adults[115,116] or in children.[109,117,118]

The possibility that the birthweight–blood pressure association has been underestimated because it is concentrated in a subset of the population receives some support from observations made in the Uppsala study, in which the relationship between low birthweight and higher mean blood pressure appeared to be particularly marked in participants with the highest body mass index in middle-age.[111] Such an observation would be consistent with other studies that have suggested that birthweight interacts with obesity in its effect on coronary risk.[119] However, many other studies, both in adults and children, have failed to find an interaction of this kind.[89]

Is it likely that the birthweight–blood pressure association among contemporary infants and children when they reach adult life will be sufficiently strong to be of great public health importance? This depends both on estimates of the birthweight–blood pressure relationships already observed in such participants in infancy and childhood and on the likelihood that these associations will become still stronger with increasing age. The strengths of association between systolic pressure and birthweight in contemporary children is of the order of −1 mm Hg/kg after adjustment for current height and −2 mm Hg/kg after adjustment for height and body mass.[96,109,112] Early overviews of cross-sectional studies at different ages[115] and longitudinal studies examining the relationship between birthweight and blood pressure at different ages in the same individuals[108] provided some support for the possibility of amplification. However, the evidence for amplification from cross-sectional study data has become less convincing as more data have accrued. The most recent systematic review of the relationship between birthweight and blood pressure, the first to provide a formal meta-analysis of the relationship, provided no consistent evidence of amplification with age.[91] Moreover, the longitudinal data on the relationships that are now available from several more recent studies[120–123] do not provide strong evidence for amplification. Thus it seems unlikely that the association between birthweight and blood pressure will be stronger than that of current estimates[91] in contemporary children when they reach adult life.

What causal pathway underlies the relationship between birthweight and blood pressure? It is likely that low birthweight is a reflection of fetal undernutrition,[124] which could then affect biological structure or function,[125] but the more important question is whether maternal nutrition is an underlying (and potentially changeable) aetiological factor—acting through (or to some extent independently of) birthweight. Animal studies have provided some support for this possibility, showing, for example, that protein restriction in pregnant rats is associated with higher blood pressure levels in offspring[126] and also raising the possibility that failure of fetal protection against maternal glucocorticoids might be important.[127] However, in humans the role of maternal nutrition is less certain. Though it is recognized that variation in birthweight is largely environmentally determined,[128,129] conventional observational studies relating maternal nutritional status to blood pressure in offspring have provided inconclusive results. Studies carried out on survivors of the Dutch famine (1944–1945) have suggested that maternal starvation during pregnancy has very limited effects on the birthweight of offspring and then only in the third trimester.[130] The effects of maternal starvation (in any trimester of pregnancy) on offspring blood pressure were small.[131,132] A study of the relationship of maternal diet and offspring blood pressure 40 years later carried out in Aberdeen provided results that were difficult to interpret, with higher mean offspring blood pressure levels associated either with a combination of high carbohydrate and low protein intakes or with a combination of low carbohydrate and high protein intakes.[133] Though maternal anaemia has also been implicated as a possible nutritional marker,[134] it is not consistently related to blood pressure.[99] Moreover, anaemia in pregnancy is closely related to physiological haemodilution, which tends to be related to higher mean birthweight,[135] so that there is a contradiction between the hypotheses that low birthweight and low maternal haemoglobin concentration during pregnancy are both risk factors for later cardiovascular risk.[99] Maternal smoking, though strongly related to lower mean birthweight, has little or no effect on offspring blood pressure[99] and does not appear to play an important role in this context.

A novel approach to the study of the influence of maternal nutrition on offspring blood pressure has been the use of twin studies. Within twin pairs it might be assumed that maternal nutrition is consistent, so that if maternal nutrition were important, the relationship between birthweight and blood pressure would be expected to be stronger between twin pairs than within twin pairs. The first two studies published (one in adults, one in children) suggested that the relationship between birthweight and blood pressure was stronger within twin pairs than between them[136,137] and was interpreted as suggesting that fetal nutrition and possibly genetic factors rather than maternal nutrition were playing a dominant role.[138] However, those studies were small and subsequent larger studies[139–141] have suggested that the relationship between birthweight and blood pressure within twin pairs is weak and inconsistent—a conclusion supported by the results of a recent meta-analysis.[91] Though detailed comparisons of within-pair and between-pair analyses are so far lacking for several studies,[142] it seems unlikely that without very much larger investigations twin studies will resolve the role of maternal nutrition.[143] However, long-term large-scale studies examining the effects of pre-conceptual maternal nutrition on the health of the offspring may provide further insights into this issue.

9.5.2 Other factors that may affect blood pressure at specific points of the life course

9.5.2.1 Infant feeding

The possibility that initial breastfeeding might be associated with lower levels of subsequent blood pressure (particularly because the sodium content of breast milk was often lower than that of bottle milk until the 1980s) has been explored in some studies. Several relatively small observational studies have suggested that breastfeeding may be associated with lower blood pressure levels, even after adjustment for potential con-founding factors such as body build and social class).[121,144] Follow-up of participants in a trial of infant feeding among preterm infants at 13–15 years also suggested that breastfeeding might be associated with lower blood pressure,[80] though this observa-tion was made on only a small proportion of the original randomized population and no overall difference between the groups had been observed at 8 years.[145] A recent 25-year follow-up of participants who participated in a dried milk supplementation trial in infancy has suggested that increased intake of dried milk is associated with higher subsequent blood pressure.[146] However, a review of published data on blood pressure levels of breast- and bottle-fed participants suggests that overall differences in blood pressure between breast- and bottle-fed participants are small and prone to publication bias.[147] A recent report suggesting that long-chain n-3 fatty acids may influence later blood pressure requires confirmation.[148]

9.5.2.2 Postnatal growth

It has been suggested that postnatal growth or weight gain at particular periods of development could have an important long-term effect on blood pressure; one specific suggestion has been the possibility that rapid growth in low birthweight infants accounts for the relationship between birthweight and blood pressure. However, several studies both in children and adults have shown that weight at 1 year has no long-term relationship with blood pressure once current weight is taken into account.[117,109] Moreover, it has recently been shown that catch-up growth in infancy standardized for regression to the mean has no important influence on blood pressure in early adult life.[116] It is however possible that later childhood growth is important. Poor height gain in childhood may be an independent determinant of raised blood pressure in later life,[149] a finding that requires further exploration. While growth later in childhood, particularly at adrenarche and at puberty, is strongly related to blood pressure rise,[13] it remains uncertain whether the timing and extent of growth at these periods have long-term effects on attained blood pressure that are independent of later growth and attained adult size. This possibility requires critical examination in future studies.

9.6 Conclusions

Blood pressure in middle and later life is the main influence on cardiovascular risk. The influence of potential determinants on blood pressure in middle-age therefore provides the main indicator of their potential importance. The differences in blood pressure seen in middle-age between individuals are apparent from childhood or infancy; those between populations probably appear during late childhood or adoles-cence. Several individual determinants of blood pressure in middle-age (particularly body mass, alcohol intake, potassium intake, and physical activity) appear to have sim-ilar effects on blood pressure at younger ages. Though their effects on blood pressure are reversible, the conditioning of dietary and exercise behaviour from childhood and adolescence onwards[150] is likely in practice to make these factors difficult to reverse in middle-age, emphasizing the importance of primary 'primordial' prevention from childhood onwards. The evidence that dietary factors operating in infancy 'pro-gramme' blood pressure is weak, though the influence of sodium intake and long chain n-3 fatty acid in the first year of life requires further examination. The potential importance of the associations between size at birth and later blood pressure is that, once established, they may represent irreversible influences on adult blood pressure. However, these associations are weak, the underlying relationships have not yet been clarified, and, in particular, the contribution of maternal nutrition remains conjectural. The conclusion that adult influences, rather than early life influences, are the dominant influence on adult blood pressure is supported by the results of studies of the influence of migration on blood pressure (see Chapter 6), which suggest that the adult environment plays the more important role. Though programming could be playing a role and could still alter our understanding of possible approaches to the prevention of hypertension in adult life (particularly on the role of maternal nutrition), further research should clarify the exact nature of the relevant causal pathways and define the scope for prevention.

References

Those marked with an asterisk are especially recommended for further reading.

1 **Pickering GW.** *High blood pressure* (2nd edn). London: Churchill, 1968.

2 **Peart WS.** Concepts in hypertension: the Croonian Lecture 1979. *J R Coll Physicians* 1979;**14**:141–52.

3 **Rose G.** Hypertension in the community. In Bulpitt CJ, ed. *Epidemiology of hypertension*. Amsterdam: Elsevier, 1985:1–14.

4 Intersalt Cooperative Research Group. Intersalt: an international study of electrolyte excretion and blood pressure. Results for 24 hour urinary sodium and potassium excretion. *Br Med J* 1988;**297**:319–28.

5 **Elliott P, Stamler J, Nichols R, Dyer AR, Stamler R, Kesteloot H** *et al.* Intersalt revisited: further analyses of 24 hour sodium excretion and blood pressure within and across populations. Intersalt Cooperative Research Group. *Br Med J* 1996;**312**:1249–53.

6 **Smith WCS, Crombie IK, Tavendale RT.** Urinary electrolyte excretion, alcohol consumption and blood pressure in the Scottish Heart Health Study. *Br Med J* 1988; **297**:329–30.

7 **Klatsky AL, Friedman GD, Armstrong MA.** The relationships between alcoholic beverage use and other traits to blood pressure: a new Kaiser Permanente study. *Circulation* 1986;**73**:628–36.

8 **Law MR, Frost CD, Wald NJ.** By how much does dietary salt reduction lower blood pressure? I —Analysis of observational data among populations. *Br Med J* 1991;**302**:811–15.

9 **Frost CD, Law MR, Wald NJ.** By how much does dietary salt reduction lower blood pressure? II —Analysis of observational data within populations. *Br Med J* 1991;**302**:815–18.

10 **Law MR, Frost CD, Wald NJ.** By how much does dietary salt reduction lower blood pressure? III—Analysis of data from trials of salt reduction. *Br Med J* 1991;**302**:819–24.

11 **Fagard RH.** Physical activity, fitness and blood pressure. In Bulpitt CJ, ed. *Handbook of hypertension Volume 20. Epidemiology of hypertension.* Amsterdam: Elsevier, 2000:191–211.

12 **Pickering TG.** Psychosocial stress and hypertension: clinical and experimental studies. In Swales JD, ed. *Textbook of hypertension.* Oxford: Blackwell Scientific, 1994:640–654.

*13 **Lever AF, Harrap SB.** Essential hypertension: a disorder of growth with origins in childhood? *J Hypertens* 1992;**10**:101–20.

*14 **Barker DJ.** *Mothers, babies and health in later life* (2nd edn). London: Churchill Livingstone, 1998.

*15 Lucas A. Programming by early nutrition in man. In Bock GR, Whelan J, eds. *The childhood environment and adult disease.* Chichester: John Wiley, 1991:38–55.

 16 Clarke R, Lewington S, Youngman L, Sherliker P, Peto R, Collins R. Underestimation of the importance of blood pressure and cholesterol for coronary heart disease mortality in old age. *Eur Heart J* 2002;**23**:286–93.

 17 Collins R, Peto R, MacMahon S, Hebert P, Fiebach NH, Eberlein KA *et al.* Blood pressure, stroke, and coronary heart disease. Part 2. Short-term reductions in blood pressure: overview of randomised drug trials in their epidemiological context. *Lancet* 1990;**335**:827–38.

*18 Prospective Studies Collaboration. Age-specific relevance of usual blood pressure to vascular mortality: one million adults in 61 prospective studies. *Lancet* 2002;**360**:1903–13.

 19 MacMahon S. Blood pressure as a risk factor. In Swales JD, ed. *Textbook of Hypertension.* Oxford: Blackwell Scientific, 1994:46–57.

 20 Paffenbarger RS Jr, Wing AL. Characteristics in youth predisposing to fatal stroke in later years. *Lancet* 1967;**1**:753–4.

 21 Paffenbarger RS Jr, Wing AL. Chronic disease in former college students. X. The effects of single and multiple characteristics on risk of fatal coronary heart disease. *Am J Epidemiol* 1969;**90**:527–35.

 22 McCarron P, Okasha M, McEwen J, Davey Smith G. Blood pressure in early life and cardiovascular disease mortality. *Arch Intern Med* 2002;**162**:610–11.

 23 Miura K, Daviglus ML, Dyer AR, Liu K, Garside DB, Stamler J *et al.* Relationship of blood pressure to 25-year mortality due to coronary heart disease, cardiovascular diseases, and all causes in young adult men: the Chicago Heart Association Detection Project in Industry. *Arch Intern Med* 2001;**161**:1501–8.

 24 Newman WP III, Freedman DS, Voors AW, Gard PD, Srinivasan SR, Cresanta JL *et al.* Relation of serum lipoprotein levels and systolic blood pressure to early atherosclerosis. The Bogalusa Heart Study. *N Engl J Med* 1986;**314**:138–44.

 25 McGill HC Jr, McMahan CA, Tracy RE, Oalmann MC, Cornhill JF, Herderick EE *et al.* Relation of a postmortem renal index of hypertension to atherosclerosis and coronary artery size in young men and women. Pathobiological Determinants of Atherosclerosis in Youth (PDAY) Research Group. *Arterioscler Thromb Vasc Biol* 1998;**18**:1108–18.

 26 Mongeau JG. Heredity and blood pressure. *Semin Nephrol* 1989;**9**:208–16.

 27 He J, Klag MJ, Whelton PK, Chen JY, Mo JP, Qian MC *et al.* Migration, blood pressure pattern, and hypertension: the Yi Migrant Study. *Am J Epidemiol* 1991;**134**:1085–101.

*28 Elford J, Phillips A, Thomson AG, Shaper AG. Migration and geographic variations in blood pressure in Britain. *Br Med J* 1990;**300**:291–5.

 29 de Swiet M, Fayers P, Shinebourne EA. Blood pressure survey in a population of newborn infants. *Br Med J* 1976;**2**:9–11.

 30 Rosner B, Hennekens CH, Kass EH, Miall WE. Age-specific correlation analysis of longitudinal blood pressure data. *Am J Epidemiol* 1977;**106**:306–13.

 31 de Swiet M, Fayers P, Shinebourne EA. Value of repeated blood pressure measurements in children—the Brompton study. *Br Med J* 1980;**280**:1567–9.

 32 Andre JL, Deschamps JP, Petit JC, Gueguen R. Change of blood pressure over five years in childhood and adolescence. *Clin Exp Hypertens A* 1986;**8**:539–45.

*33 Hofman A, Valkenburg HA. Determinants of change in blood pressure during childhood. *Am J Epidemiol* 1983;**117**:735–43.

 34 Clarke WR, Woolson RF, Lauer RM. Changes in ponderosity and blood pressure in childhood: the Muscatine Study. *Am J Epidemiol* 1986;**124**:195–206.

35 **Marmot MG.** Geography of blood pressure and hypertension. *Br Med Bull* 1984;**40**:380–6.

36 **Knuiman JT, Hautvast JG, Zwiauer KF, Widhalm K, Desmet M, De Backer G** *et al.* Blood pressure and excretion of sodium, potassium, calcium and magnesium. *Eur J Clin Nutr* 1988;**42**:847–55.

37 **Brotons C, Singh P, Nishio T, Labarthe DR.** Blood pressure by age in childhood and adolescence: a review of 129 surveys worldwide. *Int J Epidemiol* 1989;**18**:824–9.

38 **Intersalt Cooperative Research Group.** Centre specific results by age and sex. Appendix tables. *J Hum Hypertens* 1989;**3**:331–407.

39 **Whincup PH.** *A study of blood pressure in children in nine British towns.* London: London University, 1991.

40 **Beaglehole R, Eyles E, Salmond C, Prior I.** Blood pressure in Tokelauan children in two contrasting environments. *Am J Epidemiol* 1978;**108**:283–8.

41 **Beaglehole R, Eyles E, Prior I.** Blood pressure and migration in children. *Int J Epidemiol* 1979;**8**:5–10.

42 **Colhoun HM, Hemingway H, Poulter NR.** Socio-economic status and blood pressure: an overview analysis. *J Hum Hypertens* 1998;**12**:91–110.

43 **Chen E, Matthews KA, Boyce WT.** Socioeconomic differences in children's health: how and why do these relationships change with age? *Psychol Bull* 2002;**128**:295–329.

44 **Shaper AG.** Communities without hypertension. In Shaper AG, ed. *Cardiovascular disease in the tropics.* London: British Medical Association, 1974:77–83.

45 **Owen CG, Whincup PH, Cook DG.** Are fetal factors responsible for international differences in adult blood pressure? *J Pediatr Res* 2003;**53**:A31.

46 **Leon DA, Davey Smith G.** Infant mortality, stomach cancer, stroke, and coronary heart disease: ecological analysis. *Br Med J* 2000;**320**:1705–6.

47 **Salmond CE, Prior IA, Wessen AF.** Blood pressure patterns and migration: a 14-year cohort study of adult Tokelauans. *Am J Epidemiol* 1989;**130**:37–52.

48 **Poulter NR, Khaw KT, Hopwood BE, Mugambi M, Peart WS, Rose G** *et al.* The Kenyan Luo migration study: observations on the initiation of a rise in blood pressure. *Br Med J* 1990;**300**:967–72.

49 **Rosenthal T, Grossman E, Knecht A, Goldbourt U.** Blood pressure in Ethiopian immigrants in Israel: comparison with resident Israelis. *J Hypertens* 1989;**7**(**suppl**):S53–55.

50 **O'Dea K.** Interpretation of genetic versus environmental factors—lessons from the Australian aborigines when westernized. In Smith A, ed. *Hypertension as an insulin resistant disorder. Genetic factors and other mechanisms.* Amsterdam: Elsevier, 1991:69–87.

51 **Cappuccio FP.** Electrolyte intake and human hypertension: part B, calcium and magnesium. In Swales JD, ed. *Textbook of hypertension.* Oxford: Blackwell Scientific, 1994:551–66.

52 **Williams PT, Fortmann SP, Terry RB, Garay SC, Vranizan KM, Ellsworth N** *et al.* Associations of dietary fat, regional adiposity, and blood pressure in men. *J Am Med Assoc* 1987;**257**:3251–6.

53 **Smoak CG, Burke GL, Webber LS, Harsha DW, Srinivasan SR, Berenson GS.** Relation of obesity to clustering of cardiovascular disease risk factors in children and young adults. The Bogalusa Heart Study. *Am J Epidemiol* 1987;**125**:364–72.

54 **Ciba Foundation Symposium.** *No. 201: Origins and consequences of obesity.* Chichester: John Wiley, 1996.

55 **Holland FJ, Stark O, Ades AE, Peckham CS.** Birth weight and body mass index in childhood, adolescence, and adulthood as predictors of blood pressure at age 36. *J Epidemiol Commun Health* 1993;**47**:432–5.

56 **Cutler JA.** Randomized clinical trials of weight reduction in nonhypertensive persons. *Ann Epidemiol* 1991;**1**:363–70.

57 Havlik RJ, Hubert HB, Fabsitz RR, Feinleib M. Weight and hypertension. *Ann Intern Med* 1983;**98**:855–9.

58 Power C, Lake JK, Cole TJ. Measurement and long-term health risks of child and adolescent fatness. *Int J Obes Relat Metab Disord* 1997;**21**:507–26.

59 Visscher TL, Seidell JC. The public health impact of obesity. *Annu Rev Pub Health* 2001;**22**:355–75.

60 Marmot MG, Elliott P, Shipley MJ, Dyer AR, Ueshima H, Beevers DG *et al.* Alcohol and blood pressure: the INTERSALT study. *Br Med J* 1994;**308**:1263–7.

61 Bruce NG, Wannamethee G, Shaper AG. Lifestyle factors associated with geographic blood pressure variations among men and women in the UK. *J Hum Hypertens* 1993;**7**:229–38.

62 Xin X, He J, Frontini MG, Ogden LG, Motsamai OI, Whelton PK. Effects of alcohol reduction on blood pressure: a meta-analysis of randomized controlled trials. *Hypertension* 2001;**38**:1112–17.

63 Elliott P, Dyer A, Stamler R. The INTERSALT study: results for 24 hour sodium and potassium, by age and sex. INTERSALT Co-operative Research Group. *J Hum Hypertens* 1989;**3**:323–30.

64 Graudal NA, Galloe AM, Garred P. Effects of sodium restriction on blood pressure, renin, aldosterone, catecholamines, cholesterols, and triglyceride: a meta-analysis. *J Am Med Assoc* 1998;**279**:1383–91.

65 Cutler JA, Follmann D, Allender PS. Randomized trials of sodium reduction: an overview. *Am J Clin Nutr* 1997;**65**:643S–51S.

66 Hooper L, Bartlett C, Davey Smith G, Ebrahim S. Systematic review of long term effects of advice to reduce dietary salt in adults. *Br Med J* 2002;**325**:628–32.

67 Sacks FM, Svetkey LP, Vollmer WM, Appel LJ, Bray GA, Harsha D *et al.* Effects on blood pressure of reduced dietary sodium and the Dietary Approaches to Stop Hypertension (DASH) diet. DASH–Sodium Collaborative Research Group. *N Engl J Med* 2001;**344**:3–10.

68 Heino T, Kallio K, Jokinen E, Lagstrom H, Seppanen R, Valimaki I *et al.* Sodium intake of 1 to 5-year-old children: the STRIP project. The Special Turku Coronary Risk Factor Intervention Project. *Acta Paediatr* 2000;**89**:406–10.

69 Cooper R, Soltero I, Liu K, Berkson D, Levinson S, Stamler J. The association between urinary sodium excretion and blood pressure in children. *Circulation* 1980;**62**:97–104.

70 Cooper R, Liu K, Trevisan M, Miller W, Stamler J. Urinary sodium excretion and blood pressure in children: absence of a reproducible association. *Hypertension* 1983;**5**:135–9.

71 Whincup PH, Cook DG, Papacosta O, Jones SR. Relations between sodium: creatinine and potassium: creatinine ratios and blood pressure in childhood (abstract). *J Hypertens* 1992;**10**:1434.

72 Geleijnse JM, Grobbee DE, Hofman A. Sodium and potassium intake and blood pressure change in childhood. *Br Med J* 1990;**300**:899–902.

73 Cooper R, Van Horn L, Liu K, Trevisan M, Nanas S, Ueshima H *et al.* A randomized trial on the effect of decreased dietary sodium intake on blood pressure in adolescents. *J Hypertens* 1984;**2**:361–6.

74 Sinaiko AR, Gomez-Marin O, Prineas RJ. Effect of low sodium diet or potassium supplementation on adolescent blood pressure. *Hypertension* 1993;**21**:989–94.

*75 Hofman A, Hazebroek A, Valkenburg HA. A randomized trial of sodium intake and blood pressure in newborn infants. *J Am Med Assoc* 1983;**250**:370–3.

76 Hofman A. Sodium intake and blood pressure in newborns: evidence for a causal connection. In Hofman A, ed. *Children's blood pressure: report of the 88th Ross conference on paediatric research.* Columbus: Ross Laboratories, 1989.

77 Pomeranz A, Dolfin T, Korzets Z, Eliakim A, Wolach B. Increased sodium concentrations in drinking water increase blood pressure in neonates. *J Hypertens* 2002;**20**:203–7.

*78 Geleijnse JM, Hofman A, Witteman JC, Hazebroek AA, Valkenburg HA, Grobbee DE. Long-term effects of neonatal sodium restriction on blood pressure. *Hypertension* 1997;**29**:913–17.

79 Lucas A, Morley R, Hudson GJ, Bamford MF, Boon A, Crowle P *et al.* Early sodium intake and later blood pressure in preterm infants. *Arch Dis Child* 1988;**63**:656–7.

80 Singhal A, Cole TJ, Lucas A. Early nutrition in preterm infants and later blood pressure: two cohorts after randomised trials. *Lancet* 2001;**357**:413–19.

81 Beauchamp GK, Cowart BJ, Mennella JA, Marsh RR. Infant salt taste: developmental, methodological, and contextual factors. *Dev Psychobiol* 1994;**27**:353–65.

82 Whelton PK, He J, Cutler JA, Brancati FL, Appel LJ, Follmann D *et al.* Effects of oral potassium on blood pressure. Meta-analysis of randomized controlled clinical trials. *J Am Med Assoc* 1997;**277**:1624–32.

83 McGarvey ST, Zinner SH, Willett WC, Rosner B. Maternal prenatal dietary potassium, calcium, magnesium, and infant blood pressure. *Hypertension* 1991;**17**:218–24.

84 Strazzullo P, Cappuccio FP, Trevisan M, De Leo A, Krogh V, Giorgione N *et al.* Leisure time physical activity and blood pressure in schoolchildren. *Am J Epidemiol* 1988;**127**:726–33.

85 Kikuchi S, Rona RJ, Chinn S. Physical fitness of 9 year olds in England: related factors. *J Epidemiol Commun Health* 1995;**49**:180–5.

86 Paffenbarger RS Jr, Wing AL, Hyde RT, Jung DL. Physical activity and incidence of hypertension in college alumni. *Am J Epidemiol* 1983;**117**:245–57.

87 Hagberg JM, Park JJ, Brown MD. The role of exercise training in the treatment of hypertension: an update. *Sports Med* 2000;**30**:193–206.

88 Raitakari OT, Porkka KV, Taimela S, Telama R, Rasanen L, Viikari JS. Effects of persistent physical activity and inactivity on coronary risk factors in children and young adults. The Cardiovascular Risk in Young Finns Study. *Am J Epidemiol* 1994;**140**:195–205.

89 Huxley RR, Shiell AW, Law CM. The role of size at birth and postnatal catch-up growth in determining systolic blood pressure: a systematic review of the literature. *J Hypertens* 2000;**18**:815–31.

90 Nilsson PM, Ostergren PO, Nyberg P, Soderstrom M, Allebeck P. Low birth weight is associated with elevated systolic blood pressure in adolescence: a prospective study of a birth cohort of 149 378 Swedish boys. *J Hypertens* 1997;**15**:1627–31.

*91 Huxley R, Neil A, Collins R. Unravelling the fetal origins hypothesis: is there really an inverse association between birthweight and subsequent blood pressure? *Lancet* 2002;**360**:659–65.

92 Elford J, Whincup P, Shaper AG. Early life experience and adult cardiovascular disease: longitudinal and case–control studies. *Int J Epidemiol* 1991;**20**:833–44.

93 Barker DJ, Bull AR, Osmond C, Simmonds SJ. Fetal and placental size and risk of hypertension in adult life. *Br Med J* 1990;**301**:259–62.

94 Martyn CN, Barker DJ, Jespersen S, Greenwald S, Osmond C, Berry C. Growth *in utero*, adult blood pressure, and arterial compliance. *Br Heart J* 1995;**73**:116–21.

95 Whincup PH, Cook DG, Shaper AG. Early influences on blood pressure: a study of children aged 5–7 years. *Br Med J* 1989;**299**:587–91.

96 Whincup PH, Cook DG, Papacosta O. Do maternal and intrauterine factors influence blood pressure in childhood? *Arch Dis Child* 1992;**67**:1423–9.

97 Churchill D, Perry IJ, Beevers DG. Ambulatory blood pressure in pregnancy and fetal growth. *Lancet* 1997;**349**:7–10.

98 Taylor SJ, Whincup PH, Cook DG, Papacosta O. Blood pressure in pregnancy and fetal growth. *Lancet* 1997;**349**:802–3.

99 **Whincup P, Cook D, Papacosta O, Walker M, Perry I.** Maternal factors and development of cardiovascular risk: evidence from a study of blood pressure in children. *J Hum Hypertens* 1994;**8**:337–43.

100 **Paneth N, Susser M.** Early origin of coronary heart disease (the 'Barker hypothesis'). *Br Med J* 1995;**310**:411–12.

*101 **Lucas A, Fewtrell MS, Cole TJ.** Fetal origins of adult disease—the hypothesis revisited. *Br Med J* 1999;**319**:245–9.

102 **Barker DJ, Osmond C, Golding J, Kuh D, Wadsworth ME.** Growth *in utero*, blood pressure in childhood and adult life, and mortality from cardiovascular disease. *Br Med J* 1989;**298**:564–7.

103 **Law CM, Barker DJ, Bull AR, Osmond C.** Maternal and fetal influences on blood pressure. *Arch Dis Child* 1991;**66**:1291–5.

104 **Ravelli GP, Stein ZA, Susser MW.** Obesity in young men after famine exposure *in utero* and early infancy. *N Engl J Med* 1976;**295**:349–53.

105 **Whincup PH.** Fetal origins of cardiovascular risk: evidence from studies in children. *Proc Nutr Soc* 1998;**57**:123–7.

106 **Whincup PH, Cook DG, Adshead F, Taylor SJ, Walker M, Papacosta O** *et al.* Childhood size is more strongly related than size at birth to glucose and insulin levels in 10–11-year-old children. *Diabetologia* 1997;**40**:319–26.

107 **Owen CG, Whincup PH, Odoki K, Gilg JA, Cook DG.** Birthweight and blood cholesterol: a study in adolescents and a systematic review. *Pediatrics* 2002;**111**:1081–9.

108 **Whincup P, Cook D, Papacosta O, Walker M.** Birth weight and blood pressure: cross sectional and longitudinal relations in childhood. *Br Med J* 1995;**311**:773–6.

109 **Whincup PH, Bredow M, Payne F, Sadler S, Golding J.** Size at birth and blood pressure at 3 years of age. The Avon Longitudinal Study of Pregnancy and Childhood (ALSPAC). *Am J Epidemiol* 1999;**149**:730–9.

110 **Barker DJ, Godfrey KM, Osmond C, Bull A.** The relation of fetal length, ponderal index and head circumference to blood pressure and the risk of hypertension in adult life. *Paediatr Perinat Epidemiol* 1992;**6**:35–44.

111 **Leon DA, Koupilova I, Lithell HO, Berglund L, Mohsen R, Vagero D** *et al.* Failure to realise growth potential *in utero* and adult obesity in relation to blood pressure in 50 year old Swedish men. *Br Med J* 1996;**312**:401–6.

112 **Taylor SJ, Whincup PH, Cook DG, Papacosta O, Walker M.** Size at birth and blood pressure: cross sectional study in 8–11 year old children. *Br Med J* 1997;**314**:475–80.

113 **Moore VM, Miller AG, Boulton TJ, Cockington RA, Craig IH, Magarey AM** *et al.* Placental weight, birth measurements, and blood pressure at age 8 years. *Arch Dis Child* 1996;**74**:538–41.

114 **Williams S, St George IM, Silva PA.** Intrauterine growth retardation and blood pressure at age seven and eighteen. *J Clin Epidemiol* 1992;**45**:1257–63.

115 **Law CM, de Swiet M, Osmond C, Fayers PM, Barker DJ, Cruddas AM** *et al.* Initiation of hypertension *in utero* and its amplification throughout life. *Br Med J* 1993;**306**:24–7.

*116 **Law CM, Shiell AW, Newsome CA, Syddall HE, Shinebourne EA, Fayers PM** *et al.* Fetal, infant, and childhood growth and adult blood pressure: a longitudinal study from birth to 22 years of age. *Circulation* 2002;**105**:1088–92.

117 **Ley D, Stale H, Marsal K.** Aortic vessel wall characteristics and blood pressure in children with intrauterine growth retardation and abnormal foetal aortic blood flow. *Acta Paediatr* 1997;**86**:299–305.

118 Blake KV, Gurrin LC, Evans SF, Beilin LJ, Stanley FJ, Landau LI *et al.* Adjustment for current weight and the relationship between birth weight and blood pressure in childhood. *J Hypertens* 2000;**18**:1007–12.

119 Frankel S, Elwood P, Sweetnam P, Yarnell J, Davey Smith G. Birthweight, body-mass index in middle age, and incident coronary heart disease. *Lancet* 1996;**348**:1478–80.

120 Uiterwaal CS, Anthony S, Launer LJ, Witteman JC, Trouwborst AM, Hofman A *et al.* Birth weight, growth, and blood pressure: an annual follow-up study of children aged 5 through 21 years. *Hypertension* 1997;**30**:267–71.

121 Taittonen L, Nuutinen M, Turtinen J, Uhari M. Prenatal and postnatal factors in predicting later blood pressure among children: cardiovascular risk in young Finns. *Pediatr Res* 1996;**40**:627–32.

122 Koupilova I, Leon DA, Lithell HO, Berglund L. Size at birth and hypertension in longitudinally followed 50–70-year-old men. *Blood Press* 1997;**6**:223–8.

123 Moore VM, Cockington RA, Ryan P, Robinson JS. The relationship between birth weight and blood pressure amplifies from childhood to adulthood. *J Hypertens* 1999;**17**:883–8.

124 Harding JE. The nutritional basis of the fetal origins of adult disease. *Int J Epidemiol* 2001;**30**:15–23.

*125 Mackenzie HS, Brenner BM. Fewer nephrons at birth: a missing link in the etiology of essential hypertension? *Am J Kidney Dis* 1995;**26**:91–8.

126 Langley-Evans SC, Jackson AA. Increased systolic blood pressure in adult rats induced by fetal exposure to maternal low protein diets. *Clin Sci (Lond)* 1994;**86**:217–22.

127 Edwards CR, Benediktsson R, Lindsay RS, Seckl JR. Dysfunction of placental glucocorticoid barrier: link between fetal environment and adult hypertension? *Lancet* 1993;**341**:355–7.

128 Carr-Hill R, Campbell DM, Hall MH, Meredith A. Is birthweight determined genetically? *Br Med J* 1987;**295**:687–9.

129 Robson EB. The genetics of birthweight. In Falkner F, Tanner JM, eds. *Human growth. Vol I: Principles and prenatal growth.* New York: Plenum Press, 1978.

130 Stein Z, Susser M. The Dutch famine, 1944–1945, and the reproductive process. I. Effects on six indices at birth. *Pediatr Res* 1975;**9**:70–6.

131 Roseboom TJ, van der Meulen JH, Ravelli AC, van Montfrans GA, Osmond C, Barker DJ *et al.* Blood pressure in adults after prenatal exposure to famine. *J Hypertens* 1999;**17**:325–30.

132 Roseboom TJ, van der Meulen JH, van Montfrans GA, Ravelli AC, Osmond C, Barker DJ *et al.* Maternal nutrition during gestation and blood pressure in later life. *J Hypertens* 2001;**19**:29–34.

133 Campbell DM, Hall MH, Barker DJ, Cross J, Shiell AW, Godfrey KM. Diet in pregnancy and the offspring's blood pressure 40 years later. *Br J Obstet Gynaecol* 1996;**103**:273–80.

134 Godfrey KM, Redman CW, Barker DJ, Osmond C. The effect of maternal anaemia and iron deficiency on the ratio of fetal weight to placental weight. *Br J Obstet Gynaecol* 1991;**98**:886–91.

135 Gibson HM. Plasma volume and glomerular filtration rate in pregnancy and their relation to differences in fetal growth. *J Obstet Gynaecol Br Commonw* 1973;**80**:1067–74.

136 Poulter NR, Chang CL, MacGregor AJ, Snieder H, Spector TD. Association between birth weight and adult blood pressure in twins: historical cohort study. *Br Med J* 1999;**319**:1330–3.

137 Dwyer T, Blizzard L, Morley R, Ponsonby AL. Within pair association between birth weight and blood pressure at age 8 in twins from a cohort study. *Br Med J* 1999;**319**:1325–9.

138 Leon DA. Twins and fetal programming of blood pressure. Questioning the role of genes and maternal nutrition. *Br Med J* 1999;**319**:1313–14.

139 Loos RJ, Fagard R, Beunen G, Derom C, Vlietinck R. Birth weight and blood pressure in young adults: a prospective twin study. *Circulation* 2001;**104**:1633–8.

140 Christensen K, Stovring H, McGue M. Do genetic factors contribute to the association between birth weight and blood pressure? *J Epidemiol Commun Health* 2001;**55**:583–7.

141 Johansson-Kark M, Rasmussen F, De Stavola B, Leon DA. Fetal growth and systolic blood pressure in young adulthood: the Swedish Young Male Twins Study. *Paediatr Perinat Epidemiol* 2002;**16**:200–9.

142 Dwyer T, Morley R, Blizzard L. Twins and fetal origins hypothesis: within-pair analyses. *Lancet* 2002;**359**:2205–6.

143 Leon DA. The foetal origins of adult disease: interpreting the evidence from twin studies. *Twin Res* 2001;**4**:321–6.

144 Wilson AC, Forsyth JS, Greene SA, Irvine L, Hau C, Howie PW. Relation of infant diet to childhood health: seven year follow up of cohort of children in Dundee infant feeding study. *Br Med J* 1998;**316**:21–5.

145 Lucas A, Morley R. Does early nutrition in infants born before term programme later blood pressure? *Br Med J* 1994;**309**:304–8.

146 Martin RM, McCarthy A, Davey Smith G, Davies DP, Ben-Shlomo Y. Infant nutrition and blood pressure in early adulthood: the Barry Caerphilly Growth cohort study. *Am J Clin Nutr* 2003;**77**:1489–97.

147 Owen CG, Whincup PH, Gilg JA, Cook DG. Effect of breast feeding in infancy on blood pressure in later life: systematic review and meta-analysis. *Br Med J* 2003;**327**:1189–95.

148 Forsyth JS, Willatts P, Agostini C, Bissenden J, Casaer P, Boehm G. Long chain polyunsaturated fatty acid supplementation in infant formula and blood pressure in later childhood. *Br Med J* 2003;**326**:953.

149 Langenberg C, Hardy R, Kuh D, Wadsworth ME. Influence of height, leg and trunk length on pulse pressure, systolic and diastolic blood pressure. *J Hypertens* 2003;**21**:537–43.

150 World Health Organization. *Prevention in childhood and youth of adult cardiovascular diseases: time for action. 792.* Geneva, World Health Organization, 1990.

Chapter 10

A life course approach to respiratory and allergic diseases

David P. Strachan and Aziz Sheikh

Respiratory illnesses are caused by a sometimes complex interaction of infection, allergy, mucus hypersecretion, reversible bronchospasm, and irreversible airflow obstruction. Cigarette smoking is a powerful and partially reversible influence on the risk of mucus hypersecretion and reversible and irreversible airflow obstruction and should be the priority in any preventive programme. However, not all smokers appear to be prone to disabling or fatal airflow obstruction and cofactors including impaired prenatal and postnatal lung growth, genetic antitrypsin deficiency, and dietary antioxidant deficiency may determine which smokers are most susceptible. In the past, high levels of outdoor air pollution were associated with increased morbidity and mortality among bronchitic patients, but the role of outdoor or indoor air pollution as a determinant of the prevalence of obstructive lung disease remains uncertain.

As smoking becomes less common, allergic sensitization and other influences on adult asthma may attain greater relative importance. A role for dietary factors in adult asthma and chronic airflow obstruction has been suggested but not consistently confirmed by observational or experimental studies. There is suggestive but not conclusive evidence that the risk of allergy may to some extent be programmed in early childhood, by early allergen exposure and exposure to infectious illnesses (the latter being protective). Although childhood chest infections are closely associated with subsequent asthma, the direction of cause and effect here remains a matter for debate.

10.1 Introduction

Respiratory disease poses a substantial public health problem in terms of premature death, disability, hospital admissions, primary care contacts, loss of productivity, and interference with work and schooling.[1] Much of this disease burden is thought to relate to five broadly defined clinical syndromes.

1. *Respiratory infections*, often of a viral nature, affecting all ages but more severe in the very young and the elderly.

2. *Atopy*, characterized by elevated levels of circulating immunoglobulin E (IgE) and cutaneous hypersensitivity on skin prick testing with common aeroallergens.

3. *Reversible airflow obstruction*, embracing 'wheezy bronchitis' in early life, 'extrinsic asthma' of children and young adults, and 'intrinsic asthma', typically of later onset.

4. *Chronic mucus hypersecretion*, characterized by persistent cough and phlegm, used by the British Medical Research Council to define 'chronic bronchitis'.

5. *Irreversible airflow obstruction*, the main cause of death and severe disability from chronic respiratory disease[2] and an important predictor of all-cause mortality, even among lifelong non-smokers.[3,4]

These syndromes are interconnected by a complex web of associations and putative causal relationships (Fig. 10.1). Lower respiratory illnesses in infancy (1) have been proposed as a cause of a chronic wheezing tendency (3),[5,6] chronic cough and phlegm (4),[5,7] impaired ventilatory function (5),[5,8] and related mortality.[9] An alternative explanation for these associations could be that they reflect a longstanding tendency to all forms of chest illness, perhaps related to impaired lung development[10] or asthma (3).[11] Although viral infections (1) are an immediate cause of many wheezing attacks (3),[12] it has been suggested that early infection may protect against the development of allergic sensitization (2).[13]

The association between atopy (2) and extrinsic asthma (3) is well-established, but the role of atopic history in the other wheezing syndromes is less clear.[10,14] Asthma[11] and airways responsiveness (3)[15] are associated with chronic productive cough (4). Irreversible airflow obstruction (5) has been postulated as the end result of chronic airway irritation and inflammation (4)—the so-called 'English hypothesis'[16]—or related primarily to the asthmatic tendency (3)—the 'Dutch hypothesis'.[17] Although much of the excess mortality among asthmatic adults (3) is due to deaths certified as chronic bronchitis or emphysema, rather than asthma,[18] the true degree of overlap between these syndromes remains in dispute.[19]

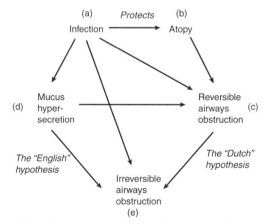

Fig. 10.1 Postulated relationships between different forms of respiratory and allergic disease.

These relationships are further complicated by interactions with causal factors. Thus, active smoking is established as a powerful cause of mucus hypersecretion (4)[16] and progressive decline of ventilatory function (5),[14,16] but asthmatics and those with non-specific airways hyperreactivity may be particularly susceptible to these effects.[14] Smoking can also trigger asthmatic attacks (3) and increase the risk of atopic sensitization to some occupational allergens (2).[20] A wide range of other factors have been related to one or more of the respiratory syndromes, including birthweight, family size and structure, passive smoking, urban air pollution, diet, occupation, and socioeconomic circumstances in childhood and adult life. A life course approach to the epidemiology of respiratory disease thus seems appropriate.

This chapter addresses the independent and combined effects of perinatal or childhood exposures and adult lifestyle on the development of both allergic and non-allergic lung disease.

10.2 Development of ventilatory function

10.2.1 Lung growth

The emergence of severe impairment of ventilatory function, as measured by marked reductions in spirometric indices such as forced expiratory volume in one second (FEV$_1$) and peak expiratory flow rate (PEFR), is the end result of many years of decline in function from maximal levels attained during early adulthood. The risk of disabling airflow obstruction in later adult life is believed to be influenced by the maximum level attained through lung growth and by the rate of functional decline throughout adulthood (Fig. 10.2).

The factors influencing lung growth are not fully understood but may include both prenatal and postnatal exposures.[21] Ventilatory function is reduced among children of low birthweight,[22,23] whether this is due to prematurity or intrauterine growth retardation. Maternal smoking during pregnancy is currently the most important remediable influence on intrauterine growth, and lung function abnormalities in the offspring of smoking mothers are apparent shortly after birth.[24] Premature infants who require prolonged artificial ventilation appear to be at particular risk of later lung function abnormalities.[25]

Maternal smoking and neonatal intensive care are unlikely to have influenced the lung development of today's adults who have survived to middle and old age. Nevertheless, low birthweight predicted both lower FEV$_1$ and mortality from chronic obstructive lung disease among men born in Hertfordshire during 1911–1930.[26] Weight at 1 year of age was less strongly associated with adult FEV$_1$, although the study had insufficient statistical power to distinguish conclusively the effects of prenatal and postnatal growth. When taken together with data from other birth cohorts however,[27] these suggest that prenatal and postnatal lung growth may negatively impact on the 'capital investment' of ventilatory function in early adult life which is subject to 'depreciation' with advancing age.

10.2.2 Functional decline

The progressive and irreversible decline in ventilatory function throughout adult life is commonly due to pulmonary emphysema, a widespread destruction of alveolar ducts and walls, which is thought to result from an imbalance between destructive and repair forces

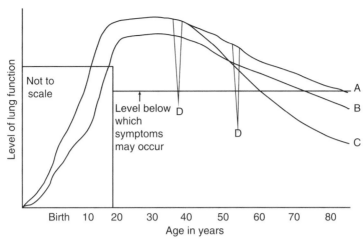

Fig. 10.2 Schematic representation of the life course of ventilatory function measurements such as forced expiratory volume in 1s. A = normal growth and decline; B = impaired prenatal or postnatal growth, leading to reduced maximal function and increased risk of later disability and death from chronic respiratory disease despite a normal rate of decline; C = normal growth but accelerated decline, leading to premature disability and risk of death from chronic respiratory disease; D = episodes of reversible airflow obstruction, which may be superimposed on any of curves A, B, or C.

in the peripheral lung and smaller airways. The environmental factors that may influence this balance favourably or unfavourably are discussed in a later section of this chapter.

Superimposed upon the irreversible component may be episodes of reversible airways narrowing related to asthma (Fig. 10.2). The propensity to asthma attacks is usually associated with measurable airflow reductions on inhalation of provocation agents such as histamine or methacholine. This non-specific bronchial hyperresponsiveness (BHR) is widely believed to relate to chronic inflammatory processes in the airways, which may be initiated or sustained in atopic individuals by allergen exposure. If this inflammation persists it is thought that remodelling of the airway tissues may lead to a degree of irreversible airflow obstruction, which may thus predispose to disabling or fatal chronic obstructive lung disease. Such a link between reversible and irreversible airways obstruction was first proposed by Dutch workers in the 1960s[17] and since termed the 'Dutch hypothesis'.

There has been considerable debate about the relationship between BHR and accelerated decline in adult ventilatory function.[14,28] Confusion arises because BHR in adults without asthma may be related to cigarette smoking, itself a powerful risk factor for rapid lung function decline. In cross-sectional studies, BHR is most closely associated with atopy and asthma in younger adults and with smoking in older age groups.[29] The increased BHR of older smokers is almost invariably associated with reduced baseline FEV_1, so it is possible that irreversible airways obstruction alone may increase BHR, perhaps through distortions of airway geometry.[30]

Burrows and colleagues have proposed that it may be useful to consider two major causes of persistent airflow obstruction in middle-aged and elderly people.[19] One type, associated with asthma and atopy mainly in non-smokers, is that to which the Dutch hypothesis applies most clearly. The other, with a worse prognosis, occurs in non-atopic cigarette smokers among whom BHR may be a consequence, rather than a cause, of accelerated lung function decline. This distinction may be relevant to the subsequent discussion of effects of childhood chest illness on chronic respiratory disease in adults.

10.3 Effects of childhood chest illness

An association between chest illness in childhood and both chronic respiratory morbidity and impaired ventilatory function in later life has emerged in several studies.[5] This could reflect lung damage due to early episodes of chest infection, a longstanding susceptibility to all forms of lung disease, or continuity of socioeconomic circumstances or environmental exposure[31] (Fig. 10.3).

Two historical cohort studies, in Hertfordshire[26] and Derbyshire,[32] suggest that lower respiratory illness in the first year of life is associated with later cough, phlegm, and impaired ventilatory function, independent of smoking habit and social class. Illnesses after the first year did not appear to pose a risk. Mortality from chronic respiratory disease was associated with early bronchitis and pneumonia in Hertfordshire.[26] These studies, together with ecological correlations[9,33] have been interpreted as evidence of persistent lung damage from chest infections in infancy. In contrast, a prospective study of the UK 1946 birth cohort found that there was no significant independent effect of bronchitis, bronchiolitis, or pneumonia before 2 years of age on PEFR at age 36, although early chest illnesses were independently associated with lower respiratory illness, phlegm, and asthma or wheeze in adulthood.[34] When all respiratory illnesses up

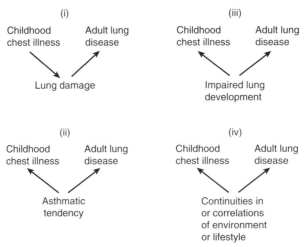

Fig. 10.3 Four possible explanations for the association of childhood chest illness and adult respiratory disease.

to 10 years of age were considered, a significant effect on PEFR was found for bronchitis and pneumonia,[8] but not for whooping cough.[35]

Asthmatic children often have a history of early chest illnesses, which in past decades might have been labelled as bronchitis or pneumonia. The direction of cause and effect is a matter of debate,[31] but it has been suggested that the asthmatic trait might form a continuity between childhood and adult life and increase the susceptibility to both early chest illness and adult morbidity (model (ii), Fig. 10.3).[11] Supporting evidence comes from studies of whooping cough—although asthmatic children are more common among those with a history of whooping cough, the onset of wheezing symptoms usually precedes the whooping cough illness.[36] Two long-term follow-up studies confirm that although the majority of wheezy children grow out of their asthma, those that do not are at increased risk of cough and phlegm in their early 20s.[11,37] An American study, of retrospective design, also suggested that the respiratory problems in childhood that were associated with adult obstructive airways disease were those in the category of 'chronic or recurrent airway disease' (consistent with childhood asthma) rather than 'severe acute respiratory illness'.[38] On the other hand, the association of early chest illness and adult respiratory symptoms in the UK 1946 birth cohort was independent of asthma history.[34] Furthermore, a nested case–control study of participants in a 30-year follow-up survey of Aberdeen school children failed to show any relationship between exposure to infections, as measured by parental reports obtained at ages 10–14 years and serological tests in adulthood, and the development of wheezing disorders in adult life.[39]

The influences of early and later onset asthma or wheezy bronchitis on adult ventilatory function were studied at ages 34–35 in the UK 1958 cohort. Of the children with a history of pneumonia by 2 years of age, 75% developed later asthma or wheezing. Ventilatory function of young adults who had 'outgrown' a childhood wheezing tendency did not differ from that of healthy control participants.[40] Young adults reporting wheeze in the past year at examination had lower levels of ventilatory function, the reduction being greater for those with childhood wheezing of earlier onset. These differences persisted after inhalation of salbutamol, suggesting a degree of irreversible airflow obstruction. Two longitudinal studies have suggested progressive deterioration in ventilatory function (as measured by FEV_1/FVC ratio) among adolescents with persistent asthma[41] or BHR.[42] These findings would be consistent with cumulative airway damage resulting from chronic inflammation in the bronchi of asthmatic individuals.

Infants with small airways are prone to early respiratory illnesses[43,44] that usually do not progress to chronic asthma.[44] It has thus been suggested that the link between early childhood chest illness and chronic respiratory disease in adults may arise from host susceptibility related to impaired prenatal lung growth, rather than from continuities in disease or lung damage from early infectious illnesses (model (iii), Fig.10.3).[10] The results of the 1958 cohort study offer only limited support for this hypothesis, in that FEV_1 at age 35 was slightly lower among children with transient early wheezing illness than among control participants, although the dominant effect was of persistent asthma (that is, model (ii)).[40]

Marked seasonal fluctuations in many respiratory viruses and the greater vulnerability of young infants together imply that babies born in the autumn are at substantially greater risk of developing viral bronchiolitis, bronchitis, and pneumonia than those born in the spring. If these early infections had direct long-term consequences for lung function or respiratory symptoms, then these outcomes should also be more common among autumn births. This was not found in several large datasets,[45] arguing that host susceptibility related to lung development (model (iii)) or airways reactivity (model (ii)), rather than lung damage (model (i)), may be the more important factor underlying the association of early chest illness with later lung disease and respiratory mortality.

10.4 Allergic sensitization

The ability to generate an IgE response to common inhaled proteins (aeroallergens) such as pollens, house dust mite faeces, or pet dander is consistently related to asthma and BHR in cross-sectional surveys of older children[46] and adults.[29] This atopic tendency may be assessed directly by skin prick tests or by measurement of serum IgE levels or imputed (less reliably) from a history of hay fever, allergic rhinitis, or eczema. Both the incidence and prognosis of asthma throughout childhood and early adult life are strongly influenced by atopy.[47]

Although there is undoubtedly a genetic component to atopy, environmental exposures are important in its expression. There is growing evidence that the process of allergic sensitization may be influenced by events during a critical period in early childhood or on the first contact with the sensitizing allergen. Three possibilities have been considered: early growth, early allergen exposure, and early infection.

Godfrey and colleagues[48] measured levels of serum IgE among men and women aged about 50 years whose weight and dimensions at birth had been recorded in unusual detail. Raised IgE levels were positively correlated with head circumference and weight at birth, independent of circumstances in adult life. Head circumference was found to be the more influential factor, with no significant effect of birthweight at any given head circumference. They speculated that prenatal undernutrition of the thymus may influence subsequent IgE production and allergic sensitization, but no consistent evidence has emerged linking neonatal head circumference or other birth measurements to allergen-specific IgE production or clinically apparent allergic disease.[49]

The relative immaturity of the immune system in early infancy has led to widespread speculation that allergen exposure in the first few months of life may enhance the risk of later sensitization. The inverse relationship between prematurity and allergic rhinitis seen in a large retrospective cohort study of Swedish conscripts provides indirect evidence to support this idea, the suggestion being that the prolonged period of immunological immaturity in such individuals increases the risk of atopic sensitization.[50] A number of studies have reported birth month variations in sensitization to grass or tree pollens but the evidence overall is inconsistent, both between and within studies.[45,51] If programming by early allergen exposure does occur, it is clearly a matter of degree, because sensitization can occur to occupational allergens encountered for the first time in adult life, as discussed in Section 10.5.4.

Several studies have shown that children from large families are at reduced risk of developing hay fever,[13,52,53] eczema,[13,53] and allergic sensitization to common aeroallergens.[51,53,54] Older siblings appear to exert a stronger protective effect than younger siblings[52–54] and offspring of more affluent families are at increased risk of hay fever and allergic sensitization.[54,55] Such observations led to speculation that infection acquired by household contact in early childhood might protect against allergic sensitization.[13,55] Further indirect evidence of the possible protective role of infections in early childhood comes from studies that have shown children of farmers and those with exposure to livestock (both of which are imputed to increase risk of exposure to bacterial agents) to be at reduced risk of developing hay fever and asthma.[56]

Recent advances in our understanding of human immunological development have suggested a possible mechanism for such a protective effect.[57] Production of IgE responses and symptomatic atopic disease are associated with the presence of allergen-specific thymus-derived helper 2 (Th2) lymphocytes, whereas in non-atopic individuals non-pathogenic responses to the same antigens are mediated by Th1 cells. Th1 and Th2 cells are thought to develop in early life from uncommitted precursors and the direction of differentiation can be influenced by the levels of cytokines prevailing at the time of challenge with antigen. The 'natural' immune response to bacterial and viral infections increases the production of cytokines, which selectively enhance the development of Th1-type lymphocytes and suppress Th2-type differentiation.[57]

Direct evidence of a protective effect of early infection is still awaited.[52,58] The critical period during which programming by infection may occur is also uncertain. The suggestion that the first month of life is especially important[59] has been tested specifically and is not supported by the epidemiological evidence.[52] It is likely that a stable pattern of allergen-specific IgE response may evolve over a number of years,[60] in relation to repeated exposures to allergen, offering multiple 'windows of opportunity' for infection acquired from siblings and playmates to influence the cytokine environment of developing thymus-derived lymphocytes.

10.5 Later influences on adult respiratory disease

10.5.1 Tobacco smoking

Tobacco smoking is the dominant influence on respiratory symptoms related to chronic mucus hypersecretion, irreversible airflow obstruction, and asthma. The evidence implicating smoking and the benefits of smoking cessation have been extensively reviewed[61,62] and only the salient points are reiterated here. Cough, phlegm, wheeze, and breathlessness are much more common among individuals and populations who smoke and are reduced when they quit the habit. The decline of ventilatory function is slowed, but not reversed, by smoking cessation. These benefits have been determined largely from observational studies but are supported by the results of two randomized controlled trials of antismoking advice.[63,64] Unfortunately, these lack the statistical power to demonstrate a reduction in respiratory mortality.

Although most smokers develop chronic mucus hypersecretion, only a minority develop disabling airflow obstruction and the rate of decline of ventilatory function throughout adult life varies greatly.[14,16,28,30] A rare but powerful risk factor for accelerated decline is genetically determined alpha$_1$-antitrypsin deficiency.[65] Smokers with the abnormal PiZ alpha$_1$-antitrypsin genotype rapidly develop severe emphysema and usually die in their thirties or forties. Non-smokers with alpha$_1$-antitrypsin deficiency have a survival curve closer to that of smokers in the general population.

10.5.2 Diet

Alpha$_1$-antitrypsin is one of several lung antiprotease enzymes that are defence mechanisms against destructive proteolytic enzymes released in the lung on exposure to tobacco smoke. These antiproteases are inactivated by oxidants and this has led to speculation that antioxidants may improve the protease–antiprotease balance and thus protect against emphysema. By analogy with genetic alpha$_1$-antitrypsin deficiency, this protective effect might be more evident in smokers. Cross-sectional studies have generally found lower levels of lung function in people consuming fewer fruit and vegetables or fewer antioxidant vitamins,[66–69] although this effect appears in both smokers and non-smokers and it has been difficult to exclude residual confounding by socioeconomic factors. Longitudinal data relating dietary changes to change in lung function are sparse but suggestive of a reversible effect.[70] This is contrary to what might be expected if antioxidants prevent emphysematous lung damage.

A link between dietary sodium and reversible airflow obstruction was first suggested from a regional correlation of asthma mortality and salt purchases in England and Wales.[71] This was supported by observations of a reduction in BHR on dietary salt restriction[72] and a double-blind randomized placebo-controlled study, which showed that large increases in dietary sodium result in significant physiological deterioration in lung function and increased morbidity in male asthmatic patients.[73] A later study did not confirm the association of BHR sodium excretion but suggested that dietary magnesium might protect against BHR and wheezing in adults.[74] Recent reports of the inverse relationship between dietary vitamin E and serum IgE concentrations[75] suggest that further studies investigating the role of nutritional factors in the aetiology of asthma and allergic disease can be expected.

10.5.3 Socioeconomic status

It has long been recognized that there is a strong association between poor socioeconomic status and both mortality and general practice consultations for adult respiratory disease in Britain.[76] Although much of this may be attributable to social class differences in smoking behaviour, population surveys have shown associations of socioeconomic status with symptoms of mucus hypersecretion[77,78] and measures of ventilatory function,[79] independent of current smoking habit. Furthermore, bronchitis mortality showed a strong social class gradient long before there was any substantial variation in smoking behaviour by social class.[80] Socioeconomic gradients may reflect upbringing and living conditions in childhood or lifestyle and environment in adult life. Indeed, continuity of socioeconomic circumstances may be a further factor underlying associations between respiratory morbidity in childhood and adult life (model (iv), Fig. 10.3). Among the UK 1946 birth cohort, strong associations emerged between indices of socioeconomic deprivation in childhood (particularly domestic crowding) and adult ventilatory function, measured as PEFR.[34] However, chronic cough and PEFR were also related to current socioeconomic circumstances, as indicated by housing tenure.[8] More specific studies of socially mobile individuals are required to distinguish reliably between influences in childhood and later life.

10.5.4 Occupational exposures

Marked social class trends are apparent in women (classified by their husband's occupation) as well as men, suggesting that specific occupational exposures play only a small part in explaining socioeconomic differentials. Nevertheless, a causal link between occupational dust exposure and mucus hypersecretion is generally acknowledged[77,81] and allergic sensitization to proteins and low-molecular-weight chemicals encountered in the workplace accounts for a small proportion of adult-onset asthma.[82] Smoking seems to promote allergic sensitization to some,[20] but not all,[83] occupational allergens. The role of dust and fumes in the aetiology of progressive airflow obstruction remains controversial. The best evidence emerges from longitudinal studies of workers in specific occupations, which suggest that exposures to a variety of inorganic dusts and to sulphur dioxide are consistently related to more rapid decline in FEV_1, whereas exposure to other fumes such as chlorine is not.[84]

10.5.5 Outdoor pollution

A more widespread source of inhaled particles and sulphur dioxide is combustion of fossil fuels and throughout the past century there has been concern that urban air pollution may initiate or exacerbate chronic respiratory disease.[85] The following discussion will concentrate on disease initiation, as it is of greater relevance to the life course approach. Historically there was a geographical correlation between particulate pollution and chronic respiratory disease mortality in the UK,[86] but this became less marked after control of pollution in the 1960s.[87] Nevertheless, studies of communities exposed to lower levels of pollution in the USA during the 1970s show correlations of particulate exposure with both reduced FEV_1[88] and physician-diagnosed bronchitis.[89] UK reviews have concluded that the possibility of chronic effects on respiratory health at levels of particulates below 100 mg/m^3 annual average cannot be excluded,[90] although it is impossible to distinguish the effects of current low-level exposure from past exposure to higher levels of air pollution.[91]

There have been few longitudinal studies addressing cumulative pollution exposure in relation to adult respiratory disease. The most comprehensive of these is the UK 1946 birth cohort, who were exposed as children to high levels of smoke and sulphur dioxide pollution in urban areas, but as adults to much lower levels. Air pollution exposure in childhood was estimated from domestic coal consumption in the area of residence during wartime coal rationing. Although childhood chest illnesses were more common in highly polluted areas,[92] the effect of early pollution on symptoms of cough and phlegm at age 21 was small.[7] At age 36, air pollution exposure from age 2 to 11 years was significantly associated with lower respiratory illnesses over the preceding 16 years, but not with phlegm, wheeze, asthma, or reduced PEFR, after adjustment for current smoking, socioeconomic status, parental history of bronchitis, and history of asthma or chest illness before age 2 years.[34] It is arguable that the last two of these might be intermediate factors, rather than confounders, but this analysis suggests that long-term consequences are difficult to demonstrate, even from days when particulate and sulphur dioxide pollution levels were orders of magnitude higher than are currently experienced in UK.

While in the past research and policy focused on the link between chronic bronchitis and smoke and sulphur dioxide ('old-fashioned winter pollutants'), more recently public concern has concentrated on asthma and the possible hazards of 'new' pollutants such as nitrogen oxides, ozone, and diesel particles, which are related to vehicle emissions. The evidence relating outdoor air pollution to asthma has been extensively reviewed.[93,94] Although other factors are likely to be more important than air pollution in the initiation of asthma, there are two lines of evidence that suggest outdoor pollution exposure should not be entirely dismissed.

Studies have shown a higher prevalence of wheezing and allergic rhinitis among non-smoking adults living close to busy roads[95] and it has been suggested that either diesel exhaust particles or nitrogen oxides, or both, may potentiate allergic sensitization.[93] On the other hand, no association with local traffic density was found in a large study of general practitioner consultations for asthma in east London[96] and no excess of respiratory symptoms has emerged in studies of groups with heavy occupational exposure to traffic fumes.[93]

Well designed cohort studies among Seventh Day Adventists in California have found a significantly higher incidence of asthma and chronic respiratory symptoms among people with high cumulative exposure to particulates and ozone.[97,98] These studies are especially valuable because the study group avoid smoking for religious reasons, removing an important potential confounding variable.

10.5.6 Indoor pollution

The Seventh Day Adventist studies[98] are among the more convincing to demonstrate an adverse effect of home or workplace exposure to environmental tobacco smoke on chronic respiratory disease in adults. This emphasizes that throughout life, indoor environments contribute a much greater proportion of personal pollutant exposure than does outdoor air; of these, environmental tobacco smoke exposure ranks as one of the most important risk factors for development of adult respiratory disease.[99] Nitrogen dioxide, although generated by motor vehicles, is often found at higher levels indoors than outdoors, due to emissions from unvented gas or paraffin appliances. Few studies have investigated the effects of indoor nitrogen dioxide on respiratory health in adults. The findings with respect to allergic sensitization, chronic cough and phlegm, and lung function are inconsistent, possibly because the presence of a gas cooker has been used as a crude surrogate for personal nitrogen dioxide exposure. In one small study where nitrogen dioxide exposure was measured, there was also a significant association with spirometric measurements in non-smoking women at entry to the study, but not with the rate of subsequent lung function decline.[100] Although a causal relationship between nitrogen dioxide exposure and respiratory disease has not been disproved, the balance of evidence suggests it is unlikely.[94] These results suggest that indoor air quality deserves greater emphasis in future studies of the chronic respiratory effects of air pollution exposure.

10.6 Trends in chronic obstructive pulmonary disease, asthma, and allergy

10.6.1 Chronic obstructive pulmonary diseases

Recent trends in mortality from chronic obstructive pulmonary disease (COPD—chronic bronchitis, emphysema, asthma, and chronic airflow obstruction) vary substantially by country and by gender.[101] Rates are generally stable or falling in men and stable or rising in women, although death rates of men have continued to rise in some west European countries, the USA, and Canada during the 1980s.[102–105] Neither current nor past trends in cigarette smoking adequately explain the international variation in the direction of trends, although within countries smoking is universally a powerful risk factor for COPD mortality.[101] This paradox may reflect inadequacy of national smoking data or may be evidence of influential factors other than smoking.

Longer-term COPD mortality trends in England and Wales are well described by a cohort-related rise and fall superimposed on a downward linear drift.[104,105] The peak of the cohort effect corresponds to generations of men born around 1900 and women born some 20–30 years later. A similar cohort pattern emerges in Canadian death rates.[106] This non-linearity is clearly related to uptake of cigarette smoking, but published age–period–cohort analyses have drawn different conclusions about whether the linear drift represents a cohort or period phenomenon.[104,105] Possible explanations considered earlier in this chapter include improved prenatal or postnatal growth, a decline in childhood respiratory infection, air pollution control, dietary changes, or introduction of antibiotics. The downward drift started in the late nineteenth century in all age groups simultaneously[107] and therefore is more likely to be a period of death effect, at least at the start. Mortality from bronchitis and pneumonia among infants and young children did not start to decline until the early years of the twentieth century, so it is unlikely that this was the key influence on adult mortality.

There is clearer evidence that trends in morbidity have been influenced by changes in smoking behaviour. Reviews of UK prevalence studies during the period 1950–1990[108,109] suggest a modest reduction in prevalence of persistent cough and phlegm in middle-aged men. The decline (from about 25% in the 1950s and 1960s to about 15% in 1990) parallels a decline in current smoking (from 75% to 30%). There was no change among middle-aged women (9–10% in the 1950s and 1960s, compared to 8–9% in the 1980s), reflecting more stable smoking habits (about 25% currently smoking in both periods). These patterns are similar to those for general practitioner contacts for chronic respiratory disease over a similar period.[109]

Marked reductions in urban smoke and sulphur dioxide air pollution over the past 30 years have reduced the daily and seasonal fluctuations in morbidity experienced by chronic bronchitic patients,[110] although the long-term effect of air pollution control on respiratory mortality remains poorly evaluated. Previously marked geographical correlations between air pollution levels and respiratory mortality[111] became weaker as air pollution levels fell during the 1960s,[112] but it is too early to assess a possible cohort-related benefit from reduced pollution exposure in childhood.

10.6.2 Asthma and allergy

The prevalence of wheeze did not fall in line with the prevalence of cough and phlegm as UK men gave up smoking during the 1960s and 1970s.[108] As smoking is strongly related to reports of wheeze in middle-age, this suggests that another factor may have been operating to increase the prevalence of wheeze. There is consistent evidence from the UK,[113] Australia,[114] and many other countries[115] of an increase in the prevalence of asthma and wheeze among children of school age, by about 50% in relative terms over the period 1965–1990. Two studies of children[116,117] have also shown an increase in non-specific BHR, suggesting that these changes are not entirely explained by changes in parental reporting or labelling of symptoms.

Much less is known about trends in asthma in adults. Hospital admission rates rose in all adult age groups in England and Wales through the 1980s and early 1990s and general practitioner contacts also became more common.[118] These trends are not entirely explained by diagnostic transfer from chronic bronchitis and related diagnoses, but they could reflect changes in the use of health services rather than a true increase in morbidity. It is salutary to note that despite widespread use of effective therapies and a decline from levels experienced in the 1960s and 1980s, asthma mortality in England and Wales in the 1990s was at a similar level to that prevailing in the 1930s.[119]

Consistent evidence of an increase in asthma prevalence in younger adults emerges from three studies of military recruits, in Sweden,[120] Finland,[121] and Israel.[122] The 20-fold increase among Finnish conscripts from 1966 to 1989 is the most remarkable—this change is too large to be plausibly explained by changes in symptom reporting or disease labelling. There is also suggestive evidence of a rising prevalence of allergic rhinitis among American college students[123] and Swedish army conscripts.[120] Two studies of adult populations report an increasing prevalence of positive skin prick tests to common aeroallergens.[124,125] In contrast, no change in skin prick positivity and a *decrease* in prevalence of non-specific BHR was found in Busselton between 1981 and 1990.[126] Although not entirely consistent, these findings suggest that the prevalence of allergic sensitization may be rising and this would be a plausible explanation for an increase in the prevalence of asthma, particularly in young adults.

The skin prick results from the longitudinal study in Tucson, Arizona[125] are particularly interesting because age-specific prevalence data are available from two examinations 8 years apart. At each survey, the proportion of adults with positive skin prick reactions declined with age from about 40 onwards, yet on follow-up, an increasing proportion of participants in each age group were prick positive. Two explanations could be advanced for this. Skin prick reagents and test methods are notoriously difficult to standardize and this may have resulted in a systematic difference between the two surveys (an artefactual period effect). Alternatively, the decline in prevalence with age in the first survey could be a manifestation of a cohort effect, with earlier born generations carrying a reduced risk of allergic sensitization throughout life.

10.6.3 Projections of future disease burden

Apart from cigarette smoking, the reasons underlying the trends in respiratory mortality and morbidity are poorly understood. Because the influence of smoking appears in mortality trends as a cohort effect, it is possible to predict with some confidence its impact on future death rates. Thus, death rates of women from COPD will tend to rise while those among men (apart from the oldest age groups) will tend to fall. Changes in the tar composition of cigarettes, inhalation behaviour, and other factors may modulate these effects and the impact of future tobacco control strategies are unknown. Superimposed on these trends is the downward drift in COPD mortality and a suspected rise in prevalence of asthma. The former is welcome but unexplained and therefore unpredictable. It is at least arguable that the increase in adult asthma is part of a more general increase in allergic diseases that may be attributable to developmental changes in the immune system related to living conditions early in life,[127] as discussed earlier in this chapter. Thus, the rising prevalence of asthma and allergy among children and adolescents may be a worrying foresight of future trends among adults.

10.7 Conclusion

Respiratory and allergic diseases are well-suited to the life course approach. It is evident that events early in the development of the lung and immune system may influence susceptibility to later infectious, allergenic, or toxic challenges to the airways. The critical periods during which these early influences may operate are poorly defined, but probably include both prenatal and postnatal development. The complex relationships between early infectious illness and later lung disease may prove particularly difficult to disentangle. While early intervention offers exciting prospects for prevention in the future, there is ample scope to modify the risk at later ages. Control of tobacco smoking remains the highest priority, but diet may also prove to be a remediable influence worthy of attention. Air pollution exposure, either indoors or outdoors, is probably less important than is generally recognized.

References

Those marked with an asterisk are especially recommended for further reading.

1 **Anderson HR, Esmail A, Hollowell J, Littlejohns P, Strachan D.** Lower respiratory disease. In Stevens A, Raftery J, eds. *Health care needs assessment. The epidemiologically based needs assessment reviews. Volume 1.* Oxford: Radcliffe Medical Press, 1994:256–340.

*2 **Peto R, Speizer FE, Cochrane AL, Moore F, Fletcher CM, Tinker CM** *et al.* The relevance in adults of airflow obstruction, but not of mucus hypersecretion, to mortality from chronic lung disease. *Am Rev Respir Dis* 1983;**128**:491–500.

3 **Lange P, Nyboe J, Appleyard M, Jensen G, Schnohr P.** Spirometric findings and mortality in never smokers. *J Clin Epidemiol* 1990;**43**:867–73.

4 **Strachan DP.** Ventilatory function, height and mortality among lifelong non-smokers. *J Epidemiol Commun Health* 1992;**46**:66–70.

*5 **Samet JM, Tager IB, Speizer FE.** The relationship between respiratory illness in childhood and chronic air-flow obstruction in adulthood. *Am Rev Respir Dis* 1983;**127**:508–23.

6 **McConnochie KM, Roghmann KJ.** Bronchiolitis as a possible cause of wheezing in childhood: new evidence. *Pediatrics* 1984;**74**:1–10.

7 **Colley JRT, Douglas JWB, Reid DD.** Respiratory disease in young adults: influence of early childhood lower respiratory tract illness, social class, air pollution and smoking. *Br Med J* 1973;**iii**:195–8.

8 **Britten N, Davies JMC, Colley JRT.** Early respiratory experience and subsequent cough and peak expiratory flow rate in 36 year old men and women. *Br Med J* 1987;**297**:1317–20.

9 **Barker DJP, Osmond C.** Childhood respiratory infection and adult chronic bronchitis in England and Wales. *Br Med J* 1986;**293**:1271–5.

 *10 Silverman M. Out of the mouths of babes and sucklings. Lessons from early childhood asthma. *Thorax* 1993;**48**:1200–4.

 11 Strachan DP, Anderson HR, Bland JM, Peckham CS. Asthma as a link between chest illness in childhood and chronic cough and phlegm in young adults. *Br Med J* 1988;**296**:890–3.

 12 Busse WW. The relationship between viral infections and onset of allergic diseases and asthma. *Clin Exp Allergy* 1989;**19**:1–9.

 13 Strachan DP. Hay fever, hygiene and household size. *Br Med J* 1989;**299**:1259–60.

 14 O'Connor GT, Sparrow D, Weiss ST. The role of allergy and nonspecific airways responsiveness in the pathogenesis of chronic obstructive pulmonary disease. *Am Rev Respir Dis* 1989;**140**:225–52.

 15 Woolcock AJ, Peat JK, Salome CM, Yan K, Anderson SD, Schoeffel RE *et al.* Prevalence of bronchial hyperresponsiveness and asthma in a rural adult population. *Thorax* 1987;**42**:361–8.

 16 Fletcher CM, Peto R, Tinker CM, Speizer FE. *The natural history of chronic bronchitis and emphysema. An 8-year study of working men in London.* Oxford: Oxford University Press, 1976.

 17 Orie NGM, Sluiter HJ, de Vries K, Tammerling GJ, Witkop J. The host factor in bronchitis. In Orie NGM, Sluiter HJ, eds. *Bronchitis.* Assen: Royal van Gorcum, 1961:43–59.

 18 Markowe HLJ, Bulpitt CJ, Shipley MJ, Rose G, Crombie DL, Fleming DM. Prognosis in adult asthma: a national study. *Br Med J* 1987;**295**:949–52.

 19 Burrows B, Bloom JW, Traver GA, Cline MG. The course and prognosis of different forms of chronic airways obstruction in a sample from the general population. *N Engl J Med* 1987;**317**:1309–14.

 20 Venables KM, Topping MD, Howe W, Luczynska CM, Hawkins R, Newman Taylor AJ. Interaction of smoking and atopy in producing specific IgE antibody against a hapten protein conjugate. *Br Med J* 1985;**290**:201–4.

 21 Sly PD, Willet K. Developmental physiology. In Silverman M, ed. *Childhood asthma and other wheezing disorders.* London: Chapman and Hall, 1995:55–66.

 22 Chan KN, Noble-Jamieson CM, Elliman A, Bryan EM, Silverman M. Lung function in children of low birth weight. *Arch Dis Child* 1989;**64**:1284–93.

 23 Rona RJ, Gulliford MC, Chinn S. Effects of prematurity and intrauterine growth on respiratory health and lung function in childhood. *Br Med J* 1993;**306**:817–20.

 24 Cook DG, Strachan DP, Carey IM. Parental smoking and spirometric indices in children. Thorax 1998;**53**:884–93.

 25 de Kleine MJK, Roos CM, Voorn WJ, Jansen HM, Koppe JG. Lung function 8–18 years after intermittent positive pressure ventilation for hyaline membrane disease. *Thorax* 1990;**45**:941–6.

 26 Barker DJP, Godfrey KM, Fall C, Osmond C, Winter PD, Shaheen SO. Relation of birth weight and childhood respiratory infection to adult lung function and death from chronic obstructive lung disease. *Br Med J* 1991;**303**:671–5.

 27 Stick S. The contribution of airway development to paediatric and adult lung disease. *Thorax* 2000;**55**:587–94.

 28 Pride NB, Burrows B. Development of impaired lung function: natural history and risk factors. In Calverley P, Pride N, eds. *Chronic obstructive pulmonary disease.* London: Chapman and Hall, 1995:69–91.

 29 Burney PGJ, Britton JR, Chinn S, Tattersfield AE, Papacosta AE, Kelson MC *et al.* Descriptive epidemiology of bronchial reactivity in an adult population: results from a community study. *Thorax* 1987;**42**:38–44.

30 Pride NB, Taylor RG, Lim TK, Joyce H, Watson A. Bronchial hyperresponsiveness as a risk factor for progressive airflow obstruction in smokers. *Bull Eur Physiopathol Respir* 1987;**23**:369–75.

31 Strachan DP. Do chesty children become chesty adults? *Arch Dis Child* 1990;**65**:161–2.

32 Shaheen SO, Barker DJP, Shiell AW, Crocker FJ, Wield GA, Holgate ST. The relationship between pneumonia in early childhood and impaired lung function in late adult life. *Am Rev Respir Dis* 1994;**149**:616–19.

33 Barker DJP, Osmond C, Law CM. The intrauterine and early postnatal origins of cardiovascular disease and chronic bronchitis. *J Epidemiol Commun Health* 1989;**43**:237–40.

*34 Mann SL, Wadsworth MEJ, Colley JRT. Accumulation of factors influencing respiratory illness in members of a national birth cohort and their offspring. *J Epidemiol Commun Health* 1992;**46**:286–92.

35 Britten N, Wadsworth J. Long term sequelae of whooping cough in a nationally representative sample. *Br Med J* 1986;**292**:441–4.

36 Johnston IDA, Anderson HR, Lambert HP, Patel S. Respiratory morbidity and lung function after whooping cough. *Lancet* 1983;**ii**:1104–8.

37 Martin AJ, Landau LI, Phelan PD. Asthma from childhood at age 21: the patient and his disease. *Br Med J* 1982;**284**:380–2.

38 Burrows B, Knudson RJ, Lebowitz MD. The relationship of childhood respiratory illness to adult obstructive lung disease. *Am Rev Respir Dis* 1977;**115**:751–60.

39 Bodner C, Anderson WJ, Reid TS, Godden DJ. Childhood exposure to infection and risk of adult onset wheeze and atopy. *Thorax* 2000;**55**:383–7.

*40 Strachan DP, Griffiths JM, Anderson HR, Johnston IDA. Ventilatory function in British adults after asthma and wheezing illness at ages 0–35. *Am J Respir Crit Care Med* 1996;**154**:1629–35.

41 Weiss ST, Tosteson TD, Segal MR, Tager IB, Redline S, Speizer FE. Effects of asthma on pulmonary function in children. A longitudinal population-based study. *Am Rev Respir Dis* 1992;**145**:58–64.

42 Sherrill D, Sears MR, Lebowitz MD, Holdaway MD, Hewitt CJ, Flannery EM *et al.* The effects of airway hyperresponsiveness, wheezing and atopy on longitudinal pulmonary function in children: a 6-year follow-up study. *Pediatr Pulmonol* 1992;**13**:78–85.

43 Tager IB, Hanrahan JP, Tosteson TD, Castille RG, Brown RW, Weiss ST *et al.* Lung function, pre- and post-natal smoke exposure, and wheezing in the first year of life. *Am Rev Respir Dis* 1993;**147**:811–17.

44 Martinez FD, Wright AL, Taussig LM, Holberg C, Halonen M, Morgan WJ (Group Health Medical Associates). Asthma and wheezing in the first six years of life. *N Engl J Med* 1995;**332**:133–8.

45 Strachan DP, Seagroatt V, Cook DG. Chest illness in infancy and chronic respiratory disease in later life: an analysis by month of birth. *Int J Epidemiol* 1994;**23**:1060–8.

46 Burrows B, Sears MR, Flannery EM, Herbison GP, Holdaway MD. Relationship of bronchial responsiveness assessed by methacholine to serum IgE, lung function, symptoms and diagnosis in 11 year old children. *J Allergy Clin Immunol* 1992;**90**:376–85.

47 Strachan DP, Butland BK, Anderson HR. The incidence and prognosis of asthma and wheezing illness from early childhood to age 33 in a national British cohort. *Br Med J* 1996;**312**:1195–9.

48 Godfrey KM, Barker DJP, Osmond C. Disproportionate fetal growth and raised IgE concentration in adult life. *Clin Exp Allergy* 1994;**24**:641–8.

49 Katz KA, Pocock SJ, Strachan DP. Neonatal head circumference, neonatal weight, and risk of hay fever, asthma, and eczema in a large cohort of adolescents from Sheffield, England. *Clin Exp Allergy* 2002;**33**:737–45.

50 Bråbäck L, Hedberg A. Perinatal risk factors for atopic disease in conscripts. *Clin Exp Allergy* 1998;**28**:936–42.

51 Björkstén B. The intrauterine and postnatal environments. *J Allergy Clin Immunol* 1999;**104**:1119–27.

52 Strachan DP, Taylor EM, Carpenter RG. Family structure, neonatal infection and hay fever in adolescence. *Arch Dis Child* 1996;**74**:422–6.

53 Golding J, Peters T. Eczema and hay fever. In Butler N, Golding J, eds. *From birth to five. A study of the health and behaviour of Britain's five-year-olds.* Oxford: Pergamon Press, 1986: 171–86.

54 Strachan DP, Harkins LS, Johnston IDA, Anderson HR. Childhood antecedents of allergic sensitisation in young British adults. *J Allergy Clin Immunol* 1997;**99**:1–12.

*55 Strachan DP. Family size, infection and atopy: the first decade of the "hygiene hypothesis". *Thorax* 2000;**55(suppl 1)**:S2–10.

56 Riedler J, Braun-Fahrländer C, Eder W, Schreuer M, Waser M, Maisch S *et al.* Exposure to farming in early life and development of asthma and allergy: a cross-sectional survey. *Lancet* 2001;**358**:1129–33.

57 Rao A, Avni O. Molecular aspects of T-cell differentiation. *Br Med Bull* 2000;**56**:969–84.

58 Backman A, Björkstén F, Ilmonen S, Juntunen K, Suoniemi I. Do infections in infancy affect sensitization to airborne allergens and development of allergic disease? *Allergy* 1984;**39**:309–15.

59 Martinez FD. Role of viral infections in the inception of asthma and allergies during childhood: could they be protective? *Thorax* 1994;**49**:1189–91.

60 Hattevig G, Kjellman B, Björkstén B. Appearance of IgE antibodies to ingested and inhaled allergens during the first 12 years of life in atopic and non-atopic children. *Pediatr Allergy Immunol* 1993;**4**:182–6.

*61 United States Department of Health and Human Services, Public Health Service. *The health consequences of smoking: chronic obstructive lung disease. A report of the Surgeon General.* Washington, DC: US Government Printing Office, 1984.

*62 United States Department of Health and Human Services, Public Health Service. *The health benefits of smoking cessation. A report of the Surgeon General.* Washington, DC: US Government Printing Office, 1990.

63 Rose G, Hamilton PJS. A randomised controlled trial of the effect on middle-aged men of advice to stop smoking. *J Epidemiol Commun Health* 1978;**32**:275–81.

64 Kuller LH, Ockene JK, Townsend M, Browner W, Meilahn E, Wentworth D. The epidemiology of pulmonary function and COPD mortality in the Multiple Risk Factor Intervention Trial. *Am Rev Respir Dis* 1989;**140**:S76–81.

65 Larsson C. Natural history and life expectancy in severe alpha-1-antitrypsin deficiency, PiZ. *Acta Med Scand* 1978;**204**:345–51.

66 Strachan DP, Cox BD, Erzinclioglu SW, Walters DE, Whichelow MJ. Ventilatory function and winter fresh fruit consumption in a random sample of British adults. *Thorax* 1991;**46**:624–9.

67 Schwartz J, Weiss ST. Relationship between dietary vitamin C intake and pulmonary function in the First National Health and Nutrition Examination Survey (NHANES I). *Am J Clin Nutr* 1994;**59**:110–14.

68 Britton JR, Pavord ID, Richards KA, Knox AJ, Wisniewski AF, Lewis SA *et al.* Dietary antioxidant vitamin intake and lung function in the general population. *Am J Respir Crit Care Med* 1995;**151**:1383–7.

69 Hu G, Cassano PA. Antioxidant nutrients and pulmonary function: the Third National Health and Nutrition Examination Survey (NHANES III). *Am J Epidemiol* 2000;**151**:975–81.

70 Carey IM, Strachan DP, Cook DG. The effects of changes in fresh fruit consumption on ventilatory function in healthy British adults. *Am J Respir Crit Care Med* 1998;**158**:728–38.

71 Burney P. A diet rich in sodium may potentiate asthma. Epidemiologic evidence for a new hypothesis. *Chest* 1987;**6(suppl)**:143–8S.

72 Burney PG, Britton JR, Chinn S, Tattersfield AE, Platt HS, Papcosta AO *et al.* Response to inhaled histamine and 24 hour sodium excretion. *Br Med J* 1986;**292**:1483–6.

73 Carey OJ, Locke C, Cookson JB. Effect of alterations of dietary sodium on the severity of asthma in men. *Thorax* 1993;**48**:714–8.

74 Britton J, Pavord I, Richards K, Wisniewski A, Knox A, Lewis S *et al.* Dietary magnesium, lung function, wheezing and airway hyperreactivity in a random adult population sample. *Lancet* 1994;**344**:357–62.

75 Fogarty A, Lewis S, Weiss S, Britton J. Dietary vitamin E, IgE concentrations and atopy. *Lancet* 2000;**356**:1573–4.

76 Strachan DP. Epidemiology: a British perspective. In Calverley P, Pride N, eds. *Chronic obstructive pulmonary disease*. London: Chapman and Hall, 1995:47–68.

77 Dean G, Lee PN, Todd GF, Wicken AJ, Sparks DN. Factors related to respiratory and cardiovascular symptoms in the United Kingdom. *J Epidemiol Commun Health* 1978;**32**:86–96.

78 Respiratory Diseases Study Group of the College of General Practitioners. Chronic bronchitis in Great Britain. *Br Med J* 1961;**ii**:973–8.

79 Cox BD. Blood pressure and respiratory function. In Cox BD, Blaxter M, Buckle ALJ, Fenner NP, Golding JF, Gore M *et al.*, eds. *The health and lifestyle survey. Preliminary report of a nationwide survey of the physical and mental health, attitudes and lifestyle of a random sample of 9003 British adults*. London: Health Promotion Research Trust, 1987:17–33.

80 Registrar-General for England and Wales. *Decennial supplement for 1921. Occupational mortality*. London: His Majesty's Stationery Office, 1931.

81 Morgan WKC. Industrial bronchitis. *Br J Ind Med* 1978;**35**:285–91.

82 Newman Taylor AJ. Occupational asthma. *Thorax* 1980;**35**:241–5.

83 Chang-Yeung M. Occupational asthma. *Chest* 1990;**98(suppl 5)**:148–61.

84 Becklake MR. Occupational exposures: evidence for a causal association with chronic obstructive pulmonary disease. *Am Rev Respir Dis* 1989;**140**:S85–9.

85 Collis EL. The general and occupational prevalence of bronchitis and its relation to other respiratory diseases. *J Ind Hyg Toxicol* 1923;**5**:264–76.

86 Gardner MJ, Crawford MD, Morris JN. Patterns of mortality in middle and old age in the county boroughs of England and Wales. *Br J Prev Soc Med* 1969;**23**:133–40.

87 Chinn S, Florey CDV, Baldwin IG, Gorgol M. The relationship of mortality in England and Wales 1969–73 to measurements of air pollution. *J Epidemiol Commun Health* 1981;**35**:174–9.

88 Chestnut LG, Schwartz J, Savitz DA, Burchfiel CM. Pulmonary function and ambient particulate matter: epidemiological evidence from NHANES I. *Arch Environ Health* 1991;**46**:135–44.

89 Schwartz J. Particulate air pollution and chronic respiratory disease. *Environ Res* 1993;**62**:7–13.

90 Department of Health Advisory Group on the Medical Aspects of Air Pollution Episodes. *Second report: sulphur dioxide, acid aerosols and particulates*. London: Her Majesty's Stationery Office, 1992.

91 Department of Health Committee on the Medical Effects of Air Pollutants. *Non-biological particles and health*. London: Her Majesty's Stationery Office, 1995.

92 Douglas JWB, Waller RE. Air pollution and respiratory infection in children. *Br J Prev Soc Med* 1966;**20**:1–8.

93 Department of Health Committee on the Medical Effects of Air Pollutants. *Asthma and outdoor air pollution.* London: Her Majesty's Stationery Office, 1995.

*94 Strachan DP. The role of environmental factors in asthma. *Br Med Bull* 2000;**56**:865–82.

95 Nitta H, Sato T, Nakai S, Maeda K, Aoko S, Ono M. Respiratory health associated with exposure to automobile exhaust. I. Results of cross-sectional studies in 1979, 1982 and 1983. *Arch Environ Health* 1993;**48**:53–8.

96 Livingstone AE, Shaddick G, Grundy C, Elliott P. Do people living near inner city main roads have more asthma needing treatment? A case–control study using routine general practice data. *Br Med J* 1996;**311**:676–7.

97 Abbey DE, Lebowitz MD, Mills PK, Petersen FF, Beeson L, Burchette RJ. Long-term ambient concentrations of particulates and oxidants and development of chronic disease in a cohort of nonsmoking California residents. *Inhalation Toxicol* 1995;**7**:19–34.

98 Greer JR, Abbey DE, Burchette RJ. Asthma related to occupational and ambient air pollutants in nonsmokers. *J Occup Med* 1993;**35**:909–15.

99 Coultas DB. Passive smoking and risk of adult asthma and COPD: an update. *Thorax* 1998;**53**:381–7.

100 Fischer P, Remjin B, Brunekreef B, van der Lende R, Schouten J, Quanjer P. Indoor air pollution and its effect on pulmonary function of adult non-smoking women. II: Associations between nitrogen dioxide and pulmonary function. *Int J Epidemiol* 1985;**14**:221–6.

101 Brown CA, Crombie IK, Tunstall-Pedoe H. Failure of cigarette smoking to explain international differences in mortality from chronic obstructive pulmonary disease. *J Epidemiol Commun Health* 1994;**48**:134–9.

102 Thom TJ. International comparisons in COPD mortality. *Am Rev Respir Dis* 1989; **140(suppl)**:S27–34.

103 Feinleib M, Rosenberg HM, Collins JG, Delozier JE, Pokras R, Chevarley FM. Trends in COPD morbidity and mortality in the United States. *Am Rev Respir Dis* 1989; **140(suppl)**:S9–18.

104 Barker DJP, Osmond C. Childhood respiratory infection and adult chronic bronchitis in England and Wales. *Br Med J* 1986;**293**:1271–5.

*105 Lee PN, Fry JS, Forey BA. Trends in lung cancer, chronic obstructive lung disease, and emphysema death rates for England and Wales 1941–85 and their relation to trends in cigarette smoking. *Thorax* 1990;**45**:657–65.

106 Manfreda J, Mao Y, Litven W. Morbidity and mortality from chronic obstructive pulmonary disease. *Am Rev Respir Dis* 1989;**140(suppl)**:S19–26.

107 Strachan DP. Trends in respiratory mortality in England and Wales. *Thorax* 1991;**46**:149.

108 Cook DG, Kussick SJ, Shaper AG. The respiratory benefits of stopping smoking. *J Smoking Related Dis* 1990;**1**:45–58.

*109 Strachan DP. Epidemiology: a British perspective. In Calverley P, Pride N, eds. *Chronic obstructive pulmonary disease.* London: Chapman and Hall, 1995:47–68.

110 Waller RE. Control of air pollution: present success and future prospect. In Bennett AE, ed. *Recent advances in community medicine I.* Edinburgh: Churchill Livingstone, 1978:59–72.

111 Gardner MJ, Crawford MD, Morris JN. Patterns of mortality in middle and old age in the county boroughs of England and Wales. *Br J Prev Soc Med* 1969;**23**:133–40.

112 Chinn S, Florey CDV, Baldwin IG, Gorgol M. The relationship of mortality in England and Wales 1969–73 to measurements of air pollution. *J Epidemiol Commun Health* 1981;**35**:174–9.

113 **Anderson HR.** Is asthma really increasing? *Paed Resp Med* 1993;**1**:6–10.

114 **Bauman A.** Has the prevalence of asthma symptoms increased in Australian children? *J Paediatr Child Health* 1993;**29**:424–8.

115 **Burr ML.** Epidemiology of asthma. In Burr ML, ed. *Epidemiology of clinical allergy*. Basel: Karger, 1993:80–102.

116 **Burr ML, Butland BK, King S, Vaughan-Williams E.** Changes in asthma prevalence: two surveys 15 years apart. *Arch Dis Child* 1989;**64**:1118–25.

117 **Peat JK, van den Berg RH, Green WF, Mellis CM, Leeder SR, Woolcock AJ.** Changing prevalence of asthma in Australian children. *Br Med J* 1994;**308**:1591–6.

*118 **Department of Health Committee on the Medical Effects of Air Pollutants.** *Asthma and outdoor air pollution.* London: Her Majesty's Stationery Office, 1995.

119 **Burney PGJ.** Asthma deaths in England and Wales 1931–85: evidence for a true increase in asthma mortality. *J Epidemiol Commun Health* 1988;**42**:316–20.

120 **Äberg N.** Asthma and allergic rhinitis in Swedish conscripts. *Clin Exp Allergy* 1989;**19**:59–63.

121 **Haahtela T, Lindholm H, Bjorkstein F, Koskenvuo K, Laitenen LA.** Prevalence of asthma in Finnish young men. *Br Med J* 1990;**301**:266–8.

122 **Laor A, Cohen L, Danon YL.** Effects of time, sex, ethnic origin and area of residence on prevalence of asthma in Israeli adolescents. *Br Med J* 1993;**307**;841–4.

123 **Hagy GW, Settipnae GA.** Bronchial asthma, allergic rhinitis and allergy skin tests among college students. *J Allergy* 1969;**44**:323–32.

124 **Sibbald B, Rink E, D'Souza M.** Is atopy increasing? *Br J Gen Pract* 1990;**40**:338–40.

*125 **Barbee RA, Kaltenborn W, Lebowitz MD, Burrows B.** Longitudinal changes in allergen skin test reactivity in a community population sample. *J Allergy Clin Immunol* 1987;**79**:16–24.

126 **Peat JK, Haby M, Spijker J, Berry G, Woolcock AJ.** Prevalence of asthma in adults in Busselton, Western Australia. *Br Med J* 1992;**305**:1326–9.

*127 **Strachan DP.** Time trends in asthma and allergy: ten questions, fewer answers. *Clin Exp Allergy* 1995;**25**:791–4.

Chapter 11

A life course approach to cancer epidemiology

Nancy Potischman, Rebecca Troisi, and Lars Vatten

Many years of epidemiologic research into the aetiology of cancers have focused on host or environmental factors in adulthood. With much of cancer aetiology yet to be explained, new research efforts have focused on earlier time periods. Although investigations of early origins of cardiovascular disease (CVD) and diabetes have proceeded rapidly since the late 1980s, such investigations have only recently begun for cancers. The data are sparse, yet emerging evidence suggests that the early environment may set the stage for later adult cancers, including breast, testicular, and perhaps prostate cancers. An increased research emphasis on factors that act during childhood and adolescence, along with evaluation of the interplay among such factors, is likely to accelerate progress and improve our understanding of how early influences may contribute to risk for adult cancers.

11.1 Introduction

Current knowledge suggests that tumours develop in stages, with extreme variation in growth velocity before clinical detection. Multiple factors over an individual's lifetime are likely to be important, but research has focused primarily on adult or adolescent risk factors. Since the early 1990s an increasing number of studies have evaluated factors that may act *in utero* or very early in life. Linking risk factors that operate at different developmental periods may advance our understanding of the origins of cancer, but the life course approach has received little attention in evaluations of cancer development. Factors could be part of a chain of biologically linked events (that is, the 'chains of risk model') that results in the development of cancer; alternatively, there could be cumulative effects of a set of independent risk factors that culminate in disease development (that is, the 'accumulation model') (see Chapter 1).

Ideally, such questions will be resolved with information from large cohorts of people with serial data. However, cohorts that exist are either too small or still too young to assess the influence of factors that operate very early in life. Researchers with record linkage capabilities, largely from the Scandinavian countries, have begun using various sources of data to obtain exposure information over substantial time frames. Large studies are needed because cancers are relatively rare compared with other chronic diseases. For example, prostate cancer, a relatively common cancer in men, has an annual incidence rate in the USA of 142/100 000,[1] whereas the US incidence of CVD is estimated to be 431/100 000.[2] Therefore, the cohort size would have to be three times as large to study prostate cancer compared with CVD and even larger to study less common cancers. Another barrier to the application of the life course approach to cancer is the lack of intermediate end-points, such as blood lipids and hypertension, which exist for CVD. This has limited the possibility of studying risk factors in young cohorts. Merging data from multiple cohort studies, with long follow-up, may create the best opportunities for investigations of the life course epidemiology of cancers.

Epidemiologic studies have evaluated a limited number of cancer sites for risk factors over the life course. This review will focus on *in utero* and perinatal factors and, to the extent possible, link these factors and motivating biology to subsequent time periods to incorporate the life course perspective. The original hypothesis put forth by Trichopoulos[3] stated that *in utero* exposure to oestrogens would influence risk of adult breast cancer. Researchers have expanded this hypothesis to other endocrine factors and other hormone-related cancers, including testicular and prostate cancers. This review will consider breast, testicular, and prostate cancers because the majority of the literature focuses on these tumours. Renal cell tumours have been related to high birthweight but data are limited at this time.[4] Malignant melanoma also may be related to early life and cumulative sun exposure but only limited data are available and this cancer has been reviewed elsewhere.[5] For each risk factor reviewed, an overall summary of the evidence is presented first, followed by more detailed descriptions of the studies.

11.2 Breast cancer

11.2.1 Pre-pubertal, adolescent, and adult risk factors

Many risk factors have been identified for breast cancer and those that operate in adolescence and adulthood[6,7] are suggested to account for about half of the disease incidence.[8,9] Reproductive factors consistently related to increased risk include late age at first birth, nulliparity, low parity, early onset of menarche, and late age at menopause. A family history of breast cancer in a first-degree relative is a strong risk factor but accounts for only approximately 5% of all breast cancers. Demographic and lifestyle risk factors include having never been married, being of upper socioeconomic status, adult weight gain, and alcohol consumption. In addition, a recent analysis of studies from a variety of countries suggests that lactation for long durations reduces risk.[10] New methods of characterizing the density and parenchymal patterns of breast tissue from mammograms should prove useful in identifying women at high risk of breast cancer.[11] Although breast densities may be valuable intermediate markers of breast cancer,[11] the necessary radiologic methods are not widely available to the public and will need to be routinely used in clinical practice to be useful for large epidemiologic studies.

A high endogenous oestrogen environment is hypothesized to underlie the observed epidemiology of breast cancer. Recently studies have suggested a role for androgens,[12] insulin, and insulin-like growth factors (IGFs)[13,14] but risks related to critical time periods and duration of hormonal exposure are unclear. It has been suggested that the developing breast during adolescence is particularly vulnerable to environmental insults,[15] and that the period between puberty and first birth may set the stage for later disease.[16] Studies to date have not addressed environmental or hormonal exposures during early adulthood in relation to later disease risk. However, body weight in the postmenarcheal period has been investigated in some studies and this may be a proxy variable for a variety of nutritional and hormonal variables.

Weight and body mass index (BMI) have been evaluated in relation to changes across distinct time periods. Weight gain from early to later adulthood has been associated with increased risk of postmenopausal breast cancer,[17–19] whereas weight loss over this time period has been associated with reduced risk.[18] A high BMI from adolescence throughout early adulthood has been associated with reduced risk both for premenopausal[20–22] and postmenopausal breast cancer.[21,23,24] The underlying mechanisms for the apparent protective effects related to high BMI during the premenopausal years remain unknown but have been attributed to anovulatory menstrual cycles[25] resulting in lower lifetime exposure to the hormonal environment. These results may suggest that the hormonal milieu during the reproductive years has lasting effects on risk of postmenopausal breast cancer.[18] Risk related to critical time periods for body weight and weight changes over the life course is complex,[26] but recent studies can evaluate breast cancer risk in relation to measurements made at multiple time points.

Several established breast cancer risk factors operate during adolescence, including early age at menarche, low adolescent body weight, and greater attained height.[6,18,27] The positive association between adult height and breast cancer risk has strengthened the hypothesis that factors that promote growth in childhood and adolescence are positively associated with breast cancer risk. Detailed information on growth patterns suggests that high growth velocity and a relatively early growth spurt are associated with a higher breast cancer risk compared with reaching maximal height at a later point during adolescent development.[28] Leg length may be a marker of growth in adolescence but the associations with breast cancer are inconsistent.[27] If prepubertal energy intake is important,[29,30] then growth velocity may be a useful proxy variable and studies that incorporate this measure may yield more informative results than studies with crude measures of diet. The few breast cancer studies that have assessed adolescent diet retrospectively from adults have been inconclusive.[31–33] Further, one study of the postmenarcheal period[34] showed no protective effect of restricted energy intake between menarche and first birth.

11.2.2 Perinatal and infant risk factors

The original Trichopoulos hypothesis[3] on oestrogen's influence on the development of breast cancer has evolved to include other endocrine factors. Nonetheless, much of the research has focused solely on variables thought to represent *in utero* oestrogens and their relationship to breast cancer and some methodologic studies have attempted to document the usefulness of these proxies in representing the *in utero* oestrogen environment. The major hormone-related variables that have been investigated include preeclampsia, birthweight, and twinship. The evidence suggests that preeclampsia is associated with reduced risk but being a twin or having had a high birthweight is associated with increased risk. Results are inconsistent for placental weight, gestational age, maternal age, birth order, and having been breastfed. The following sections review the literature for the surrogate variables for oestrogens and methodologic studies will be addressed in later sections.

11.2.2.1 Preeclampsia

Preeclampsia, a pregnancy condition characterized by hypertension, hyperuricaemia, and proteinuria, is associated also with reduced maternal urinary oestriol excretion and has been hypothesized to reduce breast cancer risk in female offspring born of these pregnancies. However, many physiologic changes occur in preeclamptic pregnancies besides alterations in oestrogen metabolism. Methodologic studies have evaluated fetal exposure based on maternal blood sampling, though few studies have measured hormones in cord blood. Because preeclamptic babies tend to be smaller for gestational age than other babies, this condition may also affect breast cancer risk through an alteration of established breast cancer risk factors, such as pubertal development and adult size. Given that there are few major reports on this risk factor, albeit with compelling risk estimates, other larger epidemiologic investigations need to verify the association while further elaboration of possible mechanisms is pursued.

The earliest investigation of this hypothesis, based on only four exposed cases, reported an *increased* breast cancer risk among women born of preeclamptic pregnancies,[35] whereas two later Swedish studies[36,37] found highly protective effects (Fig. 11.1). Investigators used cancer registry data to identify breast cancer cases born in five hospitals in one region of Sweden and obtained birth records for cases and control participants selected from the same hospital. A markedly reduced risk of breast cancer among daughters born to preeclamptic mothers was noted in the first analysis of 458 cases from one hospital[36] (odds ratio (OR) = 0.24, 95% confidence interval (CI) = 0.09–0.70) and similar results were obtained when the other four hospitals' cases were included (1068 cases, OR = 0.41, 95% CI = 0.22–0.79).[37] Both analyses were adjusted for other maternal and pregnancy factors that might be related to risk, such as maternal age, maternal parity, maternal socioeconomic status, and birthweight.

Study	No. of cases	No. of preeclampsia cases/controls	OR & 95% CI
Le Marchand *et al.*, 1988	153	4/4	
Ekbom *et al.*, 1992	458	8/45	
Ekbom *et al.*, 1997	1068	14/81	
Sanderson *et al.*, 1998	509	20/21	
Innes *et al.*, 2000[a]	402	6/39	

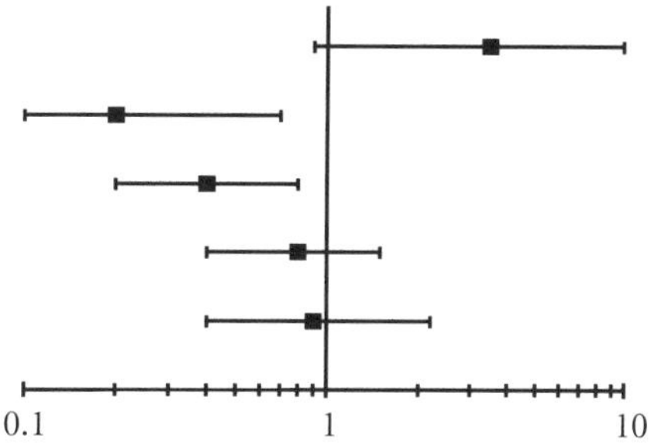

[a]premenopausal women

Fig. 11.1 Preeclampsia and subsequent risk of breast cancer (odds ratios (ORs) and 95% confidence intervals (CI)).

Data were unavailable, however, to allow evaluation of confounding or effect modification by the daughter's adult breast cancer risk factors. Additional evidence of a protective effect of preeclamptic pregnancies derives from two case–control studies, one using information from participants' mothers[38] and the other linking birth and cancer registry data in New York State.[39] Lack of detail regarding the severity of the disease, the possibility of residual differences in gestational age, and the small number of participants born of preeclamptic/eclamptic pregnancies warrants caution in interpreting these findings.

The authors of the two Swedish studies suggested that preeclampsia could be accompanied by lower intrauterine oestrogen and that this could explain the lower breast cancer risk in the female offspring. Urinary oestrogen levels are clearly reduced in women presenting with preeclampsia during pregnancy. However, it is unclear whether concentrations also are reduced in blood.[40,41] In addition, few data are available on concentrations of other, more potent oestrogens such as oestradiol,[41–44] oestrone,[42] and oestrogen precursors in preeclampsia. Cohn and coworkers[45] raised the hypothesis that greater androgen exposure due to compromises in the integrity and function of the placenta might confer long-term protection against breast cancer by antagonizing oestrogen's effects on the fetal breast.

Other biological factors that are potentially altered in preeclampsia also may play an intriguing role in breast cancer, such as alpha-fetoprotein (AFP)[44] and IGFs.[46] For example, cord levels of AFP may be higher in preeclampsia than in normotensive pregnancies,[44] and two studies have shown that high AFP levels in the circulation of pregnant women are associated with reduced subsequent risk for breast cancer in these women.[47,48] On the other hand, cord levels of IGF-I appear to be low in preeclampsia,[46] possibly as a consequence of placental dysfunction. In adult women some evidence suggests that low circulating levels of IGF-I are associated with reduced risk for premenopausal breast cancer.[14] Data on AFP and IGF-I in preeclampsia are intriguing and may represent links between preeclampsia and breast cancer for both offspring and mother.

11.2.2.2 Birthweight

Birthweight was initially investigated as a marker for the intrauterine oestrogen environment,[3] but the positive association between birthweight and breast cancer could be mediated through a high oestrogen milieu[49] or through insulin, IGFs, or other endocrine factors.[50,51] Thirteen studies to date have examined whether larger babies are at increased risk of breast cancer. Although the data are heterogeneous, there is a trend of increasing risk of breast cancer with increasing birthweights and there appears to be no threshold. The evidence thus far for high compared with low birthweight suggests an association[35,36,52–56] (Fig. 11.2), which may be limited to premenopausal breast cancer. The larger studies, with 1716 cases[57] and 1068 cases,[37] comprised mainly of older women, provide persuasive evidence for the lack of an association between birthweight and postmenopausal breast cancer.

Studies using cancer registry data and cohort studies incorporating birth record data tend to show increased risk with higher birthweights. Record linkage studies from Scandinavian countries have shown increased risks for higher birthweight babies (for example, greater than 3700 or 4000 g compared with lower weights),[36,58–60] although

Study	No. of cases	OR	Odds ratio and 95% confidence interval
Le Marchand et al., 1988	74	0.8	
Ekbom et al., 1992	458	1.2	
Michels et al., 1996	550	1.5	
Sanderson et al., 1996[a]	630	1.7	
Sanderson et al., 1996[b]	292	0.6	
Ekbom et al., 1997	1068	1.0	
Sanderson et al., 1998[a]	448	1.3	
De Stavola et al., 2000[c]	37	2.0	
Innes et al., 2000[a]	481	3.3	
Andersson et al., 2001	62	1.9	
Hilakivi-Clarke et al., 2001	177	1.9	
Hübinette et al., 2001[d]	174	1.5	
Kaijser et al., 2001[d]	180	2.0	
Sanderson et al., 2002	288	0.7	
Titus-Ernstoff et al., 2002[b]	1716	1.2	
Vatten et al., 2002	373	1.4	

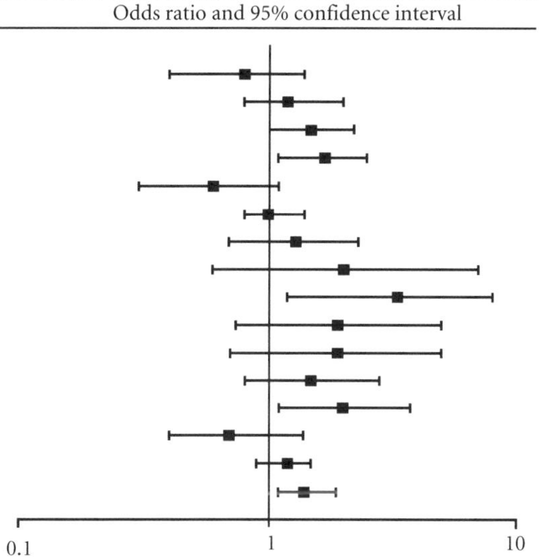

0.1   1   10

[a]premenopausal women
[b]postmenopausal women
[c]the effect measure is not OR, but incidence rate ratio (IRR)
[d]twins

Fig. 11.2 Odds ratio (OR) of breast cancer comparing women in the highest birthweight category with the reference category.

other studies have not.[35,37] A record linkage study of breast cancer at very young ages (< 37 years) found a J-shaped relationship with birthweight.[39] Increased risks were associated with birthweights less than 2500 g and higher than 4500 g. Similar to the Scandinavian results, a cohort study in the UK showed a linear increase in risk: women who weighed 4000 g or more at birth had twice the risk of women who weighed less than 3000 g.[56]

Studies using birthweight information from mothers of adult participants are considered to have higher validity than studies using birthweight from daughters' self-report.[61,62] However, as shown from comparison with birth registry data, both self-report sources are considered adequate for retrospective studies ($r = 0.8$ and $r = 0.7$, respectively). The main limitation of mothers' data is the low response among mothers. Nonetheless, in a study using mothers' information from the Nurses' Health Study,[53] a linear trend of decreasing risk was observed for decreasing birthweights compared with birthweights of 4000 g or more (OR = 0.86, 0.68, 0.66, and 0.55 for birthweights 3500–3999 g, 3000–3499 g, 2500–2999 g, and < 2500 g, respectively). Studies of premenopausal women suggested increased risk for low and high birthweight American women,[38,52] whereas data from mothers in a low-risk Chinese population suggested a reduced risk for high birthweights (4000 g plus).[63] Using self-reported birthweight in case–control studies of postmenopausal disease, a small study[52] showed a nonsignificant decreased risk for high birthweight (4000 g plus), whereas a study with 1716 cases suggested no relationship.[57]

Record linkage studies of birthweights among twins provide unique information. Compared with singletons, twins generally have shorter gestational ages and lower birthweights but potentially higher exposure to hormonal factors. Two Swedish studies demonstrated a 3.5–6-fold increased risk[54,55] for higher (>3000 g) compared with lower (<2000 g) birthweight twins. These studies provide additional evidence for a link between growth *in utero* and breast cancer risk.

Potentially confounding factors, including other maternal or pregnancy factors and daughter's adult breast cancer risk factors, do not appear to influence the birthweight findings. Risk estimates were affected slightly by maternal age, birth order, and the offspring's adult height in one study,[56] and possibly by participants' age, menopausal status, and maternal smoking in another study.[52] Nonetheless, lack of demonstrated confounding in most studies[38,39,53,58–60] increases confidence in the interpretation of record linkage studies that typically contain information only on perinatal factors.

Few studies have investigated effect modification of the birthweight and breast cancer finding by other breast cancer risk factors. Sanderson and coworkers[52] reported no significant interactions of birthweight with a variety of breast cancer risk factors assessed in the offspring. However, De Stavola and others[56] showed that high birthweight was related to breast cancer risk only for girls with high growth velocity in childhood, as indicated by height measured at age 7. A similar risk relationship between high birthweight and breast cancer was observed only in those with an earlier menarche and earlier menarche was related to greater height at age 7. It was not possible to evaluate the nature of the relationships among the three factors (birthweight, childhood growth, and age at menarche) and risk of breast cancer but they present leads to a pathway, which bears replication in other studies. Another study,[59] in fact, did not find an interactive relationship of birthweight and BMI at ages 7–15 with risk of breast cancer. These studies, using longitudinal information from birth throughout childhood and adolescence, present useful models for evaluations of the interactions among early risk factors and for potential evaluations among risk factors identified throughout the life course.

Only a few studies have evaluated the associations between birthweight and risk factors for breast cancer. Age at menopause showed no relationship with birthweight,[64,65] but was associated with weight at age 2 in a UK cohort.[65] In terms of childhood growth variables, birthweight was unrelated to BMI at ages 7, 9, 11, and 15,[59] but was modestly correlated with height in some studies ($r = 0.2$).[27]

11.2.2.3 Length of gestation

At least two hypotheses have been suggested for a mechanism mediating an effect of gestational age on breast cancer risk. One posits that the duration of time spent *in utero* equals the duration of oestrogen exposure to the breast (thus, short gestational age should be protective). The other suggests that oestrogen secretion is enhanced in pregnancies destined to prematurely deliver (thus, short gestational age is adverse). The majority of studies, however, have shown no consistent association between gestational age at birth and risk of breast cancer.[35,38,52,53]

Two Swedish studies evaluating the effect of extreme prematurity found that breast cancer risk was increased in women born at 33 weeks of gestation or earlier,[37,66] although the latter study had only three breast cancer cases. No other investigation has observed an association with having been born before term.[35,38,52,53] In contrast, lending evidence to the hypothesis that risk is elevated with longer duration *in utero*, a Swedish study of female twins found a positive association of gestational age and breast cancer and no increase in risk with preterm birth.[55] Data from singletons also showed no association for preterm birth but suggested an increased risk for gestations of 43 or more weeks.[38] Further, a linked registry study of young breast cancer showed a substantially reduced breast cancer risk in daughters born before 33 weeks after adjustment for birthweight and other pregnancy and neonatal characteristics.[39] Small numbers of participants who had been pre- or postterm and a lack of attention to the combined effects of birthweight and gestational age have limited the interpretation of findings from these studies.

11.2.2.4 Placental weight

The placenta is the main regulator of the intrauterine hormonal environment in pregnancy, making it reasonable to evaluate its size and function in relation to future breast cancer risk of female offspring. There is a positive correlation between placental weight and birthweight and the hormonal influence of a large placenta is likely to stimulate a larger birth size. However, findings for placental weight have been inconsistent. The smaller of the Swedish linked-registry studies demonstrated slightly increased risks for those with higher placental weights,[36] while two other studies showed no relationship with breast cancer risk.[37,60] In contrast, high-risk mammographic parenchymal patterns were associated with placental weight in another Swedish study.[67] Further, while variance in placental weight is great, it is likely measured with substantial error unless research staff are specifically trained and standardized procedures are in place. Additional analysis of this variable in more controlled data collection settings would be useful.

11.2.2.5 Twins

A number of investigators have suggested that twins may have different breast cancer risk than singletons and risk has been hypothesized to vary by the zygosity of the twin pair. Twins from dizygotic pregnancies have been hypothesized to be at increased risk of breast cancer, owing to a greater hormonal influence from two rather than one placenta, whereas a reduced risk may be expected among monozygotic twins who share one placenta. Overall, breast cancer risk appears to be increased in twins. Whether risk is higher in dizygotic compared with monozygotic twins and singletons, however, is not clear. The data also seem to suggest that the influence of twinning may be more pronounced in early-onset than in postmenopausal disease.

Most,[37,68–71] but not all,[52,72] studies have found an elevated risk of breast cancer among twins compared with singletons. Evidence from the Swedish twin registry indicates that compared with singletons, risk is elevated for dizygotic but not for monozygotic twins.[37,71] The results of two case–control studies that adjusted for other risk factors are consistent with this finding,[68,69] but a study among same-sex twins based on the Swedish twin registry showed a higher breast cancer risk in monozygotic than in dizygotic twins.[73] In a population-based study of twins only, risk of early-onset breast cancer was not elevated in women whose cotwin was male (representing dizygotic twins) compared with those whose cotwin was female (representing a mixture of mono- and dizygotic twins) (OR = 1.1, 95% CI 0.81–1.6).[74] In contrast, results from the case–control studies are consistent with higher risk for having a male cotwin but the issue of zygosity could not be addressed in these studies.[68,69] While the data are inconsistent, they suggest higher risk for dizygotic twins.

The data addressing the mechanism whereby cancer risk in offspring of twin pregnancies may be altered show that compared with singletons, oestrogen levels are higher in the maternal circulation as are urinary oestriol values.[75,76] Differences in urinary oestrogen levels between monozygotic and dizygotic pregnancies, however, have not been shown.[77]

11.2.2.6 Maternal age and birth order

It has been speculated that higher maternal age is associated with increased breast cancer risk in offspring and modestly increased risks have been observed for daughters born to older mothers in some,[35,78–83] but not all studies.[36,37,52,69,84,85] One study[86] also showed a weak increase in risk with increasing paternal age at the patient's birth. It has been suggested that an effect of maternal age may be modified by birth order.[87,88] However, this interaction was not supported in a study that evaluated the joint effects of older maternal age and being a first born[79] and studies that have investigated birth order as a main effect have shown no relationship with breast cancer risk.[35,52,60,78,79,81] One recent study[57] reported an inverse association between number of older sisters and risk, though not with number of older brothers, number of younger siblings, sibship, gender ratio, or total size of sibship. These investigators hypothesize that these data are consistent with a viral aetiology of breast cancer, such as from Epstein–Barr virus. Because older sisters are more likely than older brothers to be intimately involved in the care of younger siblings, the investigators suggest that early exposure to a virus may be protective.

11.2.2.7 Breastfeeding

Risk related to exposure to breast milk was evaluated in early studies of breast cancer aetiology. In these studies, investigators hypothesized that a viral agent could be transmitted through breast milk. These studies found little association of having been breastfed with risk of breast cancer.[80,89,90] One of the drawbacks of these studies was limited variability in the prevalence of breastfeeding. Further, evaluation of national and international trends of breastfeeding practices and breast cancer rates suggested a transmissible agent for breast cancer was unlikely.[91] Finally, a large case–control study[92] showed that risk was not increased in breastfed daughters whose mother later developed breast cancer, which is inconsistent with an infectious aetiology related to breastfeeding.

More recent studies have focused on a potentially protective effect of having been breastfed. Using record linkage data, investigators showed no association between having been breastfed at discharge from the hospital and risk of breast cancer.[93] In contrast, data from four case–control studies, with greater ability to categorize mothers as to breastfeeding practices, show a protective effect of ever having been breastfed.[69,92,94,95] Three other analyses, however, have not found an association.[38,92,96]

Convincing results of no relationship between having been breastfed and post-menopausal breast cancer were presented in a large case–control study in the USA.[92] Interestingly, in this study a protective effect was observed for premenopausal breast cancer (OR = 0.65, 95% CI 0.41–1.0) but the sample size in this group limited the interpretation. Results from other studies using data from mothers[38,96] or from partic-ipants[96] indicated no association for premenopausal[38,96] or postmenopausal breast cancer.[96] No studies to date have evaluated effect modification and only one study has evaluated potential confounding by other breast cancer risk factors.[96] In this large prospective study, none of the established risk factors for breast cancer was related to having been breastfed as an infant. In summary, four of seven analytical studies suggest reduced risk for breast cancer in young women,[69,92,94,95] but results for postmenopausal women suggest no association.[92,93,96]

11.2.2.8 Other factors

Several other pregnancy and neonatal factors thought to be associated with hormone levels have been assessed in relation to breast cancer risk in daughters but generally have shown little or no association. The small number of cases studied has generally limited the interpretation of findings.

A case–control study of breast cancer in young women using mothers' recall of their pregnancy experience[38] found an increased risk with a pregnancy weight gain of 25–34 pounds (11–15 kg) (OR = 1.5, 95% CI = 1.2–2.0), but no increased risk for higher weight gains. Risk of early-onset breast cancer with nausea and vomiting during the pregnancy, particularly with use of antiemetic drugs also was elevated (OR = 2.9, 95% CI = 1.1–8.1) and nonsignificantly elevated for anaemia and coffee consumption in pregnancy. No associations were observed for alcohol consumption, prepregnancy BMI, hypertension, or use of oral contraceptives or other hormones. Although diethylstilbestrol (DES), a synthetic oestrogen, was associated with an increased risk (OR = 2.3, 95% CI = 0.8–6.4), the number of exposed women was small. In another cohort of daughters[97] with documented exposure or nonexposure to DES *in utero*, subsequent risk of early-onset breast cancer was slightly elevated (Relative Risk (RR) = 2.5, CI = 1.0–6.3) but again, the number of cases was small and the cohort continues to be followed. Studies provide little evidence that maternal smoking during pregnancy[38,52,69,98] or exposure to passive smoking[38] affects daughter's risk of breast cancer. An increased risk was noted for infants who experienced jaundice in one study.[37] Several studies have assessed whether season of birth affects breast cancer risk in daughters, with some showing an increase in risk resulting from births occurring at certain times of the year. However, the effect is small and inconsistent.[99–101]

11.3 Other cancers

11.3.1 Prostate cancer

Despite more than 10-fold differences in prostate cancer incidence among different geographic areas and ethnic populations and dramatically increased risk related to migration from low- to high-risk areas, the aetiology of prostate cancer remains puzzling.[102] Hormonal factors, such as androgens and IGFs, have been implicated but no direct relationship has been established. A 'westernized' lifestyle is clearly important for prostate cancer, but specific factors convincingly associated with this cancer remain to be identified. With the rising interest in early life factors and adult diseases, six studies have reported on the relationship between perinatal factors and prostate cancer risk but the results are inconsistent. It remains unclear whether early life factors are of importance to prostate cancer risk.

11.3.1.1 Birthweight

The evidence to date does not support a strong relationship between birthweight and prostate cancer risk. Three studies were conducted among Swedish men.[103–105] Their strengths include the retrieval of perinatal information from midwives' birth charts and the collection of information on prostate cancer from cancer registries. The relationship with birthweight was first reported from a small Swedish cohort study of 366 men, in which 21 men developed prostate cancer during follow-up.[103] The results showed a strong positive association between birthweight and prostate cancer risk. Later studies, however, come to somewhat different conclusions. In a second case–control study of 250 cases of prostate cancer, results showed weak but positive associations for birthweight and for infant ponderal index.[104] The third Swedish study was a relatively large case–control study nested within a cohort of men born between 1889 and 1941.[105] Perinatal information was collected from birth charts of 834 men who had developed prostate cancer and 1880 control participants. In this study, neither birthweight nor birth length was associated with prostate cancer risk. Furthermore, in a retrospective analysis of prostate cancer risk among health professionals in the USA, in which information on birthweight was collected for a proportion of participants, no clear association emerged.[106]

11.3.1.2 Preeclampsia

Information on preeclampsia was available from midwives' birth charts in two Swedish case–control studies.[104,105] In the smaller study, prostate cancer risk was strongly reduced in men born of preeclamptic pregnancies,[104] but in the larger study, this association was attenuated and showed a nonsignificant reduction in risk.[105] However, preeclampsia is a rare condition, and even a study of 834 cases is likely to include only a small number of cases exposed to preeclampsia, suggesting that evaluation of this factor will require very large studies.

11.3.1.3 Parental age and birth order

The relationship between perinatal factors and prostate cancer risk was first studied in the context of a large case–control study of a number of cancers in the USA.[81] Results showed higher risks of prostate cancer if the parents were relatively young at the birth of the patient, whereas birth order was not associated with increased risk. In the Framingham study, 141 out of 2164 men developed prostate cancer over a 40-year period.[107] The results showed a gradual increase in risk with increasing paternal, but not maternal age, and the relationship with paternal age was stronger if prostate cancer was diagnosed relatively early, before 65 years of age. The results from the smaller of the two Swedish case–control studies suggested that high maternal age at birth was related to higher risk of prostate cancer in the offspring,[104] but this finding was not confirmed in the larger study.[105] Therefore, no convincing evidence exists that parental age or the patient's birth order is important for prostate cancer risk.

11.3.1.4 Other factors

The association between placental weight and prostate cancer risk was analysed in both case–control studies from Sweden. Again, the smaller study detected a weak but positive association that could not be confirmed in the later, larger study.[104,105] In both studies, however, a shorter length of gestation (36 weeks or shorter), indicating prematurity, was related to a substantially reduced risk of prostate cancer.[104,105] In the smaller study, the researchers also reported an increased risk related to neonatal jaundice.[104]

11.3.2 Testicular cancer

In most western countries, the incidence of testicular cancer has gradually increased over the last 50 years, but peak incidence has remained fairly stable at approximately 25–30 years of age (see Chapter 12). A time trend study from six European countries indicated that this increase is compatible with a birth cohort pattern.[108] A total of 11 reported studies have investigated the relationship between perinatal factors and the risk of testicular cancer and the results of these studies support the hypothesis that prenatal and perinatal factors associated with the hormonal environment (sex hormones, insulin, and IGF) are important for the development of testicular cancer. The evidence suggests that birthweight is positively associated and that risk is gradually reduced with increasing number of older siblings. Dizygotic twins appear to be at increased risk and the use of sex steroid medication in pregnancy is likely to increase the risk of testicular cancer in the male offspring.

11.3.2.1 Birthweight

In five studies,[109–113] the association with birthweight has been examined and in four of these studies, higher birthweights were related to increased risk of testicular cancer.[109–112] However, the study that showed no association with birthweight had nearly twice as many testicular cancer cases as any of the other studies,[113] thus weakening the evidence that birthweight is related to an increased risk.

11.3.2.2 Maternal age and birth order

Testicular cancer risk in offspring has been hypothesized to decrease with increasing maternal age, possibly through age related changes in the hormonal milieu of pregnancy. A similar effect has been proposed for increasing maternal parity. An increased risk associated with older maternal age at birth was found in two studies,[112,114] whereas in two others no association with maternal age was reported.[111,113] The results for birth order have been more consistent suggesting that testicular cancer risk is reduced with increasing number of older siblings.[114–117]

11.3.2.3 Twins

The hypothesis that hormonal factors produced by two placentas could increase the risk of testicular cancer among dizygotic twins has been investigated. In a study that linked data from the Swedish twin and cancer registries, dizygotic twins were at increased risk of testicular cancer compared with the general population.[71]

Similarly, a case–control study from the UK showed an increased risk of testicular cancer if the cotwin was a girl (all dizygotic)[118] and a reduced risk if the cotwin was a boy (a mixture of dizygotic and monozygotic). In a subsequent study that ascertained twin zygosity, the same investigators confirmed that dizygotic twins had higher risk of testicular cancer than monozygotic twins.[119]

11.3.2.4 Other factors

Increased risk of testicular cancer has been associated with higher prepregnancy maternal weight,[109] excessive nausea,[109] shorter gestational age,[113] neonatal jaundice,[111,117] and a retained placenta.[117] Evaluation of cigarette smoking during pregnancy revealed a reduced risk of testicular cancer in sons if the mother smoked.[113] Two studies have found a strongly increased risk of testicular cancer associated with use of exogenous hormones during pregnancy,[109,113] though a third found no evidence for any association.[110]

Overall, the evidence that early life factors may influence the risk of testicular cancer is stronger than for prostate cancer. In fact, the relative proximity in time from birth until the presence of clinical disease may indicate that testicular cancer originates early in life.

11.4 Methodologic issues

The life course approach to cancer epidemiology is made difficult by the lack of intermediate end-points, inadequate knowledge of the biologic mechanisms related to the development of cancers, and the relative rarity of specific cancers in populations. Approaches to using epidemiologic data for investigating early life factors and adult cancers have been innovative but have suffered from limitations. Cohort studies with lifetime information tend to have limited numbers of cases for any one particular cancer. For example, a UK cohort of 2221 women followed since 1946 yielded 37 breast cancer cases for analysis in 1997.[56] Other cohort studies have data for limited time periods that may permit investigating associations among risk factors, for example, birth size and age at menarche,[120] but without cancer outcomes. Case–control studies are limited in the types and accuracy of early life information obtainable through recall from adult participants or from birth records. Missing data due to low response rates among participants or surrogates and inability to recall exposures in the distant past present major difficulties. Mothers of participants often provide a greater variety of information on the pregnancy than could be obtained from birth records or from adult offspring. However, these studies are difficult to interpret because often less than 50% of mothers participate. Record linkage studies in the Scandinavian countries have been the most productive sources of new results, but have been limited to data from one time period, usually birth information. Although confounding by other risk factors, particularly those in the adult period, may not be an issue, effect modification may prove to be informative. Thus, data sources with large numbers of participants and information across the life course are needed.

An evaluation of pregnancy and childhood characteristics across populations that vary in cancer risk may provide leads to understanding cancer development. One such study compared pregnancy hormones in China, a population with a low incidence of breast cancer and in the USA, where incidence is high.[121] The results were provocative, with higher maternal concentrations of oestrogens, androgens, and growth hormone in the Chinese compared with the American women. This finding was unanticipated because other studies show that Chinese and Japanese women have lower levels of circulating steroid hormones in the nonpregnant state compared with Caucasian women.[122,123] Further, lower birthweights in Chinese than in Caucasian infants[121] are inconsistent with the higher oestrogen–higher birthweight hypothesis. These enigmatic findings from the study of pregnant Chinese and American women[121] warrant follow-up investigations.

Another avenue of investigation has been the evaluation of hormone levels by purported risk factors. Maternal age, initially thought to be a risk factor for breast and prostate cancers in the offspring, was hypothesized to influence risk through alterations in maternal pregnancy hormone levels. Studies, however, have shown little association,[49,124] and in particular, have failed to show that oestrogens increase with maternal age. Oestradiol levels have been shown to be higher in first compared with second pregnancies,[124,125] providing a possible mechanism for an inverse association of cancer risk with birth order as observed for testicular cancer. Studies of hormones have not evaluated maternal age and parity together nor have they assessed a variety of hormonal factors. Evidence for associations between birthweight and pregnancy oestrogens are weak for oestrone and oestradiol,[126] but stronger for oestriol.[49] Finally, most studies have evaluated pregnancy hormones in maternal samples. Assessing fetal exposure and evaluating the concordance between maternal and fetal values is an important methodologic issue to be addressed in epidemiologic studies.

One of the most promising leads for understanding the early origins of cancers comes from the observed reduced risks associated with preeclamptic pregnancies. Studies that have evaluated preeclampsia, however, have not considered the heterogeneous nature of this disorder.[127] One subtype of preeclampsia is dominated by vascular reactivity that increases blood pressure in pregnancy and appears not to substantially reduce fetal growth.[128] The other type may originate from an implantation abnormality and result in reduced utero-placental blood flow, affecting fetal nutrition and typically resulting in intrauterine growth restriction. The two types of preeclampsia are not easily distinguishable, but because these subtypes are likely to reflect different underlying causes, it would be worth exploring cancer risk by preeclampsia subtype.

11.5 Commentary

This review has emphasized the importance of perinatal determinants of breast cancer in women and of prostate and testicular cancers in men. The paucity of data evaluating early life risk factors for cancers and relationships among risk factors over time is apparent. Although the literature on breast cancer is wider than that on prostate and testicular cancers, a common emphasis in recent studies has been on birthweight. The prenatal characteristics reflected in a positive association between birthweight and these cancers are not clear. Birthweight adjusted for differences in gestational age at birth may be an appropriate indicator of fetal growth. At best, it should be recognized that birthweight is a crude indicator of endocrine factors in pregnancy and the evidence to date is compatible with a positive association for birthweight in relation to early-onset breast and testicular cancers.

The evidence from recent studies of breast cancer suggests that a chain of interrelated risk factors may originate early in life, continue into childhood and adolescence, and ultimately increase risk for cancer in adulthood. The nature of the relationship among the risk factors and time periods is unknown but may represent interactive or cumulative effects of exposure. However, most studies contain exposure information from one time period only. The importance of longitudinal information was recently demonstrated[29,56,59] and should be pursued further in amenable datasets.

Application of currently available methods and datasets may prove useful in evaluating relationships among established risk factors. For example, both tallness and an early age at menarche appear to increase breast cancer risk, but the relationship between these factors seems paradoxical, because women who become tall also tend to have a later age at menarche.[129] This may indicate the presence of a high-risk subgroup comprised of women who become tall but experience an early menarche. Exploring a possible interaction of these factors in studies that have already collected information on menarche and height would be useful.

Addressing most of these issues will require either a longitudinal approach or a large cohort because of the interrelationship between factors that act at different developmental time periods and because the ultimate end-point (cancer) is rare. For cancer aetiology, it is likely that periods of rapid growth and tissue maturation represent specific periods of susceptibility. *In utero*, early childhood, pubertal, and pregnancy periods are likely to be critical time points. It is increasingly important to collect new and more detailed information. Studies that have already been established for other purposes, but cover the intrauterine period and the first years of life, may provide new insights if the data are analysed with a cancer risk perspective. Analogously, already established studies of childhood and adolescent growth and reproductive development could be equally useful. In the meantime investigators should continue evaluating the life course epidemiology of cancer using multiple approaches, including describing the physiologic mechanisms of purported risk factors and using this information to better formulate hypotheses for cancer outcomes.

Acknowledgements

The authors wish to thank Tom Ivar Lund Nilsen for his work on the figures and Anne Rogers for review and helpful comments on previous drafts of this chapter.

References

Those marked with an asterisk are especially recommended for further reading.

1 **American Cancer Society.** *Cancer facts and figures 2002.* New York: American Cancer Society, 2002.

2 **Tunstall-Pedoe H, Kuulasmaa K, Mahonen M, Tolonen H, Ruokokoski E, Amouyel P.** Contribution of trends in survival and coronary-event rates to changes in coronary heart disease mortality: 10-year results from 37 WHO MONICA project populations. Monitoring trends and determinants in cardiovascular disease. *Lancet* 1999;**353**:1547–57.

*3 **Trichopoulos D.** Hypothesis: does breast cancer originate *in utero*? *Lancet* 1990;**335**:939–40.

4 Bergstrom A, Lindblad P, Wolk A. Birthweight and risk of renal cell cancer. *Kidney Int* 2001;**59**:1110–13.

5 Armstrong BK, English DR. Cutaneous malignant melanoma. In Schottenfeld D, Fraumeni JF Jr, eds. *Cancer epidemiology and prevention*. New York: Oxford University Press, 1996:1282–312.

6 Brinton LA, Devesa SA. Etiology and pathogenesis of breast cancer. Epidemiologic factors. In Harris JR, Morrow M, Lippman ME, Hellman S, eds. *Diseases of the breast*. Philadelphia: Lippincott-Raven, 1996:159–8.

7 Lipworth L. Epidemiology of breast cancer. *Eur J Cancer Prev* 1995;**41**:7–30.

8 Madigan MP, Ziegler RG, Benichou J, Byrne C, Hoover RN. Proportion of breast cancer cases in the United States explained by well-established risk factors. *J Natl Cancer Inst* 1995;**87**:1681–5.

9 Tavani A, Braga C, La Vecchia C, Negri E, Russo A, Franceschi S. Attributable risks for breast cancer in Italy: education, family history and reproductive and hormonal factors. *Int J Cancer* 1997;**70**:159–63.

10 Collaborative Group on Hormonal Factors in Breast Cancer. Breast cancer and breastfeeding: collaborative reanalysis of individual data from 47 epidemiological studies in 30 countries, including 50,302 women with breast cancer and 96,973 women without the disease. *Lancet* 2002;**360**:187–95.

11 Boyd NF, Lockwood GA, Byng JW, Tritchler DL, Yaffe MJ. Mammographic densities and breast cancer risk. *Cancer Epidemiol Biomarkers Prev* 1998;**7**:1133–44.

12 Liao DJ, Dickson RB. Roles of androgens in the development, growth, and carcinogenesis of the mammary gland. *J Steroid Biochem Mol Biol* 2002;**80**:175–89.

13 Bruning PF, Bonfrer JMG, van Noord PAH, Hart AAM, Jong-Bakker MD, Nooijen WJ. Insulin resistance and breast cancer risk. *Int J Cancer* 1992;**52**:511–16.

14 Hankinson SE, Willett WC, Colditz GA, Hunter DJ, Michaud DS, Deroo B *et al*. Circulating concentrations of insulin-like growth factor-1 and risk of breast cancer. *Lancet* 1998;**351**:1393–6.

15 Berkey CS, Frazier AL, Gardner JD, Colditz GA. Adolescence and breast carcinoma risk. *Cancer* 1999;**85**:2400–9.

*16 Colditz GA, Frazier AL. Models of breast cancer show that risk is set by events of early life: prevention efforts must shift focus. *Cancer Epidemiol Biomarkers Prev* 1995;**4**:567–71.

17 Friedenreich CM. Review of anthropometric factors and breast cancer risk. *Eur J Cancer Prev* 2001;**10**:15–32.

18 Willett WC. Diet and breast cancer. *J Intern Med* 2001;**249**:395–411.

19 IARC Handbooks of Cancer Prevention. *Weight control and physical activity, Volume 6*. Lyon: IARC Press, 2002:95–112.

20 LeMarchand L, Kolonel LN, Earle ME, Mi M-P. Body size at different periods of life and breast cancer risk. *Am J Epidemiol* 1988;**128**:137–52.

21 Huang Z, Hankinson SE, Colditz GA, Stampfer MJ, Hunter DJ, Manson JE *et al*. Dual effects of weight and weight gain on breast cancer risk. *J Am Med Assoc* 1997;**278**:1407–11.

22 Trentham-Dietz A, Newcomb PA, Storer BE, Longnecker MP, Baron J, Greenberg ER *et al*. Body size and risk of breast cancer. *Am J Epidemiol* 1997;**145**:1011–19.

23 Brinton LA, Swanson CA. Height and weight at various ages and risk of breast cancer. *Ann Epidemiol* 1992;**2**:597–609.

24 Barnes-Josiah D, Potter JD, Sellers TA, Himes JH. Early body size and subsequent weight gain as predictors of breast cancer incidence (Iowa, United States). *Cancer Causes Control* 1995;**6**:112–18.

25 Rich-Edwards JW, Goldman MB, Willett WC, Hunter DJ, Stampfer MJ, Colditz GA, Manson JE. Adolescent body mass index and ovulatory infertility. *Am J Obstet Gynecol* 1994;**171**:171–7.

26 Ballard-Barbash R. Anthropometry and breast cancer. Body size—a moving target. *Cancer* 1994;**74**:1090–100.

27 Gunnell D, Okasha M, Davey-Smith G, Oliver SE, Holly JMP. Height, leg length and cancer risk: a systematic review. *Epidemiol Rev* 2001;**23**:313–42.

28 Li CI, Malone KE, White E, Daling JR. Age when maximum height is reached as a risk factor for breast cancer among young U.S. women. *Epidemiology* 1997;**8**:559–65.

29 Berkey CS, Gardner JD, Frazier AL, Colditz GA. Relation of childhood diet and body size to menarche and adolescent growth in girls. *Am J Epidemiol* 2000;**152**:446–52.

30 Albanes D. Energy balance, body size, and cancer. *Crit Rev Oncol Hematol* 1990;**10**:283–303.

31 Hislop TG, Coldman AJ, Elwood JM, Brauer G, Kan L. Childhood and recent eating patterns and risk of breast cancer. *Cancer Detect Prev* 1986;**9**:47–58.

32 Pryor M, Slattery ML, Robinson LM, Egger M. Adolescent diet and breast cancer in Utah. *Cancer Res* 1989;**49**:2161–7.

33 Potischman N, Weiss HA, Swanson CA, Coates RJ, Gammon MD, Malone KE *et al.* Diet during adolescence and risk of breast cancer among young women. *J Natl Cancer Inst* 1998;**90**:226–33.

34 Dirx MJ, van den Brandt PA, Goldbohm RA, Lumey LH. Diet in adolescence and the risk of breast cancer: results of the Netherlands Cohort Study. *Cancer Causes Control* 1999;**10**:189–99.

35 Le Marchand L, Kolonel LN, Myers BC, Mi M-P. Birth characteristics of premenopausal women with breast cancer. *Br J Cancer* 1988;**57**:437–9.

*36 Ekbom A, Trichopoulos D, Adami HO, Hsieh CC, Lan SJ. Evidence of prenatal influences on breast cancer risk. *Lancet* 1992;**340**:1015–18.

37 Ekbom A, Hsieh C-C, Lipworth L, Adami H-O, Trichopoulos D. Intrauterine environment and breast cancer risk in women: a population-based study. *J Natl Cancer Inst* 1997;**89**:71–6.

38 Sanderson M, Williams MA, Daling JR, Holt VL, Malone KE, Self SG *et al.* Maternal factors and breast cancer risk among young women. *Paediatr Perinat Epidemiol* 1998;**12**:397–407.

39 Innes K, Byers T, Schymura M. Birth characteristics and subsequent risk for breast cancer in very young women. *Am J Epidemiol* 2000;**152**:1121–8.

40 Stamilio DM, Sehdev HM, Morgan MA, Propert K, Macones GA. Can antenatal clinical and biochemical markers predict the development of severe preeclampsia? *Am J Obstet Gynecol* 2000;**182**:589–94.

41 Ranta T, Stenman U-H, Unnérus H-A, Rossi J, Seppälä M. Maternal plasma prolactin levels in preeclampsia. *Obstet Gynecol* 1980;**55**:428–30.

42 Rosing U, Carlström K. Serum levels of unconjugated and total oestrogens and dehydroepiandrosterone, progesterone, and urinary oestriol excretion in pre-eclampsia. *Gynecol Obstet Invest* 1984;**18**:199–205.

43 Acromite MT, Mantzoros CS, Leach RE, Hurwitz J, Dorey LG. Androgens in preeclampsia. *Am J Obstet Gynecol* 1999;**180**:60–3.

*44 Vatten LJ, Romundstad PR, Odegard RA, Nilsen ST, Trichopoulos D, Austgulen R. Alpha-foetoprotein in umbilical cord in relation to severe pre-eclampsia, birthweight and future breast cancer risk. *Br J Cancer* 2002;**86**:728–31.

45 Cohn BA, Cirillo PM, Christianson RE, van den Berg BJ, Siiteri PK. Placental characteristics and reduced risk of maternal breast cancer. *J Natl Cancer Inst* 2001;**93**:1133–40.

46 Vatten LJ, Nilsen ST, Odegard RA, Romundstad PR, Austgulen R. Insulin-like growth factor I and leptin in umbilical cord plasma and infant birth size at term. *Pediatrics* 2002;**109**:1131–5.

47 Melbye M, Wohlfahrt J, Lei U, Norgaard-Pedersen B, Mouridsen HT, Lambe M *et al.* Alpha-fetoprotein levels in maternal serum during pregnancy and maternal breast cancer incidence. *J Natl Cancer Inst* 2000;**92**:1001–5.

48 Richardson BE, Hulka BS, Peck JL, Hughes CL, van den Berg BJ, Christianson RE *et al.* Levels of maternal serum alpha-fetoprotein (AFP) in pregnant women and subsequent breast cancer risk. *Am J Epidemiol* 1998;**148**:719–27.

49 Kaijser M, Granath F, Jacobsen G, Cnattingius S, Ekbom A. Maternal pregnancy estriol levels in relation to anamnestic and fetal anthropometric data. *Epidemiology* 2000;**11**:315–19.

50 O'Dell SD, Day IN. Insulin-like growth factor II (IGF-II). *J Biochem Cell Biol* 1998;**30**:767–71.

51 Pollack M, Blouin M-J, Zhang J-C, Kopchick JJ. Reduced mammary gland carcinogenesis in transgenic mice expressing a growth hormone antagonist. *Br J Cancer* 2001;**85**:428–30.

52 Sanderson M, Williams MA, Malone KE, Stanford JL, Emanuel I, White E *et al.* Perinatal factors and risk of breast cancer. *Epidemiology* 1996;**7**:34–7.

53 Michels KB, Trichopoulos D, Robins JM, Rosner BA, Manson JE, Hunter DJ *et al.* Birthweight as a risk factor for breast cancer. *Lancet* 1996;**348**:1542–6.

54 Kaijser M, Lichtenstein P, Granath F, Erlandsson G, Cnattingius S, Ekbom A. *In utero* exposures and breast cancer: a study of opposite-sexed twins. *J Natl Cancer Inst* 2001;**93**:60–2.

55 Hubinette A, Lichtenstein P, Ekbom A, Cnattingius S. Birth characteristics and breast cancer risk: a study among like-sexed twins. *Int J Cancer* 2001;**91**:248–51.

*56 De Stavola BL, Hardy R, Kuh D, dos Santos Silva I, Wadsworth M, Swerdlow AJ. Birthweight, childhood growth and risk of breast cancer in a British cohort. *Br J Cancer* 2000;**83**:964–68.

57 Titus-Ernstoff L, Egan KM, Newcomb PA, Ding J, Trentham-Dietz A, Greenberg ER *et al.* Early life factors in relation to breast cancer risk in postmenopausal women. *Cancer Epidemiol Biomarkers Prev* 2002;**11**:207–10.

58 Andersson SW, Bengtsson C, Hallberg L, Lapidus L, Niklasson A, Wallgren A *et al.* Cancer risk in Swedish women: the relation to size at birth. *Br J Cancer* 2001;**84**:1193–8.

59 Hilakivi-Clarke L, Forsen T, Eriksson JG, Luoto R, Tuomilehto, Osmond C *et al.* Tallness and overweight during childhood have opposing effects on breast cancer risk. *Br J Cancer* 2001;**85**:1680–4.

60 Vatten LJ, Maehle BO, Lund Nilsen TI, Tretli S, Hsieh C-C, Trichopoulos D *et al.* Birthweight as a predictor of breast cancer: a case–control study in Norway. *Br J Cancer* 2002;**86**:89–91.

61 Troy LM, Michels KB, Hunter DJ, Spiegelman D, Manson JE, Colditz GA *et al.* Self-reported birthweight and history of having been breastfed among younger women: an assessment of validity. *Int J Epidemiol* 1996;**25**:122–7.

62 Sanderson M, Williams MA, White E, Daling JR, Holt V, Malone KE *et al.* Validity and reliability of subject and mother reporting of perinatal factors. *Am J Epidemiol* 1998;**147**:136–40.

63 Sanderson M, Shu XO, Jin F, Dai Q, Gao Y-T, Zheng W. Weight at birth and adolescence and premenopausal breast cancer risk in a low-risk population. *Br J Cancer* 2002;**86**:84–8.

64 Treloar SA, Sanrzadeh S, Do K-M, Martin NG, Lambalk CB. Birthweight and age at menopause in Australian female twin pairs: exploration of the fetal origin hypothesis. *Hum Reprod* 2000;**15**:55–9.

65 Hardy R, Kuh D. Does early growth influence timing of the menopause? Evidence from a British birth cohort. *Hum Reprod* 2002;**17**:2474–9.

66 Ekbom A, Erlandsson G, Hsieh C, Trichopoulos D, Adami HO, Cnattingius S. Risk of breast cancer in prematurely born women. *J Natl Cancer Inst* 2000;**92**:840–1.

67 Ekbom A, Thurfjell E, Hsieh CC, Trichopoulos D, Adami HO. Perinatal characteristics and adult mammographic patterns. *Int J Cancer* 1995;**61**:177–80.

68 Hsieh C-C, Lan S-J, Ekbom A, Petridou E, Adami H-O, Trichopoulos D. Twin membership and breast cancer risk. *Am J Epidemiol* 1992;**136**:1321–6.

69 Weiss HA, Potischman NA, Brinton LA, Brogan D, Coates RJ, Gammon MD *et al.* Prenatal and perinatal risk factors for breast cancer in young women. *Epidemiology* 1997;**8**:181–7.

70 Holm NV. Studies of cancer etiology in the Danish Twin Population. I. Breast cancer. In *Twin research 3: epidemiological and clinical studies.* New York: Alan R. Liss, 1981:211–16.

71 Braun MM, Ahlbom A, Floderus B, Brinton L, Hoover RN. Effect of twinship on incidence of cancer of the testis, breast and other sites (Sweden). *Cancer Causes Control* 1995;**6**:519–24.

72 Kaprio J, Teppo L, Koskenvuo, Pukkala E. Cancer in the adult same-sex twins: a historical cohort study. In *Twin research 3: epidemiological and clinical studies.* New York: Alan R. Liss, 1981:217–23.

73 Ahlbom A., Lichenstein P, Malstrom H, Feychting M, Hemminki K, Pedersen NL. Cancer in twins: genetic and nongenetic familial risk factors. *J Natl Cancer Inst* 1997;**89**:287–93.

74 Swerdlow AJ, De Stavola B, Maconochie N, Siskind V. A population-based study of cancer risk in twins: relationships to birth order and sexes of the twin pair. *Int J Cancer* 1996;**67**:472–8.

75 Duff GB, Brown JB. Urinary oestriol excretion in twin pregnancies. *J Obstet Gyn (British)* 1974;**81**:695–700.

76 TambyRaja RL, Ratman SS. Plasma steroid changes in twin pregnancies. In *Twin research 3: twin biology and multiple pregnancy.* New York: Alan R. Liss, 1981:189–96.

77 Kappel B, Hansen K, Moller J, Faaborg-Andersen J. Human placental lactogen and dU-estrogen levels in normal twin pregnancies. *Acta Genet Med Gemellol (Roma)* 1985;**34**:59–65.

78 Standfast S. Birth characterisitcs of women dying from breast cancer. *J Natl Cancer Inst* 1967;**39**:33–42.

79 Rothman KJ, MacMahon B, Lin TM, Lowe CR, Mirra AP, Ravnihar B *et al.* Maternal age and birth rank of women with breast cancer. *J Natl Cancer Inst* 1980;**65**:719–22.

80 Henderson BE, Powell D, Rosario I, Keys C, Hanisch R, Young M *et al.* An epidemiologic study of breast cancer. *J Natl Cancer Inst* 1974;**53**:609–14.

81 Janerich DT, Hayden CL, Thompson WD, Selenskas SL, Mettlin C. Epidemiologic evidence of perinatal influence in the etiology of adult cancers. *J Clin Epidemiol* 1989;**42**:151–7.

82 Thompson WD, Janerich DT. Maternal age at birth and risk of breast cancer in daughters. *Epidemiology* 1990;**1**:101–6.

83 Hemminki K, Mutanen P. Birth order, family size, and the risk of cancer in young and middle-aged adults. *Br J Cancer* 2001;**84**:1446–71.

84 Baron JA, Vessey M, McPherson K, Yeates D. Maternal age and breast cancer risk. *J Natl Cancer Inst* 1984;**72**:1307–9.

85 Colditz GA, Willett WC, Stampfer MJ, Hennekens CH, Rosner B, Speizer FE. Parental age at birth and risk of breast cancer in daughters: a prospective study among US women. *Cancer Causes Control* 1991;**2**:31–6.

86 Hemminki K, Kyyronen P. Parental age and risk of sporadic and familial cancer in offspring: implications for germ cell mutagenesis. *Epidemiology* 1999;**10**:747–51.

87 Hsieh C-C, Tzonou A, Trichopoulos D. Birth order and breast cancer risk. *Cancer Causes Control* 1991;**2**:95–8.

88 Janerich DT, Thompson WD, Mineau GP. Maternal pattern of reproduction and risk of breast cancer in daughters: Results from the Utah population database. *J Natl Cancer Inst* 1994;**86**:1634–9.

89 Bucalossi P, Veronesi U. Some observations on cancer of the breast in mothers and daughters. *Br J Cancer* 1957;**11**:337–47.

90 Tokuhata GK. Morbidity and mortality among offspring of breast cancer mothers. *Am J Epidemiol* 1969;**89**:139–53.

91 Fraumeni JF, Miller RW. Breast cancer from breast-feeding. *Lancet* 1971;**2**:1196–7.

92 Titus-Ernstoff L, Egan KM, Newcomb PA, Baron JA, Stampfer M, Greenberg ER *et al.* Exposure to breast milk in infancy and adult breast cancer risk. *J Natl Cancer Inst* 1998;**90**:921–4.

93 Ekbom A, Hsieh C-C, Trichopoulos D, Yen Y-Y, Petridou E, Adami H-O. Breast-feeding and breast cancer in the offspring. *Br J Cancer* 1993;**67**:842–5.

94 Brinton LA, Hoover R, Fraumeni JF Jr. Reproductive factors in the aetiology of breast cancer. *Br J Cancer* 1983;**47**:757–62.

*95 Freudenheim JL, Marshall JR, Graham S, Laughlin R, Vena JE, Bandera E *et al.* Exposure to breastmilk in infancy and the risk of breast cancer. *Epidemiology* 1994;**5**:324–31.

96 Michels K, Trichopoulos D, Rosner B, Hunter D, Colditz G, Hankinson S *et al.* Being breastfed in infancy and breast cancer incidence in adult life: results from the two nurses' health studies. *Am J Epidemiol* 2001;**153**:275–83.

97 Palmer JR, Hatch EE, Rosenberg C, Hartge P, Kaufman RH, Titus-Ernstoff L *et al.* Risk of breast cancer in women exposed to diethylstilbestrol *in utero*: preliminary results (United States). *Cancer Causes Control* 2002;**13**:753–8.

98 Sandler DP, Everson RB, Wilcox AJ, Browder JP. Cancer risk in adulthood from early life exposure to parents' smoking. *Am J Pub Health* 1985;**75**:487–92.

99 Severson RK, Davis S. Breast cancer incidence and month of birth: evidence against an etiologic association. *Eur J Cancer Clin Oncol* 1987;**23**:1067–70.

100 Yuen J, Ekbom A, Trichopoulos D, Hsieh C-C, Adami H-O. Season of birth and breast cancer risk in Sweden. *Br J Cancer* 1994;**70**:564–8.

101 Kristoffersen S, Hartveit F. Is a woman's date of birth related to her risk of developing breast cancer? *Oncology Rep* 2000;**7**:245–7.

102 Hsing AW, Devesa SS. Trends and patterns of prostate cancer: What do they suggest? *Epidemiol Rev* 2001;**23**:3–13.

103 Tibblin G, Eriksson M, Cnattingius S, Ekbom A. High birthweight as a predictor of prostate cancer risk. *Epidemiology* 1995;**6**:423–4.

104 Ekbom A, Hsieh C-C, Lipworth L, Wolk A, Pontén J, Adami H-O *et al.* Perinatal characteristics in relation to incidence of and mortality from prostate cancer. *Br Med J* 1996;**313**:337–41.

*105 Ekbom A, Wuu J, Adami H-O, Lu C-M, Lagiou P, Trichopoulos D *et al.* Duration of gestation and prostate cancer risk in offspring. *Cancer Epidemiol Biomarkers Prev* 2000;**9**:221–3.

106 Platz EA, Giovannucci E, Rimm EB, Curhan GC, Spiegelman D, Colditz GA *et al.* Retrospective analysis of birthweight and prostate cancer in the Health Professionals Follow-up study. *Am J Epidemiol* 1998;**147**:1140–4.

107 Zhang Y, Kreger BE, Dorgan JF, Cupples LA, Myers RH, Splansky GL *et al.* Parental age at child's birth and son's risk of prostate cancer. The Framingham study. *Am J Epidemiol* 1999;**150**:1208–12.

*108 Bergström R, Adami H-O, Möhner M, Zatonski W, Storm H, Ekbom A *et al.* Increase in testicular cancer incidence in six European countries: a birth cohort phenomenon. *J Natl Cancer Inst* 1996;**88**:727–33.

*109 Depue RH, Pike MC, Henderson BE. Estrogen exposure during gestation and risk of testicular cancer. *J Natl Cancer Inst* 1983;**71**:1151–5.

110 Brown LM, Pottern LM, Hoover RN. Prenatal and perinatal risk factors for testicular cancer. *Cancer Res* 1986;**46**:4812–16.

111 Akre O, Ekbom A, Hsieh C-C, Trichopoulos D, Adami H-O. Testicular nonseminoma and seminoma in relation to perinatal characteristics. *J Natl Cancer Inst* 1996;**88**:883–9.

112 Moller H, Skakkebaek NE. Testicular cancer and cryptorchidism in relation to prenatal factors: case–control studies in Denmark. *Cancer Causes Control* 1997;**8**:904–12.

113 Weir HK, Marrett LD, Kreiger N, Darlington GA, Sugar L. Prenatal and perinatal exposures and risk of testicular germ-cell cancer. *Int J Cancer* 2000;**87**:438–43.

114 Swerdlow AJ, Huttly SR, Smith PG. Prenatal and familial associations of testicular cancer. *Br J Cancer* 1987;**55**:571–7.

115 Westergaard T, Andersen PK, Pedersen JB, Frisch M, Olsen JH, Melbye M. Testicular cancer risk and maternal parity: a population-based cohort study. *Br J Cancer* 1998;**77**:1180–5.

116 Prener A, Hsieh C-C, Engholm G, Trichopoulos D, Jensen OM. Birth order and risk of testicular cancer. *Cancer Causes Control* 1992;**3**:265–72.

117 Wanderas EH, Grotmol T, Fossa SD, Tretli S. Maternal health and pre- and perinatal characteristics in the etiology of testicular cancer: a prospective population and register-based study on Norwegian males born between 1967 and 1995. *Cancer Causes Control* 1998;**9**:475–86.

118 Swerdlow AJ, De Stavola B, Maconochie N, Siskind V. A population-based study of cancer risk in twins: relationships to birth order and sexes of the twin pair. *Int J Cancer* 1996;**67**:472–8.

119 Swerdlow AJ, De Stavola B, Swanwick MA, Maconochie N. Risks of breast and testicular cancers in young adult twins in England and Wales: evidence on prenatal and genetic aetiology. *Lancet* 1997;**350**:1723–8.

120 Adair LS. Size at birth predicts age at menarche. *Pediatrics* 2001;**107**(4):E59.

121 Lipworth L, Hsieh C-C, Wide L, Ekbom A, Yu S-S, Yu G-P *et al.* Maternal pregnancy hormone levels in an area with a high incidence (Boston, USA) and in an area with a low incidence (Shanghai, China) of breast cancer. *Br J Cancer* 1999;**79**:7–12.

122 Key TJ, Chen J, Wang DY, Pike MC, Boreham J. Sex hormones in women in rural China and in Britain. *Br J Cancer* 1990;**62**:631–6.

123 Bernstein L, Yuan J-M, Ross RK, Pike MC, Hanish R, Lobo R *et al.* Serum hormone levels in premenopausal Chinese women in Shanghai and white women in Los Angeles: results from two breast cancer case–control studies. *Cancer Causes Control* 1990;**1**:51–8.

124 Panagiotopoulou K, Katsouyanni K, Petridou E, Garas Y, Tzonou A, Trichopoulos D. Maternal age, parity, and pregnancy estrogens. *Cancer Cause Control* 1990;**1**:119–24.

125 Bernstein L, Depue RH, Ross RK, Judd HL, Pike MC, Henderson BE. Higher maternal levels of free estradiol in first compared to second pregnancy: early gestational differences. *J Natl Cancer Inst* 1986;**76**:1035–9.

126 Petridou E, Panagiotopoulou K, Katsouyanni K, Spanos E, Trichopoulos D. Tobacco smoking, pregnancy estrogens, and birthweight. *Epidemiology* 1990;**1**:247–50.

127 Ness RB, Roberts JM. Heterogeneous causes constituting the single syndrome of preeclampsia: a hypothesis and its implications. *Am J Obstet Gynecol.* 1996;**175**:1365–70.

128 Odegard RA, Vatten LJ, Nilsen ST, Salvesen KA, Austgulen R. Risk factors and clinical manifestations of pre-eclampsia. *Br J Obstet Gynaecol* 2000;**107**:1410–16.

129 Vatten LJ. Prospective studies of the risk of breast cancer. Doctoral thesis. Tapir, Trondheim: University of Trondheim, 1990.

Chapter 12

Time trends in cancer incidence and mortality

Isabel dos Santos Silva

Examination of time trends in disease risk provides a helpful means of assessing determinants of disease risk at a population rather than individual level. In this chapter we examine trends in cancer incidence and mortality for selected cancer sites in both developed and developing countries in relation to trends in known risk factors. There were strong cohort-related variations in the risk of lung cancer (which paralleled cumulative lifetime cigarette consumption in different cohorts), stomach cancer (perhaps related to cohort improvement in childhood socioeconomic conditions and declines in the prevalence of *Helicobacter pylori* infection), and cervical cancer (which paralleled cohort changes in sexual behaviour and in the prevalence of human papillomavirus (HPV) infection). There were also strong cohort effects for testicular germ cell cancer in developed countries and although its age distribution strongly suggests a prenatal/early life aetiology, the relevant exposures are yet to be identified. Interpretation of the breast cancer trends was more complex; they could not be explained by trends in prenatal factors or adult reproductive behaviour but were consistent with trends in age at menarche and adult height (as well as trends in adult body weight). The need for a life course approach to cancer aetiology is illustrated by recent evidence showing that excess adult body weight, the origins of which are known to stretch back to early life, is associated with an increased risk of developing cancer at several sites. Thus, if current trends in body weight persist we may witness a dramatic increase in the number of cancers attributed to this exposure in the near future.

12.1 Introduction

The importance of cancer as a cause of death has increased progressively during the twentieth century in many developed countries. This is partly because deaths from infections and, more recently, cardiovascular diseases have declined and partly because life expectancy has increased and, hence, people are surviving to the ages when cancer is particularly common. Improved medical diagnostic techniques have also led to better detection of cancer. In this chapter, we will begin by attempting to integrate experimental models of carcinogenesis and the life course approach into a common aetiological framework and follow with a brief overview of trends in the most common cancer sites in relation to potential risk factors. Particular emphasis will be given to breast and testicular cancers, sites for which there is evidence that their origins stretch as far back as the prenatal period.

12.2 Stages in neoplastic development: from biology to epidemiology

Several lines of evidence suggest that carcinogenesis is a multistage process.[1–3] Laboratory experiments have identified various stages in the natural history of neoplastic development including, among others, an 'initiation' stage, which results in permanent and irreversible DNA damage and a 'promotion' stage, during which there is a reversible increase in the replication of progeny of the initiated cell population. Initiated cells persist in the tissue long after the initiating agent has disappeared, remaining latent until acted upon by promoting agents. Epidemiological observations also seem to indicate that some agents would affect carcinogenesis primarily at an early stage, whereas others would affect the process at a later stage. If the agent is an 'early-stage' carcinogen, both the increase in incidence beginning with and during exposure and the decrease in incidence following cessation of exposure will be delayed. However, when a late stage is affected, responses both to starting and ceasing exposure will be much more rapid.

There is growing epidemiological evidence that multiple factors spanning across an individual's life course, not just adult life, sometimes stretching back into the prenatal period, are important in the aetiology of many cancers. The incidence of most cancers clearly increases with age. However, the weight of evidence suggests that age *per se* does not affect the rate at which tumours occur independently of the effect of prolonging exposure.[4] For instance, cumulative mesothelioma risk in humans[5] and cumulative risk of skin tumour in mice treated weekly with benzo(a)pyrene depend on time since first carcinogenic exposure but not age, suggesting an initiating effect of these carcinogens.[6,7] Lung cancer incidence in smokers depends on duration of smoking but not on age and the rapidity with which it stops increasing when smoking stops indicates both early- and late-stage effects.[4]

Paradoxically, most epidemiological research into the aetiology of cancer has, mainly for logistic reasons, relied on exposure data from one single period of life, usually adulthood. In contrast, the life course approach requires examination of factors over an individual's lifetime and, therefore, it complements the multistage carcinogenesis model derived from experimental systems by allowing examination of the cumulative and combined effect of factors operating at different stages of life and, in doing so, leads to new insights into the nature of the underlying cellular mechanisms. Conversely, the multistage model allows researchers to relate life course epidemiological features to biological events.

12.3 Interpretation of temporal variations in cancer risk

There is a long tradition of examining temporal variations in cancer incidence and mortality within a single population[8–15] or between populations.[16–27] Disease rates in any given population at any calendar time will depend on three distinct dimensions: *cohort effects*, which summarize the cumulative experience(s) of a given generation up to that point in time; *calendar period effects*, which reflect exposures occurring at that point in time; and *age effects*, as a measure of the degree of maturation an individual has achieved and, indirectly, as a measure of duration of exposure. The study of temporal variations in cancer incidence involves consideration of these three components.[28,29] Age effects can be examined by displaying rates against age. Period effects, such as those caused by the sudden introduction of an exposure in a population that affects simultaneously and equally all age groups, can be detected by plotting rates against year of occurrence (usually, taken as being the year of diagnosis for incidence data or the year of death for mortality data); a simultaneous (upward or downward) shift in rates across all age groups provides evidence in favour of a period effect.[28] By contrast, cohort (or generational) effects, such as long-term effects of prenatal and early life exposures, can be identified if there is a simultaneous shift in age-specific rates when these rates are plotted against year of birth rather than year of occurrence.[28] The first analysis of cancer trends in relation to birth cohort, using information on year of death and 5-year age group at death to estimate year of birth, were published in the 1950s.[10–13, 30] Period and cohort effects operate simultaneously and therefore it is rather difficult to ascribe temporal variations in disease risk to any of them. Complex age–period–cohort statistical models are often used to assess temporal variations in cancer risk and to try to separate cohort from period effects, but such models cannot overcome the fact that there is a linear dependency between the three time dimensions: age, calendar period, and birth cohort.[29] Thus, in spite of the recognized importance of determining birth cohort patterns when studying life course influences at a population level, the identification of such patterns has proven difficult because of the inability to separate unambiguously linear trends in birth cohort effects from linear trends in calendar period effects.

Interpretation of trends in cancer incidence and mortality also requires careful consideration of possible artefacts such as variations in case ascertainment resulting from changes in diagnostic and screening practices, variations in diagnostic classifications and registration/certification practices, and changes in the coverage and completeness of the cancer registration/death certification schemes. In addition, trends in cancer mortality are affected by temporal variations in survival from this disease.

12.4 Trends in risk for selected cancer sites and their relationship to trends in risk factors

Tobacco smoking, infections, diet, excessive body weight, and reproductive and hormonal factors jointly account for a substantial proportion of cancers worldwide.[31] We shall consider below trends in each one of these risk factors and their relationship to temporal changes in the incidence of various types of cancer.

12.4.1 Smoking-related cancers

Tobacco smoking causes one-third of all cancer deaths in developed countries and it is responsible for about 60% of all cancers among current smokers.[31] There are clear cohort-related variations in lung cancer rates that correspond to estimates of lifetime cigarette consumption in different cohorts. The large increase in male cigarette smoking in the UK during and after the First World War caused a massive epidemic of lung cancer among men born around 1900 (Fig. 12.1). Women began smoking later than men and so their lung cancer epidemic peaked a few decades later.[15] Trends in more recent cohorts have been influenced by declines in the tar content of cigarettes and in

(a)

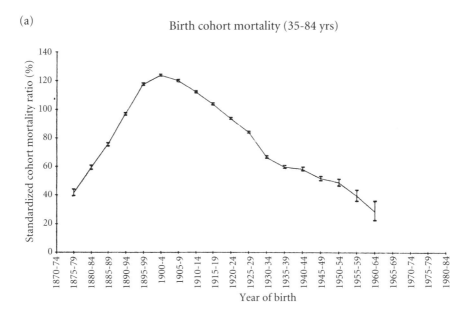

(b)

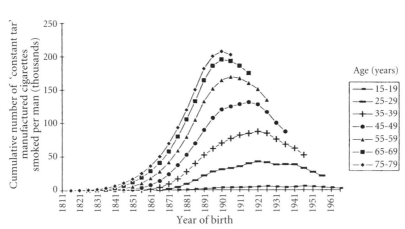

Fig. 12.1 (a) Male lung cancer mortality by year of birth, England and Wales, 1960–1999 (standardized cohort mortality ratios (SCMRs) and 95% confidence intervals (CIs)); (b) cumulative 'constant tar' manufactured cigarette consumption per men born 1816–1966, UK.[15] Reprinted by permission of Oxford University Press.

the prevalence of smoking. A similar epidemic of lung cancer occurred 20 years later in the USA and is now spreading to south and eastern European countries.[32] Tobacco smoking was introduced much later in developing countries but, if nothing is done to change current smoking trends, we will witness massive epidemics of lung cancer in these countries in the next few decades.[32]

The carcinogenic effects of tobacco smoking are not restricted to the lung, however. Smoking increases the risk of cancers of the pancreas, bladder, and kidney and (synergistically with alcohol) the larynx, mouth, pharynx (except nasopharynx), and oesophagus.[33] Trends in some of these cancer sites have paralleled, to a certain extent, the trends in smoking.[15,27] More recent evidence indicates that several other types of cancer such as those of the stomach, liver, and (probably) cervix, are also increased by smoking.[34–36] In China, where liver cancer is common, smoking causes more premature deaths from liver cancer than from heart diseases.[35]

Total male cancer mortality attributed to smoking over the period 1975–1990 increased in many developed countries, particularly in eastern Europe (Hungary, Slovakia, Poland, the Czech Republic, and the former USSR), but there were decreases in many western European countries (the UK, Finland, and the Netherlands)[32] (Fig.12.2). In females, there were substantial increases in total cancer mortality attributed to smoking in Denmark, the USA, Canada, the UK, New Zealand and, to a lesser extent, in certain Eastern European countries, while in other populations female rates remained low and constant. In each sex, however, there was little variation in rates for cancer mortality not attributed to smoking (Fig. 12.2), which seems to imply that tobacco smoking accounts for most of the between-country variation in developed countries as well as for most of the adult male and female trends in total cancer mortality.[32]

12.4.2 Infection-related cancers

About 15% of all cancers worldwide are long-term consequences of infections acquired earlier in life,[37] the most important being stomach cancer, which has been associated with chronic infection with *Helicobacter pylori*;[38] cervical cancer, which has been linked to persistent infection with certain types of HPV;[39,40] and liver cancer, which has been associated with chronic infection with hepatitis-B virus (HBV) and hepatitis-C virus (HCV).[41] Cancer is a rare outcome of infection and although the infectious agents are capable of altering the genetic makeup of the target cell (initiation) and of inducing cell division (promotion), it is clear that other cofactors play a role in tumour development.

Stomach cancer still accounts for 10% of new cancers in the world,[37] despite marked declines in incidence observed in most developed countries over the twentieth century (Fig. 12.3). Countries with historically high stomach cancer rates, such as those in eastern Asian and central America, have also experienced declines in mortality although these began later than in low-risk areas.[17,18] The major modes of transmission of *Helicobacter pylori* are still unknown but the prevalence of infection in the general population is high, particularly in developing countries (about 80–90%)[37] where infection is contracted at young ages and persists throughout life. In developed countries, the prevalence is lower in more recent birth cohorts,[42] perhaps due to improvement in social conditions early in life such as a decline in house overcrowding.[43,44] Cohort declines in the prevalence of *Helicobacter pylori* infection as well as improved food storage, notably refrigeration, and greater availability of fresh fruit and vegetables in the diet may have been responsible for the steady decline in stomach cancer rates during the twentieth century.

Cervical cancer is the second most common female cancer worldwide and the most common female cancer in many developing countries.[27] Total (all-ages) incidence of,

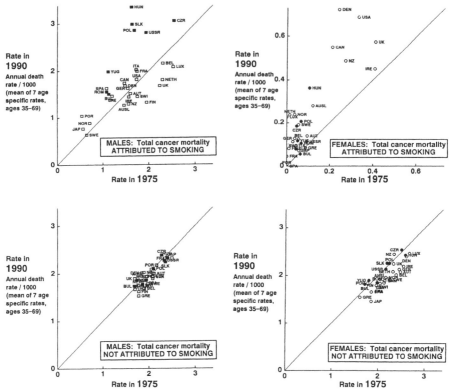

Fig. 12.2 Trends in total cancer mortality attributed to smoking and in total cancer mortality not attributed to smoking in middle-age in 30 developed countries, 1975 and 1990 (solid symbols represent former socialist economies).[32]

and mortality from, cervical cancer has declined in most developed and in the developing countries for which there are reliable data,[27,45] perhaps due to improvements in socioeconomic conditions and the introduction of effective screening practices. At young ages, however, there is evidence of recent upturns in risk,[27,45] perhaps due to changes in sexual behaviour. One of the earliest indications that cervical cancer might be a late complication of a sexually transmitted infection was the close similarity between trends in cervical cancer by birth cohort and trends in the incidence of gonorrhoea at age 20 years as a marker of sexually transmitted diseases;[46] Fig. 12.4 shows similar data for a more recent period. More recently, epidemiological studies have shown that cervical cancer is associated with certain types of HPV. Human papillomavirus infection is common in young women but in most the infection is transient. In some, however, the infection persists and may evolve to cervical cancer. Thus, it is important to differentiate between factors that increase a woman's risk of becoming infected with HPV and those which are associated with an increased risk of cervical cancer once a woman is HPV positive. A recent study[36] showed, for instance, that number of sexual partners and a relatively recent new sexual relationship were associated with an increased risk of

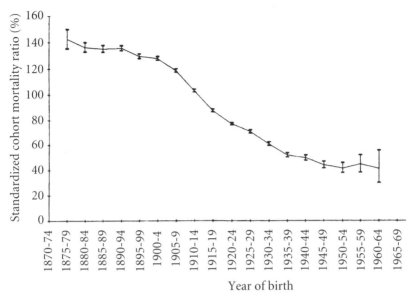

Fig. 12.3 Stomach cancer mortality in men by year of birth, England and Wales, 1960–1999 (standardized cohort mortality ratios (SCMRs) and 95% confidence intervals (CIs)).

infection with HPV whereas early age at first intercourse, large number of years since start of the latest regular sexual relationship, and cigarette smoking were associated with an increase in the risk of severe dysplasia and carcinoma *in situ* (cervical intraepithelial neoplasia, grade 3 (CIN 3)) among HPV-infected women.

Current evidence strongly supports the hypothesis that chronic infection with HBV is the most significant aetiological factor in liver cancer.[41,47] Trends in liver cancer incidence are difficult to interpret because of the potential for under-registration due to rather short survival and the potential for metastases to the liver to be misclassified as primary malignancies.[27] Nevertheless, the few studies that have examined international trends in liver cancer showed no consistent pattern.[48,49] Areas with a high HBV prevalence generally have high mortality from liver cancer,[41] with the exception of Greenland Eskimos who have low liver cancer incidence despite having high HBV prevalence.[50] Hepatitis-B virus transmission may occur at three different times in life: at birth or in early childhood (these two common routes are frequently seen in high HBV prevalence areas in Africa and Asia) or in adult life (the most common in developed countries where the prevalence of HBV is low). Early age at infection is the major determinant of whether a person becomes a carrier.[41] Perinatal transmission confers the highest probability of becoming a carrier, with about 80–100% of infected newborns becoming carriers. In children aged 1–10 years the risk is 20–40% whereas in adolescence and adult life the risk is less than 10%.[41] Other cofactors throughout life interact with chronic HBV infection to produce liver cancer, such as exposure to mycotoxins such as aflatoxin-B and

(a)

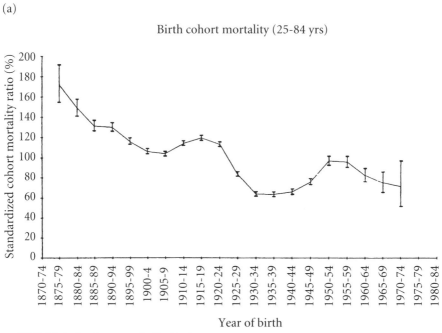

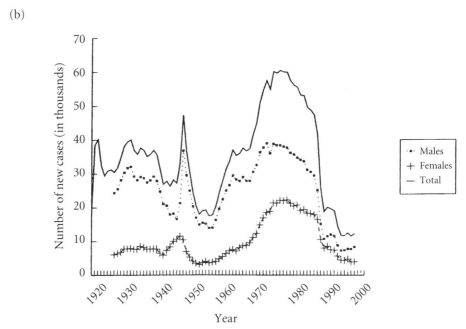

Fig. 12.4 (a) Cervical cancer mortality by year of birth, England and Wales, 1960–1999 (standardized cohort mortality ratios (SCMRs) and 95% confidence intervals (CIs)); (b) numbers of new cases of gonorrhoea seen at genitourinary medicine clinics, England and Wales, 1918–1997.[15] Reprinted by permission of Oxford University Press.

alcohol and tobacco consumption. Hepatitis-C virus, which is mainly transmitted by the parental route, is also carcinogenic.[41] It has been estimated that 77% of all liver cancers worldwide are attributable to HBV or HCV (with some of them the result of joint infections).[37]

12.4.3 Diet and body weight

Ecological studies have found moderate international correlations between rates for various cancers and average consumption of particular foods/nutrients[51] (or between trends in specific dietary factors and trends in cancer incidence within a single population group).[52] But for most foods/nutrients the evidence from individual-based studies has been far from conclusive.[52] The only exception is alcohol intake which has been associated with cancers of the oropharynx, larynx, oesophagus, liver,[52,53] and breast.[54] An individual's dietary intake is notoriously difficult to quantify, however. Moreover, although most individual-based studies have focused on diet in adult life, diet in early life could be as important.[55]

The mechanisms through which adulthood diet may influence cancer risk are not known but one possibility is that its effect may be partly mediated through body weight.[52] There is now considerable evidence that excessive body weight is associated with an increased risk of developing cancer at several sites.[56,57] An exceptionally large prospective study of more than 900 000 US adults followed for up to 16 years showed a positive association between increasing levels of body mass index (BMI) and increasing mortality from cancer of the oesophagus, colon and rectum, liver, gallbladder, pancreas, kidney, non-Hodgkin's lymphoma, and multiple myeloma in each sex.[57] Similar positive associations were also observed for mortality from stomach and prostatic cancers in men and for breast, endometrial, cervical, and ovarian cancers in women. It was estimated that excess body weight (that is, BMI greater than 24.9) may account for 14% of all deaths from cancer in men and 20% of those in women in the USA.[57] Similarly, about 5% of all incident cancers in the European Union might be prevented if nobody's BMI exceeded 25 kg/m^2.[58] As trends in overweight and obesity are rising, this proportion is likely to increase in the future. The causes of obesity-related cancers may stretch back to early life as adult obesity has been linked to patterns of growth and, in particular, to fatness in childhood.[59]

12.4.4 Reproduction-related cancers

The effects of reproductive factors on breast, ovarian, and endometrial cancers in women have been assumed to reflect underlying lifelong cumulative exposure to hormonal influences.[60–62] Hormonal mechanisms have also been postulated for prostatic and testicular cancers in men.[60,62] These hormonal factors are not regarded as genetoxic but by promoting cell division they would induce the replication of initiated cells.[62] In the rest of this section we will examine in detail trends in breast and testicular cancer in relation to trends in known and potential risk factors. Some of the breast cancer material presented here has been previously discussed in another book of this series on the life course approach to adult health.[63]

12.4.4.1 Breast cancer

Breast cancer is the most common cancer in women worldwide.[27] Breast cancer mortality increased in most developed countries for most of the twentieth century.

There was, however, considerable inter-country variability in the rate of this increase. Analysis of data for successive generations of women born in Europe since the last decades of the nineteenth century revealed that the largest proportional increases in rates occurred in countries where rates had been historically low (for example, Spain, Greece, Hungary, Poland, and Portugal) and smallest for countries where rates had historically been high (for example, the UK, Denmark, and Sweden)[64] (Fig. 12.5). In countries where rates had been high such as the UK, Sweden, Canada, and the USA there was an indication of a slight downturn or a slow down in the rate of increase for cohorts born since the 1920s[64–66] (Figs 12.5, 12.6(b), and 12.7(a and b)). The few populations in Asia and Latin America for which data are available experienced marked rises in breast cancer incidence or mortality.[27]

Although mortality data are available for a large number of populations and over longer periods of time, it is important to emphasize that incidence trends have not always paralleled mortality trends, particularly in recent years. Breast cancer mortality in England and Wales has been declining at premenopausal ages (taken to be under 50 years) since the early 1970s and at postmenopausal ages since 1985–1989; in contrast, incidence of this tumour in women at postmenopausal ages has increased throughout the period, particularly in recent years at ages 50–69, whereas at premenopausal ages the overall trend was upwards (Fig. 12.7(c and d). The decline in breast cancer mortality in recent years, but not in incidence, has been attributed to improvements in survival[67] consequent to improvements in treatment[68,69] and, more recently, to screening. The sharp rise in the incidence of this tumour at ages 50–69 years in recent years is probably due to the introduction of the national breast screening programme in 1988.[70] Similar recent diverging incidence and mortality trends were observed in the Nordic countries.[27]

There has been a shift towards early detection and treatment over the last decades in many developed countries, even in those where organized screening programmes have never been introduced. In the USA, breast physical examinations by physicians increased during the 1970s whereas mammographic screening increased substantially in the 1980s;[71] these diagnostic changes together with the introduction of better treatments seem to have accounted for some of the recent declines in breast cancer mortality in that country (Fig. 12.6).[72,73]

Risk of breast cancer in women is related to a wide range of factors that span the entire life course (see Chapter 11). These include, among others, age at menarche, adult height, age at first birth, number of children, and postmenopausal obesity. There is also some evidence that prenatal factors may affect the risk of this cancer.

Prenatal factors. Recent evidence suggests that the *in utero* environment may affect the risk of breast cancer later in life. In particular, several studies,[74–77] although not others,[78–80] have reported positive associations between high birthweight and subsequent risk of this cancer; in some,[74,75,77] the associations were particularly strong at premenopausal ages. Long-term data from several developed countries show that the rise in breast cancer rates was not paralleled by a rise in average birthweight. There were variations in birthweight with changes in socioeconomic conditions but no clear overall trend from the middle of the nineteenth century to the second half of the twentieth century,[81–83] although there is some indication of a slight upward trend since the 1970s.[84] There has been some change in the distribution of birthweight in England and Wales, with the percentage of low birthweight live births (<2.500 kg) having

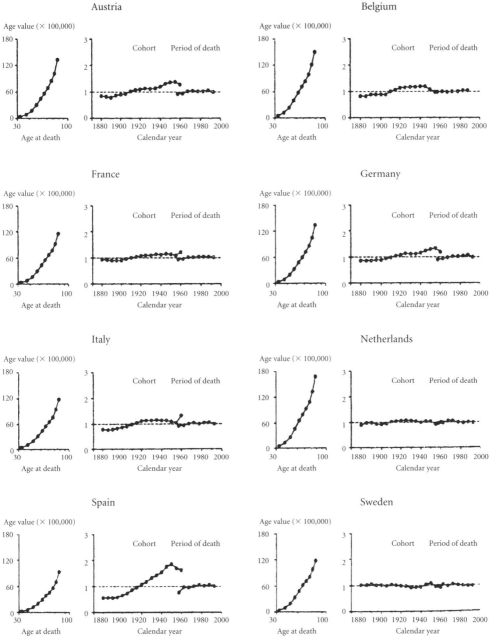

Fig. 12.5 Age-specific mortality rates (per 100 000 person-years) and period and cohort mortality ratios for female breast cancer in selected European countries. From La Vecchia et al.[64], Age, cohort-of-birth, and period-of-death trends in breast cancer mortality in Europe. *J Natl Cancer Inst*, 1997;**89**:732–3, by permission of Oxford University Press.

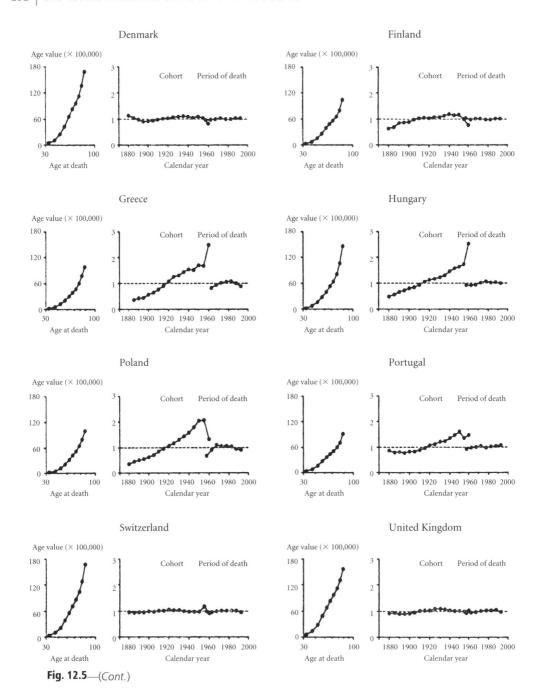

Fig. 12.5—(*Cont.*)

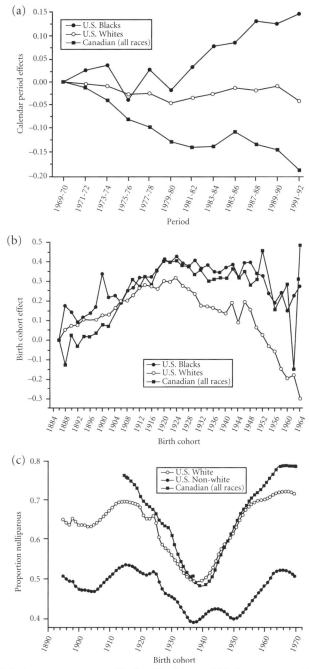

Fig. 12.6 Trends in breast cancer mortality for US white and black women and for all Canadian women, 1969–1992 and their relationship with cohort trends in nulliparity. (a) Calendar period effects; (b) cohort effects; (c) proportion of nulliparous women aged 20–24 years by year of birth (the US non-white curve closely reflects trends in nulliparity in US black women). From Tarone *et al.*[66] Birth cohort and calendar period trends in breast cancer mortality in the United States and Canada. *J Natl Cancer Inst* 1997;**89**:251–6, by permission of Oxford University Press.

(a)

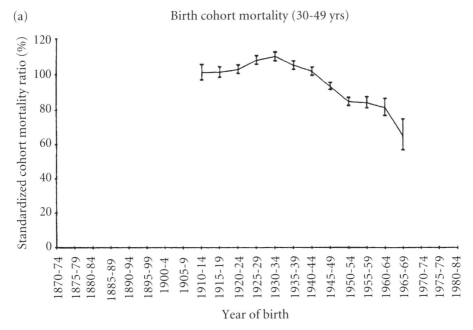

SCMR(%): Indirectly age-standardized by 5-year age-group

(b)

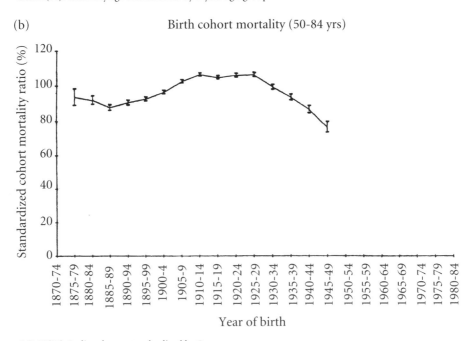

SCMR(%): Indirectly age-standardized by 5-year age-group

Fig. 12.7 Trends in breast cancer in England and Wales. (a) and (b) Mortality by age and year of birth, 1960–1999 (standardized cohort mortality ratios (SCMRs) and 95% confidence intervals (CIs));

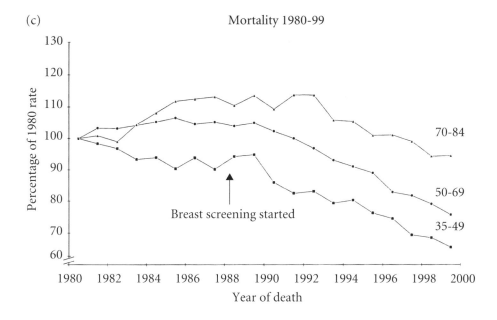

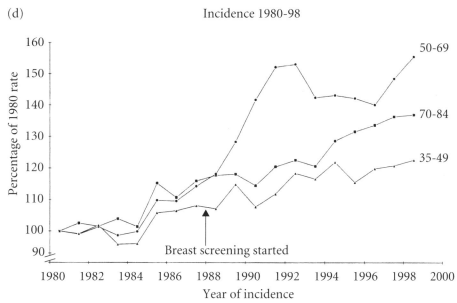

Fig. 12.7—(*Cont.*) (c) mortality by age and year of death, 1980–1999; (d) incidence by age and year of diagnosis, 1980–1998.

remained fairly constant since 1950 whereas the percentage of births weighing between 2.500 and 3.499 kg having declined slightly since 1978. In contrast, the proportion of those weighing at least 3.500 kg has increased since 1977.[15]

Childhood factors. Young age at menarche and tall adult height are risk factors for breast cancer perhaps as indicators of growth and nutrition in childhood. Age at menarche has declined by about two months per decade during the first half of the twentieth century in many developed countries.[85] This decline would be consistent with the long-term rise in breast cancer rates. There is evidence suggesting that the decline in age at menarche has slowed or even reversed in many developed countries for women born since the 1950s,[86] but these cohorts are still too young to be certain of their risk of breast cancer.

Historical data on height, mainly derived from male conscripts, show a long-term increase in adult height in many developed countries since the beginning of the nineteenth century, although in some countries there was a fall in the middle or second half of the nineteenth century during rapid industrialization or urbanization.[87–89] Equivalent historical data are not available for women but data for a more recent period show modest increases in mean adult height for successive generations of women born from 1900 to 1958.[63] This modest secular trend in height for women since the start of the twentieth century is consistent with the observed increase in breast cancer rates.

Adult life factors. The risk of developing breast cancer increases with nulliparity, late age at first birth, and low parity. The trends in these reproductive factors, however, have not always paralleled the trends in breast cancer (Figs 12.5–12.8).

The increases in breast cancer incidence and mortality for cohorts born from 1885 to 1910 in England and Wales (Figs 12.7(a and b) were paralleled by decreases in fertility at young ages (taken as a proxy for age at first birth for which there are no data for cohorts born before 1920) and completed family size, but did not accord with the lack of change in the levels of nulliparity during these cohorts (Fig. 12.8). For cohorts born in 1910–1929, breast cancer risk rose slightly despite an increase in fertility at young ages and a decline in nulliparity. The decline in breast cancer mortality, but not incidence, for cohorts born from the late 1920s to the 1940s, would accord with the marked decreases in nulliparity and in mean age at first birth as well as increases in completed family size observed for these cohorts. Similar declines in breast cancer mortality for cohorts born between the 1920s and the 1940s were observed in many other countries and in most they were paralleled by falls in nulliparity and mean age at first birth.[65] Studies in North America have also shown that the decline in breast cancer mortality in cohorts born from 1925 to 1940 coincided with low nulliparity (Fig. 12.6)[66,90] or higher fertility at ages 20–24.[91] For cohorts born in England and Wales since the Second World War mean age at first birth and nulliparity increased, which would accord with the rising incidence of breast cancer in recent years (Figs 12.7–12.8).

Risk of breast cancer is increased by older age at menopause, but there was little change in the average age at natural menopause during the twentieth century in England and Wales whereas the proportion of those who have had an artificial menopause has increased slightly (from about 1% for those born at the turn of the century to about 5% for those born in the late 1930s).[92] Similar trends were observed in the USA.[93] In Japan, where there have been marked rises in breast cancer rates, the

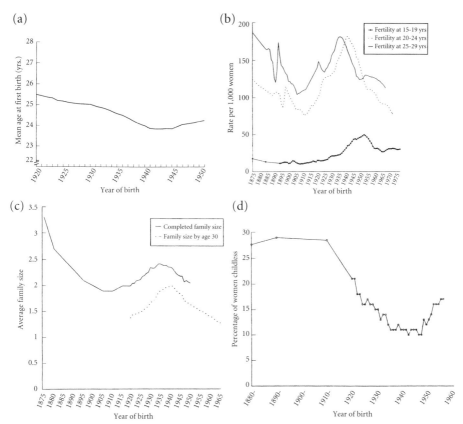

Fig. 12.8 Trends in reproductive-related factors, England and Wales. (a) Mean age at first birth for cohorts of women born 1920–1977 (not available for the most recent cohorts because they have not yet completed their reproductive years); (b) fertility at young ages for cohorts of women born 1875–1977; (c) family size by age for cohorts of women born 1875–1965; (d) nulliparity by age 40 years for cohorts of women born 1880–1956.[15] Reprinted by permission of Oxford University Press.

median age at natural menopause increased 1.2 years from the 1880–1899 cohort to the 1910–1914 cohort and the prevalence of surgical menopause from 5.0% to 8.9%.[93]

Lactation has been reported to reduce the risk of breast cancer[94] but prevalence of breastfeeding in England and Wales,[15] the USA,[95] and in many other developed countries, decreased from the beginning of the twentieth century until the 1970s. The decrease in the prevalence of breastfeeding was for cohorts in whom breast cancer incidence generally increased. Use of oral contraceptives (OCs) and of hormone replacement therapy (HRT) seems to increase the risk of breast cancer in current and recent users.[96,97] The increase in the prevalence of use of OCs and HRT among recent cohorts[15] would accord with the rises in breast cancer incidence experienced by these cohorts.

Total energy and dietary fat intake in adulthood have been found to be associated with the risk of breast cancer in population-based studies, although the evidence from person-based studies has been far from conclusive.[52] Population data on total energy intake and fat consumption over time show some parallels with breast cancer trends. The increases in total energy and fat intake in England and Wales from the turn of the century to a peak in the early 1970s, except for a fall during the Second World War,[15] paralleled the secular increase in breast cancer risk at both pre- and postmenopausal ages. However, total energy and fat consumption have fallen since then[15] whereas recorded breast cancer rates have continued to increase (although, in recent years, this may be an artefact consequent to the introduction of the national screening programme).

At postmenopausal[57,98] (but not premenopausal[99]) ages, increasing BMI is a risk factor for breast cancer, probably because adipose tissue is the main source of oestrogens after the menopause. Nationally representative data from North America,[100,101] parts of Europe,[102,103] and Japan[93] showed marked increases in the prevalence of excess body weight. These rising trends are consitent with the observed general secular increase in breast cancer incidence.

12.4.4.2 Testicular germ cell cancer

Testicular germ cell tumours have a very unusual age distribution with a peak in incidence at young adult ages.[104] Long-term data, however, show that this peak appeared during the twentieth century in many European and North American countries. These countries have now the highest rates, testicular germ cell cancer being the most common cancer in young men.[27,104,105] The reasons for this rise are not known but its magnitude is far too large to be explained by diagnostic or registration artefacts.

The young peak strongly suggests early life influences on the aetiology of these tumours. It has been hypothesized that factors that increase the bioavailability of oestrogens *in utero*, and in particular during the first trimester when the testis is being formed, play a major role in the causation of testicular germ cell cancers.[60,106] Indirect evidence to support the hypothesis that prenatal exposures may be important in the aetiology of testicular cancer also comes from the fact that men born during the Second World War in Denmark, Norway, and Sweden had a lower risk of testicular cancer than previous and subsequent generations[107] (Fig. 12.9). These falls in risk have been related to changes in diet that occurred during the war years, suggesting that dietary exposures *in utero*, probably mediated through hormonal changes, may be important risk factors for testicular cancer. No similar relationships were observed in Finland, East Germany, Poland[107] (Fig. 12.9), or England and Wales.[15]

The rise in the incidence of testicular cancer parallels an increase in the incidence of undescended testis[108] and other uro-genital malformations, the major known risk factors for cancer of the testis,[109] but these conditions are too rare to account for the entire rise in the rate of this cancer. In some studies,[106,110–112] but not all,[113] risk of testicular cancer has been associated with low birthweight but, as discussed above, the available data do not show any substantial changes in the prevalence of low birthweight. Being first born has been associated with an increased risk of testicular cancer but the proportion of live births that were first births in England and Wales decreased from 1938 to 1964[15] while testicular cancer incidence increased in these cohorts. There is some evidence that first-born men to women having this pregnancy at an early age are at an increased risk of testicular cancer and in Los Angeles County (USA) the rise in the incidence of this cancer for men born since the 1950s was paralleled by a decline in mean age at first full-term pregnancy for women born from 1910 to 1940.[114] The increase in testicular cancer incidence in England and Wales for cohorts of men born

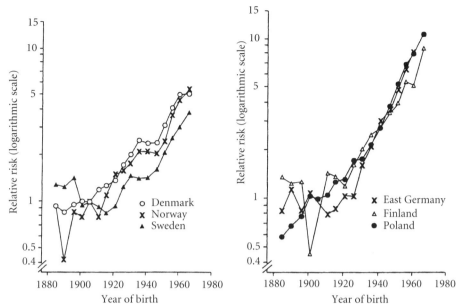

Fig. 12.9 Trends in testicular cancer by country and year of birth (men born between 1900 and 1909 taken as the reference group). From Bergström *et al.*[107] Increase in testicular cancer incidence in six European countries: a birth cohort phenomenon. *J Natl Cancer Inst* 1996;**88**:727–33, by permission of Oxford University Press.

since the 1940s was also accompanied by declines in mean age at first birth for cohorts of women born from 1920 to the 1940s (Fig. 12.8(a)). Adult height and early age at puberty, which are strongly related to childhood nutrition, have been found to be positively associated to risk of testicular cancer.[115] Mean adult height[63] and, presumably, early age at puberty in men rose in many developed countries through the period for which testicular cancer rates increased.

12.5 General conclusions

Interpretation of cancer trends should be done with caution for the reasons indicated earlier in this chapter. Cancer mortality data are available for a longer period, and from a large number of populations, than incidence data, but mortality is a good proxy for incidence only for cancer sites with high fatality rate (such as lung and stomach cancers), not for those with relatively good survival (such as breast and testicular cancers). Data on potential risk factors were also limited—often too crude and only available for short, and relatively recent, time periods.

Bearing all these caveats in mind, what do the cancer trends tells us about life course aetiology? In a rather simplistic way one might assume that trends for cancer sites whose aetiology is mainly determined by prenatal and early life influences would, at a population level, show strong birth cohort effects. This was certainly true for testicular cancer whose age distribution strongly suggests a prenatal/early life aetiology, although the relevant exposures are yet to be identified. But while birth cohort effects may reflect prenatal and/or early life influences they can also result from differences between successive generations in the adoption of later life risk factors. For instance, the strong birth cohort effects in lung cancer described above were not due to early life influences but to cohort variations in the uptake of smoking. Similarly, the observed cohort effects for cervical cancer reflected differences in sexual behaviour across successive generations of women. Moreover, trends for many cancer sites are determined by a large number of factors acting at different stages of the life course rather than just by a single one. Interactions between early and later life factors may occur and these might lead to no clear predictions regarding the importance of period and cohort effects. Breast cancer is a good illustration of this. The data presented here would suggest that the rising trend in breast cancer incidence could not be explained by trends in prenatal factors, as crudely measured by birthweight, or by trends in reproduction-related factors but would accord with trends in age at menarche and adult height (as well as trends in adult weight). However, most of the known breast cancer risk factors are likely to affect a woman's risk by affecting her cumulative exposure to underlying hormonal influences. As the prevalence of many of these risk factors changed over time, sometimes in opposite directions, it is impossible to establish what their net effect was.

Finally, although identification of cohort and/or period effects may provide some insights into the underlying aetiological pathways it is by no means crucial to the life course approach as this approach legitimately spans the contribution of influences on health acting at all ages, not just the influence of early life factors.[116] Recent evidence showing that excess adult body weight is associated with increasing risk of developing cancer at several sites[57] provides a good illustration of how a life course approach might contribute to a better understanding of the origins of cancer by helping to track down the early life social and biological origins of excess body weight in adulthood. This is of considerable public health importance as, if current trends in overweight and obesity were to persist, the proportion of cancer cases attributed to excess body weight will increase dramatically in the future in both developed and developing countries.

References

Those marked with an asterisk are especially recommended for further reading.

1 **Nordling CO.** A new theory on the cancer inducing mechanisms. *Br J Cancer* 1953;**7**:68–72.

2 **Armitage P, Doll R.** The age distribution of cancer and a multistage theory of carcinogenesis. *Br J Cancer* 1954;**8**:1–12.

3 **Hanahan D, Weinberg RA.** The hallmarks of cancer. *Cell* 2000;**100**:57–70.

4 **Doll R.** An epidemiological perspective of the biology of cancer. *Cancer Res* 1978;**38**:3573–83.

5 **Peto J.** Early- and late-stage carcinogenesis in mouse skin and in man. **In Borzsonyi M, Day NE, Lapis K, Yamasaki H, eds.** *Models, mechanisms and aetiology of tumour promotion* (International Agency for Research on Cancer (IARC) Scientific Publication No. 56). Lyon: IARC, 1984:359–71.

6 **Lee PN, O'Neill JA.** The effect both of time and dose applied on tumour incidence rates in benzpyrene skin painting experiments. *Br J Cancer* 1971;**25**:759–70.

7 **Peto R, Roe FJC, Lee PN, Levy L, Clack J.** Cancer and ageing in mice and men. *Br J Cancer* 1975;**32**:411–26.

8 **Newsholme A.** Cancer mortality. In Newshole A, ed. *The elements of vital statistics*. London: Allen and Unwin, 1923:489–500.

9 Greenwood M. *Epidemics and crowd diseases, an introduction to the study of epidemiology.* New York: Macmillan, 1935.

10 Stocks P. Studies of cancer death rates at different ages in England and Wales in 1921 to 1950: uterus, breast and lung. *Br J Cancer* 1953;**7**:283–302.

11 Case RAM. Cohort analysis of cancer mortality in England and Wales, 1911–54 by site and sex. *Br J Prev Soc Med* 1956;**10**:172–99.

12 McKenzie A, Case RAM, Pearson JT. *Cancer statistics for England and Wales 1901–1955. a summary of data relating to mortality and morbidity* Studies in Medical and Population Subjects (SMPS No. 13). London: Her Majesty's Stationery Office, 1957.

13 Haenszel W, Schimkin MB. Smoking patterns and the epidemiology of lung cancer in the United States: are they compatible? *J Natl Cancer Inst* 1956;**16**:1417–41.

14 Osmond C, Gardner MJ, Acheson ED, Adelstein AM. *Trends in cancer mortality 1951–1980. Analyses by period of birth and death* Office of Population Censuses and Surveys (OPCS Series DH1 No. 11). London: Her Majesty's Stationery Office.

*15 Swerdlow A, dos Santos Silva I, Doll R. *Cancer Incidence and mortality in England and Wales: trends and risk factors.* Oxford: Oxford University Press, 2001.

16 Segi Institute of Cancer Epidemiology. *Age-adjusted death rates for cancer for selected sites in 46 countries.* Nagova: University of Nagova Press, 1964.

17 Kurihara M, Aoki K, Tominaga S, eds. *Cancer mortality statistics in the world.* Nagoya: University of Nagoya Press, 1984.

18 Kurihara M, Aoki K, Hisamichi S, eds. *Cancer mortality statistics in the world 1950–85.* Nagoya: University of Nagoya Press, 1989.

19 Aoki K, Kurihara M, Hayakawa N, Suzuki S. *Death rates for malignant neoplasms for selected sites and 5-year age-group in 33 countries 1953–57 to 1983–87.* Nagoya: University of Nagoya Press, 1992.

20 Doll R, Payne P, Waterhouse JAH. *Cancer incidence in five continents* (Vol. I. International Union against Cancer (UICC)). Berlin: Springer, 1966.

21 Waterhouse JAH, Doll R, Muir CS, eds. *Cancer incidence in five continents* (Vol. II. UICC). Berlin: Springer, 1970.

22 Waterhouse JAH, Muir CS, Correa P, eds. *Cancer incidence in five continents* (Vol. III (IARC Scientific Publication No. 15)). Lyon: IARC, 1976.

23 Waterhouse JAH, Muir CS, Shanmugaratnam K, Powell J, eds. *Cancer incidence in five continents* (Vol. IV (IARC Scientific Publication No. 42)). Lyon: IARC, 1982.

24 Muir CS, Waterhouse J, Mack T, Powell J, Whelan S, eds. *Cancer incidence in five continents* (Vol. V (IARC Scientific Publication No. 88)). Lyon: IARC, 1987.

25 Parkin DM, Muir CS, Whelan SL, Gao YT, Ferlay J, Powell J, eds. *Cancer incidence in five continents* (Vol. VI (IARC Scientific Publication No. 120)). Lyon: IARC, 1992.

26 Parkin DM, Whelan SL, Ferlay J, Raymond L, Young J, eds. *Cancer incidence in five continents* (Vol. VI (IARC Scientific Publication No. 143)). Lyon: IARC, 1997.

27 Coleman MP, Esteve J, Damiecki P, Arslan A, Renard H. *Trends in cancer incidence and mortality.* Geneva: World Health Organization, 1993.

28 Clayton D, Schifflers E. Models for temporal variations in cancer rates. I. Age–period and age–cohort models. *Stat Med* 1987;**6**:449–67.

29 Clayton D, Schifflers E. Models for temporal variations in cancer rates. II. Age–period–cohort models. *Stat Med* 1987;**6**:469–81.

30 Case RAM. Cohort analysis of mortality rates as an historical or narrative technique. *Br J Prev Soc Med* 1956;**10**:159–71.

*31 Peto J. Cancer epidemiology in the last century and the next decade. *Nature* 2001;**411**:56–61.

*32 Peto R, Lopez AD, Boreham J, Thun M, Heath C Jr. *Mortality from smoking in developed countries 1950–2000*. Oxford: Oxford Medical Publications, 1994.

*33 Doll R, Peto R. The causes of cancer: quantitative estimates of avoidable risks of cancer in the United States today. *J Natl Cancer Inst* 1981;**66**:1191–308.

34 Doll R. Cancers weakly related to smoking. *Br Med Bull* 1996;**52**:35–49.

35 Liu B-Q, Peto R, Chen Z-M, Boreham J, Wu Y-P, Li J-Y *et al*. Emerging tobacco hazards in China: 1. Retrospective proportional mortality study of one million deaths. *Br Med J* 1998;**317**:1411–22.

36 Deacon JM, Evans CD, Yule R, Desai M, Binns W, Taylor C *et al*. Sexual behaviour and smoking as determinants of cervical HPV infection and of CIN3 among those infected: a case–control study nested within the Manchester cohort. *Br J Cancer* 2000;**83**:1565–72.

*37 Parkin DM, Pisani P, Munoz N, Ferlay J. The global burden of infection associated cancers. *Cancer Surv* 1999;**33**:5–33.

38 IARC. *Schistosomes, liver flukes and* Helicobacter pylori (IARC Monographs on Evaluation of Carcinogenic Risks to Humans, No. 61). Lyon: IARC, 1994.

39 Walboomers JM, Jacobs MV, Manos MM, Bosch FX, Kummer JA, Shah KV *et al*. Human papillomavirus is a necessary cause of invasive cervical cancer worldwide. *J Pathol* 1999;**189**:12–19.

40 IARC. *Human papillomaviruses* (IARC Monographs on Evaluation of Carcinogenic Risks to Humans, No. 64). Lyon: IARC, 1995.

41 IARC. *Hepatitis viruses* (IARC Monographs on Evaluation of Carcinogenic Risks to Humans, No. 59). Lyon: IARC, 1994.

42 Banatvala N, Mayo K, Megraud F, Jennings R, Deeks JJ, Feldman RA. The cohort effect and *helicobacter pylori*. *J Infect Dis* 1993;**168**:219–21.

43 Feldman RA, Eccersley JP, Hardie JM. Epidemiolgy of *Helicobacter pylori*: acquisition, transmission and disease-to-infection ratio. *Br Med Bull* 1998;**54**:39–53.

44 Whitaker CJ, Dubiel AJ, Galpin OP. Social and geographical risk factors in *Helicobacter pylori* infection. *Epidemiol Infect* 1993;**111**:63–70.

45 Beral V, Hermon C, Munoz N, Devesa SS. Cervical cancer. **In Doll R, Fraumeni JF, Jr., Muir CS, eds**. *Trends in cancer incidence and mortality. Cancer surveys, Vol. 19/20*. New York: Cold Spring Harbor Laboratory Press, 1994:265–85.

46 Beral V. Cancer of the cervix. A sexually transmitted infection? *Lancet* 1974;**i**:1037–40.

47 Beasley RP, Hwang L-Y, Lin C-C, Chien C-S. Hepatocellular carcinoma and hepatitis B virus: a prospective study of 22,707 men in Taiwan. *Lancet* 1981;**ii**:1129–33.

48 Stevens RG, Merkle EJ, Lustbader ED. Age and cohort effects in primary liver cancer. *Int J Cancer* 1984;**33**:453–8.

49 Munoz N, Bosch X. Epidemiology of hepatocellular carcinoma. In Okuda K, Ishak K, eds. *Neoplasms of the liver*. Tokyo: Springer, 1987:3–19.

50 Melbye M, Skinhøj P, Nielsen NH, Vestergaard BF, Ebbesen P, Hansen PPH *et al*. Virus-associated cancers in Greenland: frequent hepatitis B virus infection but low primary hepatocellular carcinoma incidence. *J Natl Cancer Inst* 1984;**73**:1267–72.

51 Armstrong BK, Doll R. Environmental factors and cancer incidence and mortality in different countries with special reference to dietary practices. *Int J Cancer* 1975;**15**:617–31.

*52 World Cancer Research Fund and American Institute for Cancer Research. *Food, nutrition and the prevention of cancer: a global perspective*. Washington: American Institute for Cancer Research, 1997.

53 Thun MJ, Peto R, Lopez AD, Monaco JH, Henley J, Heath CW *et al*. Alcohol consumption and mortality among middle-aged and elderly U.S. adults. *N Engl J Med* 1998;**279**:535–40.

*54 Collaborative Group on Hormonal Factors in Breast Cancer. Alcohol, tobacco and breast cancer. *Br J Cancer* 2002,**87**:1234–45.

55 Frankel S, Gunnell DJ, Peters TJ, Maynard M, Davey-Smith G. Childhood energy intake and adult mortality from cancer: the Boyd Orr cohort study. *Br Med J* 1998;**316**:499–504.

56 Calle EE, Thun MJ, Petrelli JM, Rodriguez C, Heath CW. Body-mass index and mortality in a prospective cohort of U.S. adults. *N Engl J Med* 1999;**341**:1097–105.

*57 Calle EE, Rodriguez C, Walker-Thurmond K, Thun MJ. Overweight, obesity, and mortality from cancer in a prospectively studied cohort of US adults. *New Engl J Med* 2003;**348**:1625–38.

58 Bergström A, Pisani P, Tenet V, Wolk A, Adami H-O. Overweight as an avoidable cause of cancer in Europe. *Int J Cancer* 2001;**91**:421–30.

59 Power C, Parsons T. Overweight and obesity from a life course perspective. In Kuh D, Hardy R, eds. *A Life course approach to women's health.* Oxford: Oxford University Press, 2002:304–19.

60 Henderson BE, Ross RK, Pike MC, Casagrande JT. Endogenous hormones as a major factor in human cancer. *Cancer Res* 1982;**42**:3232–9.

61 Moolgavkar, SH. Hormones and multistage carcinogenesis. *Cancer Surv* 1986;**5**:635–48.

62 Preston-Martin S, Pike MC, Ross RK, Jones PA, Henderson, BE. Increased cell division as a cause of human cancer. *Cancer Res* 1990;**50**:7415–21.

63 Kuh D, dos Santos Silva I, Barrett-Connor E. Disease trends in women living in established market economies: evidence of cohort effects during the epidemiologic transition. In Kuh D, Hardy R, eds. *A life course approach to women's health.* Oxford: Oxford University Press, 2002:347–73.

64 La Vecchia C, Negri E, Levi F, Decarli A. Age, cohort-of-birth, and period-of-death trends in breast cancer mortality in Europe. *J Natl Cancer Inst* 1997;**89**:732–3.

65 Hermon C, Beral V. Breast cancer mortality rates are levelling off or begining to decline in many western countries: an analysis of time trends, age–cohort and age–period models of breast cancer mortality in 20 countries. *Br J Cancer* 1996;**73**:955–60.

66 Tarone RE, Chu KC, Gaudette LA. Birth cohort and calendar period trends in breast cancer mortality in the United States and Canada. *J Natl Cancer Inst* 1997;**89**:251–6.

67 Peto R, Boreham J, Clarke M, Davies C, Beral V. UK and USA breast cancer deaths down 25% in year 2000 at ages 20–69 years. *Lancet* 2000;**355**:1822.

68 Early Breast Cancer Trialists' Collaborative Group. Systemic treatment of early breast cancer by hormonal, cytotoxic, or immune therapy: 133 randomised trials involving 31 000 recurrences and 24 000 deaths among 75 000 women. *Lancet* 1992;**339**:1–15 and 71–85.

69 Early Breast Cancer Trialists' Collaborative Group. Tamoxifen for early breast cancer: an overview of the randomised trials. *Lancet* 1998;**351**:1451–67.

70 Moss SM, Michel M, Patnick J, Johns L, Blank R, Chamberlain J. Results from the NHS breast screening programme 1990–1993. *J Med Screening* 1995;**2**:186–90.

71 Ursin G, Bernstein L, Pike MC. Breast cancer. In Doll R, Fraumeni JF Jr, Muir CS, eds. *Trends in cancer incidence and mortality. Cancer surveys, Vol. 19/20.* New York: Cold Spring Harbor Laboratory Press, 1994:241–64.

72 Tarone RE, Chu KC. Evaluation of birth cohort patterns in population disease rates. *Am J Epidemiol* 1996;**143**:85–91.

73 Chu KC, Tarone RE, Kessler LG, Ries LAG, Hankey BF, Miller BA *et al.* Recent trends in US breast cancer incidence, survival and mortality rates. *J Natl Cancer Inst* 1996;**88**:1571–8.

74 Michels KB, Trichopoulos D, Robins JM, Rosner BA, Manson JE, Hunter DJ *et al.* Birth weight as a risk factor for breast cancer. *Lancet* 1996;**348**:1542–6.

75 De Stavola BL, Hardy R, Kuh D, dos Santos Silva I, Wadsworth M, Swerdlow AJ. Birth weight, childhood growth and risk of breast cancer in a British cohort. *Br J Cancer* 2000;**83**:964–8.

76 Vatten LJ, Mæhle BO, Lund Nilsen TI, Tretli S, Hsieh C-C, Trichopoulos D *et al.* Birth weight as a predictor of breast cancer: a case-control study in Norway. *Br J Cancer* 2002;**86**:89–91.

77 McCormack VA, dos Santos Silva I, De Stavola BL, Mohsen R, Leon DA, Lithell HO. Foetal growth and subsequent risk of breast cancer: results from a long-term follow-up of a Swedish cohort of over 5000 women. *Br Med J* 2003;**326**:248–51.

78 Ekbom A, Hsieh C-C, Lipworth L, Adami H-O, Trichopoulos D. Intrauterine environment and breast cancer risk in women: a population-based study. *J Natl Cancer Inst* 1997;**88**:71–6.

79 Sanderson M, Shu X, Jin F, Dai Q, Ruan Z, Gao T-Y *et al.* Weight at birth and adolescence and premenopausal breast cancer risk in a low-risk population. *Br J Cancer* 2002;**86**:84–88.

80 Hilakivi-Clarke L, Forsén T, Eriksson JG, Luoto R, Tuomilehto J, Osmond C *et al.* Tallness and overweight during childhood have opposing effects on breast cancer risk. *Br J Cancer* 2001;**85**:1680–4.

81 Rosenberg M. Birth weights in three Norwegian cities, 1960–84. Secular trends and influencing factors. *Ann Hum Biol* 1988;**15**:275–88.

82 McCalman J. *Sex and suffering: women's health and a women's hospital.* Melbourne: Melbourne University Press, 1998.

83 Ward PW. *Birth weight and economic growth.* Chicago: University of Chicago Press, 1993.

84 Alberman E. Are our babies becoming bigger? *J R Soc Med* 1991;**84**:257–60.

85 Wyshak J. Evidence of a secular trend in age at menarche. *N Engl J Med* 1982;**306**:1033–5.

86 Whincup PH, Gilg JA, Odoki K, Taylor SJC, Cook D. Age at menarche in contemporary British teenagers: survey of girls born between 1982 and 1986. *Br Med J* 2001;**322**:1095–6.

87 Floud R, Wachter K, Gregory A. *Height, health and history. nutritional status in the United Kingdom, 1750–1980.* Cambridge: Cambridge University Press, 1990.

88 Steckl RH, Floud R. *Health and welfare during industrialisation.* Chicago: University of Chicago Press, 1997.

89 Hermanussen M, Burmeister J, Burkhardt V. Stature and stature distribution in recent West German and historic samples of Italian and Dutch conscripts. *Am J Hum Biol* 1995;**7**:507–15.

90 Blot WJ, Devesa SS, Fraumeni JF Jr. Declining breast cancer mortality among young American women. *J Natl Cancer Inst* 1987;**78**:451–4.

91 Wigle DT. Breast cancer and fertility trends in Canada. *Am J Epidemiol* 1977;**105**:428–37.

92 McKinlay S, Jefferys M, Thompson B. An investigation of the age at menopause. *J Biosoc Sci* 1972;**4**:161–73.

93 Hoel DG, Wakabayashi T, Pike MC. Secular trends in the distributions of breast cancer risk factors—menarche, first birth, menopause and weight—in Hiroshima and Nagasaki, Japan. *Am J Epidemiol* 1983;**118**:78–89.

*94 Collaborative Group on Hormonal Factors in Breast Cancer. Breast cancer and breastfeeding: collaborative reanalysis of individual data from 47 epidemiological studies in 30 countries, including 50 302 women with breast cancer and 96 973 women without the disease. *Lancet* 2002;**360**:187–95.

95 United Sates Department of Health and Human Services. Racial and educational factors associated with breastfeeding—United States, 1969 and 1980. *Morb Mortal Weekly Rep* 1984;**33**:153–4.

96 Collaborative Group on Hormonal Factors in Breast Cancer. Breast cancer and hormonal contraceptives: collaborative reanalysis of individual data on 53 297 women with breast cancer and 100 239 women without breast cancer from 54 epidemiological studies. *Lancet* 1996;**347**:1713–27.

97 **Collaborative Group on Hormonal Factors in Breast Cancer.** Breast cancer and hormone replacement therapy: collaborative reanalysis of data from 51 epidemiological studies of 52 705 women with breast cancer and 108 411 women without breast cancer. *Lancet* 1997;**350**:1047–59.

98 **van den Brandt PA, Spiegelman D, Yaun S-S, Adami H-O, Beeson L, Folsom AR** *et al.* Pooled analysis of prospective cohort studies on height, weight, and breast cancer risk. *Am J Epidemiol* 2000;**152**:514–27.

99 **Ursin G, Longnecker MP, Haile RW, Greenland S.** A meta-analysis of body mass index and risk of pre-menopausal breast cancer. *Epidemiology* 1995;**6**:137–41.

100 **Flegal KM, Carroll MD, Kuczmarski RJ, Johnson CL.** Overweight and obesity in the United States: prevalence and trends, 1960–1994. *Int J Obesity* 1998;**22**:39–47.

101 **Mokdad AH, Serdula MK, Dietz WH, Bowman BA, Marks JS, Koplan JP.** The spread of the obesity epidemic in the United States, 1991–1998. *J Am Med Assoc* 1999;**282**:1519–22.

102 **Knight I.** *The heights and weights of adults in Great Britain.* London: Her Majesty's Stationery Office, 1984.

103 **Erens B, Primatesta P, Prior G, eds.** *Health survey for England: the health of minority ethnic groups 99.* London: Her Majesty's Stationery Office, 2001. http://www.doh.gov.uk/public/hse99.htm.

104 **Ross RK, McCurtis JW, Henderson BE, Menck HR, Mack TM, Martin SP.** Descriptive epidemiology of testicular and prostatic cancer in Los Angeles. *Br J Cancer* 1979;**39**:284–92.

105 **Østerlind A.** Diverging trends in incidence and mortality of testicular cancer in Denmark, 1943–82. *Br J Cancer* 1986;**53**:501–5.

106 **Depue R, Pike M, Henderson B.** Estrogen exposure during gestation and risk of testicular cancer. *J Natl Cancer Inst* 1983;**71**:1151–5.

*107 **Bergström R, Adami H-O, Möhner M, Zatonski W, Storm H, Ekbom A** *et al.* Increase in testicular cancer incidence in six European countries: a birth cohort phenomenon. *J Natl Cancer Inst* 1996;**88**:727–33.

108 **John Radcliffe Hospital Cryptorchidism Study Group.** Cryptorchidism: an apparent substantial increase since 1960. *Br Med J* 1986;**293**:1401–4.

109 **United Kingdom Testicular Cancer Study Group.** Aetiology of testicular cancer: association with congenital abnormalities, age at puberty, infertility, and exercise. *Br Med J* 1994;**308**:1393–9.

110 **Brown LM, Pottern LM, Hoover RN.** Prenatal and perinatal risk factors for testicular cancer. *Cancer Res* 1986;**46**:4812–16.

111 **Akre O, Ekbom A, Hsieh C-C, Trichopoulos D, Adami H-O.** Testicular nonseminoma and seminoma in relation to perinatal characteristics. *J Natl Cancer Inst* 1996;**88**:883–9.

112 **Moller H, Skakkebaek NE.** Testicular cancer and cryptorchidism in relation to prenatal factors: case–control studies in Denmark. *Cancer Causes Control* 1997;**8**:904–12.

113 **Weir HK, Marrett LD, Kreiger N, Darlington GA, Sugar L.** Prenatal and perinatal exposures and risk of testicular germ cell cancer. *Int J Cancer* 2000;**87**:438–43.

114 **Henderson B, Ross RK, Yu MC, Bernstein L.** An explanation for the increasing incidence of testis cancer: decreasing age at first full-term pregnancy. *J Natl Cancer Inst* 1997;**89**:818–20.

115 **United Kingdom Testicular Cancer Study Group.** Social, behavioural and medical factors in the aetiology of testicular cancer: results from the UK study. *Br J Cancer* 1994;**70**:513–20.

116 **Leon DA.** Commentary on 'Disease trends in women living in established market economies: evidence of cohort effects during the epidemiological transition'. In Kuh D, Hardy R, eds. *A life course approach to women's health.* Oxford: Oxford University Press, 2002:366–8.

Chapter 13

A life course approach to biological ageing

Avan Aihie Sayer and Cyrus Cooper

The interpretation of findings from ageing studies can be problematic. Numerous definitions of ageing are utilized and ageing may be studied at a number of different levels, from a population approach down to studies at a molecular or cellular level in individuals. The ageing of a population is defined in terms of mortality statistics but individual ageing may be defined more broadly as the deteriorative changes with time during postmaturational life that underlie an increasing vulnerability to challenges, thereby decreasing the ability to survive. These deteriorative changes of ageing have been well described but distinguishing cause from effect has proved more difficult. Progress in understanding why ageing occurs has come from the field of evolutionary biology and there is growing support for the concept that failure of repair is central to ageing. Specific genetic and adult environmental influences are being increasingly recognized but a relatively recent development is the idea that the early environment may be important. Progress is now being made integrating the evidence from a wide range of scientific disciplines using a life course model of human ageing. In this chapter we focus on emerging evidence that early growth and nutrition may influence ageing, with particular reference to ageing in the musculoskeletal system. Taking this work forward will not only involve detailed characterization of important life course influences on ageing, particularly those occurring in early life that have yet to be fully explored, but also investigation into how they interact biologically. Perhaps this will be the key to identifying successful interventions to modify the deleterious effects of the human ageing process.

13.1 Introduction

The interpretation of findings from ageing studies can be problematic. Numerous definitions of ageing are utilized and ageing is studied at a number of different levels, from the population approach down to molecular and cellular studies in individuals. Identification of the specific aspect of ageing being studied is key to integrating the findings from different areas of ageing research.

13.2 Understanding the concept of ageing

13.2.1 Population ageing

The ageing of populations is described using mortality statistics including survival curves, maximum lifespan, and age-specific mortality rates but the utility of such measures is limited because death also reflects factors not related to ageing, such as the level of danger in the environment. However a further characteristic of the age-specific mortality rate is that it shows a postmaturational exponential increase with age regardless of environmental conditions. The relationship between age-specific mortality rate and chronological age has been summarized by a number of mathematical models including the Gompertz equation, which has also been used to calculate the mortality rate doubling time.[1] The mortality rate doubling time appears to be consistent within species and is therefore a better measure of population ageing.

In humans, the mortality rate doubling time is approximately 8 years and this appears to be fairly constant across different human populations as well as over time. For example the same 8-year mortality doubling time has been documented in US women in 1980 and in Australian civilians during the Second World War.[2] This consistency contrasts with recent increases in mid-life average life expectancy and maximum lifespan documented for countries in both the developed and developing world.[3,4] Similarly men and women appear to have similar mortality rate doubling times[5] and analysis of mortality statistics suggests that the well-documented survival advantage in women[6] reflects a lower initial mortality rate rather than gender differences in the ageing rate.

13.2.2 Ageing at the individual level

The ageing of an individual cannot be described by mortality statistics and broader definitions have been developed. For example, individual ageing has been defined as the deteriorative changes with time during postmaturational life that underlie an increasing vulnerability to challenges, thereby decreasing the ability to survive.[7] There have been many studies describing these deteriorative changes but, even at a cellular or molecular level, it has proved problematic to distinguish cause from effect.

Theories of ageing are multiple[8] but can be divided into two major groups according to whether ageing is viewed as genetically predetermined ('the biological clock') or as a response to random events over time. Distinction can also be made with regard to whether ageing is considered to have evolved as a beneficial process in its own right (the adaptive theories) or as a by-product of other processes (the non-adaptive theories). Further classification distinguishes those theories primarily concerned with molecular changes, those describing ageing at a systems level, and those viewing it as a whole body process. These groups however are not mutually exclusive (Fig. 13.1).

13.2.3 Genetic theories of ageing

The adaptive theories involve the concept that specific genes have evolved to cause ageing. For example, in the fitness of species theory, it is suggested that evolutionary pressure for such genes would arise from the beneficial effect of removing reproductively inactive old individuals from the population. However this is a circular argument, if ageing did not occur, there would be no need to remove the reproductively aged.

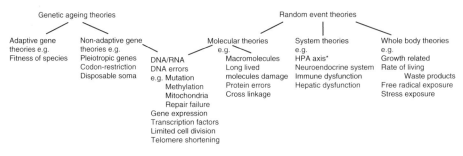

*HPA axis Hypothalamic pituitary adrenal axis

Fig. 13.1 Classification system for ageing theories.

Furthermore most deaths in natural populations occur by causes other than ageing. It is also known that natural selection does not tend to operate in favour of the species at the expense of the individual and that it is least effective at influencing characteristics in later life.[9] The existence of specific ageing genes is therefore now considered unlikely and the adaptive theories have fallen from favour.

There does, however, remain good evidence for the role of genes in ageing including the existence of species-specific lifespans, limited heritability of lifespan, and the human progeroid syndromes, such as Werner's syndrome where a rare autosomal recessive genetic disorder is associated with premature ageing changes.[10] The non-adaptive group of genetic theories suggest that natural selection for the responsible genes has occurred for reasons other than to cause ageing. For example the pleiotropic gene theory proposes that certain genes are expressed early in life to the overall benefit of the organism but at a later stage have different and potentially detrimental effects.[11] It has been argued that such change in gene expression over time would itself require an initiating event rather than be a primary cause. However it could be the gene product that has variable effect depending on whether gene expression occurs during the prevailing conditions of development or when maturity has been reached. Many candidate ageing genes have been proposed but the number of relevant genes is likely to be large and there is increasing recognition of the importance of gene–environment interactions.[12]

13.2.4 Random events and ageing

The other major group of theories regard ageing as an outcome of random events over time and the role of chance in ageing is increasingly recognized.[13] Some theories focus on molecular changes such as DNA damage,[14] others on alteration in gene expression associated with errors in transcription factors.[15] It has long been known that cultured human diploid cell strains have a limited *in vitro* life because of a finite number of cell divisions (the Hayflick limit)[16] but the relevance of this to *in vivo* ageing remains unclear.[17] More recent work has demonstrated sequential loss of telomeric DNA from chromosome ends with somatic cell division and it has been proposed that eventually a critical point is reached, which triggers cell senescence.[18] Telomere shortening may act as a mitotic ageing clock in those tissues that have actively dividing cells and explain the Hayflick limit. However whether the telomere changes cause ageing in these tissues or reflect an epiphenomenon of ageing remains unclear.

Alterations in proteins have also been investigated as cause of ageing since the error catastrophe theory proposed that accumulation of protein transcriptional errors could be a source of progressive deterioration of cells and cell lines.[19] This hypothesis has been widened to include acquired damage to all long-lived macromolecules as the cause of ageing.[20] In particular it has been suggested that ageing occurs as a result of the accumulation of cross-links in macromolecules causing structural stabilization and altered actions.[21] Other theories have implicated specific systems as fundamental to ageing, for example, the hypothalamic–pituitary axis or the immune system and a link has been proposed between psychosocial factors such as stress and ageing.[22] Hypotheses have also linked ageing to whole body processes such as growth or metabolism and a number have focused on the role of ongoing exposure to metabolic or waste products, for example, reducing sugars or free radicals, as the cause of deteriorative changes.

13.2.5 The role of repair

Many ageing theories focus on mechanisms and effects of ageing while failing to address why ageing might occur. However progress has been made in the field of evolutionary biology. The disposable soma theory suggests that ageing has evolved because of the existence of a trade-off for individual species between the rate of reproduction and essential somatic processes such as maintenance and repair.[23] These place large demands on available energy and other biological resources. For higher organisms like mammals, where somatic tissues are distinct from the germ line, it suggests that the optimal level of investment in growth, maintenance, and repair of the soma is one which provides adequate protection against endogenous and exogenous damage for survival in the short-term, but which is always less than that required for indefinite survival. A high-risk environment is likely to favour fast reproduction at the expense of tissue maintenance; a low-risk environment favours the opposite.

13.2.6 A life course model of ageing

This concept of ageing provides a framework for understanding the ageing processes operating at an individual level. It suggests that the genetic and environmental determinants of the need for maintenance and repair as well as the capacity to carry it out are likely to underlie the well-documented effects of ageing and contribute to the wide variation in rates of ageing between individuals. The aged phenotype therefore results from intrinsic and extrinsic exposures across the life course and the corresponding response in terms of regeneration, maintenance, and repair. This has been called the life course exposure response model of ageing (Fig. 13.2)[24] and differences in both exposure and individual response are likely to underlie the variation in rates of ageing seen between individuals and also possibly between systems of the same individual.

13.2.7 Ageing and age related disease

A number of attempts have been made to distinguish structural and functional ageing changes from age related disease. For example, one approach involves the recognition of age related and age-dependent diseases, where the former occur more commonly

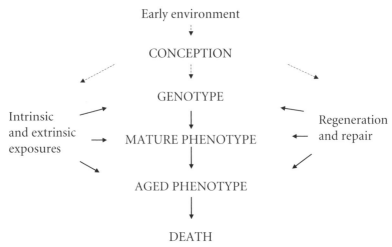

Fig. 13.2 Life course model of ageing and early environmental influences.[24]

with older age but ageing processes are not directly involved in aetiology whereas the latter are caused at least in part by ageing processes.[25] However in practice partitioning the contributory causes remains arbitrary and of questionable benefit. Ageing as defined by the life course exposure response model includes structural and functional ageing changes and age related diseases as well as length of life. If the purpose of aetiological ageing research is understanding the origins of the aged phenotype and developing beneficial interventions, distinction between ageing and age related disease is unhelpful.

13.2.8 Measuring ageing in the individual

Chronological age is the most frequently used measure of individual ageing but is not reliable because the rate of ageing varies considerably between individuals of the same age. This has led to the concept of biological age as distinct from chronological age and a number of test batteries have been developed involving a profile of physical parameters.[26–28] Unfortunately no standardized battery has been recognized and a wide range of measures have been included including muscle strength, respiratory function, blood pressure, hearing, and vision. More recently physical frailty has been recognized as a good summary marker of underlying ageing processes and considerable work has been done to develop objective measures of physical performance.[29]

Ageing is a universal human phenomenon, therefore aetiological epidemiology cannot identify causative agents but rather must focus on influences altering the rate at which ageing occurs. The approach therefore differs fundamentally from chronic disease epidemiology. Studies of population ageing have provided insights into the relationship between ageing and mortality allowing comparison between genders and across populations, but studies in individuals allow investigation of genetic and environmental factors operating across the life course to influence the rate of phenotypic ageing.

13.3 Lifetime influences on ageing

13.3.1 Early growth

The study of environmental influences on ageing has largely been confined to consideration of those operating in adult life. Recent work has started to also consider the role of the early environment including that experienced in prenatal life, infancy, and childhood. Interest in this area has stemmed from a number of epidemiological studies showing that markers of poor fetal growth, including low weight, thinness, and shortness at birth, are associated with increased mortality and morbidity from cardiovascular and other age related diseases.[30] The relevance of these findings to structural and functional ageing changes in different body systems was explored in the UK Hertfordshire Ageing Study.[31] This involved tracing men and women born in Hertfordshire between 1920 and 1930, who had stored birth records documenting weight at birth and 1 year. Markers of ageing in a number of different systems including the eye, ear, skin, and muscle were measured. Poor infant growth was associated with increased lens opacity, worse hearing, thinner skin, and reduced muscle strength whereas low birthweight was only significantly associated with reduced muscle strength (Table 13.1). This may reflect the importance of prenatal as well as postnatal factors on muscle development compared with the relative dominance of postnatal factors on the other systems studied. However confirmation of this distinction is difficult in observational studies, particularly as the postnatal growth trajectory is known to be influenced by the prenatal environment.[32]

13.3.2 Nutrition in early life

Programming is the term used to describe persisting changes in structure and function caused by environmental influences acting at critical periods during early development and these findings support the concept that the determinants of poor early growth have adverse long-term consequences on ageing processes. Inadequate prenatal and infant nutrition have been postulated to underlie these observations, however the literature on the relationship between early diet restriction and ageing is sparse. The few existing animal studies suggest that inadequate diet either *in utero* or immediately after birth and before weaning do have an opposite effect to later intervention. Early studies using a rat model, showed that maternal diet restriction resulted in progeny with permanent stunting of growth, anaemia, and reduced resistance to hypothermia in later life[33] and also demonstrated earlier age related haemoglobin decline in the offspring of restricted mothers.[34] Further work showed that reduction of nutrition in prenatal and early postnatal life resulted in increased levels of age-associated enzymes in the liver and kidney[35] and produced evidence that early growth retardation by dietary restriction could lead to a permanent reduction in muscle mass.[36,37] These findings led to the first clear formulation of the idea that diet restriction in the early stages of life may be followed by accelerated ageing in contrast to the reduction in ageing seen when this intervention is instituted in adulthood.[38]

Effects of early diet restriction on lifespan have also been demonstrated in animal models. One study on mice dating back to 1920 showed that alteration of diet shortly after birth, sufficient to slow growth, resulted in a shorter lifespan.[39] Recently, this finding has been explored further. Using a rat model the effect of prenatal exposure to

Table 13.1 Hertfordshire Ageing Study: the association between weight in early life and markers of ageing in different body systems[14]

Early weight		Mean lens opacity score (LOCS III)* (number)		Mean hearing threshold (dBA)* (number)		Mean grip strength (kg) (number)		Mean skin thickness (mm) (number)	
(g)	(lb)								
At birth									
<2500	(<5.5)	2.27	(16)	24.4	(16)	28.5	(16)	1.19	(16)
–2950	(–6.5)	2.36	(94)	29.3	(93)	30.3	(95)	1.27	(95)
–3400	(–7.5)	2.38	(224)	29.2	(231)	31.0	(231)	1.24	(231)
–3860	(–8.5)	2.38	(205)	28.7	(217)	32.2	(217)	1.24	(217)
–4310	(–9.5)	2.29	(84)	28.4	(89)	32.5	(89)	1.22	(89)
>4310	(>9.5)	2.36	(32)	28.8	(35)	32.4	(35)	1.25	(35)
Multiple regression†		P = 0.71		P = 0.97		P = 0.01		P = 0.32	
At 1 year									
(kg)	(lb)								
<8.16	(<18)	2.67	(26)	33.6	(26)	29.8	(26)	1.20	(26)
–9.07	(–20)	2.40	(133)	29.4	(134)	30.7	(134)	1.22	(134)
–9.98	(–22)	2.33	(198)	29.3	(209)	31.1	(211)	1.24	(211)
–10.89	(–24)	2.37	(187)	29.1	(194)	31.6	(194)	1.25	(194)
–11.79	(–26)	2.33	(70)	26.5	(77)	32.6	(77)	1.25	(77)
>11.79	(>26)	2.24	(41)	24.8	(41)	34.2	(41)	1.25	(41)
Multiple regression†		P = 0.003		P = 0.008		P = 0.02		P = 0.19	
All		2.36	(655)	28.8	(681)	31.5	(683)	1.24	(683)
Standard deviation		1.21		1.6		10.1		0.18	

*Logarithms used in analysis, therefore means geometric.

†Adjusted for age, sex, current social class, social class at birth, and height.

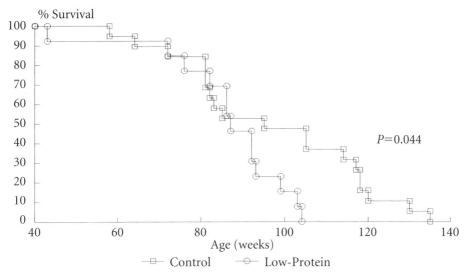

Fig. 13.3 Survival curves for female rats exposed to prenatal low-protein diet compared to control group exposed to unrestricted prenatal diet.[40]

a maternal low-protein diet on lifespan of the offspring was investigated.[40] Rat dams were fed either a control diet or a low-protein diet from conception until the end of pregnancy. The average lifespan of the female rats exposed to a low-protein diet *in utero* was reduced by 11% (Fig. 13.3). There was a similar but non-significant trend in the males. These findings are consistent with those of two recent studies, which found that prenatal diet restriction was associated with a shorter lifespan; telomere shortening has been postulated as an underlying mechanism.[41,42]

The generalizability of these findings from animal models to humans is unclear[43] and there have been no intervention studies to investigate the effects of early diet restriction on human ageing. Observational evidence comes from studies involving survivors of the Dutch Hunger Winter, which occurred from 1944 to 1945 at the end of the Second World War. During this famine, pregnant women received between 400 and 1000 calories per day. Women who had been exposed to famine in late gestation produced babies who were significantly lighter and shorter at birth.[44] Ongoing follow-up of the children has shown persisting effects into adult life. People exposed to famine in late or mid-gestation had reduced glucose tolerance. People exposed in early gestation had a more atherogenic lipid profile. Further follow-up is now underway to determine if this translates into effects on the development of age related diseases, specifically type 2 diabetes and coronary heart disease, in later life.[45]

A similar study on survivors from the siege of Leningrad, who were also exposed to undernutrition *in utero*, found that intrauterine malnutrition was not associated with glucose intolerance, dyslipidaemia, hypertension, or cardiovascular disease in adulthood. However participants exposed to malnutrition showed evidence of endothelial dysfunction and a stronger influence of obesity on blood pressure.[46] There have also been studies of the long-term effects of less extreme variation in human maternal nutrition. A study in Scotland used dietary records from 30 years ago on women who modified their diet during pregnancy. They had been advised to eat 1 pound of red meat per day and to avoid carbohydrate-rich food. This was found to be associated with increased blood pressure in their offspring.[47]

The effect of childhood nutrition on subsequent mortality has been investigated in follow-up studies of the people who took part in Lord Boyd Orr's Carnegie survey of family diet and health in pre war UK between 1937 and 1939.[48] This showed no effect on all-cause mortality, but a relationship between shorter leg length, marking adverse early diet and increased risk of adult coronary heart disease.[49] There was also evidence that both reduced childhood energy intake and possibly shorter leg length may be associated with subsequent reduced cancer risk.[50] This contrasts with the findings from the animal literature that suggest that only diet restriction instituted in later life (after weaning) has beneficial effects.[51]

13.3.3 Nutrition in later life

Nutrition in later life remains the best studied environmental influence on ageing. Laboratory rats placed on energy-restricted diets after weaning age slower and live longer than their *ad libitum*-fed counterparts. In fact, diet restriction is the only intervention consistently shown to extend both median and maximal lifespan in mammals. The beneficial effects of lower food consumption extend to animals given freedom of dietary choice, where longevity can be predicted entirely on the basis of dietary and growth responses in early postweaning life.[52] Recent research has focused on identifying the mechanisms responsible for the beneficial effects of energy restriction in animals. Hypotheses include changes in stress hormones, altered characteristics of glucose utilization, reduced glycation of macromolecules, decreased oxygen radical damage, and changes in gene expression. There is evidence that ageing is associated with selective up-regulation of the synthesis of proteins associated with inflammation and oxidative stress.[53]

Little is known about the effects of selective energy restriction on human ageing. Some of the most detailed data have arisen from the natural experiment of Biosphere 2, a closed self-sustaining ecological space near Tuscon, Arizona, USA, containing seven biomes including habitat for human participants.[54] In 1991, four men and four women were sealed inside for 2 years. During this time the daily intake of energy was less than anticipated due to crop failure. The low-energy nutrient-dense character of the diet resembled in principle that which has been shown to retard ageing in other species. Physiological variables including blood pressure, blood glucose, and insulin levels were closely monitored during the 2 years of closure and for 30 months after release. Weight loss in the biosphere was associated with a reduction in blood pressure, glucose, and insulin levels, which were not sustained after returning to a normal diet. The human physiological responses closely resembled those seen in rodents and monkeys, but the identification of effects on human ageing await longer follow-up. There has been one small study of diet restriction and longevity in humans where the intervention was initiated in late life.[55] Healthy participants over 65 years of age living in a religious institution for the aged were either given a balanced diet containing 2300 calories on odd days and 1 litre of milk with 500 g of fruit on even days or given a balanced diet every day. Those given the restricted diet spent significantly less time in an infirmary than control participants and six died compared with the 13 fed more, but this difference did not reach statistical significance.

13.3.4 Antioxidants

Oxidative damage accumulates with age.[56] This reflects ongoing exposure to free radicals from both the external environment and through the normal metabolic pathways necessary for sustaining life. The body has several mechanisms for detoxifying free radicals, including the enzymes superoxide dysmutase, catalase, and glutathione peroxidase as well as vitamin E, vitamin C, uric acid, and β-carotene[57] but there is some evidence that these mechanisms become less efficient in older age. One of the best characterized results of age related accumulation of free radical damage is seen in the increased concentration of oxidized proteins that may reflect their slower removal from ageing cells. This can be associated with a marked decline in enzyme activity.[58] There is also observational evidence linking lower intake of antioxidant vitamins with a number of age related diseases.[59] However interventional studies have failed to show benefit of antioxidant supplementation in human[60,61] or in animal models.[62]

13.3.5 Physical activity

There is growing evidence for systemic effects and therapeutic benefits of exercise training for older people. Certainly some of the age related decline in cardiovascular, metabolic, and musculoskeletal function appears to be mediated by decreases in physical activity and changes in body composition associated with ageing. Physiological benefits from regular physical exercise in older people include augmented aerobic capacity, increased muscle strength, reduced blood pressure, lower plasma lipids, improved glucose tolerance, and insulin sensitivity.[63] However the role of weight loss and the other mechanisms by which physical conditioning operates to attenuate ageing changes in the cardiovascular, metabolic, and musculoskeletal systems remain unclear.

13.4 Musculoskeletal ageing

Musculoskeletal ageing is a key contributor to the development of physical frailty, disability, and dependency in later life. The three main components of the musculoskeletal system are muscle, bone, and cartilage, and ageing is associated with the loss of muscle mass and strength (sarcopenia), thinning of bone (osteoporosis), and changes in cartilage (osteoarthritis). Environmental influences operating in adult life include physical activity, hormonal status, and diet and some genetic factors have been identified.[64–66] However there remains considerable unexplained variation in rates of ageing between individuals and recent work has utilized a life course approach to investigate the role of early environmental influences.[67]

13.4.1 Muscle

The relationship between birthweight and muscle strength in later life, first described in the Hertfordshire Ageing Study,[31] has been replicated using a prospective national birth cohort of 1371 men and 1404 women, aged 53 years (Fig. 13.4).[68] This study was also able to investigate the effect of childhood growth on adult muscle function and demonstrated that there was no interaction between birthweight and later body size. A potential underlying mechanism is that birthweight is related to an individual's

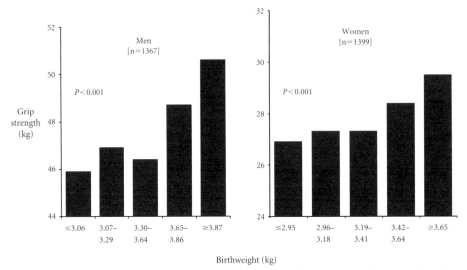

Fig. 13.4 Grip strength at 53 years according to birthweight in the National Survey of Health and Development 1946 birth cohort.[68]

number of muscle fibres that are established by birth and that even in middle-age, compensating hypertrophy may be inadequate.

The relationship between birthweight and muscle strength may reflect a common genetic mechanism but this has been little explored. One study investigated the role of polymorphism in the insulin-like growth factor 2 (IGF2) gene.[69] The product of this gene, insulin-like growth factor II, is central to fetal growth and has a proliferative action in adult muscle. However the study showed that birthweight and polymorphism of the IGF2 gene had independent effects on grip strength in men suggesting that this polymorphism did not explain the observed association between early growth and grip.

Adult muscle mass, as estimated by urinary creatinine excretion, is also related to early size independent of adult size.[70] A study of men and women aged 50 years showed that muscle mass was predicted by low birthweight and small head circumference, but not by thinness at birth. A study of adult body composition in 143 people aged 65–75 years using whole body dual X-ray absorptiometry confirmed that low birthweight was associated with significantly lower adult lean mass in both men and women. About 25% of the variation in whole body lean mass was explained by birthweight. There was no significant relationship with fat mass but low birthweight was related to lower bone mass (Fig. 13.5).[71] This suggests that allocation of cells to different body compartments (muscle, bone, and fat) during critical periods of development may be influenced by early growth and nutrition.

13.4.2 **Bone**

Ageing is associated with bone loss and osteoporosis, a skeletal disorder characterized by low bone mass and microarchitectural deterioration of bony tissue. Osteoporosis is a major cause of morbidity and mortality through its association with age related fracture.[72] These fractures typically occur at the hip, spine, and distal forearm.

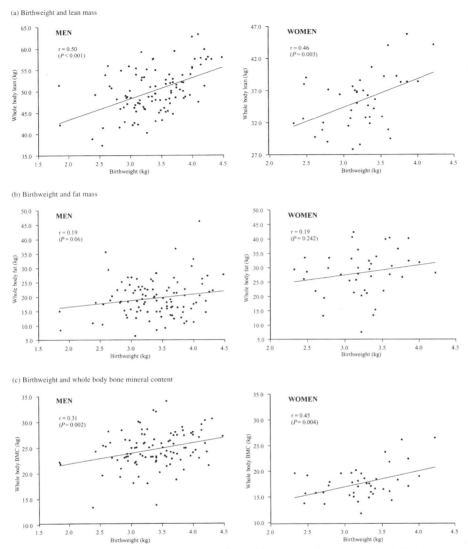

Fig. 13.5 The relationship between birthweight and lean mass, fat mass, and whole body bone mineral content after adjustment for age, in men and women.[71]

The frequency of fracture at all three sites increases with age and fracture pathogenesis depends upon both bone strength and propensity to trauma. Bone strength is directly related to bone mass; the bone mass of an individual in later life depends upon the peak attained during skeletal growth and the subsequent rate of bone loss. Although there is evidence to suggest that peak bone mass is inherited, current genetic markers are unable to explain more than a small proportion of the variance in individual bone mass[65] and determinants of bone loss are incompletely understood. However, evidence is accumulating that early environmental influences also modulate peak bone mass and fracture risk.

Several epidemiological studies have addressed the relationship between birthweight, weight in infancy, and bone mass in adulthood.[73] In the first of these, 153 women born in Bath, UK during 1968–69 were followed up at age 21 years; data on childhood growth were obtained from linked birth and school records.[74] Statistically significant associations were documented between weight at 1 year and bone mineral content, but not density, at the lumbar spine and femoral neck. These relationships were independent of adult body mass index. The findings were replicated in an older cohort of 238 men and 201 women aged 60–75 years in Hertfordshire.[75] Again, the relationship remained after adjustment for later environmental determinants of bone loss such as physical activity, dietary calcium intake, cigarette smoking, alcohol consumption, and age at menopause among women. In these studies, evidence has emerged that the early environment might interact with the genome in influencing bone mass.[76] Thus, polymorphism in the gene for the vitamin D receptor (a putative genetic marker of osteoporosis risk) was shown to relate to bone mineral density in opposite directions among individuals of varying birthweight. Among individuals with the 'BB' genotype, lumbar spine bone mineral density was increased in those of lower birthweight but reduced in those of higher birthweight ($P<0.05$ for the interaction between birthweight and VDR genotype on bone density). Such findings suggest that genetic influences on adult bone size and mineral density may be modified by undernutrition *in utero*.

Confirmation of these observations in the USA,[77] Scandinavia,[78] and Australia[79] has permitted an amalgamation of data relating growth in infancy with adult bone mass.[73] This demonstrates that the strongest association is found between weight in infancy and adult bone mass, with around 50% of this relationship observable by birth.

Of course, the clinically important consequence of reduced bone mass is fracture and data are now becoming available that directly link growth rates in childhood and adolescence with the risk of later hip fracture.[80] Studies of a Finnish cohort in whom birth and growth data were linked to later hospital discharge records for hip fracture have permitted follow-up of around 7000 men and women who were born in Helsinki University Central Hospital during 1924–1933. Around ten measurements of height and weight throughout childhood were recorded on each participant and hip fracture incidence was ascertained using the Finnish hospital discharge registration system. The two main determinants of hip fracture risk were tall maternal stature and low rate of weight gain between 7 and 15 years. In addition, fracture participants were found to be shorter at birth, but of average height by age 7 years, suggesting that hip fracture risk might be particularly elevated among children in whom growth of the skeletal envelope was forced ahead of the capacity to mineralize. Extrapolation from the epidemiological studies of bone mass to those of hip fracture suggest that programming of bone mass alone would be insufficient to explain the hip fracture risk. It is likely that programming of muscle size and function (see above) contributes to frailty in individuals born light and thereby adds to the risk of fracture conferred by reduced bone mass.

13.4.3 Osteoarthritis

Osteoarthritis is the commonest disorder of ageing joints. The characteristic pathological changes include focal loss of articular cartilage and a hypertrophic reaction in the subchondral bone and joint margin but the underlying causes of these changes are not well understood. Little consideration has been given to the effects of the prenatal environment on long-term joint ageing although it has long been recognized that embryological events may provide insights into the study of mature joints and their diseases.[81] There is rapid development and differentiation of the musculoskeletal system during the embryonic period and all bones and joints can be observed by the seventh week. Alteration in shape is clearly one of the critical events in embryological development and the shape of joints continues to be important particularly in the development of osteoarthritis at the hip.

Adult obesity is one of the strongest risk factors for osteoarthritis but the relationship to weight in earlier life has not been previously considered. However new work, utilizing a UK national cohort of men and women with records of weight from birth through to middle-age, has identified that low birthweight as well as increased adult weight is associated with the development of clinical hand osteoarthritis in men at the age of 53 years.[82] A similar study in an older cohort of people with detailed birth records will involve radiological ascertainment of osteoarthritis.

13.4.4 Mechanisms of programming musculoskeletal ageing

The associations between small size in early life and increased ageing in muscle and bone have been clearly demonstrated. However the underlying mechanisms are only just starting to be elucidated. Detailed physiological studies have been used to investigate hormonal influences and the role of the hypothalamic–pituitary–adrenal axis. Profiles of circulating cortisol and growth hormone were obtained in groups of men and women and related to both size in early life and adult bone density. These studies showed that low birthweight predicted increased adult cortisol levels[83] and low weight in infancy was associated with decreased growth hormone levels in later life.[84] The levels of these two skeletally active hormones were also found to be determinants of prospective bone loss.[85] The data are compatible with the hypothesis that environmental stressors, such as undernutrition, occurring during intrauterine or early postnatal life, may alter the sensitivity of the growth plate to cortisol and growth hormone. The consequence of this endocrine programming would be to reduce peak skeletal size and perhaps also mineral density, as well as to predispose individuals to an accelerated rate of bone loss during later life. Similar studies are underway to investigate the role of hormonal influences in programming muscle strength.

The determinants of neonatal bone mass have also been explored in a study looking at anthropometric and lifestyle characteristics of a series of mothers through pregnancy.[86] After adjustment for sex and gestational age, neonatal bone mass was found to be strongly, positively associated with birthweight, birth length, and placental weight. Other determinants included maternal and paternal birthweight and maternal triceps skinfold thickness at 28 weeks. Maternal smoking and maternal energy intake at 18 weeks gestation were negatively associated with neonatal bone mineral content at both the spine and whole body. The independent effects of maternal and paternal birthweight on fetal skeletal development support the notion that paternal influences, possibly through the imprinting of growth-promoting genes such as IGF2, contribute strongly to the establishment of the early skeletal growth trajectory, while maternal nutrition and body build modify fetal nutrient supply and subsequent bone accretion. The influences on neonatal lean mass are now being investigated.

13.5 **Conclusions**

There is growing evidence of early life influences on ageing and in ageing of the musculoskeletal system in particular. Taking this research forward, within a life course model of ageing, will not only involve detailed characterization of important life course influences on ageing, especially those occurring in early life which have yet to be fully explored, but also investigation into how they interact biologically. Perhaps this will be the key to identifying successful interventions to modify the deleterious effects of the human ageing process.

References

Those marked with an asterisk are especially recommended for further reading.

1 Finch CE. *Longevity, senescence and the genome.* Chicago: University of Chicago Press, 1990.

*2 Austad SN. *Why we age.* New York: John Wiley, 1997.

3 Guralnik JM, Fried LP, Salive ME. Disability as a public health outcome in the aging population. *A Rev Pub Health* 1996;**17**:25–46:25–46.

4 Kinsella K, Velkoff VA. *An aging world: 2001* (US Census Bureau, Series P95/01–1). Washington, DC: US Government Printing Office, 2001.

5 Gee EM, Veevers JE. Accelerating sex differentials in mortality: an analysis of contributing factors. *Soc Biol* 1983;**30**:75–85.

6 Hazzard WR. Biological basis of the sex differential in longevity. *J Am Geriatr Soc* 1986;**34**:455–471.

*7 Masoro EJ. Aging: current concepts. In Masoro E, ed. *Handbook of physiology Section 11: aging.* New York: Oxford University Press, 1995:3–21.

8 Medvedev ZA. An attempt at a rational classification of theories of ageing. *Biol Rev* 1990;**65**:375–98.

*9 Kirkwood TBL. Evolution of ageing. *Nature* 1977;**270**:301–4.

10 Lebel M. Werner syndrome: genetic and molecular basis of a premature aging disorder. *Cell Mol Life Sci* 2001;**58**:857–67.

11 Williams G. Pleiotropy, natural selection, and the evolution of senescence. *Evolution* 1957;**11**:398–411.

12 Miller RA. Kleemeier award lecture: are there genes for aging? *J Gerontol A Biol Sci Med Sci* 1999;**54**:B297–307.

13 Finch CE, Kirkwood TBL. *Chance, development and aging.* New York: Oxford University Press, 2000.

14 Vijg J. Somatic mutations and aging: a re-evaluation. *Mutat Res* 2000;**447**:117–35.

15 Richardson A, Cheung HT. The relationship between age-related changes in gene expression, protein turnover and the responsiveness of an organism to stimulus. *Life Sci* 1982;**31**:605–13.

16 Hayflick L. The limited *in vitro* lifetime of human diploid cell strains. *Exp Cell Res* 1965;**37**:614–36.

17 Cristofalo V. Aging in cell culture: relevance to human aging? *Biogerontology* 2003;**4**:56.

18 Vaziri H, Dragowska W, Allsopp RC, Thomas TE, Harley CB, Lansdorp PM. Evidence for a mitotic clock in human hematopoietic stem cells: loss of telomeric DNA with age. *Proc Nat Acad Sci USA* 1994;**91**:9857–60.

19 Orgel LE. The maintenance of the accuracy of protein synthesis and its relevance to ageing. *Proc Nat Acad Sci USA* 1963;**49**:517–21.

20 Sell D, Monnier VM. Aging of long-lived proteins: extra-cellular matrix (collagens, elastins, proteoglycans) and lens crystallins. In Masoro EJ, ed. *Handbook of physiology Section 11 aging.* New York: Oxford University Press, 1995:235–305.

21 Bjorksten J. A common molecular basis for the aging syndrome. *J Am Geriatr Soc* 1958;**6**:740–8.

22 Nilsson PM. Premature ageing: the link between psychosocial risk factors and disease. *Med Hypoth* 1996;**47**:39–42.

23 Kirkwood TBL, Austad SN. Why do we age? *Nature* 2000;**408**:233–8.

*24 Aihie Sayer A, Cooper C. Early undernutrition: good or bad for longevity? In Watson RR, ed. *Handbook of nutrition in the aged*. Boca Raton: CRC Press, 2000:97–106.

25 Brody JA, Schneider EL. Diseases and disorders of aging: an hypothesis. *J Chron Dis* 1986;**39**:871–6.

26 Borkan GA, Norris AH. Assessment of biological age using a profile of physical parameters. *J Gerontol* 1980;**35**:177–84.

27 Hochschild R. Improving the precision of biological age determinations. Part 1: a new approach to calculating biological age. *Exp Gerontol* 1989;**24**:289–300.

28 Hochschild R. Improving the precision of biological age determinations. Part 2: automatic human tests, age norms and variability. *Exp Gerontol* 1989;**24**:301–16.

29 Guralnik JM, Branch LG, Cummings SR, Curb JD. Physical performance measures in aging research. *J Gerontol* 1989;**44**:M141–6.

*30 Barker DJP. *Mothers, babies and health in later life* (2nd edn). Edinburgh: Churchill Livingstone, 1998.

*31 Sayer AA, Cooper C, Evans JR, Rauf A, Wormald RPL, Osmond C *et al*. Are rates of ageing determined *in utero*? *Age Ageing* 1998;**27**:579–83.

32 Barker DJP, Gluckman PD, Godfrey K, Harding JE, Owens JA, Robinson JS. Fetal nutrition and cardiovascular disease in adult life. *Lancet* 1993;**341**:938–41.

33 Chow BF, Lee C-J. Effect of dietary restriction of pregnant rats on body weight gain of the offspring. *J Nutr* 1964;**82**:10–18.

34 Kahn AJ. Embryogenic effect on post-natal changes in hemoglobin concentration with time. *Growth* 1968;**32**:13–22.

35 Roeder LM. Effect of the level of nutrition on rates of cell proliferation and of RNA and protein synthesis in the rat. *Nutr Rep Int* 1973;**7**:271–88.

36 McCance RA, Widdowson EM. Nutrition and growth. *Proc Roy Soc Lond (Biol)* 1962;**156**:326–37.

37 Winick M, Noble A. Cellular response in rats during malnutrition at various ages. *J Nutr* 1966;**89**:300–6.

38 Roeder LM, Chow BF. Maternal undernutrition and its long-term effects on the offspring. *Am J Clin Nutr* 1972;**25**:812–21.

39 Brailsford Robertson T, Ray LA. On the growth of relatively long lived compared with that of relatively short lived animals. *J Biol Chem* 1920;**42**:71–7.

40 Aihie Sayer A, Dunn R, Langley-Evans S, Cooper C. Prenatal exposure to a maternal low protein diet shortens life span in rats. *Gerontology* 2001;**47**:9–14.

41 Jennings BJ, Ozanne SE, Dorling MW, Hales CN. Early growth determines longevity in male rats and may be related to telomere shortening in the kidney. *FEBS Lett* 1999;**448**:4–8.

42 Vehaskari VM, Aviles DH, Manning J. Prenatal programming of adult hypertension in the rat. *Kidney Int* 2001;**59**:238–45.

43 Harding JE. The nutritional basis of the fetal origins of adult disease. *Int J Epidemiol* 2001;**30**:15–23.

44 Stein Z, Susser M. The Dutch famine, 1944–1945, and the reproductive process. I. Effects on six indices at birth. *Pediatr Res* 1975;**9**:70–6.

45 Roseboom TJ, van der Meulen JH, Ravelli AC, Osmond C, Barker DJ, Bleker OP. Effects of prenatal exposure to the Dutch famine on adult disease in later life: an overview. *Mol Cell Endocrinol* 2001;**185**:93–8.

46 Stanner SA, Bulmer K, Andres C, Lantseva OE, Borodina V, Poteen VV *et al.* Does malnutrition *in utero* determine diabetes and coronary heart disease in adulthood? Results from the Leningrad siege study, a cross sectional study. *Br Med J* 1997;**315**:1342–8.

47 Shiell AW, Campbell-Brown M, Haselden S, Robinson S, Godfrey KM, Barker DJ. High-meat, low-carbohydrate diet in pregnancy: relation to adult blood pressure in the offspring. *Hypertension* 2001;**38**:1282–8.

48 Gunnell DJ, Frankel S, Nanchahal K, Braddon FE, Davey Smith G. Lifecourse exposure and later disease: a follow-up study based on a survey of family diet and health in pre-war Britain (1937–1939). *Pub Health* 1996;**110**:85–94.

49 Gunnell DJ, Davey Smith G, Frankel S, Nanchahal K, Braddon FE, Pemberton J *et al.* Childhood leg length and adult mortality: follow up of the Carnegie (Boyd Orr) Survey of Diet and Health in Pre-war Britain. *J Epidemiol Commun Health* 1998;**52**:142–52.

50 Frankel S, Gunnell DJ, Peters TJ, Maynard M, Davey Smith G. Childhood energy intake and adult mortality from cancer: the Boyd Orr Cohort Study. *Br Med J* 1998;**316**:499–504.

51 Aihie Sayer A, Cooper C. Undernutrition and aging. *Gerontology* 1997;**43**:203–5.

52 Ross MH, Lustbader E. Dietary practices and growth responses as predictors of longevity. *Nature* 1976;**262**:548–53.

53 Kayo T, Allison DB, Weindruch R, Prolla TA. Influences of aging and caloric restriction on the transcriptional profile of skeletal muscle from rhesus monkeys. *Proc Natl Acad Sci USA* 2001;**98**:5093–8.

54 Walford RL, Mock D, MacCallum T, Laseter JL. Physiologic changes in humans subjected to severe, selective calorie restriction for two years in biosphere 2: health, aging, and toxicological perspectives. *Toxicol Sci* 1999;**52(suppl)**:61–5.

55 Vallejo EA. La dieta de hambre a dias alternos in la alimentacion de los viejos. *Rev Clin Exp* 1957;**63**:25.

56 Stadtman ER. Protein oxidation and aging. *Science* 1992;**257**:1220–4.

57 Pacifici RE, Davies KJ. Protein, lipid and DNA repair systems in oxidative stress: the free-radical theory of aging revisited. *Gerontology* 1991;**37**:166–80.

58 Cabiscol E, Levine RL. Carbonic anhydrase III. Oxidative modification *in vivo* and loss of phosphatase activity during aging. *J Biol Chem* 1995;**270**:14742–7.

59 Byers T, Guerrero N. Epidemiologic evidence for vitamin C and vitamin E in cancer prevention. *Am J Clin Nutr* 1995;**62(suppl)**:1385–92S.

60 Clarke R, Armitage J. Antioxidant vitamins and risk of cardiovascular disease. Review of large-scale randomised trials. *Cardiovasc Drugs Ther* 2002;**16**:411–15.

61 Shoulson I. DATATOP: a decade of neuroprotective inquiry. Parkinson Study Group. Deprenyl and Tocopherol Antioxidative Therapy of Parkinsonism. *Ann Neurol* 1998; **44(suppl 1)**:S160–6.

62 Yu BP. Putative interventions. In Masoro EJ, ed. *Handbook of physiology Section 11 aging.* New York: Oxford University Press, 1995:613–31.

63 Goldberg AP, Hagberg JM. Physical exercise in the elderly. In Schneider EL, Rowe JW, eds. *Handbook of the biology of aging.* San Diego: Academic Press, 1990:407–28.

64 Roubenoff R. Sarcopenia and its implications for the elderly. *Eur J Clin Nutr* 2000;**54(suppl 3)**:S40–7.

65 Walker-Bone K, Dennison E, Cooper C. Osteoporosis. In Silman AJ, Hochberg MC, eds. *Epidemiology of the rheumatic diseases.* Oxford: Oxford University Press, 2001:259–92.

66 Felson DT. Epidemiology of osteoarthritis. In Brandt KD, Doherty M, Lohmander LS, eds. *Osteoarthritis.* Oxford: Oxford University Press, 1998:13–22.

67 Ben-Shlomo Y, Kuh D. A life course approach to chronic disease epidemiology: conceptual models, empirical challenges and interdisciplinary perspectives. *Int J Epidemiol* 2002;**312**:85–93.

*68 Kuh D, Bassey J, Hardy R, Aihie Sayer A, Wadsworth M, Cooper C. Birth weight, childhood size, and muscle strength in adult life: evidence from a birth cohort study. *Am J Epidemiol* 2002;**156**:627–33.

69 Sayer AA, Syddall H, O'Dell SD, Chen XH, Briggs PJ, Briggs R *et al.* Polymorphism of the IGF2 gene, birth weight and grip strength in adult men. *Age Ageing* 2002;**31**:468–70.

70 Phillips DIW. Relation of fetal growth to adult muscle mass and glucose tolerance. *Diab Med* 1995;**12**:686–90.

*71 Gale CR, Martyn CN, Kellingray S, Eastell R, Cooper C. Intrauterine programming of adult body composition. *J Clin Endocrinol Metab* 2001;**86**:267–72.

72 Melton LJ, Cooper C. Magnitude and impact of osteoporosis and fractures. In Marcus R, Feldman D, Kelsey J, eds. *Osteoporosis*. San Diego: Academic Press, 2001:557–67.

73 Javaid MK, Cooper C. Prenatal and childhood influences on osteoporosis. *Best Pract Res Clin Endocrinol Metab* 2002;**16**:349–67.

74 Cooper C, Cawley M, Bhalla A, Egger P, Ring F, Morton L *et al.* Childhood growth, physical activity, and peak bone mass in women. *J Bone Min Res* 1995;**10**:940–7.

75 Cooper C, Fall C, Egger P, Hobbs R, Eastell R, Barker D. Growth in infancy and bone mass in later life. *Ann Rheum Dis* 1997;**56**:17–21.

76 Dennison EM, Arden NK, Keen RW, Syddall H, Day IN, Spector TD *et al.* Birthweight, vitamin D receptor genotype and the programming of osteoporosis. *Paediatr Perinat Epidemiol* 2001;**15**:211–19.

77 Yarbrough DE, Barrett-Connor E, Morton DJ. Birth weight as a predictor of adult bone mass in postmenopausal women: the Rancho Bernardo Study. *Osteoporos Int* 2000;**11**:626–30.

78 Duppe H, Cooper C, Gardsell P, Johnell O. The relationship between childhood growth, bone mass, and muscle strength in male and female adolescents. *Calcif Tiss Int* 1997;**60**:405–9.

79 Jones G, Dwyer T. Birth weight, birth length, and bone density in prepubertal children: evidence for an association that may be mediated by genetic factors. *Calcif Tiss Int* 2000;**67**:304–8.

*80 Cooper C, Eriksson JG, Forsen T, Osmond C, Tuomilehto J, Barker DJP. Maternal height, child-hood growth and risk of hip fracture in later life: a longitudinal study. *Osteoporos Int* 2001;**12**:623–9.

81 van den Berg R. The embryology of the musculoskeletal system. In Klippel JH, Dieppe PA, eds. *Rheumatology*. St Louis: Mosby, 1994:1–4.

*82 Sayer AA, Poole J, Cox V, Kuh D, Hardy R, Wadsworth M *et al.* Weight from birth to 53 years: a longitudinal study of the influence on clinical hand osteoarthritis. *Arthritis Rheum* 2003;**48**:1030–3.

83 Phillips DI, Walker BR, Reynolds RM, Flanagan DE, Wood PJ, Osmond C *et al.* Low birth weight predicts elevated plasma cortisol concentrations in adults from 3 populations. *Hypertension* 2000;**35**:1301–6.

84 Fall C, Hindmarsh P, Dennison E, Kellingray S, Barker D, Cooper C. Programming of growth hormone secretion and bone mineral density in elderly men: a hypothesis. *J Clin Endocrinol Metab* 1998;**83**:135–9.

85 Dennison E, Hindmarsh P, Fall C, Kellingray S, Barker D, Phillips D *et al.* Profiles of endoge-nous circulating cortisol and bone mineral density in healthy elderly men. *J Clin Endocrinol Metab* 1999;**84**:3058–63.

86 Godfrey K, Walker-Bone K, Robinson S, Taylor P, Shore S, Wheeler T *et al.* Neonatal bone mass: influence of parental birthweight, maternal smoking, body composition, and activity during pregnancy. *J Bone Miner Res* 2001;**16**:1694–1703.

Chapter 14

A life course approach to neuropsychiatric outcomes

Pam Factor-Litvak and Ezra Susser

The scope of neuropsychiatric outcomes ranges from subtle deficits in cognitive, behavioural and social functioning to frank disorders such as autism, schizophrenia and Alzheimer's disease. Recent evidence strongly suggests that such outcomes are associated with insults during critical times of brain development and with exposures over the life course. We examine how specification of the hypothesized nature and timing of exposures is important to understand the aetiology of these disorders. Three models are discussed. First the model of a prenatal insult resulting in defined outcomes over the life course, exemplified by prenatal nutritional deprivation, neural tube defects and schizophrenia. Second, the model of a severe prenatal exposure (maternal thyroid hormone deficiency resulting from iodine deficiency) leading to a frank disorder (cretinism) but a lesser prenatal exposure (maternal subclinical thyroid hormone deficiency) leading to a subtle deficit (cognition). Finally, we consider the model of cumulative exposure (pre and postnatal lead exposure) leading to subtle deficits. We also discuss the complexity of determinants at multiple organizational levels that influence the occurrence of neuropsychiatric outcomes. To date, much of the work has focused on birth cohorts through middle age; as these cohorts age, it will be possible to fully explicate the effects of early exposures on ageing populations.

14.1 Introduction

Emerging evidence suggests that neuropsychiatric outcomes over the life course may be associated with exposures during critical times of brain development and with cumulative exposures over the life course. Indeed, in the USA, research in this arena has led the development of life course research. This is illustrated by the history of the two large US pregnancy cohorts initiated in the 1950s and 1960s: one as a multisite study focused on neurodevelopmental disorders[1] and the other at a single site, with a somewhat broader focus on child development.[2] Both of the cohorts were followed into early childhood at which point the funding for follow-up was terminated. In the 1990s, the follow-up of these cohorts resumed with neuropsychiatric outcomes as the central focus.[3] Later, the cohorts were taken up for life course research in many domains, including cardiovascular, cancer, and other outcomes (for example, References 4–7). Along with the creation of these and other databases, neuropsychiatric researchers have been formulating a conceptual framework for life course research, sometimes referred to as developmental epidemiology.[8,9]

Neuropsychiatric outcomes range from subtle deficits in cognitive, behavioural, and social functioning to frank disorders such as autism, schizophrenia, and Alzheimer's disease. Neuropsychiatric disorders can be loosely defined as those with psychiatric symptoms stemming from an injury to the nervous system and particularly to the brain. While applications of new technologies of structural and functional neuroimaging, neuropsychological approaches, and neuropathological approaches allow for more precise definitions of the pathophysiology of many of the disorders, careful clinical histories remain at the core of diagnosis.

A life course approach to understanding the aetiology of these disorders and of more subtle neuropsychiatric outcomes does not rely solely on the longitudinal collection of data. Rather, it is based on specification of a longitudinal model that sequentially orders exposures, background variables and potential mediators, and moderating variables.[10] A central issue that demands attention in these investigations is the hypothesized nature and timing of exposure. Exposure can occur at a single 'critical' point in development, with consequences over the rest of the life course. As an example, consider maternal exposure to thalidomide during specified days of pregnancy and of phocomelia in the infants.[11] Exposure can also be cumulative over the life course. For example, prenatal exposure to environmental lead is associated with deficits in childhood intelligence; the deficits become greater with continued exposure.[12] For the neuropsychiatric outcomes, in particular, the model of timing must be put into context with the specific disorder or deficit.

In this chapter, we will exemplify three models of the relationship of exposure timing to neuropsychiatric outcomes. First, we consider prenatal nutritional deprivation and its potential effects on neural tube defects and schizophrenia, an example that could be consistent with a model of a prenatal insult and defined outcomes over the life course. Second, we choose an example where a severe prenatal insult (maternal thyroid hormone deficiency due to a lack of iodine in the diet) leads to a frank disorder (cretinism) and a lesser prenatal insult (maternal suboptimal thyroid function) leads to a more subtle deficit (cognitive deficit). Third, we choose an example of cumulative exposure (prenatal and postnatal exposure to environmental lead) that leads to subtle deficits in neuropsychological function. We close the chapter with a broad discussion of the complexity of neuropsychiatric development over the life course.

14.2 Prenatal nutritional deprivation, neural tube defects, and schizophrenia

Among the best studied of the neuropsychiatric disorders is schizophrenia.[13–15] From its earliest descriptions, schizophrenia was noted to have a developmental trajectory, ranging from physical anomalies to subtle prodromal symptoms.[16,17] In the 1980s, Murray and Lewis[15] and Weinberger[18] proposed a neurodevelopmental model of schizophrenia in which an early insult during brain development (due to an environmental stressor or genetic factor) predisposed the nervous system to developing psychosis at a later point in the life cycle. The model gains credence from birth cohort and other studies (reviewed in Reference 19) that find abnormalities in cognitive, behavioural, and social functioning in children who are later diagnosed with a schizophrenia spectrum disorder. These include gross and fine motor dysfunction, lower scores on cognitive tests, being described as 'antisocial', not getting along with peers, parents, or teachers, low self-esteem, and having poor communication skills. Thus the emphasis shifted from psychological explanations (for example, poor upbringing) of schizophrenia to biological early life factors in causation.[20]

14.2.1 The Dutch famine study

The investigations of the sequelae of the Dutch famine represent an early example of the life course approach to the study of neuropsychiatric disorders. Indeed, the investigators conceptualized a life course model to study both early and late effects of this prenatal exposure. The following was written by one of them a decade before the study: 'In the individual organism, some external injuries produce immediate and observable effects, while others are embodied in it to produce effects which are continuing or deferred' (p. 2).[21] Prenatal nutritional deficiencies were hypothesized causes of mental deficiency (and even schizophrenia[22]) as early as the 1950s. Data to adequately test this hypothesis, however, were difficult to obtain. It was crucial both to characterize maternal nutrition during pregnancy in a systemized fashion and to have access to neuropsychological evaluations of the children.

One of the lesser known atrocities of the Second World War occurred during the winter of 1944–1945. As retaliation for a railroad strike to halt movement of German troops, the German occupation force of the Netherlands imposed an embargo on all transport, including food supplies, to the western portion of the country. Already in short supply, the restriction of food was devastating and became even more so with an early and unusually severe winter. The famine increased in intensity throughout the winter and at the height of the famine the average daily ration was below 1000 kcal, comprising mainly bread, potatoes, and sugar beets. The famine continued until the time of liberation, 5 May 1945.

The famine has several unique aspects for a life course natural experiment. First, the timing was delineated and because the Dutch kept ration records, the actual rations for each week of the famine were available. Second, the famine had well-described effects on fertility[23] and well-described effects on birthweight, particularly on fetuses exposed during the third trimester of gestation (the effects on fertility, in particular, were less pronounced among the upper social classes, presumably because they had more access to food from black market sources).

In the late 1960s, Stein and colleagues[23] designed a cohort study to examine whether exposure to the famine during fetal development had an impact on the mental development of offspring when they reached maturity. To accomplish this, they capitalized on the Dutch military draft, where all men at the age of 18 are subject to a battery of physical and developmental examinations. Because date and place of birth were available, the investigators were able to determine whether each man was born in a famine or non-famine city and to estimate the relative caloric deprivation of his mother during each week of pregnancy. Thus the timing and severity of exposure was defined.

The major finding of the original study was that no detectable effects on cognition, measured by IQ or by other tests of performance, were attributed to the famine. This finding was consistent among all social strata. Thus, the result did not support the hypothesis that nutritional deprivation during pregnancy was a major explanatory factor for the social distribution of mental performance in high-income societies. Because the famine was acute and situated in an otherwise well-nourished population, the results were not generalized to populations with chronic nutritional deficiency persisting in the postnatal period.

A second finding, which provided the impetus for the study of nutritional deprivation and schizophrenia, was an excess of congenital anomalies of the central nervous system. This excess was only observed among births conceived at the height of the famine, suggesting an effect of exposure in early gestation. Some of the congenital anomalies were neural tube defects. Indeed, this finding provided an important rationale to research prenatal nutrition and neural tube defects, which ultimately proved that folate supplements reduce the risk of neural tube defects.[24–27] In addition, as this finding demonstrated that the famine affected fetal brain development, it also suggested that in births exposed early and severely to nutritional deprivation, there may be other neurodevelopmental anomalies that were manifest later in the life course.

The subsequent studies of schizophrenia in the Dutch famine cohort were performed with an explicit rationale and hypothesis built on the findings of the original study.[28] The *a priori* hypothesis was that the risk of schizophrenia would be increased in offspring conceived at the height of the famine—the same group exhibiting an excess of neurological congenital anomalies. As noted above, precise specification of hypotheses will give greater credence to causal inferences.

Three separate analyses produced complementary results. The first used the Dutch National Psychiatric Registry to ascertain hospitalized cases of schizophrenia between 1970 and 1992—that is, when the individuals in the original birth cohort were 24–48 years of age.[29,30] Schizophrenia was narrowly defined using International Classification of Disease (ICD)-8/ICD-9 codes for paranoid, hebephrenic, residual, and catatonic schizophrenia. Risk of schizophrenia was elevated in both males (relative risk (RR) = 2.0) and females (RR = 2.2) in exactly the same groups that displayed elevated risks of central nervous system anomalies.

The second analysis broadened the outcome to include schizophrenia-spectrum personality disorders. These may be aetiologically related to schizophrenia via two non-mutually exclusive mechanisms; first, a genetic vulnerability may express itself as either a frank disorder or as a personality disorder, depending on the presence or absence of other exposures and second, a prenatal insult may confer a vulnerability which also may manifest on a causal continuum. This analysis used schizoid personality disorder identified at the time of military conscription and was therefore restricted to males. Once again, the group conceived at the height of the famine had an increased risk (RR = 2.01) of the disorder.[31]

The third analysis combined cases of schizoid personality among male military conscripts at age 18 years and of schizophrenia among men at age 24–48 years. This analysis found a more precise estimate of the increased risk (RR = 2.7) in the same group of male offspring.[32]

The Dutch famine studies represent a story of reproductive casualty, in which vulnerability is conferred by a prenatal insult. The same exposure—early prenatal nutritional deprivation—appears to have had an effect on neuropsychiatric disorders at three points in the life course, that is, central nervous system anomalies at birth, schizoid personality disorder at age 18 years, and schizophrenia in adulthood (note that while this exposure resulted in frank disorders, it did not affect the average cognitive performance of the exposed as measured in military conscripts at age 18 years). Of course, only a small fraction of the exposed developed any neuropsychiatric disorder and we can assume that to produce the outcome, the exposure had to combine with genetic factors and other exposures either in the prenatal or postnatal periods.

14.2.2 Biological mechanisms linking nutritional deprivation with schizophrenia

Is there a biological explanation for the association? Ongoing follow-up of the Dutch famine cohort with technologically advanced neuroimaging and other neuropsychiatric work-ups has turned up clues,[33] but the numbers of cases are too small to provide any definite answers. In the absence of further results, we can turn to basic science and animal data to consider the effect of famine on brain morphology and neurotransmitter functioning and assess whether abnormalities identified can be mapped to behavioural changes that mimic schizophrenia.

Although this is a complex field (reviewed in detail elsewhere, see Reference 34), we can illustrate the relevance of these studies for interpreting the epidemiologic data. Neuroimaging and post-mortem pathological studies in schizophrenic people find diminished hippocampal size, possibly resulting from a failure of neuronal proliferation and migration during development. Studies of brain morphology following prenatal protein deprivation consistently find decreased neurogenesis in the hippocampus, an area associated with behavioural changes that 'mimic' aspects of schizophrenia. In the rat, the neurogenesis of the hippocampus occurs during postnatal days 0–24 (which correspond to the latter half of pregnancy in humans), however the groundwork is laid during the prenatal period, suggesting that protein deprivation can permanently alter hippocampal morphology. Similarly, total calorie deprivation during rat gestation and lactation is associated with decreased neurogenesis of specific cell types in the hippocampus, which may alter the flow of information to and from this brain area. Collectively, both animal evidence and evidence from limited human studies suggest that nutritional deprivation during the first half of gestation is associated with alterations in hippocampal morphology, which is then associated with behavioural changes such as those found in the schizophrenia spectrum disorders.

14.3 Prenatal exposure to thyroid hormone and childhood development

Several lines of evidence suggest deficits in neuropsychiatric function following deprivation of thyroid hormone either *in utero* or in the perinatal period. This evidence derives from studies of children born in iodine-deficient areas (iodine is essential for the synthesis of active thyroid hormones), children born with congenital hypothyroidism, premature infants with transient hypothyroxinaemia, and children born to mothers with suboptimal thyroid function. Collectively the data suggest a spectrum of reproductive casualty, depending on the severity and timing of the deprivation. Indeed, because it is not clear whether these effects persist throughout the life course and because potentially moderating variables/exposures have not been identified, this topic lends itself to a life course approach of study.

Thus, it is well documented that maternal iodine deficiency during pregnancy leads to a lowered production of iodinated thyroid hormone and an increased risk of cretinism.[35] Cretinism is a neurodevelopmental disorder resulting in serious retardation of physical and mental development; if the condition is left untreated, growth is stunted and the physical stature attained is that of a dwarf. In addition, the skin is thick, flabby, and waxy in colour, the nose is flattened, the abdomen protrudes, and there is a general slowness of movement and speech. Deficient intake of iodine is also associated with a variety of other disorders including goiter, pregnancy wastage, and hypothyroidism. The degree, timing, and duration of iodine deficiency determine the severity and pattern of these disorders. In geographic areas with severe iodine deficiency (for example, New Guinea, Java, parts of South America), the prevalence of endemic cretinism is high. Lesser forms of neurological deficits are endemic in areas of lesser iodine deficiency[36] and these are correlated with maternal thyroid hormone concentration. Intervention studies suggest that supplementation of pregnant women prior to and during the early part of gestation improved neurologic and cognitive outcomes, while supplementation later in pregnancy did not.[37–39]

Frank cretinism is rare in the developed world due to iodine supplementation in salt. However, recent research suggests that less severe deficiencies of thyroid hormone during *in utero* and early childhood development may also have long-term consequences. Congenital hypothyroidism and transient hypothyroidism of prematurity are associated with deficits in cognition in early life and it is not clear if they are reversible with replacement thyroid hormone. Some studies suggest associations between more subtle deficits in prenatal thyroid hormone exposure and mild deficits in cognition and increased reports of behaviour problems.[40,41] To date, it is not clear whether these deficits persist into adulthood. Because adequate and timely *in utero* exposure to thyroid hormone is critical for brain development to proceed in an orderly fashion, the study of subadequate exposure represents, perhaps, a new area of neuropsychiatric research. The study of deficient *in utero* exposure to thyroid hormone is emerging as a fertile area of life course research.

14.3.1 Neuropsychiatric manifestations of reduced thyroid hormone *in utero* or in early life

Below we consider four scenarios of reduced thyroid exposure during *in utero* development or in the perinatal period. These are congenital hypothyroidism, transient hypothyroxinemia of prematurity, frank maternal hypothyroidism, and suboptimal maternal hypothyroidism. Each has implications for studying the timing of exposure in relation to fetal brain development.

The inability to produce adequate amounts of thyroid hormone at birth (congenital hypothyroidism) may be due either to the presence of a defective thyroid gland or to inadequate iodine. Congenital hypothyroidism is usually detected at birth or shortly after birth in developed countries and corrected by administering replacement hormone. Although supplemented children score in the normal range on tests of cognitive development, various studies raise the possibility of deficits in specific neuropsycholog-ical domains, including speech and language, neuromotor function, perceptuomotor function, and visuospatial ability.[42–50] Additionally, these difficulties persist into the school years, as some studies,[51] but not all,[52] report lower academic achievement in these children compared to either classroom control children or siblings. Inconsistencies in the results of these studies may be attributed to the causes of hypothyroidism, stage of gestation at which the deficiency arises, and childhood thyroid function.[53] Taken together, these studies suggest that hypothyroidism beginning early in gestation is asso-ciated with more severe deficits than hypothyroidism beginning after birth.

The fetal thyroid gland begins to produce active hormone during the second trimester of pregnancy; production of adequate amounts of hormone occurs during the later part of the third trimester. Thus, preterm infants may be born before they are able to produce sufficient thyroid hormone on their own and experience a transient reduction of active hormone after birth. Three large studies[54–59] examined the associa-tion between transient hypothyroxinaemia of preterm infants and neurodevelopmen-tal outcomes in infancy and childhood. Collectively, they find an excess of neurodevelopmental deficits in infants, including reduced scores on tests of cognition and increased rates of motor dysfunction. These deficits persist into the school years.[55,57] Inference from these studies is limited, however, because severe illness and hypothyroxinaemia in preterm infants are closely related. The few randomized placebo-controlled clinical trials of replacement hormone either *in utero* or shortly after birth indicate no differences in development between those treated and those not treated; however, the sample sizes of these studies were small (reviewed in Reference 60). Although these studies do not address *in utero* exposure to maternal hormone, they do indicate that reduced exposure to thyroid hormone in the early postnatal period was associated with subsequent neurodevelopmental deficits.

Recent evidence also suggests that infants and children born to mothers with frank or subclinical hypothyroidism also exhibit deficits in neurodevelopment. Pregnancy in women with frank hypothyroidism is a relatively new phenomenon because hypothy-roidism is frequently associated with anovulation and increased risks of spontaneous abortion, stillbirth, preterm delivery, and complications of pregnancy (such as pregnancy-induced hypertension). Early case series[61,62] report severe neurological and develop-mental deficits in children born to hypothyroid mothers. More recent observations comparing women with overt (treated or untreated) hypothyroidism and subclinical hypothyroidism suggest that these complications occur more frequently in women who are either not treated or inadequately treated.[63,64]

More subtle maternal suboptimal thyroid function during pregnancy is associated with deficits in psychomotor development in infancy and cognition in chil-dren.[40,41,65–68] Among 246 children born to participants in the National Collaborative Perinatal Project in Providence, Rhode Island,[66] those born to mothers with inade-quately treated hypothyroidism performed significantly lower on verbal, performance, and full-scale IQ tests and on tests of visuomotor coordination.[67] In a more recent study of full-term births in the Netherlands, the risk of impaired development at 10 months was increased almost six-fold in children of mothers in the lower tenth per-centile of thyroid hormone at 12 weeks of gestation.[41] In contrast, thyroid hormone concentrations measured at gestational week 32 were not associated with outcome, suggesting that deficits are important early, but not later in gestation. Drawing on a prenatal screening programme for pregnant women, Haddow and colleagues[40] compared 62 women with thyroid-stimulating hormone levels at gestational week 17 above the 98th percentile to 124 matched control participants. Children born to women in the hypothyroid group performed less well on a neuropsychological battery, administered at age 8 years, than the children of control participants. Deficits were found in full-scale IQ, measures of attention, language development, academic performance, and visual motor performance. Further analysis of data in the control group suggested a (non-significant) dose–response relationship between thyroid-stimulating hormone levels in the normal range and performance on the test battery.[65] It is not known whether these deficits persist into adulthood or whether there are any early or late factors that mitigate the associations.

14.3.2 Biological mechanisms

There are strong biological underpinnings for a biological relationship between prenatal (and postnatal) thyroid function and development.[69] Because the fetal thyroid gland does not fully develop the capacity to accumulate iodine and synthesize thyroid hormone until approximately 10–12 weeks of gestation and because the fetal hypothalamic–pituitary axis does not mature until week 16, all thyroid hormone requirements are fulfilled by maternal hormone until this time. In the later half of gestation, there is continued fetal exposure to maternal hormone and continuously increasing levels of fetal hormone, such that in fetuses with normal thyroid development, the relative proportion of fetal to maternal thyroid hormone shifts to the fetus by 32 weeks. Maternal thyroid hormone crosses the placenta during all three trimesters.

Animal data suggest that deficits in exposure to thyroid hormone at critical points in development result in abnormal proliferation of axons and dendrites, synapse formation, gliogenesis and myelination in the cerebrum and cerebellum, and abnormal cellular proliferation in the cerebellum. In animal models,[69–75] associations are reported between maternal thyroid function and cognition and behaviour. Adult progeny of thyroidectomized rat dams, for example, exhibit impaired motor performance, cognition, and learning ability, perhaps due to perturbed development of the brain resulting in an asynchrony of developmental events. Reduced thyroid hormone levels during development are also associated with disrupted neurotransmitter levels, which also may contribute to the retarded developmental processes and behavioural changes.

In sum, the evidence strongly suggests that inadequate exposure to maternal thyroid hormone during *in utero* development or to thyroid hormone shortly after birth results in neuropsychiatric manifestations. The precise manifestation likely depends on the timing and severity of the deficit. There is also some, but not conclusive, biological evidence to support this assertion. The constellation of symptoms lends itself to a life course approach, especially in identifying variables that mitigate the adverse effects.

14.4 Cumulative exposure to environmental lead, neuropsychological deficits, and behaviour problems

Exposure to environmental lead represents a novel application of life course methods. Lead is a ubiquitous environmental contaminant. That frank encephalopathy was due to excessive lead exposure was known for decades. In the 1940s, Byers and Lord[76] reported a case series of children with cognitive deficits purportedly attributable to lead exposure. This study laid the foundation for numerous cross-sectional and longitudinal studies of more moderate levels of lead exposure. Collectively, these studies find small deficits in cognition and increased reports of behaviour problems, perhaps beginning at the lowest levels of exposure. Emerging evidence suggests that chelation therapy for undue lead exposure is not associated with increases in cognitive performance or with alleviation of behaviour problems. These deficits are also reported to last into late adolescence and adulthood. Data also suggest that beneficial social and environmental variables may mitigate some of the adverse association. Thus, these lead-related deficits also lend themselves to a life course approach.

14.4.1 The strength of the association

Although numerous cross-sectional and cohort studies report small associations between exposure to environmental lead and neurodevelopmental outcomes, including cognition,[77–87] motor function,[88] behaviour problems,[89,90] and academic achievement,[90] the timing of exposure and the biological mechanisms underlying the associations are not fully elucidated. Three meta-analyses[91–93] estimate deficits of approximately 2–6 points on tests of intelligence for every 10 μg/dl increase in blood lead concentration. However, the shape of the dose–response curve is not well described at exposure levels below 5 μg/dl[94] because few children in that range are included in the studies. More recent evidence[95,96] suggests that the slope of the blood lead concentration–IQ relationship is steepest for very low exposure levels, that is, blood lead concentrations less than 5 μg/dl. Increased blood lead concentration is associated with small deficits in fine motor coordination.[88] Finally, several studies find small associations between increases in blood lead concentrations and behaviour problems,[89,90,97,98] especially relating to attentional disorders.

14.4.2 Timing of exposure

In most children, exposure to environmental lead peaks in early life; maximum blood lead concentrations are usually found at age 2 in populations not unduly exposed to environmental sources. In Boston, increased blood lead concentration measured at age 2 was associated with an estimated 5.3 point decrease in 10-year IQ measures, after adjustment for confounders.[90] Although not formally tested, associations were strongest for verbal functioning.

Cumulative exposure in early life, assessed using serial measures of blood lead concentration to measure 'average lifetime' exposure, has been associated with decreased IQ scores at later ages.[80–82,86,90,99] For example, in Port Pirie, Australia, an estimated increase in average lifetime blood lead concentration from 10 μg/dl to 20 μg/dl was associated with a 3-point decrease in IQ scores at age 11–13, after adjustment for a range of potentially confounding variables.[99] The strongest deficits were in subscales measuring 'visual-motor coordination, attention, concentration and memory',[99] that is, the information, arithmetic, block design, and mazes subscales.

In the Yugoslavia Prospective Study of Environmental Lead and Child Development,[100] blood lead concentration measured at age 2 *and* average lifetime blood lead concentration were examined. Both average lifetime blood lead concentration *and* blood lead at age 2 were associated with modest decrements in intellectual functioning at ages 2, 4, and 7 years, with stronger associations consistently noted for perceptual-motor functioning.[101] At age 7 years, an increase in lifetime blood lead concentration from $10 \mu g/dl$ to $20 \mu g/dl$ was associated with an estimated 4.3-point decrease in full-scale IQ and an estimated 4.5 decrease in performance IQ.

The Yugoslavia study has suggested that the timing of environmental lead exposure is important in determining the magnitude of IQ loss.[85] In sum, these results find that early exposures (that is, in the prenatal period and up to age 2 years) have larger impacts on IQ than later exposures, although these exposures are also important. In a longitudinal analysis of children followed from the prenatal period to age 7, they found consistent associations between increases in *prenatal* blood lead concentration and small decrements in IQ scores, after adjustment for social variables. After adjustment for both social factors and prenatal blood lead concentrations, elevations in *postnatal* blood lead concentration, whether early or late in childhood, were associated with small additional decrements in IQ scores. While elevations that occurred before the age of 2 and continued afterward were associated with the largest decrements, elevations in blood lead concentrations occurring past age 2 were also associated with IQ decrements. These results were then extended to age 10–12.[96] Indeed the persistence of effects in this cohort and in a cohort in Boston[93,102] is troubling because the educational demands of the teen years involve synthesis and abstraction in the processing and use of information.

The Yugoslavia investigators also measured the concentration of lead in bone.[96,103] The importance of this measure is that it reflects cumulative exposure over the life course. The primary reservoir of lead in the body is skeletal, accounting for approximately 90–95% of lead in adults and for approximately 70–80% of lead in children;[104–106] the half-life of lead in bone is years to decades.[107] Lead in the bone primarily reflects cumulative exposure; the mobilization of lead from bone during times of rapid bone turnover (for example, childhood, pregnancy, and senescence) may represent a source of lead to target organs. Associations between bone lead concentration and several health outcomes including elevated blood pressure,[108] decreased renal function,[109] decreased haemoglobin concentration,[110] and deficits in adult neurobehavioural function[111] are stronger than the same associations between blood lead concentration and these same outcomes. Indeed, in the Yugoslavia study, the adverse associations were strongest relating bone lead concentration to IQ scores, even after controlling for blood lead concentration.[96]

These results suggest that both prenatal and postnatal exposures to environmental lead are likely to be associated with small deficits in later IQ scores. The investigators originally hypothesized that peak vulnerability to environmental lead would correspond to periods of early and rapid brain growth, especially during times of synaptogenesis, arborization, and dendritic pruning; however, these results do not correspond to any of these periods. It may be that either genetic or other prenatal or early life factors mitigate these associations. For example, quality of the childrearing environment, parental education, and parental intelligence are all more important predictors of childhood IQ than environmental lead. Indeed, Bellinger and colleagues[78–80,90] in their studies of lead exposure and childhood intelligence, found that both gender and childhood social class variables mitigate the adverse association.

14.4.3 Biological mechanisms linking lead exposure and cognitive development

Proposed biological mechanisms focus on the effects of lead on the blood–brain barrier[112] and on neurotransmitter function[113] and posit that lead produces 'synaptic noise' and inappropriate pruning of the synaptic connections. Regarding the blood–brain barrier, lead is thought to disrupt the structural components by injury to astrocytes and to the endothelial vasculature. Within the brain, lead preferentially may damage the prefrontal cerebral cortex, hippocampus, and cerebellum; these sites are related to specific cognitive and behavioural deficits found in exposed children. On a neurochemical level, lead may enhance the background release of specific neurotransmitters while concurrently impairing stimulated release. Additionally, lead may block *N*-methyl-D-aspartate glutamate receptor activity, which is a primary receptor at approximately 50% of synapses in the brain. Drugs that block this receptor are associated with deficits in learning and memory in animals. Indeed, a case report of magnetic resonance imaging results in two cousins, one with undue lead exposure and one without, residing in the same household found a reduction in the *N*-acetylaspartate: creatine ratio in both grey and white matter in the exposed child.[114] Finally, 'synaptic noise' may be increased by lead-induced activation of protein kinase C, an intracellular messenger protein that plays a role in the potentiation of signals.

Our group is currently exploring an additional biological mechanism—that is a lead-induced inability of thyroid hormone to adequately reach critical areas of the brain. Our model focuses on the choroid plexus, the site of cerebrospinal fluid production and a possible pathway for neuroendocrine communication between the brain and peripheral tissues.[115] It is the site of synthesis and secretion of a form of transthyretin, the protein that transports and distributes thyroid hormone within the brain. Synthesis of transthyretin begins early in development and continues throughout the life course, implying that damage from environmental exposures early in development as well as later in life may affect thyroid hormone transport to the developing and mature brain, respectively.

There is an increasing body of evidence that the choroid plexus sequesters heavy metals, including lead, from transport to the brain.[116,117] Further there appears to be a threshold for this sequestration—at concentrations greater than 27 mg lead/kg the choroid plexus becomes saturated. Studies in animal models suggest that lead interferes with choroid plexus function by impeding the synthesis of transthyretin and reducing the amount of thyroid hormone that reaches the brain tissue.[118,119] These observations led us to hypothesize that at least part of the association between environmental lead exposure and neurodevelopment might result from the inability of adequate thyroid hormone to reach the brain. We are currently testing this hypothesis using data from the Yugoslavia cohort study, which includes sequential measures of blood lead concentration, stored serum to measure thyroid hormone, and neurodevelopmental outcomes.

14.5 Neuropsychiatric disorders over the life course

The examples above only skim the surface of the complex interplay of variables that influence the development of frank neuropsychiatric disorders and more subtle neuropsychological deficits. In fact, the examples only consider the first half of the life course. Nevertheless, both the exposures and outcomes may be important for neuropsychiatric disorders in the second half of the life course. For example, lead exposure and the resulting decreases in IQ may lead to decreased cognitive reserve and ultimately, to an increased risk of dementia. The theory of cognitive reserve suggests that decline of cognitive ability can be mitigated and delayed by enhancing 'brain reserve capacity',[120–122] which refers to the capacity of the brain to protect against cognitive impairment. The level of protection varies among individuals because its major determinants are educational attainment[123] and intelligence.[124] Reserve capacity may also be augmented by factors throughout the life course and have important implications for the mitigation of neurodevelopmental deficits.

In addition, we have not provided any framework for considering how the social context may modify the effects of early life exposures over the life course. The context of a person's social environment may be as important to health outcomes as biological risk factors. That the social environment may play an especially large role in neuropsychiatric disorders is evidenced by numerous studies relating contextual social variables to cognitive reserve.

For instance, the neighbourhood environment at different times during the life course plays an important role in shaping multiple characteristics of an individual, including socioeconomic status, attitudes towards education, and health status.[125] Neighbourhoods influence the circumstances in which individuals live, function, and interact, both with peers and with macro-level forces that shape societies.[126]

The household reflects the most proximal social context of an individual. The family structure forms a social environment and for children, this is probably a more important context than the neighborhood.[127,128] Indeed, the most important predictors of childhood IQ scores are quality of the childrearing environment (measured using the Home Observation for the Measurement of the Environment (HOME)[129]), parental education, and parental intelligence. The prospective studies of environmental lead exposure, for example, consistently find these variables to be more important than lead exposure in predicting childhood IQ.[96]

A range of individual variables influence health outcomes, either by direct pathways to the outcome, or through mediation of the effects of other variables. Accumulating evidence from the UK 1946 birth cohort, for example, suggests that the long-term cognitive effects of early exposures are largely mediated by cognition in childhood and adolescence.[130] Our view is to consider these multiple levels over the life course and from this wider angle of vision, choose a particular focus for study.

14.6 Conclusion

Recent interest has focused on prenatal and early life predictors of neuropsychiatric disorders. Such predictors include both potentially harmful environmental exposures and contextual variables such as neighbourhood quality and quality of the childrearing environment. In this chapter, we have provided a framework for considering neuropsychiatric disorders over the life course. Thus, we propose three models: a point exposure with defined outcomes over the life course; an exposure with differing degrees of intensity leading to a continuum of outcomes; and an exposure that accumulates over the life course with implications for neuropsychiatric deficits. We exemplified each model with a specific early life exposure and its manifestations over the life course. We also indicated the complexity of determinants at multiple levels that influence the unfolding of these manifestations over time. We consider the life course approach to neuropsychiatric disorders to be in middle-childhood; as established birth cohorts age it will be possible to fully explicate the effects of early exposures on the ageing population.

References

Those marked with an asterisk are especially recommended for further reading.

1 Niswander KRGM. *The women and their pregnancies* (NIH 73–379). Washington DC: US Department of Health, Education and Welfare, 1972.

*2 van den Berg BJ, Christianson RE, Oechsli FW. The California child health and development studies of the School of Public Health, University of California at Berkeley. *Paediatr Perinat Epidemiol* 1988;**2**:265–82.

3 Wyatt RJ, Susser ES. U.S. birth cohort studies of schizophrenia: a sea change. *Schizophr Bull* 2000;**26**:255–6.

4 Cohn BA, Cirillo PM, Christianson RE, van den Berg BJ, Siiteri PK. Placental characteristics and reduced risk of maternal breast cancer. *J Natl Cancer Inst* 2001;**93**:1133–40.

5 Richardson BE, Peck JD, Wormuth JK. Mean arterial pressure, pregnancy-induced hypertension, and preeclampsia: evaluation as independent risk factors and as surrogates for high maternal serum alpha-fetoprotein in estimating breast cancer risk. *Cancer Epidemiol Biomarkers Prev* 2000;**9**:1349–55.

6 Seltzer CC, Oechsli FW. Psychosocial characteristics of adolescent smokers before they started smoking: evidence of self-selection. A prospective study. *J Chronic Dis* 1985;**38**:17–26.

7 Zhang J, Troendle JF, Levine RJ. Risks of hypertensive disorders in the second pregnancy. *Paediatr Perinat Epidemiol* 2001;**15**:226–31.

8 Buka SL, Tsuang MT, Lipsitt LP. Pregnancy/delivery complications and psychiatric diagnosis. A prospective study. *Arch Gen Psychiat* 1993;**50**:151–6.

*9 Costello EJ, Angold A. Developmental epidemiology. In Cicchetti D, Toth S, eds. *Rochester symposium on developmental psychopathology*. Hillsdale: Lawrence Erlbaum, 1991:23–56.

*10 Ben Shlomo Y, Kuh D. A life course approach to chronic disease epidemiology: conceptual models, empirical challenges and interdisciplinary perspectives. *Int J Epidemiol* 2002;**31**:285–93.

11 McBride WG. Teratogenic action of thalidomide. *Lancet* 1978;**1**:1362.

12 Wasserman GA, Liu X, Popovac D, Factor-Litvak P, Kline J, Waternaux C *et al.* The Yugoslavia Prospective Lead Study: contributions of prenatal and postnatal lead exposure to early intelligence. *Neurotoxicol Teratol* 2000;**22**:811–18.

13 Carpenter WT Jr, Buchanan RW. Schizophrenia. *N Engl J Med* 1994;**330**:681–90.

14 Waddington JL. Schizophrenia: developmental neuroscience and pathobiology. *Lancet* 1993;**341**:531–6.

15 Murray RM, Lewis SW. Is schizophrenia a neurodevelopmental disorder? *Br Med J* 1987;**295**:681–2.

16 Kraepelin E. *Dementia Praecox. Psychiatrie*. Leipzig: Barth, 1896.

17 Bleuler E. Die Prognose der Dementia Praecox—Schizophreniegruppe. *Allgemeine Zeitschrift fur Psychiatrie* 1908;**65**:436–64.

18 Weinberger DR. Implications of normal brain development for the pathogenesis of schizophrenia. *Arch Gen Psychiat* 1987;**44**:660–9.

19 Cannon MC, Tarrant CJ, Huttunen MO, Jones P. Childhood development and later schizophrenia: evidence from genetic high-risk and birth cohort studies. In Murray R, Jones P, Susser E, van Os, Cannon M, eds. *The epidemiology of schizophrenia*. Cambridge, UK: Cambridge University Press, 2003:100–23.

*20 Jones PB. Longitudinal approaches to the search for the causes of schizophrenia: past, present and future. In Gattaz WF, Hafner H, eds. *Searches for the causes of schizophrenia. Volume IV, Balance of the century*. Darmstadt: Steinkopf and Berlin: Springer, 1999:91–119.

21 Susser MW, Watson W. *Sociology in medicine*. London: Oxford University Press, 1962.

22 Pasamanick B, Rogers ME, Lilienfeld AM. Pregnancy experience and the development of behavior disorder in children. *Am J Psychiat* 1956;**12**:613–18.

23 Stein ZA, Susser M, Saenger G, Marolla F. *Famine and human development: the Dutch hunger winter of 1944–1945*. New York: Oxford University Press, 1975.

24 Prevention of neural tube defects: results of the Medical Research Council Vitamin Study. MRC Vitamin Study Research Group. *Lancet* 1991;**338**:131–7.

25 Rosano A, Smithells D, Cacciani L, Botting B, Castilla E, Cornel M *et al.* Time trends in neural tube defects prevalence in relation to preventive strategies: an international study. *J Epidemiol Commun Health* 1999;**53**:630–5.

26 Smithells RW, Sheppard S, Schorah CJ. Vitamin dificiencies and neural tube defects. *Arch Dis Child* 1976;**51**:944–50.

27 Wild J, Seller MJ, Schorah CJ, Smithells RW. Investigation of folate intake and metabolism in women who have had two pregnancies complicated by neural tube defects. *Br J Obstet Gynaecol* 1994;**101**:197–202.

28 Susser E, Hoek HW, Brown A. Neurodevelopmental disorders after prenatal famine: the story of the Dutch Famine Study. *Am J Epidemiol* 1998;**147**:213–16.

29 Susser ES, Lin SP. Schizophrenia after prenatal exposure to the Dutch Hunger Winter of 1944–1945. *Arch Gen Psychiat* 1992;**49**:983–8.

30 Susser E, Neugebauer R, Hoek HW, Brown AS, Lin S, Labovitz D *et al.* Schizophrenia after prenatal famine. Further evidence. *Arch Gen Psychiat* 1996;**53**:25–31.

31 Hoek HW, Susser E, Buck KA, Lumey LH, Lin SP, Gorman JM. Schizoid personality disorder after prenatal exposure to famine. *Am J Psychiat* 1996;**153**:1637–9.

32 Hoek HW, Brown AS, Susser E. The Dutch famine and schizophrenia spectrum disorders. *Soc Psychiat Psychiatr Epidemiol* 1998;**33**:373–9.

33 Hulshoff Pol HE, Hoek HW, Susser E, Brown AS, Dingemans A, Schnack HG *et al.* Prenatal exposure to famine and brain morphology in schizophrenia. *Am J Psychiat* 2000;**157**:1170–2.

34 Butler PD, Printz D, Klugewicz D, Brown AS, Susser ES. Plausibility of early nutritional deficiency as a risk factor for schizophrenia. In Susser ES, Brown AS, Gorman JM, eds. *Prenatal exposures in schizophrenia*. Washington DC: American Psychiatric Press, 1999:163–93.

35 Kline J, Stein Z, Susser M. *Conception to birth: epidemiology of prenatal development*. New York: Oxford University Press, 1989.

36 Pharoah PO, Connolly KJ. Relationship between maternal thyroxine levels during pregnancy and memory function in childhood. *Early Hum Dev* 1991;**25**:43–51.

37 Stanbury JB. Iodine and human development. *Med Anthropol* 1992;**13**:413–23.

38 Pharoah PO, Buttfield IH, Hetzel BS. Neurological damage to the fetus resulting from severe iodine deficiency during pregnancy. *Lancet* 1971;**1**:308–10.

39 Cao XY, Jiang XM, Dou ZH, Rakeman MA, Zhang ML, O'Donnell K *et al.* Timing of vulnerability of the brain to iodine deficiency in endemic cretinism. *N Engl J Med* 1994;**331**:1739–44.

*40 Haddow JE, Palomaki GE, Allan WC, Williams JR, Knight GJ, Gagnon J *et al.* Maternal thyroid deficiency during pregnancy and subsequent neuropsychological development of the child. *N Engl J Med* 1999;**341**:549–55.

41 Pop VJ, Kuijpens JL, van Baar AL, Verkerk G, van Son MM, de Vijlder JJ *et al.* Low maternal free thyroxine concentrations during early pregnancy are associated with impaired psychomotor development in infancy. *Clin Endocrinol (Oxf)* 1999;**50**:149–55.

42 Rickards AL, Ford GW, Kitchen WH, Doyle LW, Lissenden JV, Keith CG. Extremely-low-birthweight infants: neurological, psychological, growth and health status beyond five years of age. *Med J Aust* 1987;**147**:476–81.

43 Rovet J, Ehrlich R, Sorbara D. Intellectual outcome in children with fetal hypothyroidism. *J Pediatr* 1987;**110**:700–4.

44 Rovet JF, Ehrlich RM, Sorbara DL. Neurodevelopment in infants and preschool children with congenital hypothyroidism: etiological and treatment factors affecting outcome. *J Pediatr Psychol* 1992;**17**:187–213.

45 Gottschalk B, Richman RA, Lewandowski L. Subtle speech and motor deficits of children with congenital hypothyroid treated early. *Dev Med Child Neurol* 1994;**36**:216–20.

46 Fuggle PW, Grant DB, Smith I, Murphy G. Intelligence, motor skills and behaviour at 5 years in early-treated congenital hypothyroidism. *Eur J Pediatr* 1991;**150**:570–4.

47 Rochiccioli P, Roge B, Alexandre F, Tauber MT. School achievement in children with hypothyroidism detected at birth and search for predictive factors. *Horm Res* 1992;**38**:236–40.

48 Grant DB, Fuggle P, Tokar S, Smith I. Psychomotor development in infants with congenital hypothyroidism diagnosed by neonatal screening. *Acta Med Austriaca* 1992;**19 (suppl 1)**:54–6.

49 Kooistra L, Laane C, Vulsma T, Schellekens JM, van der Meere JJ, Kalverboer AF. Motor and cognitive development in children with congenital hypothyroidism: a long-term evaluation of the effects of neonatal treatment. *J Pediatr* 1994;**124**:903–9.

50 Virtanen M, Santavuori P, Hirvonen E, Perheentupa J. Multivariate analysis of psychomotor development in congenital hypothyroidism. *Acta Paediatr Scand* 1989;**78**:405–11.

51 Rovet JF, Ehrlich R. Psychoeducational outcome in children with early-treated congenital hypothyroidism. *Pediatrics* 2000;**105**:515–22.

52 New England Congenital Hypothyroidism Collaborative. Elementary school performance of children with congential hypothyroidism. *J Pediatr* 1990;**116**:27–62.

53 Heyerdahl S, Kase BF, Lie SO. Intellectual development in children with congenital hypothyroidism in relation to recommended thyroxine treatment. *J Pediatr* 1991;**118**:850–7.

54 Lucas A, Rennie J, Baker BA, Morley R. Low plasma triiodothyronine concentrations and outcome in preterm infants. *Arch Dis Child* 1988;**63**:1201–6.

55 Lucas A, Morley R, Fewtrell MS. Low triiodothyronine concentration in preterm infants and subsequent intelligence quotient (IQ) at 8 year follow up. *Br Med J* 1996;**312**:1132–3.

56 Meijer WJ, Verloove-Vanhorick SP, Brand R, van den Brande JL. Transient hypothyroxinaemia associated with developmental delay in very preterm infants. *Arch Dis Child* 1992;**67**:944–7.

57 Den Ouden AL, Kok JH, Verkerk PH, Brand R, Verloove-Vanhorick SP. The relation between neonatal thyroxine levels and neurodevelopmental outcome at age 5 and 9 years in a national cohort of very preterm and/or very low birth weight infants. *Pediatr Res* 1996;**39**:142–5.

58 Reuss ML, Paneth N, Pinto-Martin JA, Lorenz JM, Susser M. The relation of transient hypothyroxinemia in preterm infants to neurologic development at two years of age. *N Engl J Med* 1996;**334**:821–7.

59 Paneth N. Does transient hypothyroxinemia cause abnormal neurodevelopment in premature infants? *Clin Perinatol* 1998;**25**:627–43.

60 Van Wassenaer AG, Kok JH, de Vijlder JJ, Briet JM, Smit BJ, Tamminga P *et al.* Effects of thyroxine supplementation on neurologic development in infants born at less than 30 weeks' gestation. *N Engl J Med* 1997;**336**:21–6.

61 Carr E, Beierwaltes W, Raman G, Dodson V, Tanton J, Betts J *et al.* The effect of maternal thyroid function on fetal thyroid function and development. *J Clin Endocrinol Metab* 1959;**19**:1–18.

62 Greenman G, Gabrielson M, Howard-Flanders J, Wessel M. Thyroid dysfunction in pregnancy. *N Engl J Med* 1962;**267**:426–31.

63 Wasserstrum N, Anania CA. Perinatal consequences of maternal hypothyroidism in early pregnancy and inadequate replacement. *Clin Endocrinol (Oxf)* 1995;**42**:353–8.

64 Leung AS, Millar LK, Koonings PP, Montoro M, Mestman JH. Perinatal outcome in hypothyroid pregnancies. *Obstet Gynecol* 1993;**81**:349–53.

65 Haddow JE, Klein RZ, Mitchell M. Letter. *N Engl J Med* 1999;**341**:2017.

66 Man EB, Holden RH, Jones WS. Thyroid function in human pregnancy. VII. Development and retardation of 4-year-old progeny of euthyroid and of hypothyroxinemic women. *Am J Obstet Gynecol* 1971;**109**:12–19.

67 Man EB, Serunian SA. Thyroid function in human pregnancy. IX. Development or retardation of 7-year-old progeny of hypothyroxinemic women. *Am J Obstet Gynecol* 1976;**125**:949–57.

68 Man EB, Brown JF, Serunian SA. Maternal hypothyroxinemia: psychoneurological deficits of progeny. *Ann Clin Lab Sci* 1991;**21**:227–39.

*69 Porterfield SP, Hendrich CE. The role of thyroid hormones in prenatal and neonatal neurological development—current perspectives. *Endocr Rev* 1993;**14**:94–106.

70 Morreale dE, Pastor R, Obregon MJ, Escobar dR. Effects of maternal hypothyroidism on the weight and thyroid hormone content of rat embryonic tissues, before and after onset of fetal thyroid function. *Endocrinology* 1985;**117**:1890–1900.

71 Hendrich CE, Jackson WJ, Porterfield SP. Behavioral testing of progenies of Tx (hypothyroid) and growth hormone-treated Tx rats: an animal model for mental retardation. *Neuroendocrinology* 1984;**38**:429–37.

72 Sinha AK, Pickard MR, Kim KD, Ahmed MT, al Yatama F, Evans IM *et al.* Perturbation of thyroid hormone homeostasis in the adult and brain function. *Acta Med Austriaca* 1994;**21**:35–43.

73 Pickard MR, Sinha AK, Ogilvie L, Ekins RP. The influence of the maternal thyroid hormone environment during pregnancy on the ontogenesis of brain and placental ornithine decarboxylase activity in the rat. *J Endocrinol* 1993;**139**:205–12.

74 Evans IM, Sinha AK, Pickard MR, Edwards PR, Leonard AJ, Ekins RP. Maternal hypothyroxinemia disrupts neurotransmitter metabolic enzymes in developing brain. *J Endocrinol* 1999;**161**:273–9.

75 Attree E, Sinha A, Davey M, Pickard M, Rose F, Ekins R. Effects of maternal hypothyroxinemia on activity, emotional responsiveness and exploratory behaviour in adult rat progeny. *Med Sci Res* 1992;**20**:197–9.

76 Byers RK, Lord EE. Late effects of lead poisoning on mental development. *Am J Dis Child* 1943;**66**:471–94.

77 Baghurst PA, McMichael AJ, Wigg NR, Vimpani GV, Robertson EF, Roberts RJ *et al.* Environmental exposure to lead and children's intelligence at the age of seven years. The Port Pirie Cohort Study. *N Engl J Med* 1992;**327**:1279–84.

78 Bellinger D, Leviton A, Waternaux C, Needleman H, Rabinowitz M. Longitudinal analyses of prenatal and postnatal lead exposure and early cognitive development. *N Engl J Med* 1987;**316**:1037–43.

79 Bellinger D, Leviton A, Waternaux C, Needleman H, Rabinowitz M. Low-level lead exposure, social class, and infant development. *Neurotoxicol Teratol* 1988;**10**:497–503.

80 Bellinger D, Sloman J, Leviton A, Rabinowitz M, Needleman HL, Waternaux C. Low-level lead exposure and children's cognitive function in the preschool years. *Pediatrics* 1991;**87**:219–27.

81 Dietrich KN, Succop PA, Berger OG, Hammond PB, Bornschein RL. Lead exposure and the cognitive development of urban preschool children: the Cincinnati Lead Study cohort at age 4 years. *Neurotoxicol Teratol* 1991;**13**:203–11.

82 Dietrich KN, Berger OG, Succop PA, Hammond PB, Bornschein RL. The developmental consequences of low to moderate prenatal and postnatal lead exposure: intellectual attainment in the Cincinnati Lead Study Cohort following school entry. *Neurotoxicol Teratol* 1993;**15**:37–44.

83 Wasserman G, Graziano JH, Factor-Litvak P, Popovac D, Morina N, Musabegovic A *et al.* Independent effects of lead exposure and iron deficiency anemia on developmental outcome at age 2 years. *J Pediatr* 1992;**121**:695–703.

84 Wasserman GA, Graziano JH, Factor-Litvak P, Popovac D, Morina N, Musabegovic A *et al.* Consequences of lead exposure and iron supplementation on childhood development at age 4 years. *Neurotoxicol Teratol* 1994;**16**:233–240.

85 Wasserman GA, Liu X, Popovac D, Factor-Litvak P, Kline J, Waternaux C *et al.* The Yugoslavia Prospective Lead Study: contributions of prenatal and postnatal lead exposure to early intelligence. *Neurotoxicol Teratol* 2000;**22**:811–18.

86 McMichael AJ, Baghurst PA, Wigg NR, Vimpani GV, Robertson EF, Roberts RJ. Port Pirie Cohort Study: environmental exposure to lead and children's abilities at the age of four years. *N Engl J Med* 1988;**319**:468–75.

87 Ernhart CB, Morrow-Tlucak M, Wolf AW, Super D, Drotar D. Low level lead exposure in the prenatal and early preschool periods: intelligence prior to school entry. *Neurotoxicol Teratol* 1989;**11**:161–70.

88 Wasserman GA, Musabegovic A, Liu X, Kline J, Factor-Litvak P, Graziano JH. Lead exposure and motor functioning in 4(1/2)-year-old children: the Yugoslavia prospective study. *J Pediatr* 2000;**137**:555–61.

89 Wasserman GA, Staghezza-Jaramillo B, Shrout P, Popovac D, Graziano J. The effect of lead exposure on behavior problems in preschool children. *Am J Publ Health* 1998;**88**:481–6.

90 Bellinger DC, Stiles KM, Needleman HL. Low-level lead exposure, intelligence and academic achievement: a long-term follow-up study. *Pediatrics* 1992;**90**:855–61.

91 Pocock SJ, Smith M, Baghurst P. Environmental lead and children's intelligence: a systematic review of the epidemiological evidence. *Br Med J* 1994;**309**:1189–97.

*92 Schwartz J. Low-level lead exposure and children's IQ: a meta-analysis and search for a threshold. *Environ Res* 1994;**65**:42–55.

93 Needleman HL, Gatsonis CA. Low-level lead exposure and the IQ of children. A meta-analysis of modern studies. *J Am Med Assoc* 1990;**263**:673–8.

*94 Wasserman GA, Factor-Litvak P. Methodology, inference and causastion. Environmental lead exposure and childhood intelligence. *Arch Clin Neuropsych* 2000;**16**:343–52.

95 Canfield RL, Henderson CR Jr, Cory-Slechta DA, Cox C, Jusko TA, Lanphear BP. Intellectual impairment in children with blood lead concentrations below 10 microg per deciliter. *N Engl J Med* 2003;**348**:1517–26.

96 Wasserman GA, Factor-Litvak P, Liu X, Todd AC, Kline JK, Slavkovich V *et al.* The relationship between blood lead, bone lead and child intelligence. *Neuropsychol Dev Cogn Sect C Child Neuropsychol* 2003;**9**:22–34.

97 Needleman HL, Gunnoe C, Leviton A, Reed R, Peresie H, Maher C *et al.* Deficits in psychologic and classroom performance of children with elevated dentine lead levels. *N Engl J Med* 1979;**300**:689–95.

98 Yule W, Urbanowicz M, Landsdown R, Miller I. Teachers' ratings of children's behavior in relation to blood lead levels. *Br J Dev Psychol* 1984;**2**:295–305.

99 Tong S, Baghurst P, McMichael A, Sawyer M, Mudge J. Lifetime exposure to environmental lead and children's intelligence at 11–13 years: the Port Pirie cohort study. *Br Med J* 1996;**312**:1569–75.

*100 Factor-Litvak P, Wasserman G, Kline JK, Graziano J. The Yugoslavia Prospective Study of environmental lead exposure. *Environ Health Perspect* 1999;**107**:9–15.

101 Wasserman GA, Liu X, Lolacono NJ, Factor-Litvak P, Kline JK, Popovac D *et al.* Lead exposure and intelligence in 7-year-old children: the Yugoslavia Prospective Study. *Environ Health Perspect* 1997;**105**:956–62.

102 Needleman HL, Riess JA, Tobin MJ, Biesecker GE, Greenhouse JB. Bone lead levels and delinquent behavior. *J Am Med Assoc* 1996;**275**:363–9.

103 Todd AC, Buchanan R, Carroll S, Moshier EL, Popovac D, Slavkovich V *et al.* Tibia lead levels and methodological uncertainty in 12-year-old children. *Environ Res* 2001;**86**:60–5.

104 Barry PS. Concentrations of lead in the tissues of children. *Br J Ind Med* 1981;**38**:61–71.

105 Leggett RW. An age-specific kinetic model of lead metabolism in humans. *Environ Health Perspect* 1993;**101**:598–616.

106 Schroeder HA, Tipton IH. The human body burden of lead. *Arch Environ Health* 1968;**17**:965–78.

107 Todd AC, McNeill FE, Palethorpe JE, Peach DE, Chettle DR, Tobin MJ *et al.* In vivo X-ray fluorescence of lead in bone using K X-ray excitation with 109Cd sources: radiation dosimetry studies. *Environ Res* 1992;**57**:117–32.

108 Cheng Y, Schwartz J, Sparrow D, Aro A, Weiss ST, Hu H. Bone lead and blood lead levels in relation to baseline blood pressure and the prospective development of hypertension: the Normative Aging Study. *Am J Epidemiol* 2001;**53**:164–71.

109 Bernard AM, Vyskocil A, Roels H, Kriz J, Kodl M, Lauwerys R. Renal effects in children living in the vicinity of a lead smelter. *Environ Res* 1995;**68**:91–5.

110 Hu H, Watanabe H, Payton M, Korrick S, Rotnitzky A. The relationship between bone lead and hemoglobin. *J Am Med Assoc* 1994;**272**:1512–17.

111 Stewart WF, Schwartz BS, Simon D, Bolla KI, Todd AC, Links J. Neurobehavioral function and tibial and chelatable lead levels in 543 former organolead workers. *Neurology* 1999;**52**:1610–17.

112 Finkelstein Y, Markowitz ME, Rosen JF. Low-level lead-induced neurotoxicity in children: an update on central nervous system effects. *Brain Res Rev* 1998;**27**:168–76.

113 Johnston MV, Goldstein GW. Selective vulnerability of the developing brain to lead. *Curr Opin Neurol* 1998;**11**:689–93.

114 Trope I, Lopez-Villegas D, Lenkinski RE. Magnetic resonance imaging and spectroscopy of regional brain structure in a 10-year-old boy with elevated blood lead levels. *Pediatrics* 1998;**101**:E7.

115 Chanoine JP, Alex S, Fang SL, Stone S, Leonard JL, Korhle J *et al.* Role of transthyretin in the transport of thyroxine from the blood to the choroid plexus, the cerebrospinal fluid, and the brain. *Endocrinology* 1992;**130**:933–8.

116 Manton WI, Kirkpatrick JB, Cook JD. Does the choroid plexus really protect the brain from lead? *Lancet* 1984;**2**:351.

117 Zheng W, Perry DF, Nelson DL, Aposhian HV. Choroid plexus protects cerebrospinal fluid against toxic metals. *FASEB J* 1991;**5**:2188–93.

118 **Zheng W, Blaner WS, Zhao Q.** Inhibition by lead of production and secretion of transthyretin in the choroid plexus: its relation to thyroxine transport at blood–CSF barrier. *Toxicol Appl Pharmacol* 1999;**155**:24–31.

119 **Zheng W, Shen H, Blaner WS, Zhao Q, Ren X, Graziano JH.** Chronic lead exposure alters transthyretin concentration in rat cerebrospinal fluid: the role of the choroid plexus. *Toxicol Appl Pharmacol* 1996;**139**:445–50.

120 **Mortimer JA.** Brain reserve and the clinical expression of Alzheimer's disease. *Geriatrics* 1997;**52 (suppl 2)**:S50–3.

121 **Katzman R.** Education and the prevalence of dementia and Alzheimer's disease. *Neurology* 1993;**43**:13–20.

122 **Satz P, Morgenstern H, Miller EN, Selnes OA, McArthur JC, Cohen BA *et al.*** Low education as a possible risk factor for cognitive abnormalities in HIV-1: findings from the multicenter AIDS Cohort Study (MACS). *J Acquir Immune Defic Syndr* 1993;**6**:503–11.

*123 **Stern Y.** What is cognitive reserve? Theory and research application of the reserve concept. *J Int Neuropsychol Soc* 2002;**8**:448–60.

124 **Schmand B, Smit JH, Geerlings MI, Lindeboom J.** The effects of intelligence and education on the development of dementia. A test of the brain reserve hypothesis. *Psychol Med* 1997;**27**:1337–44.

125 **Kaplan GA.** People and places: contrasting perspectives on the association between social class and health. *Int J Health Serv* 1996;**26**:507–19.

126 **Barnett E, Casper M.** A definition of "social environment". *Am J Pub Health* 2001;**91**:465.

127 **Hughes ME, Waite LJ.** Health in household context: living arrangements and health in late middle age. *J Health Soc Behav* 2002;**43**:1–21.

128 **Storch SA, Whitehurst GJ.** The role of family and home in the literacy development of children from low-income backgrounds. *New Dir Child Adolesc Dev* 2001;**92**:53–71.

129 **Caldwell BM, Bradley RH.** *Revised administration manual for the home observation for measurements of the environment.* Little Rock: University of Arkansas, 1984.

130 **Richards M, Sacker A.** Lifetime antecedents of cognitive reserve. *J Clin Exp Neuropsychol* 2003;**25**:614–24.

Part III

Biological and social processes

Chapter 15

Fetal growth and development: the role of nutrition and other factors

Ivan J. Perry and L.H. Lumey

The risk of cardiovascular disease (CVD) and diabetes in adult life may be programmed *in utero* by specific patterns of abnormal fetal growth associated with maternal undernutrition. This nutritional programming hypothesis raises fundamental questions about patterns and determinants of fetal growth *in utero,* including the role of factors other than maternal nutrition in fetal growth and development. In developing and testing specific predictions from the nutritional programming hypothesis we need to consider the mother's diet, her growth and development in childhood, as well as her diet during pregnancy and we should distinguish between maternal nutrition and fetal nutrition. The concept of *in utero* nutritional programming of chronic disease is undoubtedly plausible in biological terms. However, we need a less discrete and deterministic model of programming. We are moving away from a simple critical period model of programming focused on nutritional deficits *in utero* towards a broader, life course model of programming, involving interactions between a range of early life factors acting at different levels. These include (1) the maternal and fetal genotype, (2) the mother's environment and lifestyle (including diet) before and during pregnancy, (3) her prepregnancy nutritional status, metabolism, and physiology, (4) the hormonal, metabolic, and circulatory milieu during pregnancy, which sustains fetal nutrition and growth, and (5) the infant's postnatal environment. The effects of prenatal nutrition on fetal growth in people depend on the timing of nutritional exposures in relation to critical periods of development and on interactions with the mother's prepregnancy nutritional status and aspects of the mother's metabolism and physiology such as glucose tolerance and blood pressure. Given an environment with adequate nutrition to sustain optimal growth in a girl's childhood and adolescence, dietary intake during pregnancy probably accounts for a small amount of variation in fetal growth. However there is a need for additional studies of prenatal diet, fetal growth rates during pregnancy, and pregnancy outcome that address problems of measurement error and explore interactions between dietary exposures and the mother's metabolism and physiology. Although a general hypothesis regarding the impact of maternal nutrition on fetal growth and *in utero* programming has been formulated and has inspired a large number of studies, there have been few attempts to test component parts of the theory. Further advances in the field therefore await research designs that address specific and critical predictions from well-defined hypotheses.

15.1 Introduction

The health of mothers and infants is a central public health concern and the notion that poor nutrition at critical periods of development in fetal life is a key determinant of health in childhood and adult life[1,2] has considerable resonance. Thus, the nutritional programming hypothesis has helped refocus interest in the role of maternal nutrition in fetal growth and development. This work, which has provided such a valuable millennial fillip for chronic adult disease epidemiology, also raises fundamental questions about patterns of fetal growth *in utero* and about the role of factors other than nutrition in fetal growth and development. It has become clear that nutrition needs to be placed in context within the broader framework of other maternal, fetal, and uterine/placental factors that are known to influence fetal growth.[3–6] In particular we need to distinguish between maternal nutrition, the mother's nutritional status and diet during pregnancy, and fetal nutrition, the net supply of metabolic substrate to the fetus.[7]

15.1.1 Fetal origins: a conceptual framework

Various markers of fetal growth are consistently associated with CVD risk.[1,2,8–11] It remains unclear however, as to whether these associations are primarily a manifestation of intrauterine 'programming' of CVD risk due to poor maternal nutrition or 'programming' due to other influences *in utero* unrelated to maternal undernutrition, such as defective placentation, maternal glucose intolerance, hypertension, or other aspects of the maternal hormonal, metabolic, or circulatory milieu. Alternatively, the associations between low birthweight and later disease may be merely statistical or artefactual and without biological meaning, confounded by genetic factors related to both low birthweight and CVD, or confounded by prenatal or postnatal environmental factors (notably poverty and social disadvantage) that link mother and infant.[12,13] In this context it is noteworthy that we now have evidence from a systematic review to suggest that we may have substantially overestimated the magnitude of the association between birthweight and blood pressure, one of the more exciting findings from the early work on the Barker hypothesis. The size of the birthweight–blood pressure effect falls with increasing study sample size, raising concerns about publication bias.[14] The dependence of the birthweight–blood pressure association on adjustment for current body weight is an additional source of concern, raising the possibility that increased postnatal 'catch-up' growth is the critical factor.[14,15]

The focus of this review is on sources of variation in fetal growth, in particular the role of nutrition (and markers of maternal nutritional status including height, pregravid weight, and gestational weight gain) in the context of the fetal nutritional programming hypothesis.[12] This hypothesis has relied heavily on specific assumptions about the effects on fetal growth of maternal undernutrition at critical periods of fetal development. However the hypothesis is largely based on studies showing associations between size at birth and risk of CVD and diabetes. These associations are linked only through the (untested) general hypothesis that maternal nutrition during specific periods in pregnancy drives size/form/proportionality at birth, which in turn drives risk of CVD and diabetes. This remains largely speculative. In 'normal' human populations it would be hard to find empirical data to refute or support this general hypothesis because variations in exposure are limited and ill defined. Relevant data are available from two so-called 'natural experiments', the Dutch famine and Leningrad siege studies. Here exposures are better defined, and offer some chance to clarify the role of nutrition *per se* on adult health.[16–19] Contrary to predictions from the fetal nutritional programming hypothesis as initially formulated by Barker,[2,20] these studies have clarified that even in maternal starvation conditions, fetal growth is only affected in the third trimester of pregnancy. However the famine studies do not provide information on the growth rate of particular organs relative to overall size. These issues need further exploration.[7] It should also be noted that the current formulation of the nutritional programming hypothesis is more cautious and no longer includes specific effects of fetal undernutrition in different trimesters in pregnancy.[21]

Against this background, there is clearly a need to broaden the concept of fetal/nutritional programming, to consider a wider canvas, such as that in Fig. 15.1, which includes

1. the fetal genotype;
2. the maternal genotype;
3. the mother's social and physical environment;
4. the mother's prepregnancy nutritional status, metabolism, and physiology;
5. her diet, lifestyle, and behaviour during pregnancy;
6. the resultant hormonal, metabolic, and circulatory milieu that sustains fetal growth;
7. the infant's postnatal environment, including factors influencing early growth rates.

Within this framework, the influence of the fetal and maternal genotype on fetal growth will be considered and it will be set in the context of non-genetic intergenerational influences on birthweight such as the mother's height and her own birthweight. The concept of programming will be considered both with reference to nutritional programming and a wider view of programming (as set out in Fig 15.1) with particular reference to the hormonal, metabolic, and circulatory milieu to which the fetus is exposed. The role of wider social, behavioural, and environmental influences on fetal growth, such as cigarette smoking[22] and physical work load during pregnancy[23] will not be reviewed. Given a life course perspective, there is a continuum of genetic, intrauterine, and postnatal influences on adult disease. Clearly therefore, in the context of links between growth and development *in utero* and adult disease, there is a potentially important role for a wide range of adverse social, behavioural, and environmental factors that plausibly link maternal health, fetal growth, and chronic disease in adult life. However, discussion of these factors is beyond the scope of this chapter.

At the outset, the need for clear concepts and definitions of both 'maternal nutrition' and 'retarded or abnormal fetal growth' is paramount.

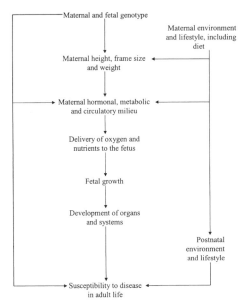

Fig. 15.1 Fetal origins of adult disease: a conceptual framework.

15.2 **Methodological issues and definitions**

15.2.1 **Maternal nutrition**

The reliable measurement of nutrition and nutritional status, however defined, presents formidable problems.[24] A broad concept of maternal nutrition may be used, such as that advanced by Barker:[25]

> ... I mean nutrients including oxygen. The nutrients that get to the fetus are clearly related to the many aspects of the mother's physiology, her preconceptual stores, her competence to sustain fetal growth and maybe to a minor extent what she eats in pregnancy, and whether the mother exercises in pregnancy. Delivery of nutrients to the fetus is a very complicated agenda. (p. 238)

Although it is difficult to quibble with such a comprehensive and all-embracing concept of maternal nutrition, there is potential for confusion between maternal nutritional intake/nutritional status and other factors further along the fetal supply line[7] that critically influence fetal nutrition, such as the mother's level of blood pressure or glucose tolerance and factors influencing placental function. It is not clear whether such a broad concept of nutrition facilitates the testing of precisely formulated hypotheses. Here, the term maternal nutrition refers to nutritional intake during pregnancy, that is, intake of calories and of macro- and micronutrients and nutritional status as measured by markers such as prepregnancy weight and height.

15.2.2 **Fetal growth**

The fertilized ovum faces three interrelated challenges *in utero*: (1) implantation and survival, (2) differentiation or the development of new structures, and (3) growth.

These challenges correspond approximately to the blastogenic, embryonic, and fetal phases of development. Growth during the blastogenic and embryonic phases of development, which span the first 8 postovulatory weeks, consists of an increase in cell numbers (hyperplasia). By the end of this period, the embryo is only about 3 cm long and weighs approximately 6 g but has already developed several thousand structures.[26] The fetal phase of development, from the third through the ninth month, is characterized by both hyperplasia, an increase in the number of cells and by hypertrophy, an increase in the size of existing cells, with the latter gradually becoming predominant.[27] In the first half of pregnancy the length of the fetus increases rapidly with peak length growth velocity before 20 weeks. By contrast, the rate of increase in fetal weight does not peak until the third trimester, between 30 and 32 weeks.[28,29]

The definition of normal and abnormal fetal growth has long been beset by confusion and controversy. For obvious reasons, work in this area has focused on the identification of a minority of infants at high risk of morbidity and mortality in the neonatal period. Birthweight is consistently and reliably recorded and is a good predictor of neonatal death and other adverse outcomes.[30] Early work focused on 'maturity' at birth and the concept of *in utero* growth failure did not emerge until the 1940s.[3] Infants weighing 2.5 kg or less are at substantially increased risk of adverse outcomes and until the 1960s, such infants were described as 'premature'. Work in the early 1960s highlighted the fact that low birthweight infants are a mixture of those born too soon ('preterm') and those born too small ('small for dates'). The concept of 'small for dates' or 'growth retardation', which then emerged, was based on the distribution of birthweight by gestational age in various reference populations[31] with an arbitrary cut-off point, usually at the 10th or 3rd percentile. Although theoretically attractive, adjustment of birthweight for gestational age was not a major advance in efforts to identify fetal growth retardation, as gestational age at birth is measured with low reliability relative to birthweight. Moreover, different populations have different fetal growth norms, depending on factors such as ethnic origin,[6] maternal height,[32] and altitude.[33] These differences, which highlight the important distinctions between 'statistically normal', 'clinically normal', and 'biologically ideal' fetal growth, provide the basis for the development of customized birthweight standards based on factors such as maternal height, weight, parity, gestation at delivery, and fetal sex.[34–36] Compared with population-based standards, customized birthweight standards improve prediction of adverse outcomes probably due to improved identification of fetal growth restriction relative to biological potential.[36] However it needs to be emphasized that the distinction between being born 'too soon' and 'too small' is often blurred. Preterm and 'small for gestational age' births share many common antecedents such as maternal short stature[30] and in studies of placental morphology a number of similar histopathological abnormalities are documented in these syndromes.[37] Thus fetal growth norms based on infants born at 34 weeks' gestation do not provide an unbiased reflection of normal fetal growth at this gestation. Similarly, studies of fetal growth retardation at 'term' probably exclude a severely affected subgroup of infants, those born too soon and too small.

15.2.2.1 Birthweight: a complex variable

The work on customized birthweight standards emphasizes the complexity of birthweight as a variable and the limitations of absolute birthweight data. Wilcox has described birthweight as 'one of the most accessible and most misunderstood variables in epidemiology'.[38] The frequency distribution of birthweight is normal with an extended lower tail (Fig. 15.2).[38] The normal component of the distribution, called the 'predominant' distribution, corresponds to the birthweight distribution of term births (≥37 weeks gestation) whereas the majority of births in the 'residual' distribution are small and preterm, a group of infants at particularly high risk. The predominant and residual distributions are at least partially independent of each other as exposures that affect fetal growth will not necessarily affect preterm births to the same extent and vice versa. Thus small changes in population mean birthweight will not invariably lead to more pronounced changes in the proportion of individuals in the lower tail of the frequency distribution. Birthweight has a reverse-J relationship with neonatal and infant mortality, observed in all populations and unchanged over time, despite falling mortality rates (Fig. 15.3).[38] If birthweight is treated as an absolute measure, certain groups of infants known to have higher neonatal mortality, such as those born to smokers, are found (contrary to expectation) to have better outcomes at low birthweight relative to lower risk groups, such as those born to non-smokers. This so-called birthweight paradox is resolved by transformation of birthweights to within-population z-scores, a relative scale. In analyses of the transformed data, the infants of smokers have higher mortality at all relative birthweights. In the context of these data, Wilcox has argued that we must be cautious in ascribing a mediating and causal role to birthweight in assessing the relationship between an adverse exposure in pregnancy (smoking in this instance) and neonatal mortality. This argument has clear implications for the Barker hypothesis in which it is assumed that reduced birthweight mediates the effect of fetal malnutrition on adult disease outcomes.[38]

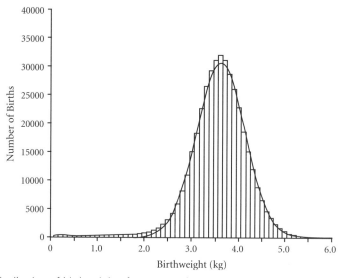

Fig. 15.2 Distribution of birthweights for 405 676 live and still births, Norway, 1992–1998.[38]

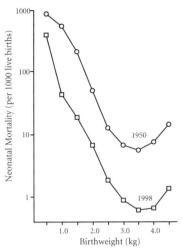

Fig. 15.3 Weight-specific neonatal mortality, USA, 1950 and 1998.[38]

15.2.2.2 Symmetrical and asymmetrical growth retardation

Much work in recent decades has addressed the need to further 'disaggregate' low birthweight with a view to elucidating specific aetiological factors. In a series of post-mortem studies on infants with birthweight below two standard deviations for gestation, Gruenwald highlighted the extent to which the effects of growth retardation are uneven or 'asymmetrical' in the majority of such infants.[39] These infants tend to have relatively large heads, a modest reduction in length relative to the reduction in weight, and thinner skinfolds. The greatest reduction in weight occurs in organs such as the liver and thymus and the least in brain weight. It is suggested that such disproportionate fetal growth reflects an inadequate supply of oxygen or nutrients (failure of the supply line) at the time of rapid increase in fetal weight in middle to late gestation but after the peak in fetal length growth velocity.[3,28,29] By contrast, it is suggested that symmetrical growth retardation, with equal reduction in brain and body size and normal skinfold thickness, is either a normal variant, reflecting low genetic growth potential or is due to adverse influences acting in early pregnancy, during the phase of cellular hyperplasia,[27] which set the fetus on a low growth trajectory. While this is a plausible model of fetal growth, we cannot necessarily assume that Gruenwald's findings apply to infants of normal birthweight.

This concept of early down-regulation of fetal growth leading to 'proportionate' fetal growth retardation was central to the development of the nutritional programming (or fetal origins) hypothesis, particularly in its early incarnation.[20] It was suggested for instance that coronary heart disease (CHD) is not associated with proportionate fetal growth arising from nutritional insults in early gestation but with disproportionate growth due to nutritional deprivation in mid and late gestation.[20] This allowed the nutritional programming hypothesis to accommodate historical and geographical trends in CHD rates that would otherwise seem inconsistent with a major aetiological role for fetal growth retardation. For example, in most Western industrialized countries CHD mortality was lower at the turn of the century than in the 1950s and it is difficult to reconcile these trends with changes in fetal nutrition and growth. Similarly, it is suggested that the relatively low rates of CHD in developing countries such as China, despite evidence of suboptimal maternal nutrition extending over a prolonged period, reflect 'proportionate' fetal growth retardation.[2]

Unsurprisingly, this model of fetal growth has attracted sceptical commentary.[40] Kramer has argued that fetal growth retardation is largely a third-trimester phenomenon, as fetal growth in early pregnancy requires relatively little nutritional support and therefore the notion of an early nutritional insult, which determines body proportions, is implausible.[40] These observations are primarily based on births under war-time famine conditions, in which the timing of nutrition deprivation relative to the stage of pregnancy can be determined.[16,41] It will be a challenge to test this model of fetal growth in 'normal' populations with a limited range of nutritional and other exposures. In this context it should also be noted that many populations in developing countries have mean birthweights that are similar to those in industrialized countries and growth failure in these environments is largely a postnatal phenomenon.[42]

The concept that an *in utero* insult in the third trimester produces disproportionate fetal growth seems more plausible, although in practice, reliable differentiation between symmetrical and asymmetrical growth retardation is often difficult.[4] In particular, the concept of brain sparing in asymmetrical growth retardation has proved difficult to document in all but the most extreme cases.[43] Examination of large human data sets has revealed a continuum of changes in body proportions as opposed to two distinct populations of infants with symmetrical and assymetrical growth restriction.[44] Moreover there is no evidence from studies involving serial ultrasound measurements in pregnancy that symmetric and asymmetric growth retardation are associated with clear temporal differences in patterns of fetal growth.[45] Ponderal index at birth (weight/length^3) is advanced as a continuous measure of fetal growth asymmetry. Ponderal index, essentially a measure of fatness/thinness at birth, is undoubtedly more sensitive to intrauterine adversity than birthweight[46] and is predictive of poor neonatal outcome.[47–49] Unfortunately, the usefulness of ponderal index and other indices such as the ratio of head circumference to length is constrained by measurement error, in particular measurement of length at birth. Ponderal index is reported to be a poor predictor of skinfold thickness at birth[50] and in a study of high-risk pregnancies it has been shown not to predict fetal growth velocity (based on serial ultrasound scans from 27 weeks) after adjustment for birthweight and gestational age.[51] Moreover, as ponderal index is highly correlated with birthweight[52] it needs to be evaluated in relation to birthweight rather than against a single absolute standard for the whole population. Thus the lower end of the normal range of ponderal index for infants weighing 3500 g is higher than for infants weighing 2500 g. This highlights the difficulty of identifying infants with birthweight and length within the normal range but with fetal growth retardation relative to their genetic growth potential. The use of postnatal catch-up growth[53] represents an interesting approach to this problem, although clearly the use of this measure raises concerns about variation in the rate of catch-up growth depending on the underlying cause and interactions with the level of nutritional and emotional support in the postnatal environment. In studies of the late effects of fetal growth retardation in adults, the use of birthweight relative to attained adult height[9] represents a similar approach to this problem, which although elegant is clearly imprecise. Thus, reliable measures of fetal growth retardation, which represent a substantial advance on birthweight combined with accurate gestational age, remain elusive. Ultimately, longitudinal studies from early pregnancy using advances in ultrasonographic biometry and fetal Doppler technology combined with relatively hard endpoints such as postnatal catch-up growth under highly standardized, optimal conditions may allow more reliable definition and characterization of fetal growth retardation.[54]

15.3 Sources of variation in fetal growth and fetal programming

Size at birth is clearly a complex outcome that depends on a host of different influences. Classification is arbitrary and difficult and inevitably incomplete (Table 15.1). Broadly, we need to consider:

1. the fetal genotype;
2. the maternal genotype;
3. other stable maternal characteristics such as height, pelvic frame size, other indirect markers of lifelong nutritional status, and maternal birthweight;
4. a range of specific influences related to placental function and the uterine environment such as defective placentation, which is linked to both 'idiopathic' intrauterine growth retardation, preeclampsia, and preterm birth;
5. maternal characteristics that vary between pregnancies such as age, parity, prepregnancy weight, gestational weight gain, smoking, and diet;
6. factors in the general environment, of which altitude is an obvious example, with a fall in mean birthweight of 100 g per 1000 m above sea level.[33]

Estimates of the proportion of variation in birthweight explained by these different factors in a Western industrialized setting vary. The data from a birthweight variance modelling study[55] suggest that between 10% and 15% is explained by the fetal genotype, approximately 25% by maternal genotype and other stable characteristics of the mother, some 20% by maternal factors that vary between pregnancies, with the remainder due to ill-defined factors related to placental function and the uterine environment. In the US Collaborative Perinatal Project on births between 1959 and 1960, only 30% of the variance in birthweight could be accounted for by factors observable at birth. Of these, pregnancy weight gain, maternal prepregnant weight, birth of a previous low birthweight infant, and maternal smoking combined accounted for 19% of birthweight variance.[56] There is evidence that mean birthweight has increased in some developed and developing countries over the last quarter century.[57–59] For instance, Kramer and colleagues have described significant increases in mean birthweight among infants of ≥37 weeks gestation in a hospital-based cohort of over 60 000 births, between 1978 and 1996. This temporal trend in fetal growth was largely explained by increases in prepregnancy body mass index, gestational weight gain, and gestational diabetes and reductions in maternal cigarette smoking and postterm delivery.[59]

Table 15.1 Factors known to influence fetal growth

Fetal and maternal genotype

Maternal factors

Age
Parity
Height/frame size, 'maternal constraint of fetal growth'
Maternal birthweight
Prepregnancy weight
Weight gain during pregnancy
Obstetric history (including previous still birth and birthweight of previous infants)
Hypertension and preeclampsia
Glucose tolerance and diabetes
Other chronic maternal disease, for example, renal impairment, antiphospholipid syndrome
Maternal anaemia
Cigarette smoking
Ethnic origin
Socioeconomic status
Social support
Physical activity level
Physical work load during pregnancy
Alcohol consumption
Illicit drug use
Nutrition

Fetal factors

Sex
Multiple pregnancy
Chromosomal anomalies
Inborn errors of metabolism

Placental factors/uterine environment

Reduced placental blood flow (uteroplacental hypoperfusion)
Other placental and cord abnormalities
Intrauterine infections

General environment factors

Altitude
Environmental pollution, for example, lead

15.3.1 Fetal and maternal genotype and familial clustering of birthweight

There is a strong tendency for consecutive births to the same mother to have similar birthweights. The birthweight correlation coefficient (r) between full siblings range from 0.36 to 0.62, with a median of approximately 0.5.[55] However, paternal half-siblings (that is, same father but different mother) show a much lower correlation ($r=0.1$) than maternal half siblings ($r=0.5$).[55] This suggests that the fetal genotype makes a relatively small contribution to variation in birthweight unless there is a marked effect of mitochondrial DNA that is only transmitted on the maternal side, which seems unlikley. Indeed it is clear that familial clustering of birthweight is largely determined by maternal factors, including the maternal genotype, but mainly by non-genetic factors, including maternal size and the mother's own birthweight.[60,61] The importance of maternal size was demonstrated by Walton and Hammond's classic cross-mating study of Shire horses and Shetland ponies.[62] The mares of these breeds differ four fold in size. The hybrid foal from the Shetland mare was small, Shetland-sized, whereas the Shire mare's foal from the same hybridization was three times larger. These observations, which have been replicated in other animals, including cattle and mice, suggest that 'maternal or uterine constraint' is an important determinant of fetal growth. However, studies in mice and other evidence, such as the late pregnancy tapering of growth in twin human pregnancies, suggest that 'constraint' of fetal growth is mainly a late-gestation phenomenon.[3]

There is considerable evidence that the mother's own birthweight contributes to non-genetic familial clustering of birthweight, interacting with other maternal factors.[61,63] In the US 1988 National Maternal and Infant Health Survey, the risk of delivering a low birthweight infant (< 2.5 kg) was increased over 14 fold (in multivariate analysis) among mothers who themselves were low birthweight and had a history of a previous low birthweight child relative to a baseline group of mothers of normal birthweight and with a previous child of normal birthweight. The relative risk (RR) of low birth-weight was intermediate among mothers with low birthweight but with a previous infant of normal birthweight (RR = 2.6) and among those of normal birthweight but with a previous low birthweight infant (RR = 5.4). These effects were seen clearly in white and black mothers and in smokers and non-smokers and were independent of a wide range of covariates, including maternal height, prepregnancy weight, education, parity, and pregnancy interval.[63] Wang and colleagues hypothesize that these intergen-erational effects are due to *in utero* programming of postnatal reproductive function.[63] As with the general programming hypothesis, this is arguably a speculative leap from birth to child bearing across a considerable expanse of potential confounders. It also raises the questions of what is meant by programming and whether the concept of pro-gramming is biologically plausible. Before addressing these questions, it is worth noting that the magnitude of the relationship between maternal and offspring birthweights was little affected by the sharp decrease in maternal birthweights during the Dutch famine of 1944–1945.[64] This observation argues against the hypothesis put forward by Wang and colleagues. On the other hand, programming of reproductive function not related to maternal birthweight could be operating because women born following first-trimester famine exposure were themselves of normal birthweight but their children, in the next generation, did not show the usual birthweight increase with parity.[65] This suggests that the timing of the insult is of critical importance.

15.3.2 **Programming**

Programming is said to occur when an early stimulus or insult, operating at a critical or sensitive period, results in a permanent or long-term change in the structure or function of the organism.[15] Nature is replete with examples of programming.[2] A clear example of the phenomenon is the lifelong effect of early exposure to sex hormones on sexual physiology. For example, a female rat injected with testosterone on the 5th day after birth will develop normally until puberty but will fail to ovulate or show normal patterns of female sexual behaviour thereafter. The release of gonadotropin by the hypothalamus has been irreversibly altered from the cyclical female pattern to the tonic male pattern. The same injection of testosterone given a few days later has little effect on reproductive function.[66] In the American alligator, the temperature at which eggs are hatched determines not only the sex of the offspring but also postnatal growth rate, skin pigmentation, and the animal's preferred temperature in adult life, with alligators gravitating towards an environment that has the same temperature as the one in which they were hatched.[67]

15.3.3 Programming and nutrition

Closer to the current discussion, Winick and Noble, in the late 1960s, studied rats severely deprived of protein at different stages of early brain development and subsequently rehabilitated. In early gestation, when the cells were rapidly multiplying (hyperplastic growth) there was evidence from biochemical measures of DNA and RNA that the number of cells was irreversibly depleted and the effects of dietary restriction were permanent, whereas in later gestation, when the cells were enlarging but were no longer hyperplastic, the effects of diet were reversible.[27] On the basis of similar experiments in the 1960s, McCance and Widdowson postulated a critical period early in development when the regulating centres of the hypothalamus are being coordinated with rate of growth.[68] They showed, for instance, that rats undernourished from 3 to 6 weeks after birth remained permanently small whereas similar deprivation between 9 and 12 weeks was followed by catch-up growth.[69] Apart from effects on growth, there is evidence from animal models of programming effects of maternal nutrition on specific aspects of the offspring's physiology. For instance, pregnant rats starved in early pregnancy and then nutritionally rehabilitated produce obese offspring[70] and rats born to mothers given a low-protein diet before and during pregnancy have been shown to have persistently raised blood pressure.[71] The data from human studies are more limited. Belizan and colleagues have followed a cohort of over 500 children whose mothers were randomly assigned during pregnancy to receive 2 g/day of elemental calcium or placebo. At age 7 years, mean systolic blood pressure was lower in the calcium group although the effect was largely confined to children of above-average weight.[72] Overnutrition at critical periods can also have long-term consequences. Using data from Lucas's nutritional intervention studies, it has been shown that adolescents born preterm who were randomized to a lower-nutrient diet, now recognized to be suboptimal in terms of growth, had lower fasting 32–33 split proinsulin concentrations—markers of insulin resistance—than those given a nutrient-enriched diet.[73] These findings, which are consistent with animal experimental data, were largely explained by differences in rates of catch-up growth between the two groups of children. The relationship between birthweight and markers of insulin resistance in this study was displaced by postnatal weight gain. The data from this study extend and broaden the nutritional programming hypothesis from the original critical period model.[74] In particular they provide further evidence of the importance of postnatal 'catch-up' growth in interpreting associations between markers of fetal growth and adult health outcomes.

15.3.3.1 Programming and the maternal uterine milieu

Diet during pregnancy influences the maternal uterine milieu, interacting with the mother's prepregnancy nutritional status, metabolism, and physiology. There is evidence from animal experiments and in humans that the hormonal, metabolic, and circulatory milieu in which the fetus finds itself can exert long-term effects on physiology and risk of disease in adult life. In the rat, it has been shown that changes in the glucose concentrations to which the fetus is exposed produce effects on glucose tolerance in the offspring that persist through several generations, mimicking genetic transmission.[75] While these are fascinating data, they should (as with all data from animal models) be interpreted cautiously, given the marked differences in nutritional requirements and rates of development between different species.[7] However, in the Pima Indian community, the children of mothers with diabetes during pregnancy were found to have a substantially higher prevalence of diabetes (45%) at age 20–24 years than the children of women who developed diabetes after pregnancy (8.4%).[76] Freinkel suggests that various factors associated with the diabetic intrauterine environment, such as elevated concentrations of glucose, ketones, amino acids, and lipids, exert direct effects on the developing fetus ('fuel mediated teratogenesis'), which confer a higher risk of obesity, insulin resistance, and abnormal glucose tolerance in childhood and early adult life.[77]

These observations further extend the notion of programming from a narrow focus on the effects of nutritional deprivation in pregnancy or on the effects of other well-circumscribed insults[78] to a broader concept, which includes wide ranging but often more subtle perturbations of the uterine environment. This broader concept however, raises questions about the feasibility of isolating specific programming effects in human populations, particularly 'nutritional programming' effects from the wider canvas of potential modulators of the uterine environment in which the pregnancy is sustained, as summarized in Fig. 15.1. In particular, the opportunity to evaluate several hypothesized programming effects in experimental studies among human populations will be limited. The difficulty we face in attempting to isolate specific 'nutritional programming' effects is well illustrated when we consider the effects of maternal blood pressure on fetal growth and the interrelations between preeclampsia, maternal hypertension, preterm birth, and idiopathic fetal growth retardation.

15.3.3.2 Preeclampsia, maternal hypertension, and idiopathic fetal growth retardation

Preeclampsia is a syndrome peculiar to human pregnancy, characterized clinically by hypertension and proteinuria. Preeclampsia, especially if severe, poses a significant threat to the health and well-being of the mother and is associated with marked derangement of uteroplacental blood flow (uteroplacental ischaemia) with high risk of fetal growth retardation.[79] Women with established essential hypertension at the outset of pregnancy are at increased risk of developing preeclampsia[79,80] and they are at substantially increased risk of giving birth to a growth retarded infant regardless of whether they develop preeclampsia. It has been assumed that aside from these specific hypertensive syndromes, maternal blood pressure levels do not influence fetal growth. However there is now evidence, from studies involving measurements of 24 h ambulatory blood pressure in pregnancy, that there is a continuous inverse association between blood pressure across the normal and the hypertensive range and fetal growth as reflected by birthweight, ponderal index, and infant's head circumference.[81,82] Thus there is evidence that both pathological and 'high normal' blood pressure are associated with reduced fetal growth. These observations raise the possibility that the reported associations between retarded fetal growth and adult hypertension are confounded by maternal blood pressure, which is associated with both fetal growth retardation via placental vascular insufficiency and with hypertension in the offspring via the shared genes and environment that link a mother and her child. In this particular case it is not clear that one needs to invoke a specific hypothesis involving maternal nutrition and intrauterine programming.

15.3.3.3 Preeclampsia, preterm birth, and diopathic fetal growth retardation

In a significant minority of cases of fetal growth retardation no predisposing maternal or fetal factors are identified. Although this is a heterogenous group, there is considerable evidence that abnormal or defective placentation is an important element in the pathogenesis of idiopathic fetal growth retardation.[83,84] The key placental changes are failure of placental trophoblastic invasion of the uterine spiral arteries with failure to convert these arteries into low resistance utero-placental vessels and 'acute atherosis' of the spiral arteries supplying the placenta. This latter term refers to fibrinoid necrosis of the arterial wall with an intramural accumulation of fat laden macrophages and a perivascular mononuclear cell infiltrate.[83] The pathogenesis of acute atherosis is unknown but an immunological basis is suspected. These placental changes however are not specific to idiopathic intrauterine growth retardation but are also observed in cases of preeclampsia[83,84] and to a lesser extent in cases of preterm birth.[37] Idiopathic intrauterine growth retardation and preeclampsia share similar haemodynamic abnormalities in pregnancy, including a relative failure of the early pregnancy expansion of the maternal vascular compartment, which normally leads to a fall in blood pressure and increased cardiac output in anticipation of the higher demands for flow, nutrients, and oxygen in late pregnancy.[85] This suggests that some cases of idiopathic intrauterine growth retardation form part of a broader syndrome or spectrum of disorders (including preeclampsia and preterm birth), characterized by failure of maternal circulatory adaptation to the presence of trophoblastic tissue.[85,86] The ultimate causes of this syndrome are unknown. A derangement of maternal–fetal immunological tolerance is likely to emerge as an important factor.[87] There is also considerable evidence that the development of preeclampsia is substantially influenced by maternal factors linked to CVD, including obesity, dyslipidaemia, and insulin resistance[80,88,89] and possibly diet[90] and infection.[91] It is also clear that women who develop preeclampsia are at increased risk of CVD in later adult life.[92] Moreover, women with low birthweight offspring are at increased risk of subsequent CVD[93] and insulin resistance.[94] These observations provide further support for the hypothesis that associations between the birthweight of individuals and their subsequent risk of CVD and diabetes may be explained, at least in part, by genetic and environmental factors shared between mothers and infants. The 'fetal insulin hypothesis'[95] emphasizes the genetic component of these shared common causal factors. Hattersley and Tooke have suggested that genetic factors related to both insulin resistance and birthweight explain part of the relationship between birthweight and risk of adult CVD and diabetes.[95]

15.3.3.4 Programming: mechanisms and caveats

It is clear that in biological terms the concept that an insult or stimulus at a critical period of development can produce (or programme) lasting effects on the organism is plausible, although at this point most supporting evidence is derived from experimental studies in animals. Different mechanisms have been proposed to explain the durability of programming effects including, at the cellular level, permanent effects of nutritional deprivation on cell numbers (as suggested by the work of Winick and Noble),[27] alteration of gene expression, and selective survival or 'natural selection' of particular clones of cells.[96] As discussed above, higher-level effects are also plausible, including effects on the structure and function of particular organs,[97] up- or down-regulation of hormone receptors and Freinkel's concept of 'fuel mediated teratogenesis'.[77] However, with regard to programming effects on specific organs, such as the kidney and the heart, our current models may be overly simplistic. The evidence from some animal models suggests that nutrient limitation at the stage of rapid organ growth in pregnancy may be associated with an increase rather than a decrease in organ size.[7] Unfortunately in the context of work on the aetiology of chronic disease in adult life such as CHD, the term 'programming' has mechanistic and deterministic connotations, which sit uneasily with a multifactorial, component cause model of aetiology.[98] Moreover, a degree of scepticism about the permanence or irreversibility of many programming effects on the function of the organism and the expression of disease is warranted. There is clearly a broad spectrum of programming scripts ranging from those apparently written in stone by a single author, such as egg hatching temperature in the American alligator, to those written in less durable material by a committee, such as in the case of a child born to a mother who smokes cigarettes and has gestational diabetes. In the latter instance, the child's risk of developing CVD and type 2 diabetes in adult life will depend at least as much (and arguably more) on genetic and postnatal lifestyle factors such as obesity, diet, smoking, and levels of exercise, as on putative *in utero* programming effects. Despite these caveats, the notion of critical periods of development has undoubtedly been helpful in work on maternal nutrition and fetal growth.

15.3.4 Maternal nutrition and fetal growth

Interest in prenatal nutrition has waxed and waned over the last 100 years as succinctly reviewed by Susser and Stein.[17] The late nineteenth century movement to promote improvement in the diet of pregnant women, led by Budin in France and Ballantyne in the UK, faltered when animal experimentalists failed to detect important effects of diet on pregnancy outcome. Interest was restored during the Great Depression in the 1930s by the efforts of nutritionists such as Boyd-Orr and in the early 1940s a number of studies reporting positive effects of food or vitamins on pregnancy outcomes were reported.[99,100] The effects of war-time starvation and privation on fetal growth and mortality, such as that associated with the 18-month Leningrad siege[101] and the 6-month Dutch famine[17] further emphasized the importance of diet in pregnancy. However two major observational studies published in the 1950s again cast doubt on the importance of nutrition during pregnancy (above a critical threshold) for fetal growth.[102,103] Thomson measured the food intake of 479 Aberdeen primigravidae during the seventh month of pregnancy using weighed food intakes and food diaries and found no significant associations between birthweight and either calorie intake or the intake of specific nutrients after adjustment for maternal height and weight. He concluded that 'within the range of diets in this survey, the influence of diet on birthweight must be small, indeed negligible'.[103]

While the effects of starvation and severe malnutrition on fetal growth are not seriously disputed,[101,104] the effect of less severe malnutrition on fetal growth is relatively small, as evidenced by the data from randomized controlled trials of maternal dietary supplementation on fetal growth.[105] Much of the earlier controversy in this area reflects the fact that the effects of prenatal nutrition on fetal growth in people are critically dependent on both the timing of nutritional exposures in relation to critical periods of development (as suggested by the programming model) and on interactions with the mother's prepregnancy nutritional status, metabolism, and physiology. As indicated earlier, maternal nutritional status is generally inferred indirectly from measures such as maternal height, pregravid weight, and skinfold thickness.

15.3.4.1 The timing of the nutritional insult

The importance of the timing of the nutritional exposure in people is illustrated by the data from the Dutch famine.[17] This famine, which was due to a Nazi-imposed transport embargo in western Holland, lasted 6 months from November 1944 to May 1945, when Holland was liberated from occupation. Clear effects of third-trimester famine exposure were seen on birthweight and placental weight and to a lesser extent on length and head circumference. Recovery of birthweight and other indices of fetal growth after the famine ended was rapid, indicating that exposure to severe malnutrition in early pregnancy had little evidence on fetal growth. Although these data provide unequivocal evidence of the effects of nutritional deprivation at a critical period of gestation, there was no evidence in these data of the setting of fetal growth on a low trajectory by early exposure to severe malnutrition.[17] In this context it is noteworthy that although famine exposure was associated with long-term effects on obesity (and other adverse outcomes[106,107]) among survivors, with more obesity among those exposed in early gestation and less in those exposed in late gestation,[108] no permanent effect of famine exposure at any stage of gestation was detectable on height at age 19 years in this economically developed country.[17] It is often assumed that short stature in adult life, such as that commonly seen in economically underdeveloped countries, largely reflects the growth trajectory set *in utero*.[2] However it is clear that there are substantial postnatal influences on both adult height and (surprisingly) body shape, principally the levels of nutrition and the incidence of infectious disease in childhood. Even minor illness in childhood is associated with slowing of growth and the nutritional requirements to sustain catch-up growth are high. Thus, the large secular trend in height in Japan between 1950 and 1980 was almost entirely due to increases in leg length, related to improved social conditions in childhood rather than improved diet in pregnancy.[42] These observations emphasize the need for caution in extrapolating data from programming experiments in animals to humans.

15.3.4.2 Interactions with prepregnancy nutritional status

A short interval between pregnancies has been linked with low birthweight, via effects on both fetal growth[109] and risk of preterm birth and there is some evidence that this may reflect, at least partially, the need for the mother to restore nutrient reserves depleted in the course of the previous pregnancy. We have already alluded to the importance of maternal height and 'frame size', regarded as markers of lifelong nutritional status, as determinants of fetal growth, especially in the third trimester. Data from a large number of studies indicate a strong relationship between maternal pregravid weight, gestational weight gain (which mainly reflects calorie intake during pregnancy), and infant birthweight.[110,111] Essentially, birthweight increases steadily with increasing pregravid weight and with increasing gestational weight gain. As shown in Table 15.2[26,112] these effects are independent of each other, additive in their combined effects, and are seen in smokers and non-smokers. As one would expect the effect of gestational weight gain on birthweight is most marked in underweight women, an observation consistent with findings from intervention studies.

There is evidence that the distribution of maternal body fat also influences fetal growth independently of pregravid weight and gestational weight gain. Brown and colleagues have described independent associations between the mother's waist-to-hip ratio measured before conception or in early pregnancy and the infant's birthweight, length, and head circumference.[113] In this study, a 0.1 unit increase waist-to-hip ratio predicted a 120 g greater birthweight, a 0.2 inch greater length, and a 0.3 cm greater head circumference. Central obesity is associated with a number of metabolic changes that may influence fetal growth, including elevated circulating levels of triglycerides[114] and free fatty acids,[115] insulin resistance, hyperinsulinaemia, and higher fasting glucose levels.[116] Insulin and insulin-like growth factors, which are also influenced by maternal nutrient intake, are particularly important regulators of fetal growth.[117] Pregnancy itself induces insulin resistance and hyperinsulinaemia in the mother,[118] which facilitates the transfer of nutrients from mother to fetus. This phenomenon (and other

Table 15.2 Mean birthweight (g) of term live births by maternal pregravid weight, gestational weight gain, and smoking status

Pregravid weight and smoking	Weight gain (lbs)					% change (<16 lb versus ≥36 lb gain)
	<16	16–20	21–25	26–35	≥36	
Underweight						
Non-smoker	2927	3100	3276	3374	3483	19.0
Smoker	2631	2821	3069	3174	3314	26.0
Normal weight						
Non-smoker	3097	3231	3428	3471	3606	16.4
Smoker	2918	3065	3135	3292	3398	16.4
Overweight						
Non-smoker	3330	3458	3526	3581	3665	10.0
Smoker	3258	3365	3379	3384	3519	8.0

Adapted from Luke[26] and Taffel.[112]

adverse maternal sequelae of pregnancy such as preeclampsia) has been interpreted in terms of 'maternal–fetal genetic conflict', that is, meeting the fetal requirements to maximize delivery of nutrients and oxygen at the expense of the mother's interest in maintaining her health and well-being.[119] Further discussion of the range of possible genetic[95] and maternal and placental hormonal and metabolic influences on fetal growth is clearly beyond the scope of this review.[120] However the associations between maternal waist-to-hip ratio and fetal growth emphasize the extent to which maternal nutrition (however defined) and the maternal hormonal–metabolic milieu are mutually interdependent and again they suggest a broader, less rigidly deterministic programming model.

15.3.4.3 Nutritional deficits and fetal/placental growth in economically developed countries

Inadequate folic acid intake has been clearly linked with malformations of the developing embryo in early pregnancy.[121] However the importance of other common nutritional deficits on fetal growth in developed countries is uncertain. Dietary restriction in previously well-nourished pregnant sheep is associated with placental hypertrophy,[122] which is interpreted as a compensatory phenomenon.[123] Godfrey and colleagues have suggested that in humans, placental hypertrophy, which results in discordance between birth and placental weight with an elevated placental ratio, is a relatively sensitive marker of inadequate nutrition such as that associated with iron deficiency anaemia.[123] This group have reported a striking association between an elevated placental ratio at birth and essential hypertension in middle-age.[124] Using data from the Oxford record linkage system, Godfrey and colleagues have described a specific association between low maternal haemoglobin combined with a fall in mean cell volume during pregnancy and elevated placental ratio.[123] By contrast, Perry and colleagues found that maternal obesity was the dominant predictor of an elevated placental ratio, in a study of European, Asian, and Afro-Caribbean women from a relatively deprived UK inner city community.[125] No associations with indices of iron deficiency anaemia, including serum ferritin, were detected. Similarly, Whincup and colleagues detected no consistent relationship between indices of iron deficiency anaemia and placental ratio in a study of over 600 children, nor was there evidence in this study of an association between maternal anaemia during pregnancy and blood pressure at ages 9–11 years.[126]

Godfrey and colleagues examined the effects of diet on fetal and placental growth in a prospective study involving a group of over 500 mothers who delivered at term in Southampton.[127] Diet was assessed using food frequency questionnaires administered in early and late pregnancy. A complex pattern of associations and interactions emerged. High carbohydrate intake in early pregnancy was associated with reduced birth and placental weight and lower protein intake in late pregnancy was also associated with reduced birth and placental weight. Although data from experimental studies in sheep are advanced to support the biological plausibility of these findings,[122] the findings have not been consistently replicated. In a further observational study, Campbell and colleagues found evidence of an inverse association between dietary protein intake and birthweight,[128] a finding which is inconsistent with the data from intervention studies when protein supplementation alone is used[129] (reviewed in Chapter 17). It is noteworthy that in neither of these studies was there evidence of placental hypertrophy in response to suboptimal nutrition. In the data from Campbell and colleagues in Aberdeen, associations were detected between the mother's intake of animal protein and carbohydrate during pregnancy and blood pressure in the offspring at age 40 years.[128] At relatively low-protein intake (below 50 g/day) there was a positive association between carbohydrate intake and blood pressure whereas above 50 g/day an inverse association was found. Unfortunately, in the absence of a clearly formulated a priori hypothesis, interpretation of these intriguing findings is difficult. Indeed, we have no firm evidence to date suggesting that maternal intake of either total energy or macronutrients during pregnancy (or maternal body composition) exerts substantial effects of offspring risk of chronic disease.[130] It should be noted, however, that we have extremely limited data from studies in humans on the effects on fetal growth rates and organ development of the balance of protein and carbohydrate in the diet and the intake of specific nutrients (such as amino acids) and micronutrients.[7]

In summary, fetal growth depends on the mother's nutritional status before conception, her diet during pregnancy, and interactions between these factors and aspects of the mother's metabolism and physiology such as glucose tolerance and blood pressure. In communities that provide adequate nutrition to sustain optimal growth in childhood and adolescence, dietary intake during pregnancy probably accounts for a relatively small amount of variation in fetal growth. Aspects of the mother's metabolism and physiology that determine the maternal uterine milieu are influenced by a range of genetic and environmental factors that are potentially important confounders in studies of associations between fetal growth and adult disease.

15.4 **Conclusions**

The fetal origins hypothesis has opened up an important and exciting agenda on the patterns and determinants of fetal growth and development. Barker and colleagues have set work in this area on a high growth trajectory and progress will be limited only by our collective imagination and our ability to develop narrowly focused hypotheses that make specific and testable predictions.[13,131–133] It is suggested that funding bodies should focus resources on research designs that seek to refute the programming hypothesis via the severest of challenges.[134] The formulation of testable hypotheses will depend critically on improvements in methods used to both measure maternal nutrition in pregnancy and fetal growth rates from early gestation and to derive quantitative, *in utero* indices of asymmetry and other abnormal patterns of fetal growth. Work on the distribution and determinants of fetal growth rates and patterns within and between populations using robust and reliable methods should then attract high priority. Further observational studies, with appropriate controls, are needed of prenatal diet, fetal growth, and pregnancy outcome, which address problems of measurement error with adequate sample size and repeated measures and which explore interactions between diet and the mother's metabolism and physiology. Because observational studies in particular are likely to be confounded by self-selection and by unmeasured socioeconomic attributes of early nutrition, research designs that use suitable control participants (including siblings) or that include interventions beyond the control of the study participants should be developed so that the effects of relevant exposures can be separated from the effects of the concomitant social, economic, and family conditions that may be associated with these exposures. In this context, the findings from twin studies have been particularly helpful in isolating genetic versus non-genetic effects (in analyses of monozygotic versus dizygotic twins) and in separating possible programming effects of maternal nutrition and nutritional status (identical for each member of a twin pair) from fetal nutrition (which can vary between twins).[135] Databases from nutrition intervention studies of pregnant women should also be used where possible for the follow-up of infants prenatally exposed to different nutrition regimens. Valuable data are now emerging from these studies.[72,73] Ultimately, detailed and long-term follow-up of the offspring from all such studies and their parents will help place nutritional programming within the broader canvas of the genetic, intrauterine, and postnatal determinants of adult morbidity and premature mortality.

Postscript

A recent analysis of birth records from the Dutch Famine of 1944-1945[136] suggests that even under famine conditions, birth size and body proportions vary only with late pregnancy exposure. In addition, estimates of head growth in relation to body size vary drastically depending on the choice of measure. The use of birth size or body proportions as a proxy for fetal nutrition is therefore not recommended in the study of adult disease.

References

Those marked with an asterisk are especially recommended for further reading.

*1 **Barker D.** *Fetal and infant origins of adult diseases.* London: British Medical Journal Publishing Group, 1992.

2 **Barker D.** *Mothers, babies and disease in later life.* London: British Medical Journal Publishing Group, 1994.

3 **Trudinger B.** Fetal growth disorders. In T Moore, Reiter R, Rebar R, Backer V, eds. *Gynecology and obstetrics: a longitudinal approach.* Edinburgh: Churchill Livingstone, 1993:487–98.

4 **Cunningham F, MacDonald P, Gant N.** Preterm and postterm pregnancy and inappropiate fetal growth. In Williams J, ed. *Williams obstetrics.* East Norwalk, Connecticut: Appleton and Lange, 1989:741–77.

5 **Robinson J.** Fetal growth. In Turnbull A, Chamberlain G, eds. *Obstetrics.* Edinburgh: Churchill Livingstone, 1989:141–50.

6 **McFadyen I.** Fetal growth. In Studd J, ed. *Progress in obstetrics and gynaecology.* Edinburgh: Churchill Livingstone, 1985:58–77.

*7 **Harding JE.** The nutritional basis of the fetal origins of adult disease. *Int J Epidemiol* 2001;**30**:15–23.

8 **Lithell HO, McKeigue PM, Berglund L, Mohsen R, Lithell UB, Leon DA.** Relation of size at birth to non-insulin dependent diabetes and insulin concentrations in men aged 50–60 years. *Br Med J* 1996;**312**:406–10.

9 **Leon DA, Koupilova I, Lithell HO, Berglund L, Mohsen R, Vagero D.** Failure to realise growth potential *in utero* and adult obesity in relation to blood pressure in 50 year old Swedish men. *Br Med J* 1996;**312**:401–6.

10 **Leon DA, Johansson M, Rasmussen F.** Gestational age and growth rate of fetal mass are inversely associated with systolic blood pressure in young adults: an epidemiologic study of 165,136 Swedish men aged 18 years. *Am J Epidemiol* 2000;**152**:597–604.

11 Eriksson JG, Forsen T, Tuomilehto J, Osmond C, Barker DJ. Early growth and coronary heart disease in later life: longitudinal study. *Br Med J* 2001;**322**:949–53.

12 Ben-Shlomo Y, Davey Smith G. Deprivation in infancy or in adult life: which is more important for mortality risk? *Lancet* 1991;**337**:530–4.

13 Kramer MS. Invited commentary: association between restricted fetal growth and adult chronic disease: Is it causal? Is it important? *Am J Epidemiol* 2000;**152**:605–8.

*14 Huxley R, Neil A, Collins R. Unravelling the fetal origins hypothesis: is there really an inverse association between birthweight and subsequent blood pressure? *Lancet* 2002;**360**:659.

*15 Lucas A, Fewtrell MS, Cole TJ. Fetal origins of adult disease–the hypothesis revisited. *Br Med J* 1999;**319**:245–9.

*16 Stein Z. *Famine and human development: the Dutch hunger winter of 1944/45.* Oxford: Oxford University Press, 1985.

17 Susser M, Stein Z. Timing in prenatal nutrition: a reprise of the Dutch Famine Study. *Nutr Rev* 1994;**52**:84–94.

18 Stanner SA, Bulmer K, Andres C, Lantseva OE, Borodina V, Poteen VV. Does malnutrition *in utero* determine diabetes and coronary heart disease in adulthood? Results from the Leningrad siege study, a cross sectional study. *Br Med J* 1997;**315**:1342–8.

19 Stanner SA, Yudkin JS. Fetal programming and the Leningrad Siege study. *Twin Res* 2001;**4**:287–92.

20 Barker DJ. Fetal origins of coronary heart disease. *Br Med J* 1995;**311**:171–4.

*21 Barker D. *Mothers, babies and disease in later life* (2nd edn). London: British Medical Journal Publishing Group, 1998.

22 Brooke OG, Anderson HR, Bland JM, Peacock JL, Stewart CM. Effects on birthweight of smoking, alcohol, caffeine, socioeconomic factors, and psychosocial stress. *Br Med J* 1989;**298**:795–801.

23 Launer LJ, Villar J, Kestler E, de Onis M. The effect of maternal work on fetal growth and duration of pregnancy: a prospective study. *Br J Obstet Gynaecol* 1990;**97**:62–70.

24 Caggiula A, Orchard T, Kuller L. Epidemiological studies of nutrition and heart disease. In Feldmad E, ed. *Nutrition and heart disease.* Edinburgh: Churchill Livingstone, 1983:1–27.

25 Barker D. The placenta in intrauterine growth retardation. Discussion. In Ward R, Smith S, Donnai D, eds. *Early fetal and growth development.* London: Royal College of Obstetricians and Gynaecologists Press, 1994:238.

26 Luke B. Nutritional influences on fetal growth. *Clin Obstet Gynecol* 1994;**37**:538–49.

27 Winick M, Noble A. Cellular response in rats during malnutrition at various ages. *J Nutr* 1966;**89**:300–6.

28 Tanner J. *Fetus into man.* Boston: Havard University Press, 1978.

29 Falkner F, Holzgreve W, Schloo RH. Prenatal influences on postnatal growth: overview and pointers for needed research. *Eur J Clin Nutr* 1994;**48(suppl 1)**:S15–22 and discussion S22–4.

30 Lumley J. Epidemiology of prematurity. In Yu V, Wood E, eds. *Prematurity.* Edinburgh: Churchill Livingstone, 1987:1–24.

31 Battaglia FC, Lubchenco LO. A practical classification of newborn infants by weight and gestational age. *J Pediatr* 1967;**71**:159–63.

32 Thomson AM, Billewicz WZ, Hytten FE. The assessment of fetal growth. *J Obstet Gynaecol Br Commonw* 1968;**75**:903–16.

33 McCullough RE, Reeves JT. Fetal growth retardation and increased infant mortality at high altitude. *Arch Environ Health* 1977;**32**:36–9.

34 de Jong CL, Gardosi J, Dekker GA, Colenbrander GJ, van Geijn HP. Application of a customised birthweight standard in the assessment of perinatal outcome in a high risk population. *Br J Obstet Gynaecol* 1998;**105**:531–5.

35 Pang MW, Leung TN, Sahota DS, Lau TK, Chang AM. Development of a customised birth-weight standard for ethnic Chinese subjects. *Aust NZ J Obstet Gynaec* 2000;**40**:161–4.

36 Clausson B, Gardosi J, Francis A, Cnattingius S. Perinatal outcome in SGA births defined by customised versus population-based birthweight standards. *Br J Obstet Gynaecol* 2001;**108**:830–4.

37 Salafia CM, Vogel CA, Vintzileos AM, Bantham KF, Pezzullo J, Silberman L. Placental patho-logic findings in preterm birth. *Am J Obstet Gynecol* 1991;**165**:934–8.

*38 Wilcox AJ. On the importance—and the unimportance—of birthweight. *Int J Epidemiol* 2001;**30**:1233–41.

39 Gruenwald P. Pathology of the deprived fetus and its supply line. In Elliott K, Knight J, eds. *Size at birth.* Amsterdam: Associated Scientic Publishers, 1974:3–9.

40 Kramer M. Early nutrition and lifelong health. Sixteenth Marabou Symposium. Discussion. *Nutr Rev* 1996;**54**:56–73.

*41 Lumey LH, Stein AD, Ravelli AC. Timing of prenatal starvation in women and offspring birthweight: an update. *Eur J Obstet Gynecol Reprod Biol* 1995;**63**:197.

42 Eveleth P, Tanner J. Environmental influences on growth. In Eveleth P, Tanner J, eds. *Worldwide variation in human growth.* Cambridge: Cambridge University Press, 1991:191–207.

43 Crane JP, Kopta MM. Comparative newborn anthropometric data in symmetric versus asymmet-ric intrauterine growth retardation. *Am J Obstet Gynecol* 1980;**138**:518–22.

44 Kramer MS, McLean FH, Olivier M, Willis DM, Usher RH. Body proportionality and head and length 'sparing' in growth-retarded neonates: a critical reappraisal. *Pediatrics* 1989;**84**:717–23.

45 Vik T, Vatten L, Jacobsen G, Bakketeig LS. Prenatal growth in symmetric and asymmetric small-for-gestational-age infants. *Early Hum Dev* 1997;**48**:167–76.

46 Perry IJ, Beevers DG. The definition of pre-eclampsia. *Br J Obstet Gynaecol* 1994;**101**:587–91.

47 Colley NV, Tremble JM, Henson GL, Cole TJ. Head circumference/abdominal circumference ratio, ponderal index and fetal malnutrition. Should head circumference/abdominal circumfer-ence ratio be abandoned? *Br J Obstet Gynaecol* 1991;**98**:524–7.

48 Patterson RM, Pouliot MR. Neonatal morphometrics and perinatal outcome: who is growth retarded? *Am J Obstet Gynecol* 1987;**157**:691–3.

49 Fay RA, Dey PL, Saadie CM, Buhl JA, Gebski VJ. Ponderal index: a better definition of the 'at risk' group with intrauterine growth problems than birth-weight for gestational age in term infants. *Aust NZ J Obstet Gynaec* 1991;**31**:17–9.

50 Frisancho AR, Compton A, Matos J. Ineffectiveness of body mass indices for the evaluation of neonate nutritional status. *J Pediatr* 1986;**108**:993–5.

51 Petersen S, Larsen T, Greisen G. Judging fetal growth from body proportions at birth. *Early Hum Dev* 1992;**30**:139–46.

52 Chard T, Costeloe K, Leaf A. Evidence of growth retardation in neonates of apparently normal weight. *Eur J Obstet Gynecol Reprod Biol* 1992;**45**:59–62.

53 Bates JA, Evans JA, Mason G. Differentiation of growth retarded from normally grown fetuses and prediction of intrauterine growth retardation using Doppler ultrasound. *Br J Obstet Gynaecol* 1996;**103**:670–5.

54 Craigo SD. The role of ultrasound in the diagnosis and management of intrauterine growth retardation. *Semin Perinatol* 1994;**18**:292–304.

55 Robson E. The genetics of birthweight. Principles and prenatal growth. In Falkner F, Tanner J, eds. *Human growth.* New York: Plenum Press, 1978:285–97.

56 Niswander KR, Singer J, Westphal M Jr, Weiss W. Weight gain during pregnancy and prepreg-nancy weight. Association with birthweight of term gestation. *Obstet Gynecol* 1969;**33**:482–91.

57 **Power C.** National trends in birthweight: implications for future adult disease. *Br Med J* 1994;**308**:1270–1.

58 **Singhal PK, Paul VK, Deorari AK, Singh M, Sundaram KR.** Changing trends in intrauterine growth curves. *Indian Pediatr* 1991;**28**:281–3.

59 **Kramer MS, Morin I, Yang H, Platt RW, Usher R, McNamara H.** Why are babies getting bigger? Temporal trends in fetal growth and its determinants. *J Pediatr* 2002;**141**:538–42.

60 **Ounsted M, Ounsted C.** Maternal regulation of intrauterine growth. *Nature* 1966;**212**:995–7.

61 **Klebanoff MA, Graubard BI, Kessel SS, Berendes HW.** Low birthweight across generations. *J Am Med Assoc* 1984;**252**:2423–7.

62 **Walton A, Hammond J.** The maternal effects on growth and conformation in Shire-horse–Shetland-pony crosses. *Proc R Soc Lond (Biol)* 1938;**125**:311–35.

63 **Wang X, Zuckerman B, Coffman GA, Corwin MJ.** Familial aggregation of low birthweight among whites and blacks in the United States. *N Engl J Med* 1995;**333**:1744–9.

*64 **Stein AD, Lumey LH.** The relationship between maternal and offspring birthweights after maternal prenatal famine exposure: the Dutch Famine Birth Cohort Study. *Hum Biol* 2000;**72**:641–54.

65 **Lumey LH, Stein AD.** Offspring birthweights after maternal intrauterine undernutrition: a comparison within sibships. *Am J Epidemiol* 1997;**146**:810–9.

66 **Barraclough C.** Production of anovulatory, sterile rats by a single injection of testosterone propianate. *Endocrinology* 1961;**68**:62–7.

67 **Fergunson M.** Overview of mechanisms in embryogenesis. In Ward R, Smith S, Donnai D, eds. *Early fetal growth and development.* London: Royal College of Obstetricians and Gynaecologists Press, 1994:1–19.

68 **McCance RA, Widdowson EM.** The determinants of growth and form. *Proc R Soc Lond B Biol Sci* 1974;**185**:1–17.

69 **Widdowson E, McCance R.** The effect of finite periods of undernutrition at different ages on the composition and subquent development of the rat. *Proc R Soc Lond (Biol)* 1963;**158**:329–42.

70 **Anguita RM, Sigulem DM, Sawaya AL.** Intrauterine food restriction is associated with obesity in young rats. *J Nutr* 1993;**123**:1421–8.

71 **Langley SC, Jackson AA.** Increased systolic blood pressure in adult rats induced by fetal exposure to maternal low protein diets. *Clin Sci* 1994;**86**:217–22 and discussion 121.

72 **Belizan JM, Villar J, Bergel E, del Pino A, Di Fulvio S, Galliano SV.** Long-term effect of calcium supplementation during pregnancy on the blood pressure of offspring: follow up of a randomised controlled trial. *Br Med J* 1997;**315**:281–5.

73 **Singhal A, Fewtrell M, Cole TJ, Lucas A.** Low nutrient intake and early growth for later insulin resistance in adolescents born preterm. *Lancet* 2003;**361**:1089–97.

74 **Ben-Shlomo Y, Kuh D.** A life course approach to chronic disease epidemiology: conceptual models, empirical challenges and interdisciplinary perspectives. *Int J Epidemiol* 2002;**31**:285–93.

75 **van Assche FA, Aerts L.** Long-term effect of diabetes and pregnancy in the rat. *Diabetes* 1985;**34**:S116–8.

76 **Pettitt DJ, Bennett PH, Saad MF, Charles MA, Nelson RG, Knowler WC.** Abnormal glucose tolerance during pregnancy in Pima Indian women. Long-term effects on offspring. *Diabetes* 1991;**40(suppl 2)**:126–30.

77 **Freinkel N.** Banting Lecture 1980. Of pregnancy and progeny. *Diabetes* 1980;**29**:1023–35.

78 **Gilbert T, Lelievre-Pegorier M, Merlet-Benichou C.** Immediate and long-term renal effects of fetal exposure to gentamicin. *Pediatr Nephrol* 1990;**4**:445–50.

79 **Taylor D.** The epidemiology of hypertension during pregnancy. In Rubin P, ed. *Handbook of hypertension.* Amsterdam: Elsevier, 1988:223–40.

80 Eskenazi B, Fenster L, Sidney S. A multivariate analysis of risk factors for preeclampsia. *J Am Med Assoc* 1991;**266**:237–41.

81 Churchill D, Perry IJ, Beevers DG. Ambulatory blood pressure in pregnancy and fetal growth. *Lancet* 1997;**349**:7–10.

82 Waugh J, Perry IJ, Halligan AW, De Swiet M, Lambert PC, Penny JA. Birthweight and 24-hour ambulatory blood pressure in nonproteinuric hypertensive pregnancy. *Am J Obstet Gynecol* 2000;**183**:633–7.

83 Fox H. The placenta in intrauterine growth retardation. In Ward R, Smith S, Donnai D, eds. *Early fetal growth and development*. London: Royal College of Obstetricians and Gynaecologists Press, 1988:223–35.

84 Fox H. The placenta in pregnancy hypertension. In Rubin P, ed. *Handbook of hypertension*. Amsterdam: Elsevier, 1994:16–37.

85 Peeters LL. The effect of early maternal maladaptation on fetal growth. *J Perinat Med* 1994;**22(suppl 1)**:9–17.

86 Khong TY, De Wolf F, Robertson WB, Brosens I. Inadequate maternal vascular response to placentation in pregnancies complicated by pre-eclampsia and by small-for-gestational age infants. *Br J Obstet Gynaecol* 1986;**93**:1049–59.

87 Robillard PY, Hulsey TC, Perianin J, Janky E, Miri EH, Papiernik E. Association of pregnancy-induced hypertension with duration of sexual cohabitation before conception. *Lancet* 1994;**344**:973–5.

88 Wolf M, Sandler L, Munoz K, Hsu K, Ecker JL, Thadhani R. First trimester insulin resistance and subsequent preeclampsia: a prospective study. *J Clin Endocrinol Metab* 2002;**87**:1563–8.

89 Solomon CG, Seely EW. Brief review: hypertension in pregnancy: a manifestation of the insulin resistance syndrome? *Hypertension* 2001;**37**:232–9.

90 Chappell LC, Seed PT, Briley AL, Kelly FJ, Lee R, Hunt BJ. Effect of antioxidants on the occurrence of pre-eclampsia in women at increased risk: a randomised trial. *Lancet* 1999;**354**:810–6.

91 von Dadelszen P, Magee LA. Could an infectious trigger explain the differential maternal response to the shared placental pathology of preeclampsia and normotensive intrauterine growth restriction? *Acta Obstet Gynecol Scand* 2002;**81**:642–8.

92 Irgens HU, Reisaeter L, Irgens LM, Lie RT. Long term mortality of mothers and fathers after pre-eclampsia: population based cohort study. *Br Med J* 2001;**323**:1213–7.

93 Davey Smith G, Hart C, Ferrell C, Upton M, Hole D, Hawthorne V. Birthweight of offspring and mortality in the Renfrew and Paisley study: prospective observational study. *Br Med J* 1997;**315**:1189–93.

94 Lawlor DA, Davey Smith G, Ebrahim S. Birthweight of offspring and insulin resistance in late adulthood: cross sectional survey. *Br Med J* 2002;**325**:359.

*95 Hattersley AT, Tooke JE. The fetal insulin hypothesis: an alternative explanation of the association of low birthweight with diabetes and vascular disease. *Lancet* 1999;**353**:1789–92.

96 Lucas A. Programming by early nutrition in man. In Bock G, Whelan J, eds. *The childhood environment and adult disease*. Chichester: John Wiley, 1991:38–55.

97 Mackenzie HS, Lawler EV, Brenner BM. Congenital oligonephropathy: The fetal flaw in essential hypertension? *Kidney Int Suppl* 1996;**55**:S30–4.

98 Rothman K. Causes. *Am J Epidemiol* 1976;**104**:587–92.

99 Ebbs J, Tisdall F, Scott W. The influence of prenatal diet on the mother and child. *J Nutr* 1991;**22**:515–26.

100 **Cameron C, Graham S.** Antenatal diet and its influence on stillbirths and prematurity. *Glasgow Med J* 1944;**142**:1–7.

101 **Antonow A.** Children born during the siege of Leningrad in 1942. *J Pediatr* 1947;**30**:250–9.

102 **McGanity W, Cannon R, Bridgfort E, Martin MP, Densen PM, Newbill JA et al.** The Vanderbilt cooperative study of maternal and infant nutrition. V. Description and outcome of obstetrics sample. *Am J Obstet Gynecol* 1954;**67**:491–500.

103 **Thomson A.** Diet in relation to the course and outcome of pregnancy. *Br J Nutr* 1959;**13**:509–25.

104 **Treasure JL, Russell GF.** Intrauterine growth and neonatal weight gain in babies of women with anorexia nervosa. *Br Med J (Clin Res Ed)* 1988;**296**:1038.

*105 **Kramer MS.** Balanced protein/energy supplementation in pregnancy. *Cochrane Database Syst Rev* 2000(2):CD000032.

106 **Roseboom TJ, van der Meulen JH, Ravelli AC, Osmond C, Barker DJ, Bleker OP.** Effects of prenatal exposure to the Dutch famine on adult disease in later life: an overview. *Twin Res* 2001;**4**:293–8.

107 **Ravelli AC, van der Meulen JH, Michels RP, Osmond C, Barker DJ, Hales CN.** Glucose tolerance in adults after prenatal exposure to famine. *Lancet* 1998;**351**:173–7.

108 **Ravelli GP, Stein ZA, Susser MW.** Obesity in young men after famine exposure *in utero* and early infancy. *N Engl J Med* 1976;**295**:349–53.

109 **Rawlings JS, Rawlings VB, Read JA.** Prevalence of low birthweight and preterm delivery in relation to the interval between pregnancies among white and black women. *N Engl J Med* 1995;**332**:69–74.

110 **Eastman NJ, Jackson E.** Weight relationships in pregnancy. I. The bearing of maternal weight gain and pre-pregnancy weight on birthweight in full term pregnancies. *Obstet Gynecol Surv* 1968;**23**:1003–25.

111 **Thomson A.** Fetal growth and size at birth. In Barron S, Thomson A, eds. *Obstetrical epidemiology*. London: Academic Press, 1983:89–142.

112 **Taffel S.** Maternal weight gain and the outcome of pregnancy, United States 1980 (Publication PHS 86–1922). Washington DC: US Department of Health and Human Services. Vital and Health Statistics, Series 21, No. 44, 1986.

113 **Brown JE, Potter JD, Jacobs DR Jr, Kopher RA, Rourke MJ, Barosso GM.** Maternal waist-to-hip ratio as a predictor of newborn size: results of the Diana Project. *Epidemiology* 1996;**7**:62–6.

114 **McKeigue PM, Pierpoint T, Ferrie JE, Marmot MG.** Relationship of glucose intolerance and hyperinsulinaemia to body fat pattern in south Asians and Europeans. *Diabetologia* 1992;**35**:785–91.

115 **Campaigne BN.** Body fat distribution in females: metabolic consequences and implications for weight loss. *Med Sci Sports Exerc* 1990;**22**:291–7.

116 **McKeigue PM, Shah B, Marmot MG.** Relation of central obesity and insulin resistance with high diabetes prevalence and cardiovascular risk in South Asians. *Lancet* 1991;**337**:382–6.

117 **Fowden AL.** The role of insulin in prenatal growth. *J Dev Physiol* 1989;**12**:173–82.

118 **Cousins L.** Insulin sensitivity in pregnancy. *Diabetes* 1991;**40(suppl 2)**:39–43.

119 **Haig D.** Genetic conflicts in human pregnancy. *Q Rev Biol* 1993;**68**:495–532.

120 **Evain-Brion D.** Hormonal regulation of fetal growth. *Horm Res* 1994;**42**:207–14.

121 **Daly LE, Kirke PN, Molloy A, Weir DG, Scott JM.** Folate levels and neural tube defects. Implications for prevention. *J Am Med Assoc* 1995;**274**:1698–702.

122 **Robinson J, Owens J, Barro TD, Lok F, Chidzanja S.** Maternal nutrition and fetal growth. In Ward R, Smith S, Donai D, eds. *Early fetal growth and development.* London: Royal College of Obstetricians and Gynaecologists Press, 1994:317–34.

123 **Godfrey KM, Redman CW, Barker DJ, Osmond C.** The effect of maternal anaemia and iron deficiency on the ratio of fetal weight to placental weight. *Br J Obstet Gynaecol* 1991;**98**:886–91.

124 **Barker DJ, Bull AR, Osmond C, Simmonds SJ.** Fetal and placental size and risk of hypertension in adult life. *Br Med J* 1990;**301**:259–62.

125 **Perry IJ, Beevers DG, Whincup PH, Bareford D.** Predictors of ratio of placental weight to fetal weight in multiethnic community. *Br Med J* 1995;**310**:436–9.

126 **Whincup P, Cook D, Papacosta O, Walker M, Perry I.** Maternal factors and development of cardiovascular risk: evidence from a study of blood pressure in children. *J Hum Hypertens* 1994;**8**:337–43.

127 **Godfrey K, Robinson S, Barker DJ, Osmond C, Cox V.** Maternal nutrition in early and late pregnancy in relation to placental and fetal growth. *Br Med J* 1996;**312**:410–4.

128 **Campbell DM, Hall MH, Barker DJ, Cross J, Shiell AW, Godfrey KM.** Diet in pregnancy and the offspring's blood pressure 40 years later. *Br J Obstet Gynaecol* 1996;**103**:273–80.

*129 **Kramer MS.** Effects of energy and protein intakes on pregnancy outcome: an overview of the research evidence from controlled clinical trials. *Am J Clin Nutr* 1993;**58**:627–35.

*130 **Gillman MW.** Epidemiological challenges in studying the fetal origins of adult chronic disease. *Int J Epidemiol* 2002;**31**:294–9.

131 **Paneth N, Susser M.** Early origin of coronary heart disease (the 'Barker hypothesis'). *Br Med J* 1995;**310**:411–2.

132 **Lumey LH.** Reproductive outcomes in women prenatally exposed to undernutrition: a review of findings from the Dutch famine birth cohort. *Proc Nutr Soc* 1998;**57**:129–35.

133 **Kramer MS, Joseph KS.** Enigma of fetal/infant-origins hypothesis. *Lancet* 1996;**348**:1254–5.

134 **Anon.** An overstretched hypothesis? *Lancet* 2001;**357**:405.

*135 **Leon DA.** Twins and fetal programming of blood pressure. Questioning the role of genes and maternal nutrition. *Br Med J* 1999;**319**:1313–4.

136 **Stein AD, Zybert PA, van de Bor M, Lumey LH.** Intrauterine famine exposure and body proportions at birth: the Dutch Hunger Winter. *Int J Epidemiol* (in press).

Chapter 16

Socioeconomic pathways between childhood and adult health

Diana Kuh, Chris Power, David Blane,
and Mel Bartley

There are two main ways that aspects of the childhood socioeconomic environment affect adult health and disease risk. First, they affect exposures to known or suspected causal factors during gestation, infancy, childhood, adolescence, or young adulthood that are part of long-term biological chains of risk. Thus differential effects on disease risk of timing and duration of exposure to a poor socioeconomic environment can provide clues to aetiology. Second, they form part of social chains of risk or protective chains that operate throughout life partly via educational and other learning experiences and lead to adult socioeconomic circumstances that affect disease risk through exposures to causal factors in later life. Causal factors at each life stage include physical hazards and behaviours with known or suspected biological pathways, but may also include stressful life conditions that affect biological resources through psychosocial processes that are only beginning to be understood. Thus evidence from two types of studies are reviewed. We discuss aetiological studies that examine how variations in adult disease outcomes are related to socioeconomic factors at different stages of life in order to understand biological chains of risk better. We also review studies of social chains of risk that have investigated either the extent to which individuals experience continuity in their socioeconomic environment or how they interact with their environment in ways that lead to socially patterned exposures that may develop or damage personal and health capital.

16.1 Introduction

Previous chapters have focused on biological risk factors at different stages of the life course and their independent and combined effects on adult disease. This chapter develops the idea that aspects of the socioeconomic environment throughout life affect adult health and disease risk. This is because health-damaging exposures or health-enhancing opportunities are socially patterned and because an individual's response, which may modify their impact or alter the risk of future exposures, will be powerfully affected by their social and economic experience. The term 'socially patterned' implies resources and opportunities are constrained by social class, ethnicity, and gender and by the nature of the roles associated with social institutions such as the family, educational institutions, or occupational groups. These, in turn, change over time and differ between societies.

Social epidemiology has documented strong and graded associations between adult socioeconomic position and mortality, morbidity, other health outcomes, and behaviours in the UK,[1–3] USA,[4–6] and other developed countries.[7–9] These are discussed in Chapter 4 and reviewed elsewhere and are not the focus of this chapter. Rather we review the evidence that socially patterned exposures during childhood, adolescence, or early adult life influence adult health and disease risk and adult socioeconomic position and social roles and thus may partly account for these observed health inequalities in adult life.

Current competing explanations for social inequalities in health reflect different traditions within social epidemiology.[10,11] One tradition studies health in relation to social class or living standards and emphasizes the role of economic resources and material conditions. The other tradition studies health in relation to social integration and social roles and emphasizes psychosocial factors generated by human interaction. A life course approach extends both these traditions by investigating whether the effects of various adverse material conditions or types of psychosocial stress that are associated with socioeconomic position vary by timing or duration of exposure. Differential effects provide clues to aetiology and suggest whether insults act cumulatively or interactively on disease risk, or have a marked effect during a particular life stage. Exposures during childhood may be particularly damaging if they impair developmental processes and become 'embedded' in bodily structures or functions, threatening long-term health. Life course explanations for gender[12,13] and ethnic[14] inequalities in health are growing areas of research but are not discussed in this chapter.

Historically, UK literature has focused on occupational measures of social class and on documenting the class gradient in health.[15] In Europe and North America educational measures have been more commonly used to study the relationship between socioeconomic factors and health.[5,8] In the North American literature there has been a long-term focus on the health and social effects of poverty and social mobility and less attention was paid, until the middle of the 1980s, to the socioeconomic gradient in health.[16] What unites these different traditions today is a common interest in understanding the underlying social and biological processes that link health to social and economic factors. Some of these processes begin early in life. Aetiological models of health inequalities need to be disease and cohort specific because of marked heterogeneity in strength and direction of the associations between socioeconomic position and different diseases and changes in these associations over time.[17]

16.2 Studying the socioeconomic environment

A similar precision needs to be applied to social and economic phenomena if we are to understand how they shape health and disease risks. We need to distinguish, for example, different dimensions of socioeconomic position[18,19] and the particular adverse or protective experiences that are socially patterned and have long-term effects on adult health or health behaviour.[20] In practice, constructs such as social class and socioeconomic status have been used loosely and interchangeably in studies of health and represented by various classifications of occupation or educational qualifications, levels of income or years of schooling, or ownership of assets. Assets are usually measured by ownership of homes or cars and more inclusive measures of wealth are uncommon in studies of health. Conceptually, social class refers to the social relationships that govern the economic structure of industrialized societies; an individual being assigned to a social group based on their control of economic resources, whether these are capital assets or their own or others' skills and knowledge.[19,21] The control of economic resources determines conditions of employment and is strongly related to the level of monetary rewards and prestige/status. Each of these dimensions of social inequality affects health and disease risk in different but overlapping ways. Conditions of work affect level of exposure to physical and psychological hazards. Monetary rewards underpin 'standard of living', that is, the provision of material resources needed to maintain the health of individuals and their families or to protect them from environmental hazards. The level of social standing, whether based on an individual's own perceptions or those of others, may affect health through exposure of the individual or other family members to stressful or protective social interactions and opportunities. Individual skills and knowledge are not only an economic resource that affects occupation, they also shape current and future attitudes, expectations, and behaviours that protect or damage the health of self or others.

Studies reviewed in this chapter use a variety of measures of socioeconomic position and often do not specify which dimension of social inequality is being investigated. We use the term 'socioeconomic position' as an aggregate term to cover measures based on occupation, education, income, or wealth and the wider terms 'socioeconomic environment' or 'socioeconomic circumstances' to cover any measure of socioeconomic position or associated dimension of social inequality.

Use of more recent theoretically based measures of social class (such as the Wright schema[19] and the National Statistics SocioEconomic Classification (NS-SEC)[22]) is becoming more common. The NS-SEC is now the official class schema for government publications in the UK. Life course studies in the UK generally still rely on the Registrar General's social class, a generic measure based on occupation and developed by Stevenson in 1913. While the criteria were never explicit, Stevenson described his classification both as a marker of 'living conditions' and of 'social standing'.[15,23] Conventional educational measures can be used as indicators of socioeconomic position because they have a close relationship to living standards and social status as well as indexing skills and knowledge.

A fundamental question for life course research is how far all these measures of adult socioeconomic position are associated with adult health because they reflect childhood socioeconomic circumstances. This applies particularly to educational measures as the highest level of education is generally achieved in adolescence and young adulthood; indeed educational characteristics are often used as a measure of childhood rather than adult socioeconomic circumstances.[24]

16.3 Pathways between the childhood socioeconomic environment and adult health

Figure 16.1 provides a simplified framework that shows the hypothesized major pathways via which aspects of the childhood socioeconomic environment affect later life health.

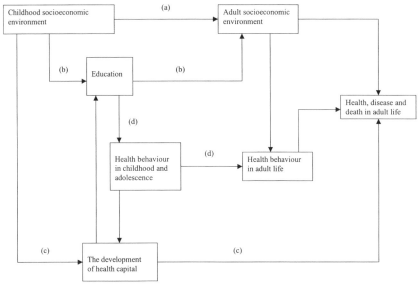

Fig. 16.1 Pathways between childhood and adult health: a simplified framework.

First, parental socioeconomic position constrains adult socioeconomic position by influencing access to social and economic resources (route a), especially opportunities for educational and other learning experiences (route b). Adult socioeconomic circumstances in turn affect disease risk by determining exposure to causal factors in later life. Second, the childhood socioeconomic environment affects exposures to known or suspected causal factors during gestation, infancy, childhood, and adolescence, which are part of long-term biological processes and are generally associated with various aspects of development (route c). We have used the term 'health capital' to mean the accumulation of biological resources, inherited and acquired during earlier stages of life, which determine current health and future health potential, including resilience to future environmental insults. This concept of health capital is analogous to the notion of constitution used in the interwar years (see Chapter 2). Third, the childhood socio-economic environment shapes the development of behaviours that endure and have long-term effects on disease risk, operating either interdependently, cumulatively, or interactively with later risk exposures (route d). A simple classification of life course models of health[25] distinguishes between early life factors that affect long-term health because they add to the cumulative damage to biological systems, act during critical periods of growth and development, or are part of social, biological, or psychological chains of risk (a sequence of linked exposures that raise disease risk because one bad experience or exposure tends to lead to another and then another). Longitudinal studies such as the UK birth cohorts[26,27] with prospective social and biological information collected in childhood and adulthood provide particularly valuable sources of life course data with which to test these models.

16.3.1 Continuity in the socioeconomic environment over the life course

There is plenty of evidence from intergenerational studies that those from more favoured family backgrounds have a much better chance of achieving a high socioeconomic position or earnings in adult life.[28–33] In the 1958 cohort, a man whose father was in social class I or II was twice as likely to be in the same class position himself at 33 years than one whose father had been a skilled manual worker and nearly three times more likely than one whose father had been in social class IV or V.[34] These results are almost identical for the 1946 cohort.[35] Conversely, the risk of unemployment in the 1958 cohort was greatest for those whose fathers suffered unemployment. Whereas almost 10% of men were unemployed, this was true of over 19% of those whose fathers had themselves been unemployed in 1974 (when the cohort member was age 16 years) and 50% of those whose fathers had also been unemployed when they were 7 and 11 years of age in 1965 and 1969. The risk of unemployment for a year or more, and of low income, was also higher for those with fathers in the lower fifths of the income distribution.[34]

The extent of intergenerational social mobility may be associated with the level of industrialization and vary with changes in the social and economic context.[36] Research from the USA in the 1960s and 1970s on intergenerational social mobility suggested that the effects of family background (at least in terms of parental schooling and occupations) on adult socioeconomic position were declining over time.[28] In contrast recent studies have revealed stronger correlations between parental income and the income of adult offspring than shown in previous studies. They are based on more representative national samples (such as the Panel Study of Income Dynamics) and employ new research methods that take into account, for example, income at multiple time points. New research from the UK also shows that there has been less intergenerational mobility in earnings in the 1970 birth cohort than in the 1958 cohort.[37]

Recent studies have also shown that long-term childhood poverty is strongly associated with the risk of poverty in early adulthood.[28,38] Childhood poverty has been increasing since the 1970s in most industrialized countries.[39] In North America, for example, poverty affects one in three children between 0 and 15 years and one in six children experience poverty for 10 years or more.[40]

How much of the continuity between child and adult socioeconomic position is mediated by educational experience (see Fig.16.1)? There is substantial evidence from cohort studies of a powerful effect of family background (in terms of parental education, income, social class, and other parental and household characteristics) on educational opportunity and attainment.[35,38,41–43] In turn, educational attainment is a powerful predictor of adult income and occupation.[31–33] The strength of these relationships are context specific and vary by place and over time.[36,44] The recent fall in intergenerational mobility in the UK was partly accounted for by an unequal increase in educational attainment with young people from more favoured backgrounds benefiting more than those from less privileged backgrounds from the rapid educational upgrading of the population.[37] Findings from the 1946 birth cohort show that father's social class still had additional effects on male mid-life earnings[31] and maternal education still had additional effects on women's earnings,[32] even after allowing for own educational experience. It is likely that besides the powerful influence that well-educated middle-class parents have on their children's educational achievement, they also develop social and personal skills in their offspring (such as motivation and self-direction, manners of speech, and peer identification) and provide financial backing and social contacts that help prepare their child for a similar class position and capacity for earning.[45,46]

Early studies of intergenerational mobility in North America indicated that the effects of family background on adult socioeconomic position operated mainly through education. Recent North American research shows most of the effects of parental poverty are independent of education.[28] This has prompted the exploration of other models of the intergenerational transmission of poverty using more detailed information on parental and neighbourhood disadvantages and the child's developmental characteristics collected in the more recent longitudinal studies. Structural models emphasize the lack of material resources within the family or the neighbourhood whereas cultural models focus on parental disadvantages associated with poverty in terms of knowledge, attitudes, and health conditions that limit parenting skills and may be negatively reinforced by welfare distribution at the family and neighbourhood level. Corcoran's review[28] concludes that there is still an independent effect of parental poverty on adult economic outcomes even after allowing for parental and neighbourhood structural and cultural disadvantages. One pathway increasingly being investigated is how the effects of poverty on economic outcomes may be mediated through deficits and delays in the child's physical, cognitive, and social development.[47] This research direction on adult economic outcomes parallels the research on adult health outcomes, which investigates how childhood socioeconomic circumstances are inscribed onto body functions and structures.[18,48,49]

16.3.2 Importance of lifetime socioeconomic circumstances for adult health

Although it is well documented that adults in the poorest socioeconomic circumstances have the worst health, only a few studies have looked at the effect of timing or duration of exposure or whether later favourable or adverse circumstances can modify the effects of earlier circumstances. A Scottish cohort study with data on social class in adulthood and retrospective data on father's occupation and own occupation at labour market entry found that those who remained in the manual classes throughout life experienced the highest mortality risk.[50] A 25-year follow-up of children in the UK from the Office of National Statistics longtudinal study also found that health and survival in young adult life was poorest among those with persisting socioeconomic disadvantage.[51] A study of self-rated health in relation to prospective measures of social class at birth and at 16, 23, and 33 years in the 1958 cohort[52] showed that duration of exposure was strongly associated with self-rated health at 33 years and was not accounted for by educational level. These and other[53,54] studies suggest that risks to health from poor socioeconomic circumstances accumulate over the life course. This is supported by research showing that measures of socioeconomic position in early old age[55] and prospective measures of childhood social disadvantage[56] are strongly related to cumulative exposure to environmental health hazards over the life course as estimated from information recalled from participants using a lifegrid interview method.

A number of studies have looked at the effects of timing of exposure to poor socioeconomic circumstances on subsequent mortality and disease. In contrast to the mixed results of earlier studies (reviewed by Elo and Preston[57]), more recent studies[58–65] have generally found that both childhood and adult socioeconomic circumstances are associated with all-cause mortality and with cardiovascular mortality or morbidity (see Chapter 4). Childhood effects are particularly apparent for mortality from stroke and stomach cancer in men even after further adjustment for conventional adult risk factors,[63] suggesting that underlying causes for these diseases have their effect in early life. Retrospective adult reports of childhood socioeconomic circumstances[50,60–63,65,66] may have weakened the observed effect on mortality. Indeed, results from the prospective 1946 birth cohort study[58] show particularly strong effects on all-cause mortality in men and women between 26 and 54 years. Studies are mostly limited to Caucasian males. An imaginative study that linked a cohort of African-Americans to the US censuses of 1900 and 1910 when they were children found that early characteristics previously found to be associated with childhood survival, such as parental literacy and growing up on a farm, were also associated with the chance of survival to age 85.[67]

Reliance on recall of childhood conditions has also limited studies that show effects of childhood conditions independent of adult conditions on some conventional risk factors for adult cardiovascular and respiratory diseases,[65,68–71] mental health outcomes,[72] cognitive function,[73] psychosocial function such as cynical hostility and hopelessness,[74] or self-reported health.[75,76] Evidence from longitudinal studies with prospective measures of childhood socioeconomic position strengthens this literature. It shows, for example, that adult central or total obesity,[54,77,78] depression,[79,80] timing of menopause,[81] cognitive function, and certain health behaviours[20]are associated with childhood socioeconomic position independent of adult socioeconomic position. This is not observed for other outcomes such as physical disability[82] and may vary when different scales, thresholds, or cut-points are applied to health indicators. For example, in the 1946 cohort, adult socioeconomic factors were better predictors than father's social class of those in the poorest health at 36 years but father's social class and level of education were better predictors of those in the best of health at 36 years, regardless of the later social environment.[83]

Fewer studies have assessed the extent to which the childhood socioeconomic environment contributes to adult socioeconomic inequalities in health although the potential importance of a life course approach is recognized.[84,85] In the 1958 cohort, socioeconomic circumstances prevailing at each stage of childhood and adolescence were found to be relevant to reported health differences[86,87] and psychological distress[88] among young adults. Two European studies in general adult populations,[89,90] which have investigated self-reported health in relation to recalled parental occupation, maternal education, and childhood financial situation, support these findings. Further research is needed to examine the extent to which childhood socioeconomic circumstances account for socioeconomic, gender, and ethnic differences in adult health and whether the effect of childhood conditions on adult health differs by gender, ethnicity, time, or place.

In summary, there is evidence from a growing number of studies that the childhood socioeconomic environment has long-term influences on various adult health outcomes. While the findings of these studies provide clues to the timing of potential causal factors, the specific nature of the underlying physiological and psychological processes is still to be clarified. Studies discussed in other chapters implicate mechanisms related to nutrition, infectious disease, chronic illness, and stress and these factors need to be studied jointly with the socioeconomic measures. Similarly more specific markers of childhood adversity, behaviour, and temperament need to be incorporated. These are the focus of the following two sections.

16.3.3 Childhood socioeconomic circumstances, the acquisition of health capital, and adult health

Growing up in a socially disadvantaged family where there is poverty, unemployment, and low levels of parental education is associated with many aspects of impaired physical, psychological, and cognitive function that are associated with a raised adult disease risk.[91–95] These include low birthweight and premature birth,[96] impaired postnatal growth[97,98] and final adult height,[99] lower respiratory infection,[100] and inadequate nutrition.[97,101] Intergenerational links, although not shown in Fig. 16.1, are suggested by research that has shown that poor social circumstances during gestation or childhood affect a young women's subsequent reproductive performance and pregnancy outcome (see Chapter 15).[102–106] Possible mediators of the effect of childhood socioeconomic position on childhood health are increasingly being explored. For example, studies suggest that maternal cigarette smoking, low gestational weight gain, short maternal height, bacterial vaginosis, and maternal stress mediate the relationship between poverty and pregnancy outcome (such as intrauterine growth restriction and preterm birth).[96] However, no study has yet been able to fully explain the association with socioeconomic position.[107]

How do the independent or cumulative socioeconomic experiences of the previous generation and of the individual in infancy, childhood, and adolescence affect the acquisition of health capital with long-term effects on disease risk? Extensive research, reviewed in other chapters in this book and in other books in the series,[13] has examined the role of prenatal and postnatal growth on adult disease risk. The associations between early physical growth and development and later health that have been observed may be due to social as well as biological pathways. This is because low birthweight babies are more likely to be born into poor families and to remain in disadvantaged circumstances during childhood[108] and adult life.[86,87] Recent studies have been able to examine the relationship between birthweight and cardiovascular risk and take account of lifetime socioeconomic position. They suggest that associations between weight at birth or infancy and cardiovascular disease and blood pressure remain after adjusting for childhood socioeconomic conditions.[109–111] Whether body weight or size in early life accounts for the observed effects of childhood socioeconomic position depends on the outcome considered.[81,112,113] Even if the adverse sequelae of impaired fetal growth are primarily biological in origin, evidence suggests they may still be modified by social influences[114] in childhood[111] or adult life.[112]

There is a well-documented relationship between adult height and cardiovascular morbidity and mortality.[115–120] Height is both a marker of child health and development[121,122] and of childhood socioeconomic conditions.[123] Although this evidence has been used to support the idea that the early environment influences adult health, an alternative interpretation is that height influences adult health through its effect on adult socioeconomic position. This is because social mobility, in terms of occupation and marriage, is selective with respect to height.[117,124–128] Another interpretation is that the relationship between height and mortality is due to differential rates of shrinkage according to health.[129] The follow-up of the Carnegie survey of diet and health in pre war UK showed that childhood height was associated with adult cardiovascular mortality[130] and pulse pressure[131] independently of later socioeconomic circumstances and adult risk factors. This provides stronger support for the role of the early socioeconomic environment. Leg length rather than trunk length, whether measured in childhood[130] or adult life,[132] is more strongly related to adult cardiovascular mortality. Leg length reflects early nutritional intake[133] and possibly infection, particularly in the first 2 years.[134] New findings from the 1946 birth cohort show that at age 53 years leg length but not trunk length was inversely related to pulse pressure.[135] While this may be due to causal factors associated with the early socioeconomic environment operating in childhood, physiological mechanisms related to arterial haemodynamics in adult life may also be involved.[135]

Overweight and obesity are risk factors for adult health (see Chapter 8) but they also predict an individual's social and economic trajectory, particularly for women.[136–138] For example, one study found that fatter women were less likely to marry, had poorer job opportunities, and lower incomes than other women.[136]As the findings were independent of baseline socioeconomic position they appear to reflect the socioeconomic consequences of being overweight. Thus both biological and social pathways over the life course may explain the relationship between being overweight and adult health.

Biological and social pathways also operate for those with serious or chronic childhood illnesses. There are socioeconomic differences in serious illness, disability, and other aspects of child health,[139–141] particularly in the first few years of life.[93,126] Childhood illness and disability have long-term consequences for adult morbidity,[83,142,143] disability,[82] and handicap.[144] This may be due to the biological sequelae associated with a specific disorder or because individual and societal expectations and opportunities are lowered (for example, through educational disruption and underachievement, poor self-esteem, or stigmatization). For example, children with chronic illness in the 1946 birth cohort study compared with other cohort members were at increased risk of unemployment in adult life, possibly because the disruption of education reduced their chances of educational attainment. They were less likely to be homeowners and had reduced social support due to higher parental death rates.[145]

Further understanding of the underlying mechanisms would be gained if reports of findings more regularly showed how the effects of childhood socioeconomic position on adult health changed after taking account of possible mediating factors. Generally the focus of research is whether the associations between these other risk factors and adult health are confounded by socioeconomic circumstances. The extent to which they account for the associations between socioeconomic circumstances at different life stages and adult health are often not discussed. One exception is the US Nurses' Health Study: this study showed that the observed small but significant excess of cardiovascular disease in women from blue-collar backgrounds was not explained by birthweight or adult height.[61]

16.4 **Extending the framework: the early psychosocial environment and the development of personal capital**

The framework in Fig. 16.1 is a simple representation of the social and economic constraints and opportunities that link the socioeconomic environment in childhood to adult health. Childhood socioeconomic disadvantage is associated with various psychological and behavioural problems in childhood and adult life.[20,74,146–148] These in turn are associated with later less successful economic[149] and disease outcomes.[150,151] Adverse coping styles and negative personality profiles may explain part of these associations.[76] Once psychosocial or behavioural explanations are invoked the framework has to be extended to allow for the reciprocal nature of interactions between the individual and their environment.

Within a given set of social and economic constraints, an individual's behaviour will help to shape both their current circumstances and future life trajectory. In turn, behaviour is an observable outcome of an individual's capacity to mobilize available resources, exploit opportunities, and be resilient to adversity. This capacity reflects the accumulation of social and cognitive skills, self-esteem, coping strategies, attitudes, and values and its development is a major function of childhood and adolescence. We originally called this capacity 'social capital'[152] but the alternative and now more common use of this term is to refer to the level of social cohesion in communities.[153] We prefer to use the term personal capital (or behavioural capital[20]), which still captures the cumulative nature of these resources, which are characteristics of the individual rather than their environment. Educational attainment, beyond being simply a mediator between, or a good marker of, childhood and adult material advantage, may be associated with later health because it is a marker of personal capital.[154]

The development of personal capital and the resulting behaviours are shaped primarily by characteristics of the family, neighbourhood, and school and all are influenced by the wider social, economic, and cultural context.[43] Recent evidence from the 1958 cohort identifies some of the pathways through which social class has effects on children's psychosocial adjustment and educational achievement. Proximal determinants include material circumstances, school characteristics, and parental involvement and aspirations for their child. The relative importance of these factors on educational and psychosocial outcomes change as a child grows up.[43] In adolescence, family influences become less important and social contexts beyond the family become more important.

Childhood and adolescence are particularly important life stages for health-related behavioural development. Decisions about diet and physical activity become increasingly the responsibility of the young person and cigarette smoking and alcohol consumption are usually initiated in adolescence. The relative influence of parents and peers on adolescent smoking and drinking is controversial but their effects are not mutually exclusive; parental factors may modify peer influence and vice versa.[155,156] Some behaviour, like smoking, is addictive and tracks strongly into adult life. Others, such as physical activity, diet, and alcohol use demonstrate more moderate levels of tracking.[20]

Adolescence and young adulthood are sensitive periods because many important 'life transitions' may be negotiated during this time (decisions about training, careers, marital partners, and childbearing), which may act as key links in chains of advantage and adversity.[157] During these transitional periods 'springboards' as well as safety nets are needed to help shift an individual onto or back onto a more advantageous trajectory or break the links in chains of risk.[158]

Many interventions to promote positive social, educational, behavioural, and health outcomes across the life course have focused on the preschool stage. In North America in the 1960s, for example, hundreds of thousands of children took part in preschool enrichment programmes such as Head Start and the Perry Preschool Program. The initial results in terms of IQ gain were very encouraging[159] and a recent systematic review concluded that these programmes prevented delay of cognitive development and increased readiness to learn, as assessed by reductions in retentions in grade and placement in special education.[160] The long-term effects have been mixed but several evaluative studies revealed long-term benefits in terms of percentage of years spent in special education, better educational and employment experiences, and less criminal behaviour.[161–164] As the individuals in these early childhood development programmes are followed into mid-life, the results so far suggest that the intervention group will show subsequent health gains.

The interpretation of these evaluative studies of early intervention centred around whether the experience 'inoculated' the children against failure, as initially expected, or began 'a chain of events in which each positive school experience made the next more likely' (p. 5).[165] The idea of inoculation suggests there is a critical period for the acquisition of personal capital. Generally the evidence is more in favour of a sensitive rather than critical period (see definitions in Chapter 1). Although particular cognitive, emotional, and social abilities are more easily acquired at different developmental stages, Hertzman and Wiens argue that there is 'consistent evidence, relating to a variety of areas of function, that if the appropriate stimulation is missed at a specific time in early childhood, the function can be developed through other forms of stimulation later on in life. It may just be harder to do' (p.1088).[114]

16.4.1 Early psychosocial environment and adult health

In this extended framework that models the dynamic interaction between the individual and their environment over the life course, parents are much more than the sum of material resources they supply or the role models they offer. Parental personal capital affects the care of their offspring in very early life and may influence growth and development[166] and later adult health, perhaps through psychoendocrine mechanisms.[167] Positive parenting practices have demonstrable effects in the short- and long-term on the development of offspring's personal capital and positive health behaviours.[20] Conversely, adverse experiences such as family or parental conflict, parental mental health and social problems, and child abuse are related to poor adult health behaviours[168] and other health risk factors and chronic disease conditions[169] in the offspring, independent of education.

There is a substantial body of evidence to show that offspring of divorced parents have more short-term health and behavioural problems, less successful educational, occupational, and marital careers, and poorer mental health and health habits in adult life than offspring from intact families.[170–175] They may even die earlier.[176] There appears to have been no closing of the well-being gap between the offspring of divorced and intact families during the 1990s, despite the experience of parental divorce having become more common.[175] Parental conflict rather than divorce as such appears to increase the risk of poor psychosocial adjustment.[171,177] Both psychosocial and socio-economic chains of risk are likely to be operating, both of which could impact on physical health.

Outside the divorce literature, studies linking the quality of social relationships within the family of origin with long-term follow-up of health and disease in offspring are rare.[178] In a general sample of the Swedish population, family conflict (based on retro-spective recall 10 years earlier) was associated with adult physical illness and mortality, independent of retrospective measures of childhood socioeconomic conditions.[179] In a US study, perceptions of parental care provided by male Harvard undergraduate students were associated with diagnosed chronic diseases up to 35 years of follow-up, after adjusting for various confounders.[180] Studies of adolescents with short-term follow-ups of 5 years or less have shown that physical symptoms are linked to poor relationships or family conflict (see, for example References 181–183).

Early relationships between young children and their parents and siblings may have lifelong effects on social integration and social support through the quantity and quality of social relationships.[184] In the 1946 cohort, survey members with parents who provided low levels of care and high levels of control (based on retrospective assessments by adult offspring) had significantly less social support in adult life.[185] A 36-year prospective study showed that having a warm or affectionate parent was associated with adult social accomplishment in terms of having a long, happy marriage, children, and relationships with close friends in mid-life.[186] In turn, marriage and other aspects of social integration have been linked to better adult health and lower mortality risk.[175,187–189]

The 1958 birth cohort study provides several examples of possible psychosocial processes that link childhood adversity to adult health and economic outcomes. Childhood psychosocial adjustment (as measured by the Rutter behaviour score) accounted for some of the class inequalities in self-reported health at 23 years and affected future social mobility[86] and the risk of unemployment between 23 and 33 years.[128] Other life course studies have shown that early positive psychosocial characteristics are related to better health outcomes in adult life and it would be of interest to know whether the experience of less adversity across the life course was an important linking mechanism. In the Terman study, for example, conscientiousness in childhood was related to longevity.[176] In the Oakland Growth Study, those with greater psychological health in adolescence (as assessed by a clinician-reported aggregate index) showed more improvement in their psychological health between 30 and 62 years of age.[190]

16.4.2 Resilience to adversity

The notion of resilience is an important concept in the life course perspective on adult health. Resilience is a dynamic process that secures positive outcomes in the face of adversity. The focus of research has been on the intrinsic and extrinsic factors associated with educational, emotional, and behavioural resilience of children.[191] There has been less focus on health outcomes and physiological resilience or on long-term resilience to adversity in childhood or earlier adult life. An exception is research by Ryff and colleagues who examined pathways to resilience in a group of middle-aged women who had high levels of psychological well-being despite a history of depression.[192] They identified various life course pathways involving one or more of the following: good starting resources, quality social relationships, realization of desired life trajectories, and positive social comparisons.

Fundamental questions from a life course perspective are whether resilience at one stage of life (and the protective factors associated with it) has long-term benefits or costs at another stage. For example, the fetal origins hypothesis assumes that fetal physiological adaptations to environmental adversity to ensure survival raise the risk of chronic disease risk in later life. Similarly, economic and social success in the face of adversity may involve psychological adaptations or levels of commitment that ultimately may have long-term health costs. This is a potentially fruitful area for further research.

16.5 **Adult factors**

According to the argument presented so far in this chapter, individuals entering adult life may bring with them a number of sources of risk for later health, such as a poor growth and development, a greater risk of exposure and vulnerability to psychosocial stress, and behaviours, such as cigarette smoking. All these have been influenced by the early social environment. The extent to which these sources of risk in early life account for variations in individual risk or social class gradients in health is as yet unknown. The individual then incurs additional sources of risk due to the constraints and opportunities afforded by adult socioeconomic position, which, as has been shown, is itself the outcome of earlier socioeconomic processes. The impact of these risks may be exacerbated if they affect those who are already most vulnerable. The question of whether a good start to life protects against the impact of poor adult circumstances has been little studied.

Adults in less advantaged socioeconomic groups have less healthy diets,[193,194] are more likely to smoke,[195] and are less likely to engage frequently in sports activities[196] than those in more privileged groups. Although some of these relationships may be accounted for by early life influences, health behaviours are strongly associated with adult socioeconomic position.[20,197] For example, current financial constraints and living in poor neighbourhoods are likely to restrict diet[198] and reduce social participation, including such things as membership of sports clubs. Similarly, smoking may be an effective coping strategy in low-income households.[199] The impact of these behaviours on health should not be overstated. They only explain some of the social inequalities in adult health or coronary heart disease mortality (see Chapter 11)[200] and even when people are successful at changing their behaviour, the effect has often been less than expected.[201]

Exposure to physical hazards and stressful life conditions are socially stratified. Manual socioeconomic groups are at higher risk of exposure to a range of physical hazards in their residential and occupational environments.[202] Persistent low income in adult life leads to poorer physical, psychological, and cognitive functioning[203] and is a strong predictor of mortality.[204] Risk of chronic limiting illness in those who accumulate the largest amount of labour market disadvantage in terms of low social class and unemployment in adult life is four times greater than in those with no exposure.[205] During the economic recessions of the 1970s and 1980s, adults in less advantaged socioeconomic groups were more likely to experience unemployment than the more privileged.[206] Unemployment carries significant risks to health.[207] Manual workers with health problems were more likely to lose their jobs and withdraw permanently from the labour market where their health may deteriorate more rapidly because of a lower standard of living.[206] In the 1946 cohort, the socioeconomic consequences of disability were shown to be more severe for manual compared with non manual workers.[82]

Material disadvantages are often combined with social exclusion associated with experiences such as unemployment or economic inactivity.[208] The low status attached to occupying a position at or near the bottom of a social hierarchy may itself be a source of stress, particularly in times of rising social expectations and growing social inequality, as witnessed in the UK and North America and many other developed countries in the last 20 years.[177,208]

Labour market experience in adult life, insofar as it affects the ability to build up an occupational pension, has a powerful affect on the standard of living after retirement, with implications for health in old age.[209] This is likely to increase with the erosion of state pensions and a greater reliance on occupational pensions. As the birth cohort studies mature it will be possible to study how socioeconomic factors in childhood, adolescence, and adult life accumulate and impact on the ageing process.

In adult life, the individual's personal capital will influence their response to the socioeconomic environment, moderating its effects on disease risk, the ageing process, and mortality at older ages when the great majority of deaths occur and modifying the risk of further exposure to adversity. Although this chapter has focused on the ways in which personal capital is influenced by early life experiences, mid-life is thought to be a developmental stage in its own right,[210,211] with opportunities to acquire new social and personal skills and coping strategies.

16.6 Social change

The twentieth century has witnessed radical changes in living conditions and family patterns in the UK, North America, and other developed countries.[177,212,213] These have affected each birth cohort at a different stage of the life course, providing a unique generational experience with different implications for health and other life chances. For example, studies have shown how growing up during the Great Depression affected the development of boys and girls in different ways[148] or how the experience of US military service allowed some men to break the chain of risk associated with early disadvantage by reshaping their life course.[214] Career opportunities expanded for many young people in the postwar period with the growth of non manual occupations and the associated expansion in secondary and further education. In contrast, young people entering the labour market during the 1970s and 1980s were at a greatly increased risk of unemployment and more restricted career opportunities.[177] Growing inequality in the distribution of income and the experience of unemployment in the developed countries over the last 20 years has increased the proportion of the population living in relative poverty.[177,208] Children have been particularly affected by this increase in relative poverty, particularly those living with single parents or whose parents have divorced.[39] These trends have worrying implications for the development of personal and health capital in these younger generations and for their health in later life.

16.7 **Conclusions**

Many studies of the effect of the childhood socioeconomic environment on adult health rely on mortality or broadly defined morbidity outcomes. Health is increasingly being considered more specifically in terms of disease outcomes, physiological, cognitive, and psychosocial functioning, and measures of positive health and resilience. A similar precision is also being applied to social and economic phenomena. These are welcome developments.

Evidence is accumulating rapidly from prospective as well as retrospective studies that childhood socioeconomic circumstances affect a range of adult health outcomes, additional to any effects of adult socioeconomic circumstances. Despite a plethora of different approaches in this interdisciplinary field, there is a common interest in understanding the underlying social, biological, and psychosocial processes that may explain these associations. So far we would conclude that there is increasing evidence for long-term biological processes related to the development of health capital during fetal life and early childhood. Social chains of risk linking childhood socioeconomic position to adult socioeconomic position are also clearly involved. There is growing interest and increasing evidence for long-term psychosocial processes that affect adult health. Social and psychosocial explanations generally have a broad focus on the whole of childhood when the acquisition of personal capital is rapid and on late adolescence and young adulthood when key life transitions are made. These processes may run in parallel and interact.[215] Childhood adversity, for example, may physiologically stunt physical growth[166] and socially set the individual on a life trajectory that includes increased risk of exposure, during the years of working life, to unemployment[128] and low job control.[56] The former is a critical period effect, the latter represents risk accumulation; and these can interact to influence subsequent health— blood pressure in this example.[131] Further research should test whether timing and duration of socioeconomic exposures have differential effects on adult health. It should also continue to exploit the maturing birth cohort studies and the follow-ups of historical cohorts with prospective information on growth and development, early temperament and behaviour, and more specific measures of early physical and social environments.

References

Those marked with an asterisk are especially recommended for further reading.

1　Townsend PN, Davidson N, Whitehead M. *Inequalities in health.* London: Penguin, 1988.

2　Drever F, Whitehead M. Health inequalities (Series DS No. 15). London: The Stationery Office, 1997.

3　Harding S, Brown J, Rosato M, Hattersley L. Socio-economic differentials in health: illustrations from the Office for National Statistics Longitudinal Study. *Health Stat Q* 1999;**1**:5–15.

4　Kitagawa EM, Hauser PM. Differential Mortality in the United States: *A study in socioeconomic epidemiology.* Cambridge, Massachusetts: Harvard University Press, 1973.

5　Elo IT, Preston SH. Educational differentials in mortality: United States, 1979–85. *Soc Sci Med* 1996;**42**:47–57.

6　Pappas G, Queen S, Hadden W, Fisher G. The increasing disparity in mortality between socio-economic groups in the United States, 1960 and 1986. *N Engl J Med* 1993;**329**:103–8.

7 **Kunst AE, Mackenbach HP.** The size of mortality differences associated with educational level in nine industrialized countries. *Am J Pub Health* 1994;**84**:932–7.

8 **Cavelaars AEJM, Kunst EE, Geurts JJM, Crialesi R, Grotvedt L.** Differences in self reported morbidity by educational level: A comparison of 11 Western European countries. *J Epidemiol Commun Health* 1998;**52**:219–27.

9 **Lahelma E, Kivela K, Roos E, Tuominen T, Dahl E, Diderichsen F** *et al.* Analysing changes of health inequalities in the Nordic welfare states. *Soc Sci Med* 2002;**55**:609–25.

10 **Krieger N.** Theories for social epidemiology in the 21st century: an ecosocial perspective. *Int J Epidemiol* 2001;**30**:668–77.

11 **Berkman LF, Kawachi I.** *Social epidemiology.* New York: Oxford University Press, 2000.

12 **Zierler S, Krieger N.** Reframing women's risk: social inequalities and HIV infection. *Annu Rev Pub Health* 1997;**18**:401–36.

13 **Kuh D, Hardy R.** *A life course approach to women's health.* Oxford: Oxford University Press, 2002.

14 **Hertzman C.** *The life course contribution to ethnic disparities in health.* In Anderson N *et al.*, eds. *Critical perspectives on racial and ethnic differentials in health in late life.* Washington DC: National Academy Press, 2004.

15 **MacIntyre S.** The Black report and beyond. What are the issues? *Soc Sci Med* 1997;**44**:723–45.

16 **Adler NE, Ostrove JM.** Socioeconomic status and health: what we know and what we don't. *Ann NY Acad Sci* 1999;**896**:3–15.

*17 **Davey Smith G, Gunnell D, Ben-Shlomo Y.** Life-course approaches to socio-economic differentials in cause-specific adult mortality. In Leon D, Walt G, eds. *Poverty, inequality and health.* Oxford: Oxford University Press, 2001:88–124.

18 **Blane D.** Socio-economic health differentials. *Int J Epidemiol* 2001;**30**:292–3.

19 **Krieger N, Williams DR, Moss NE.** Measuring social class in US public health research: concepts, methodologies, and guidelines. *Annu Rev Publ Health* 1997;**18**:341–78.

*20 **Schooling M, Kuh D.** A life course perspective on women's health behaviours. In Kuh D, Hardy R, eds. *A life course approach to women's health.* Oxford: Oxford University Press, 2002:279–303.

21 **Bartley M, Sacker A, Firth D, Fitzpatrick R.** Understanding social variation in cardiovascular risk factors in women and men: the advantage of theoretically based measures. *Soc Sci Med* 1999;**49**:831–45.

22 **Sacker A, Firth D, Fitzpatrick R, Lynch K, Bartley M.** Comparing health inequality in men and women: prospective study of mortality 1986–96. *Br Med J* 2002;**320**:1303–7.

23 **Szreter SRS.** The genesis of the Registrar General's social classification of occupations. *Br J Sociol* 1984;**35**:522–46.

24 **Davey Smith G, Hart C, Hole D, MacKinnon P, Gillis C, Watt G** *et al.* Education and occupational social class: which is the more important indicator of mortality risk? *J Epidemiol Commun Health* 1998;**52**:153–60.

25 **Ben-Shlomo Y, Kuh D.** A life course approach to chronic disease epidemiology: conceptual models, empirical challenges, and interdisciplinary perspectives. *Int J Epidemiol* 2002;**31**:285–93.

26 **Wadsworth MEJ, Kuh DJL.** Childhood influences on adult health: a review of recent work in the British 1946 national birth cohort study, the MRC National Survey of Health and Development. *Paediat Perinat Epidemiol* 1997;**11**:2–20.

27 **Power C.** A review of child health in the 1958 cohort: National Child Development Study. *Paediat Perinat Epidemiol* 1992;**6**:91–110.

*28 **Corcoran M.** Rags to rags: poverty and mobility in the United States. *Annu Rev Sociol* 1995;**21**:237–67.

29 **Heath A, Payne C.** Social mobility. In Halsey AH, Webb J, eds. *Twentieth-century British social trends.* Basingstoke: MacMillan, 2002:254–80.

30 **Solon G.** Intergenerational mobility in the labor market. In Ashenfelter O, Card D, eds. *Handbook of labor economics. Volume 3A.* Amsterdam: Elsevier, 1999.

31 **Kuh D, Wadsworth M.** Childhood influences on adult male earnings in a longitudinal study. *Br J Sociol* 1991;**42**:537–55.

32 **Kuh D, Head J, Hardy R, Wadsworth M.** The influence of education and family background on women's earnings in midlife: evidence from a British national birth cohort study. *Br J Sociol Educat* 1997;**18**:385–405.

33 **Gregg P, Machin S.** Childhood experiences, educational attainment and adult labour market performance. In Vleminckx K, Smeeding TM, eds. *Child well-being, child poverty and child policy in modern nations.* Bristol: Policy Press, 2001:129–50.

34 **Johnson P, Reed H.** *Two nations? The inheritance of poverty and affluence* (Commentary No. 53). London: Institute for Fiscal Studies, 1996.

*35 **Wadsworth MEJ.** *The imprint of time: childhood, history and adult life.* Oxford: Oxford University Press, 1991.

36 **Buchmann C, Hannum E.** Education and stratification in developing countries: a review of theories and research. *Annu Rev Sociol* 2001;**27**:77–102.

37 **Blanden J, Goodman A, Gregg P, Machin S.** Changes in intergenerational mobility in Britain. *Int J Soc Econom* 2003;**2**:105–17.

*38 **Duncan GJ, Brooks-Gunn J.** *Consequences of growing up poor.* Russel Sage Foundation: New York, 1997.

39 **Bradbury B, Jenkins SP, Micklewright J.** *The dynamics of child poverty in industrialised countries.* Cambridge: Cambridge University Press, 2001.

40 **Corcoran ME, Chaudry A.** The dynamics of child poverty. *Future Child* 1997;**7**:40–54.

41 **Halsey AH, Heath AF, Ridge JM.** *Origins and destinations: family, class and education in modern Britain.* Oxford: Clarendon Press, 1980.

42 **Ferri E, Bynner J, Wadsworth M.E.J.** *Changing Britain: changing lives. Three generations at the turn of the century.* London: Bedford Way Press, 2003.

*43 **Sacker A, Schoon I, Bartley M.** Social inequality in educational achievement and psychosocial adjustment throughout childhood: magnitude and mechanisms. *Soc Sci Med* 2002;**55**:863–80.

44 **Shavit Y, Mueller W.** *From school to work: a comparative study of educational qualifications and occupational destinations.* Oxford: Oxford University Press, 2002.

45 **Bowles S.** Understanding unequal economic opportunity. In Atkinson AB, ed. *Wealth, income and inequality.* Oxford: Oxford University Press, 1980:173–85.

46 **Kohn ML.** *Class and conformity: a study in values.* Chicago: University of Chicago Press, 1977.

47 **Keating D, Hertzman C.** Developmental health and the wealth of nations: social, biological and educational dynamics. New York: Guilford Press, 1999.

48 **Najman JM, Davey Smith G.** The embodiment of class-related and health inequalities: Australian policies. *Aust J NZ Pub Health* 2000;**24**:3.

49 **Krieger N.** A glossary for social epidemiology. *J Epidemiol Commun Health* 2001;**55**:693–700.

50 **Davey Smith G, Hart C, Blane D, Gillis C, Hawthorne V.** Lifetime socioeconomic position and mortality: prospective observational study. *Br Med J* 1997;**314**:547–52.

51 **Harding S, Rosato M, Brown J, Smith J.** Social patterning of health and mortality: children, aged 6–15 years, followed up for 25 years in the ONS Longitudinal Study. *Health Stat Q* 1999;**3**:30–4.

52 Power C, Manor O, Matthews S. The duration and timing of exposure: effects of socioeconomic environment on adult health. *Am J Pub Health* 1999;**89**:1059–65.

53 Wamala SP, Lynch J, Kaplan GA. Women's exposure to early and later life socioeconomic disadvantage and coronary heart disease risk: the Stockholm Female Coronary Risk Study. *Int J Epidemiol* 2001;**30**:275–84.

54 Langenberg C, Hardy R, Brunner E, Wadsworth MEJ. Central and total obesity in middle aged men and women in relation to lifetime socioeconomic status: evidence from a national birth cohort. *J Epidemiol Commun Health* 2003;**57**:778–83.

55 Berney L, Blane D, Davey Smith G, Gunnell DJ, Holland P, Montgomery SM. Socioeconomic measures in early old age as indicators of previous lifetime exposure to environmental health hazards. *Sociol Health Illness* 2000;**22**:415–30.

56 Holland P, Berney L, Blane D, Davey Smith G, Gunnell DJ, Montgomery SM. Life course accumulation of disadvantage: childhood health and hazard exposure during adulthood. *Soc Sci Med* 2000;**50**:1285–95.

*57 Elo IT, Preston SH. Effects of early-life conditions on adult mortality: a review. *Pop Index* 1992;**58**:186–212.

*58 Kuh D, Hardy R, Langenberg C, Richards M, Wadsworth MEJ. Mortality in adults aged 26–54 years related to socioeconomic conditions in childhood and adulthood: a post war birth cohort study. *Br Med J* 2002;**325**:1076–80.

59 Vagero D, Leon D. Effect of social class in childhood and adulthood on adult mortality. *Lancet* 1994;**343**:1224–5.

60 Nystrom Peck M. The importance of childhood socio-economic group for adult health. *Soc Sci Med* 1994;**39**:553–62.

61 Gliksman MD, Kawachi I, Hunter D, Colditz GA, Manson JE, Stampfer MJ *et al.* Childhood socioeconomic status and risk of cardiovascular disease in middle aged US women: a prospective study. *J Epidemiol Commun Health* 1995;**49**:10–15.

62 Wannamethee SG, Whincup PH, Shaper G, Walker M. Influence of fathers' social class on cardiovascular disease in middle-aged men. *Lancet* 1996;**348**:1259–63.

63 Davey Smith G, Hart C, Blane D, Hole D. Adverse socioeconomic conditions in childhood and cause specific adult mortality: prospective observational study. *Br Med J* 1998;**316**:1631–5.

64 Frankel S, Davey Smith G, Gunnell D. Childhood socioeconomic position and adult cardiovascular mortality: the Boyd Orr cohort. *Am J Epidemiol* 1999;**150**:1081–4.

65 Heslop P, Davey Smith G, Macleod J, Hart C. The socioeconomic position of employed women, risk factors and mortality. *Soc Sci Med* 2001;**53**:477–85.

66 Lynch JW, Kaplan GA, Cohen RD, Kauhanen J, Wilson TW, Smith NL *et al.* Childhood and adult socioeconomic status a predictors of mortality in Finland. *Lancet* 1994;**343**:524–7.

67 Preston SH, Hill ME, Drevenstedt GL. Childhood conditions that predict survival to advanced ages among African-Americans. *Soc Sci Med* 1998;**47**:1231–46.

68 Blane D, Hart CL, Davey Smith G, Gillis CR, Hole DJ, Hawthorne WM. The association of cardiovascular risk factors with socioeconomic position during childhood and during adulthood. *Br Med J* 1996;**313**:1434–8.

69 Kreiger N, Chen JT, Selby JV. Class inequalities in women's health: combined impact of childhood and adult social class—a study of 630 US women. *Pub Health* 2001;**115**: 175–85.

70 Brunner E, Shipley MJ, Blane D, Smith GD, Marmot MG. When does cardiovascular risk start? Past and present socioeconomic circumstances and risk factors in adulthood. *J Epidemiol Commun Health* 1999;**53**:757–64.

71 van de Mheen H, Stronks K, Looman CWN, Mackenbach JP. Does childhood socio-economic status influence adult health through behavioural factors? *Int J Epidemiol* 1998;**27**:431–7.

72 Kessler RC, Magee WJ. Childhood adversities and adult depression: basic patterns of association in a US national survey. *Psychol Med* 1993;**23**:679–90.

73 Kaplan GA, Turrell G, Lynch JW, Ererson SA, Itelkala G-L, Salonen JT. Childhood socioeconomic position and cognitive function in adulthood. *Int J Epidemiol* 2001;**30**:256–63.

74 Harper S, Lynch J, Hsu W-L, Everson SA, Hillemeier MM, Raghunathan TE *et al.* Life course socioeconomic conditions and adult psychosocial functioning. *Int J Epidemiol* 2002;**31**:395–403.

75 Rahkonen O, Lahelma E, Huuhka M. Past or present? Childhood living conditions and current socioeconomic status as determinants of adult health. *Soc Sci Med* 1997;**44**:327–36.

76 Bosma H, van de Mheen HD, Mackenbach JP. Social class in childhood and general health in adulthood: questionnaire study of contribution of psychological attributes. *Br Med J* 1999;**318**:18–22.

77 Power C, Parsons T. Overweight and obesity from a life course perspective. In Kuh D, Hardy R, eds. *A life course approach to women's health.* Oxford: Oxford University Press, 2002, 304–38.

78 Hardy R, Wadsworth MEJ, Kuh D. The influence of childhood weight and socioeconomic status on change in adult body mass index in a British national birth cohort. *Int J Obesity* 2000;**24**:1–10.

79 Gilman SE, Kawachi I, Fitzmaurice GM, Buka SL. Socioeconomic status in childhood and the lifetime risk of major depression. *Int J Epidemiol* 2002;**31**:359–67.

80 Sadowski H, Ugarte B, Kaplan C, Barnes J. Early life family disadvantages and major depression in adulthood. *Br J Psychol* 1999;**174**:112–20.

81 Hardy R, Kuh D. Does early growth influence timing of the menopause? *Hum Reprod* 2002;**17**:2474–9.

82 Kuh DJL, Wadsworth MEJ, Yusuf EJ. Burden of disability in a post war birth cohort. *J Epidemiol Commun Health* 1994;**48**:262–9.

83 Kuh DJL, Wadsworth MEJ. Physical health status at 36 years in a British national birth cohort. *Soc Sci Med* 1993;**37**:905–16.

84 Davey Smith G, Ben-Shlomo Y, Lynch J. Life-course approaches to inequalities in coronary heart disease risk. In Stansfeld S, Marmot MG, eds. *Stress and the heart: psychosocial pathways to coronary heart disease.* London: British Medical Journal Books, 2002:20–49.

*85 Graham H. Building an inter-disciplinary science of health inequalities: the example of life-course research. *Soc Sci Med* 2002;**55**:2005–16.

86 Power C, Manor O, Fox AJ. *Health and class: the early years.* London: Chapman Hall, 1991.

87 Power C, Matthews S, Manor O. Inequalities in self-rated health: explanations from different stages of life. *Lancet* 1998;**351**:1009–14.

*88 Power C, Stansfeld SA, Matthews S, Manor O, Hope S. Childhood and adulthood risk factors for socio-economic differentials in psychological distress: evidence from the 1958 British birth cohort. *Soc Sci Med* 2002;**55**:1989–2004.

89 van der Mheen H, Stronks K, van den Bos J, Mackenbach JP. The contribution of childhood environment to the explanation of socio-economic inequalities in health in adult life: a retrospective study. *Soc Sci Med* 1997;**44**:13–24.

90 Lundberg O. Causal explanations for class inequality in health—an empirical analysis. *Soc Sci Med* 1991;**32**:385–93.

91 Wadsworth MEJ. Family and education as determinants of health. In Blane D, Brunner E, Wilkinson RJ, eds. *Social organisation and health.* London: Routledge, 1996:152–70.

92 Wadsworth MEJ. Health inequalities in the life course perspective. *Soc Sci Med* 1997;**44**:859–70.

93 Seguin L, Kantiebo M, Xu Q, Zunzunegui M-V, Potvin L, Frohlich KL *et al. Longitudinal study of child development in Quebec (ELDEQ 1998–2002) Volume 1, Number 3.* Quebec: Institut de la statistique du Quebec, 2001.

94 Brooks-Gunn J, Duncan GJ. The effects of poverty on children. The future of children. *Children Poverty* 1997;**7**:55–71.

95 Aber JL, Bennett NG. The effects of poverty on child health and development. *Annu Rev Pub Health* 1997;**18**:463–83.

96 Kramer MS, Seguin L, Lydon J, Goulet L. Socio-economic disparaities in pregnancy outcomes: why do the poor fare so poorly. *Paediat Perinat Epidemiol* 2000;**14**:194–211.

97 Gunnell DJ, Smith GD, Frankel SJ, Kemp M, Peters TJ. Socio-economic and dietary influences on leg length and trunk length in childhood: a reanalysis of the Carnegie (Boyd Orr) survey of diet and health in prewar Britain (1937–39). *Paediat Perinat Epidemiol* 1998; **12(suppl 1)**:96–113.

98 dos Santos Silva I, De Stavola BL, Mann V, Kuh D, Hardy R, Wadsworth MEJ. Prenatal factors, childhood growth trajectories and age at menarche. *Int J Epidemiol* 2001;**31**:405–12.

99 Kuh D, Wadsworth MEJ. Parental height, childhood environment and subsequent adult height in a national birth cohort. *Int J Epidemiol* 1989;**18**:663–8.

100 Douglas JWB. Health and survival of infants in different social classes. *Lancet* 1951;**ii**:440–6.

101 Batty D, Leon DA. *Socio-economic position and coronary heart disease risk factors in children and young people—evidence from UK epidemiological studies.* British Heart Foundation, 2002.

102 Drillien CM. The social and economic factors affecting the incidence of premature birth. *J Obstet Gynaecol Br Empire* 1957;**64**:161–84.

103 Baird D. The epidemiology of low birth weight: changes in incidence in Aberdeen 1948–72. *J Biosoc Sci* 1974;**6**:323–41.

104 Lumey LH, Van Poppel FWA. The Dutch famine of 1944–5: mortality and morbidity in past and present generations. *Soc Hist Med* 1994;229–46.

105 Hart N. Famine, maternal nutrition and infant mortality: a re-examination of the Dutch Hunger Winter. *Pop Stud* 1993;**47**:27–46.

106 Emanuel I. Intergenerational studies of human birth weight from the 1958 birth cohort. I. Evidence for a multigenerational effect. *Br J Obstet Gynaecol* 1992;**99**:67–74.

107 Rich-Edwards J. A life course approach to women's reproductive health. In Kuh D, Hardy R, eds. *A life course approach to women's health.* Oxford: Oxford University Press, 2002:23–43.

108 Bartley M, Power C, Blane D, Davey Smith G. Birthweight and later socio-economic disadvantage: evidence from the 1958 British cohort study. *Br Med J* 1994;**309**:1475–9.

109 Leon DA, Lithell HO, Vagero D, Koupilova I, Mohsen R, Berglund L *et al.* Reduced fetal growth rate and increased risk of ischaemic heart disease mortality in 15 thousand Swedish men and women born 1915–29. *Br Med J* 1998;**317**:241–5.

110 Leon DA, Koupilova I. Birth weight, blood pressure, and hypertension. In Barker DJP, ed. *Fetal origins of cardiovascular and lung disease.* New York: Marcel Dekker, 2001:23–48.

111 Hardy R, Wadsworth MEJ, Langenberg C, Kuh D. Birth weight, childhood growth and blood pressure at 43 years in a British birth cohort. *Int J Epidemiol* (in press).

112 Barker DJP, Forsen T, Uutela A, Osmond C, Eriksson JG. Size at birth and resilience to effects of poor living conditions in adult life: longitudinal study. *Br Med J* 2001;**323**:1–5.

113 Kuh D, Hardy R, Chaturvedi N, Wadsworth M. Birth weight, childhood growth and abdominal obesity in adult life. *Int J Obesity* 2002;**26**:40–7.

114 **Hertzman C, Wiens M.** Child development and long-term outcomes: a population health perspective and summary of successful interventions. *Soc Sci Med* 1996;**43**:1083–95.

115 **Waaler HTH.** Height, weight and mortality. The Norwegian experience. *Acta Med Scand Suppl* 1984;**679**:1–56.

116 **Marmot MG, Rose GA, Shipley MJ, Hamilton PJS.** Employment grade and coronary heart disease in British civil servants. *J Epidemiol Commun Health* 1978;**32**:244–9.

117 **Nystrom Peck AM.** Childhood environment, intergenerational mobility, and adult health— evidence from Swedish data. *J Epidemiol Commun Health* 1992;**46**:71–4.

118 **Yarnell JWG, Limb ES, Layzell JM, Baker IA.** Height: a risk marker for ischaemic heart disease: prospective results from the Caerphilly and Speedwell heart disease studies. *Eur Heart J* 1992;**13**:1602–5.

119 **Rich EJW, Manson JE, Stampfer MJ, Colditz GA, Willett WC, Rosner B** *et al.* Height and the risk of cardiovascular disease in women. *Am J Epidemiol* 1995;**142**:909–17.

120 **McCarron P, Okasha M, McEwen J, Smith GD.** Height in young adulthood and risk of death from cardiorespiratory disease: a prospective study of male former students of Glasgow University, Scotland. *Am J Epidemiol* 2002;**155**:683–7.

121 **Floud R, Wachter K, Gregory A.** *Height, health and history. Cambridge studies in population; economy and society in past time. Nutritional status in the United Kingdom 1750–1980.* Cambridge: Cambridge University Press, 1990.

122 **Power C, Manor O.** Asthma, enuresis and chronic illness: long term impact on height. *Arch Dis Child* 1995;**73**:298–304.

123 **Fogel RW.** Physical growth as a measure of the economic well-being of populations: the eighteenth and nineteenth centuries. In Falkner F, Tanner JM, eds. *Human growth: a comprehensive treatise, Volume 3. Methodology; ecological, genetic and nutritional effects on growth.* New York: Plenum Press, 1986:263–305.

124 **Illsley R.** Social class selection and class differences in relation to stillbirths and infant deaths. *Br Med J* 1955;**2**:1520–4.

125 **Illsley R, Kincaid JC.** Social correlations of perinatal mortality. In Butler NR, Bonham DG, eds. *Perinatal mortality.* Edinburgh: Churchill Livingstone, 1963:270–86.

126 **Wadsworth MEJ.** Serious illness in childhood and its association with later life achievements. In Wilkinson RG, ed. *Class and health.* London: Tavistock Publications, 1986:50–74.

127 **Power C, Fogelman K, Fox AJ.** Health and social mobility during the early years of life. *Q J Soc Affairs* 1986;**2**:397–413.

128 **Montgomery SM, Bartley MJ, Cook DG, Wadsworth MEJ.** Health and social precursors of unemployment in young men in Great Britain. *J Epidemiol Commun Health* 1996;**50**:415–22.

129 **Leon D, Davey Smith G, Shipley M, Strachan D.** Height and mortality in London: early life influences, socio-economic confounding or shrinkage? *J Epidemiol Commun Health* 1995;**49**:5–9.

130 **Gunnell DJ, Davey Smith G, Frankel SJ, Nanchqhal K, Braddon FEM, Peters TJ.** Childhood leg length and adult mortality—follow up of the Carnegie survey of diet and growth in pre-war Britain. *J Epidemiol Commun Health* 1998;**52**:142–52.

131 **Montgomery SM, Berney LR, Blane D.** Prepubertal stature and blood pressure in early old age. *Arch Dis Child* 2000;**82**:358–63.

132 **Davey Smith G, Greenwood R, Gunnell D, Sweetnam P, Yarnell J, Elwood P.** Leg length, insulin resistance, and coronary heart disease risk: the Caerphilly Study. *J Epidemiol Commun Health* 2001;**55**:867–72.

133 Wadsworth MEJ, Hardy RJ, Paul AA, Marshall SF, Cole TJ. Leg and trunk length at 43 years in relation to childhood health, diet and family circumstances; evidence from the 1946 national birth cohort. *Int J Epidemiol* 2002;**31**:383–90.

134 Cole TJ. Secular trends in growth. *Proc Nutr Soc* 2000;**59**:317–24.

135 Langenberg C, Hardy R, Kuh D, Wadsworth MEJ. Influence of height, leg and trunk length on pulse pressure, systolic and diastolic blood pressure. *J Hypertens* 2003;**21**:537–43.

136 Gortmaker SL, Must A, Perrin JM, Arthur MS, Dietz WH. Social and economic consequences of overweight in adolescence and young adulthood. *N Engl J Med* 1993;**329**:1008–12.

137 Sonne-Holm S, Sorenson TIA. Prospective study of attainment of social class of severely obese subjects in relation to parental social class, intelligence, and education. *Br Med J* 1986;**292**:586–9.

138 Sargent ID, Blanchflower DG. Obesity and stature in adolescence and earnings in young adulthood. *Arch Pediat Adolesc Med* 1994;**148**:681–7.

139 Newachek PW, Jameson J, Halfon N. Prevalence and impact of chronic conditions in childhood. *Am J Pub Health* 1994;**88**:610–17.

140 Bor W, Najman J-M, Andersen M, Morrison J, Williams G. Socioeconomic disadvantage and child morbidity: an Australian Longitudinal Study. *Soc Sci Med* 1993;**36**:1053–61.

141 Cooper H, Arber S, Smaje C. Social class or deprivation? Structural factors and children's limiting longstanding illness in the 1990s. *Sociol Health Illness* 1998;**20**:289–311.

142 Power C, Peckham C. Childhood morbidity and adulthood ill health. *J Epidemiol Commun Health* 1990;**44**:69–74.

143 Blackwell DL, Hayward MD, Crimmins EM. Does childhood health affect chronic morbidity in later life? *Soc Sci Med* 2001;**52**:1269–84.

144 Kuh D, Lawrence C, Tripp J, Creber G. Work and work alternatives for disabled young people. *Disability Handicap Soc* 1988;**3**:3–26.

145 Pless IB, Cripps HA, Davies JMC, Wadsworth MEJ. Chronic physical illness in childhood and psychological and social circumstances in adolescence and early adult life. *Dev Med Child Neurol* 1989;**31**:746–55.

146 Lynch JW, Kaplan GA, Salonen JT. Why do people behave poorly? Variation in adult health behaviours and psychosocial characteristics by stages of the socioeconomic lifecourse. *Soc Sci Med* 1997;**44**:809–19.

147 Caspi A. Social selection, social causation, and developmental pathways: empirical strategies for better understanding how individuals and environments are linked across the life-course. In Pulkkinen L, Caspi A, eds. *Paths to successful development.* Cambridge: Cambridge University Press, 2002:281–301.

148 Elder GHJ, Caspi A. Economic stress in lives: developmental perspectives. *J Soc Issues* 1988;**44**:25–45.

149 Furgusson DM, Horwood LJ. Early conduct problems and later life opportunities. *J Child Psychol Psychiat* 1998;**39**:1097–108.

150 Kubzansky L, Kawachi I. Affective states and health. In Berkman LF, Kawachi I, eds. *Social epidemiology.* New York: Oxford University Press, 2000:213–41.

151 Hemingway H, Marmot M. Psychosocial factors in the aetiology and prognosis of coronary heart disease: systematic review of prospective cohort studies. *Br Med J* 1999;**318**:1460–7.

152 Kuh D, Power C, Blane D, Bartley M. Social pathways between childhood and adult health. In Kuh D, Ben-Shlomo Y, eds. *A life course approach to chronic disease epidemiology: tracing the origins of ill-health from early to adult life,* Oxford: Oxford University Press, 1997:169–200.

153 Putnam R. Tuning in, tuning out: the strange disappearance of social capital in America. *Political Sci Politics* 2002;**28**:664–83.

154 Winkleby MA, Jatulis DE, Frank E, Fortmann SP. Socioeconomic status and health: how education, income, and occupation contribute to risk factors for cardiovascular disease. *Am J Pub Health* 1992;**82**:816–20.

155 Bogenschneider K, Wu MY, Raffaelli M, Tsay JC. Parent influences on adolescent peer orientation and substance use: the interface of parenting practices and values. *Child Dev* 1998;**69**:1672–88.

156 Glendinning A, Hendry L, Shucksmith J. Lifestyle, health and social class in adolescence. *Soc Sci Med* 1995;**41**:235–48.

157 Shanahan MJ. Pathways to adulthood in changing societies: variability and mechanisms in life course perspective. *Ann Rev Sociol* 2000;**26**:667–92.

158 Bartley M, Blane D, Montgomery S. Health and the life course: why safety nets matter. *Br Med J* 1997;**314**:1194–6.

159 Bronfenbrenner V. Is early intervention effective? Facts and principles of early intervention: a summary. In Clarke AM, Clarke ADB, eds. *Early experience: myth and evidence*. New York: Free Press, 1976.

160 Anderson LM, Shinn C, Fullilove MT, Scrimshaw SC, Fielding JE, Normand J *et al*. The effectiveness of early childhood developmental programs; a systematic review. *Am J Prev Med* 2003;**24**:32–46.

161 Brown B. *Found: Long-term gains from early intervention*. American Association for the Advancement of Science, Selected Symposia Series. Boulder, Colorado: Westview Press, 1978.

162 Berrueta-Clement JR, Schweinhart LJ, Barnett WS, Epstein AS, Weikart DP. *Changed lives: the effects of the Perry Preschool Program through age 19*. Ypsilanti, Michigan: High/Scope Press, 1984.

163 Washington V, Oyemade OJ. *Project head start. Past, present, and future trends in the context of family needs*. New York and London: Garland, 1987.

164 Schweinhart LJ, Barnes HV, Weikart DP. *Significant benefits. The High/Scope Perry preschool study through age 27*. Monograph of the High/Scope Educational Research Foundation 10. Ypsilanti, Michigan: High/Scope Press, 1993.

165 Clapp G. *Child study research: current perspectives and applications*. Lexington, Massachusetts: Lexington Books, Heath and Company, 1988.

166 Montgomery SM, Bartley MJ, Wilkinson RG. Family conflict and slow growth. *Arch Dis Child* 1997;**77**:326–30.

167 Francis DD, Champagne FA, Liu D, Meaney MJ. Maternal care, gene expression, and the development of individual differences in stress reactivity. *Ann NY Acad Sci* 1999;**896**:66–84.

168 Anda RF, Croft JB, Felitti VJ, Nordenberg D, Giles WH, Williamson DF *et al*. Adverse childhood experiences and smoking during adolescence and adulthood. *J Am Med Assoc* 1999;**282**:1652–8.

169 Felitti VJ, Anda RF, Nordenberg D, Williamson DF, Spitz AM, Edwards V *et al*. Relationship of childhood abuse and household dysfunction to many of the leading causes of death in adults. *Am J Prev Med* 1998;**14**:245–58.

170 Amato PR, Keith B. Parental divorce and the well-being of children: a meta-analysis. *Psychol Bull* 1991;**110**:26–46.

171 Amato PR, Keith B. Parental divorce and adult well-being: a meta-analysis. *J Marriage Fam* 1991;**53**:43–58.

172 Amato PR, Booth A. The legacy of parents' marital discord: consequences for children's marital quality. *J Pers Soc Psychol* 2001;**81**:627–38.

173 Rodgers B, Power C, Hope S. Parental divorce and adult psychological distress. Evidence from a national birth cohort. *J Child Psychol Psychiat* 1997;**38**:867–72.

174 Wadsworth MEJ, Maclean M, Kuh D, Rodgers B. Children of divorced parents: a summary and review of findings from a national long-term follow-up study. *Fam Pract* 1990;**7**:104–9.

175 **Amato PR.** The consequences of divorce for adults and children. *J Marriage Fam* 2000;**62**:1269–87.

176 **Schwartz JE, Friedman HS, Tucker JS, Tomlinson-Keasey C, Wingard DL, Criqui MH.** Sociodemographic and psychosocial factors in childhood as predictors of adult mortality. *Am J Pub Health* 1995;**85**:1237–45.

177 **Hess LE.** Changing family patterns in Western Europe: opportunity and risk factors for adolescent development. In Rutter M, Smith DJ, eds. *Psychosocial disorders in young people: time trends and their causes.* Chichester: John Wiley, 1995:104–93.

178 **Stewart Brown S, Shaw R, Morgan L, Mockford C.** The roots of social capital: a systematic review of longitudinal studies linking relationships in the home with health and disease. Oxford: Health Services Research Unit, Department of Public Health, University of Oxford, 2002.

179 **Lundberg O.** The impact of childhood living conditions on illness and mortality in adulthood. *Soc Sci Med* 1993;**36**:1047–52.

180 **Russek LG, Schwartz GE.** Perceptions of Parental Caring Predict Health Status in Midlife: A 35-Year Follow-up of the Harvard Mastery of Stress Study. *Psychosom Med* 2002;**59**:144–9.

181 **Mechanic D, Hansell S.** Divorce, family conflict, and adolescents'well-being. *J Health Soc Behav* 1989;**30**:105–16.

182 **Sweeting H, West P.** Family life and health in adolescence: a role for culture in the health inequalities debate? *Soc Sci Med* 1995;**40**:163–75.

183 **Wickrama KAS, Conger RD, Lorenz FO, Elder GH Jr.** Parental education and adolescent self-reported physical health. *J Marriage Fam* 1998;**60**:967–78.

184 **Marks NF, Ashleman K.** Life course influences on women's social relationships at midlife. In Kuh D, Hardy R, eds. *A life course approach to women's health.* Oxford: Oxford University Press, 2002:255–78.

185 **Rodgers B.** Reported parental behaviour and adult affective symptoms 2: mediating factors. *Psychol Med* 1996;**26**:63–77.

186 **Franz CE, McClelland DC, Weinberger J.** Childhood antecedents of conventional social accomplishment in midlife adults: a 36-year prospective study. *J Pers Soc Psychol* 1991;**60**:586–95.

187 **Berkman LF, Glass T.** Social integration, networks and health. In Berkman LF, Kawachi I, eds. *Social epidemiology.* New York: Oxford University Press, 2000:137–73.

188 **Ben-Shlomo Y, Davey Smith G, Shipley M, Marmot MG.** Magnitude and causes of mortality differences between married and unmarried men. *J Epidemiol Commun Health* 1993;**47**:200–5.

189 **Wyke S, Ford G.** Competing explanations for associations between marital status and health. *Soc Sci Med* 1992;**34**:523–32.

190 **Jones CJ, Meredith W.** Developmental paths of psychological health from early adolescence to later adulthood. *Psychol ageing* 2000;**15**:351–60.

*191 **Luthar SS, Cicchetti D, Becker B.** The construct of resilience: a critical evaluation and guidelines for future work. *Child Dev* 2000;**71**:543–62.

192 **Ryff CD, Singer B, Love GD, Essex MJ.** Resilience in adulthood and later life. Defining features and dynamic processes. In Lomranz J, ed. *Handbook of aging and mental heath.* New York: Plenum Press, 1998:69–96.

193 **Irala-Estevez JD, Groth M, Johansson L, Oltersdorf U, Prattala R, Martinez-Gonzales MA.** A systematic review of socio-economic differences in food habits in Europe: consumption of fruit and vegetables. *Eur J Clin Nutr* 2000;**54**:706–14.

194 **Li R, Serdula M, Bland S, Mokdad A, Bowman B, Nelson D.** Trends in fruit and vegetable consumption among adults in 16 US states: Behavioral Risk Factor Surveillance System, 1990–1996. *Am J Pub Health* 2000;**90**:777–81.

195 Wald N, Kiryluk S, Barby S, Doll R, Pike M, Peto R. *UK smoking statistics.* Oxford: Oxford University Press, 1988.

196 Crespo CJ, Ainsworth BE, Keteyian SJ, Heath GW, Smit E. Prevalence of physical inactivity and its relation to social class in U.S. adults: results from the Third National Health and Nutrition Examination Survey, 1988–1994. *Med Sci Sports Exerc* 1999;**31**:1821–7.

197 Blane D, Hart CL, Davey Smith G, Gillis CR, Hole DJ, Hawthorne VM. The association of cardiovascular disease risk factors with socioeconomic position during childhood and during adulthood. *Br Med J* 1997;**7**:385–91.

198 Sooman A, MacIntyre S, Anderson A. Scotland's health—a more difficult challenge for some? The price and availability of healthy foods in socially contrasting localities in the West of Scotland. *Health Bull* 1993;**51**:276–84.

199 Graham H. *When life's a drag.* London: Her Majesty's Stationery Office, 1994.

200 Davey Smith G, Shipley MJ, Rose G. The magnitude and causes of socioeconomic differentials in mortality:further evidence from the Whitehall Study. *J Epidemiol Commun Health* 1990;**44**:265–70.

201 Ebrahim S, Smith GD. Systematic review of randomised controlled trials of multiple risk factor interventions for preventing coronary heart disease. *Br Med J* 1997;**314**:1666–74.

202 Blane D, Bartley M, Davey Smith G. Disease aetiology and materialist explanations of socio-economic mortality differentials. *Eur J Pub Health* 1998;**8**:259–60.

203 Lynch JW, Kaplan GA, Shema SJ. Cumulative impact of sustained economic hardship on physical, cognitive, psychological, and social functioning. *N Engl J Med* 1997;**337**:1889–95.

204 McDonough P, Duncan GJ, Williams D, House J. Income dynamics and adult mortality in the United States, 1972 through 1989. *Am J Pub Health* 1997;**87**:1476–83.

205 Bartley M, Plewis I. Accumulated labour market disadvantage and limiting long-term illness: data from the 1971–1991 Office for National Statistics' Longitudinal Study. *Int J Epidemiol* 2002;**31**:336–41.

206 Bartley M, Owen C. Relation between socioeconomic status, employment, and health during economic change, 1973–93. *Br Med J* 1996;**313**:445–59.

207 Morris JK, Cook DG, Shaper AG. Loss of employment and mortality. *Br Med J* 1994;**308**:1135–9.

208 Wilkinson RG. *Unhealthy societies. The affliction of inequality.* London: Routledge, 1996.

209 Hancock R, Weir P. *More ways than means: a guide to pensioners' incomes in Great Britain during the 1980s.* London: Age Concern Institute of Gerontology, Kings College, London, 1994.

210 Baltes PB, Baltes NM. *Successful Aging: perspectives from the behavioural sciences.* Oxford: Oxford University Press, 1990.

211 Lachman M, James JB. *Multiple paths of midlife development.* Chicago: University of Chigaco Press, 1997.

212 Smith DJ. Living conditions in the twentieth century. In Rutter M, Smith DJ, eds. *Psychosocial disorders in young people: time trends and their causes.* Chichester: John Wiley, 1995:194–295.

213 Halsey AH. *British social trends since 1900. A Guide to the changing social structure of Britain.* Basingstoke: Macmillan, 1988.

214 Elder GH. Military times and turning points in men's lives. *Dev Psychol* 1986;**22**:233–45.

215 Hallqvist J, Lynch J, Bartley M, Blane D. Accumulation, critical periods and social mobility: evidence from SHEEP study. *Soc Sci Med* (in press).

Part IV

Implications for policy and future research

Chapter 17

Should we intervene to improve fetal and infant growth?

K.S. Joseph and Michael S. Kramer

Numerous studies have demonstrated associations between suboptimal patterns of fetal and infant growth and coronary heart disease (CHD). This chapter examines the potential long-term health impacts of interventions to improve fetal and infant growth.

The effects of available interventions to improve fetal and infant growth are likely to be modest, at least in terms of their impact on subsequent CHD. The mean birthweight reduction among mothers who smoke is approximately 150 g, while interventions to reduce smoking in pregnancy result in a mean birthweight increase of approximately 28 g. Similarly, nutritional supplementation in pregnancy has modest effects on fetal growth (mean birthweight increase of approximately 25 g). Increases in infant growth could be achieved through formula feeding, although this would be at the cost of reversing current recommendations regarding breastfeeding.

About one-third of CHD deaths would be averted if all live births weighed between 9 and 9.5 pounds (3969–4422 g). Simulations with more realistic assumptions show a marginal impact on subsequent CHD deaths, however. A 100 g increase in birthweight would result in a 2% decrease in CHD deaths in Canada. Other issues that must be considered before intervening to improve fetal and infant growth include the potential for unintended effects. Increases in caesarean delivery and maternal obesity would be important maternal concerns, while possible increases in the occurrence of cancers of the prostate, breast, and ovary would constitute long-term threats to the health of the offspring.

Interventions designed to improve fetal and infant growth would lead to marginal reductions in the occurrence of adult chronic diseases and may have adverse effects. Furthermore, such interventions could detract from the contemporary obstetric focus on preventing preterm, very low birthweight infants by shifting the emphasis to normal weight infants born at term.

17.1 Introduction

Numerous recent studies have reported associations between suboptimal fetal and infant growth and CHD and other adult chronic diseases. These studies have served as the basis for the hypothesis that physiologic or metabolic 'programming' during gestation and infancy substantially determines the occurrence of various pathological phenomena in later life (see Chapter 3).[1–13] If the evidence and arguments supporting the programming hypothesis are valid, they carry important implications for both clinical practice and public health policy. In this chapter we examine the potential impact that interventions in pregnancy and early childhood might have on diseases in adult life, assuming that the documented associations are in fact causal (our viewpoints on the fetal/infant origins hypothesis are documented elsewhere).[14–17] We first review the current literature with regard to the efficacy of interventions for improving fetal growth. The next section describes the possible unintended effects that such interventions may have on the mother and the infant. We then use findings from the Hertfordshire (UK) studies and more recent publications from Finland to estimate the magnitude of CHD that could be prevented by improving fetal growth. In the final section, we discuss the implications of intervening to improve fetal growth in terms of changes in public health policy and clinical practice.

17.2 Interventions to improve fetal and infant growth

Of the various recognized determinants of fetal growth, several offer potential avenues for intervention. These interventions must be considered according to the strength of the evidence that they do indeed increase fetal growth and, if so, the magnitude of the fetal growth effect. In this section, we review the evidence regarding four potential areas for intervention: (1) nutritional advice or supplementation prior to pregnancy; (2) nutritional advice or supplementation during pregnancy; (3) interventions to reduce smoking during pregnancy; and (4) other aspects of prenatal care (see Table 17.1 for summary). For each of these, we will focus primarily on the results of controlled clinical trials. In the final subsection, we briefly discuss issues related to improving growth rates in infancy.

17.2.1 Prepregnancy nutrition

Meta-analysis indicates an extremely strong relationship between prepregnancy weight or body mass index and fetal growth.[18–20] Each additional kg of prepregnancy weight increases gestational age-adjusted birthweight by approximately 10 g.[18] Thus, infants of women with a prepregnancy weight of 75 kg have a birthweight that is about 100 g greater than that of infants born to women with a prepregnancy weight of 65 kg (assuming the same height and gestational duration). Prepregnancy weight below 50 kg increases the risk for a small-for-gestational-age infant by about 80%.[18]

To our knowledge, the only evidence from controlled clinical trials on prepregnancy nutritional status comes from the Taiwan trial of balanced energy/protein supplementation.[21,22] In that trial, supplementation was begun following the birth of a previous child and thus included the entire interpregnancy interval in addition to the index pregnancy. Although this intervention was not compared with an intervention provided during pregnancy only, the magnitude of the overall effect on fetal growth was no greater than in trials in which supplementation was restricted to pregnancy itself.[23]

17.2.2 Nutrition during pregnancy

Strong evidence from both observational studies and controlled clinical trials indicates that gestational weight gain (which reflects increases in both nutritional stores and

Table 17.1 Summary of the results of various randomized trials on the effects of intervention for improving fetal growth[23–34]

Intervention	Outcome	Results
Balanced energy and protein supplementation	Birthweight	Mean difference, range = –60 to 263 g; weighted average = 25 g (95% CI, –4–55)
	Small-for-gestational-age	Weighted odds ratio = 0.64 (95% CI, 0.53–0.78)
	Birth length	Mean difference, range = 0.0–1.8 cm; weighted average = 0.15 cm (95% CI, 0.06–0.35)
	Head circumference	Mean difference, range = –0.4–0.2 cm; weighted average = 0.07 cm (95% CI, –0.06–0.20)
High protein supplementation	Birthweight	Mean difference = –58 g (95% CI, –146–29)
Smoking reduction/cessation	Birthweight	Mean difference, range = –12 to 92 g; weighted average = 28 g (95% CI, 9–49)
	Low birthweight	Odds ratio = 0.80 (95% CI, 0.67–0.95)
Antiplatelet agents in women at risk for preeclampsia	Low birthweight	Relative risk = 0.94 (95% CI, 0.84–1.05)
	Small-for-gestational-age	Relative risk = 0.92 (95% CI, 0.84–1.01)
Intensive prenatal care	Birthweight	No difference compared with standard
Social support	Birthweight	Mean difference, range = –85–101 g; weighted average = –50 g (95% CI, –102–2)
	Low birthweight	Odds ratio = 0.96 (95% CI, 0.84–1.08)
	Small-for-gestational-age	Odds ratio = 1.06 (95% CI, 0.86 –1.30)

CI, confidence interval.

non-nutritional components, such as plasma volume and oedema fluid) and energy intake during pregnancy are important determinants of fetal growth.[18–20] Each kg of total gestational weight gain increases gestational age-adjusted birthweight by approximately 20 g; weight gains below 7 kg are associated with an approximate doubling of the risk of a growth restricted infant.[18] Moreover, the effect of weight gain on fetal growth appears to be conditional, with greater effects in women with low prepregnancy weight or body mass index and smaller effects in those who are well-nourished prior to pregnancy.

The importance of energy intake on fetal growth is apparent from the results of the Dutch famine study, which demonstrated that extreme restriction of energy intake during the third trimester can have a substantial impact on fetal growth, with a reduction in mean birthweight of approximately 300 g.[24] Nutritional advice to increase energy and protein intake succeeds in increasing pregnant women's energy and protein intake and gestational weight gain.[25] The effects on fetal growth, however, are small and statistically non-significant. Actual energy and protein supplementation during pregnancy results in more consistent (and statistically significant) effects on fetal growth, but the magnitude of the effect is again modest, with an increase in mean birthweight of 25 g and a pooled odds ratio for the occurrence of small-for-gestational-age (<10th percentile) live births of 0.64 (95% confidence interval (CI), 0.53–0.78).[23] Protein supplementation alone appears to have no beneficial effect on fetal growth independent of the energy content of the supplement.[23]

As for micronutrients, it seems clear that iron intake is unrelated to fetal growth.[26] The data are somewhat less clear with respect to folate[27] and zinc[28] intake, although most of the interest in these micronutrients focuses on their effects on preterm delivery, rather than fetal growth.

17.2.3 Interventions to reduce smoking during pregnancy

The previously cited meta-analysis[18] clearly indicates a large effect of maternal cigarette smoking during pregnancy on fetal growth; this effect has been detected in virtually every epidemiologic study that has investigated the issue. Moreover, a clear dose–response effect has been observed; larger deficits in fetal growth are associated with additional numbers of cigarettes smoked per day.[18] The mean birthweight reduction in smoking mothers is approximately 150 g or approximately 11 g per cigarette smoked per day.[18] Smokers have a 2.5-fold increased risk of giving birth to a growth-restricted infant.[18]

Intensive interventions to reduce smoking during pregnancy appear to reduce smoking and also have a beneficial effect on fetal growth.[29] Smoking cessation interventions lead to an increase in mean birthweight (weighted mean difference 28 g; 95% CI, 9–49 g). The overall magnitude of the effect of these interventions on fetal growth is not entirely clear, however, because the results of the Cochrane meta-analysis are reported according to mean birthweight and risk of low birthweight, rather than gestational age-adjusted mean birthweight or small-for-gestational-age.[29] Nonetheless, considering the comparatively modest effect of smoking on preterm delivery,[18] the pooled odds ratio of 0.80 (95% CI, 0.67–0.95) for low birthweight can be taken as a rough proxy of the effect of a smoking cessation program on reduction in small-for-gestational-age. It should be noted, however, that the pooled odds ratio and 95% CI for reduction in preterm birth from these smoking reduction strategies (odds ratio 0.83; 95% CI, 0.69–0.99) is quite similar to the corresponding values for low birthweight and thus the specific effect of these interventions on fetal growth is unclear.

17.2.4 Other aspects of prenatal care

Controlled clinical trials of 'intensive' prenatal care (as a combined package) and social support have mostly been aimed at reducing preterm delivery and the results have been disappointing.[30–33] In addition, the results of these trials do not suggest that more frequent or longer contact with providers of prenatal care or social support leads to any beneficial effect on fetal growth. Other than nutritional counselling and supplementation and interventions to reduce smoking during pregnancy, the main interventions that could potentially have such a beneficial impact include low-dose aspirin or other antiplatelet agents for the prevention of preeclampsia and small-for-gestational-age. The Cochrane meta-analysis suggests that antiplatelet agents lead to an 8% reduction (nominally significant) in small-for-gestational-age live births among women at risk of developing preeclampsia.[34]

17.2.5 Infant growth

Studies from Guatemala[35,36] on the effect of nutritional supplementation during infancy and early childhood suggest that such supplements can result in substantial increases in growth velocity, at least in a developing country with a high prevalence of childhood malnutrition. During the first year of life, each 100 kcal per day of supplement resulted in a 350 g increase in weight.[36] Similar, though smaller, effects have been reported from studies in Colombia, with supplemented infants gaining an additional 110 g between 9 and 12 months.[37]

The applicability of these studies to infants from developed countries is probably limited, at least among the majority of children. Nevertheless, a decision to intervene in infancy based on the programming hypothesis would have implications for clinical practice and public health policy in developed countries. For instance, studies have shown that infants who are breastfed up to 12 months of age (solid foods introduced after 4 months) are leaner than their formula-fed counterparts, even in populations of high socioeconomic status.[38–40] Among girls, statistically significant differences of 373, 733, and 185 g have been observed at 6, 12, and 18 months of age, respectively.[38,41] Similar though smaller differences have also been observed among boys. A decision to increase infant weight gain (based on the programming hypothesis) could reverse current recommendations regarding breast- and formula feeding. This would mean foregoing the beneficial effects of breastfeeding including those on infant morbidity and on obesity.[42–44] In this context, it is worth noting the strength of the infant weight–CHD association relative to the strength of the birthweight–CHD association; a 2 pound (908 g) increase in infant weight would be required to achieve the same reduction in CHD mortality as a 1 pound (454 g) increase in birthweight.[3]

17.3 Risks and costs of intervention

17.3.1 Risks for the mother

Perhaps the single most important, immediate consequence of an increase in fetal growth would be a rise in caesarean delivery rates.[45–47] Studies have shown that rates of caesarean delivery for dystocia increase as a function of increasing birthweight.[45] Caesarean delivery rates for dystocia are more than four times as high among deliveries involving babies weighing 4000–4499 g than with those of babies in the 3000–3499 g range. Similar increases have also been seen in the requirements for forceps deliveries for dystocia and also in the need for oxytocin to augment labour.[45]

Overall rates of caesarean delivery (that is, irrespective of indication), however, do not show as simple a relationship with birthweight. Overall rates of caesarean delivery are relatively high for mothers delivering babies weighing under 2500 g and a positive dose–response relationship between birthweight and overall caesarean delivery rates is seen only among babies with a birthweight of 2500 g or more.[46] Caution is required in interpreting these findings, however, because reverse causality is inherent in the birthweight–overall caesarean delivery relationship; preterm caesarean delivery is used to terminate pregnancies where fetal or maternal well-being is compromised and this can be responsible for a lower birthweight. Nevertheless, the birthweight–caesarean delivery relationship above 2500 g implies that an across-the-board increase in fetal growth will raise the overall rate of caesarean delivery, because births over 2500 g constitute about 95% of all births in industrialized countries.

Increased prevalence of maternal obesity is another potential adverse consequence of attempts to increase fetal growth. Although dietary and nutritional interventions for improving fetal growth are likely to have only modest effects in terms of enhancing fetal growth, the same cannot be said for their impact on mothers. Studies have shown that a significant proportion of maternal weight gain during pregnancy is likely to be retained postpartum, thereby putting some women at risk of obesity.[48–51] In one study, women with high rates of gestational weight gain (greater than 0.68 kg/week) weighed 7.9 kg more than their pregravid weight at 6 months postpartum, compared with a 3.2 kg and a 3.8 kg difference for women with low (less than 0.34 kg/week) and moderate (0.34–0.68 kg/week) rates of gestational weight gain, respectively.[49]

17.3.2 Risks for the offspring

Even if fetal growth is negatively associated with adult cardiovascular end-points, several studies have demonstrated positive associations between birthweight (or other early growth indices) and ovarian, prostate, breast, and other cancers (see Chapter 11).[52–63] The strength of the association between birthweight and these cancers is generally similar to that between birthweight and heart disease. To the extent that these associations are causal (negative studies notwithstanding),[64–67] potential reductions in heart disease that occur secondary to increases in birthweight will be attended by simultaneous increases in cancer rates.

Direct associations have also been reported between birthweight, on the one hand and atopy, acute lymphoblastic leukaemia, and obesity on the other.[68–72] A high weight gain in early life has been associated with an increased risk of type 1 diabetes mellitus in other studies.[73–76] These possible unintended effects of intervention, though relatively less frequent than CHD and type 2 diabetes mellitus, must be balanced against potential benefits when evaluating the desirability of intervention.

17.4 Potential magnitude of the effects of intervention

17.4.1 Blood pressure

The relationship between birthweight and blood pressure in later life is one of the most widely studied associations in the fetal origins literature. Given the inverse association between birthweight and subsequent blood pressure, should we contemplate intervening to increase birthweight in order to ensure reductions in the occurrence of hypertension later in life? Reviews[16,17,77,78] of studies on the relationship between birthweight and blood pressure show that systolic blood pressure (in later life) is approximately 1–3 mm Hg lower for each kg increase in birthweight. Birthweight is not significantly associated with diastolic blood pressure.[17] A 15 mm Hg increase in systolic blood pressure is required to produce a 50% increase in CHD.[79,80] On the other hand, the 1 kg increase in birthweight required to yield a mere 1–3 mm Hg decrease in systolic blood pressure is unattainable by any known intervention.

17.4.2 Coronary heart disease

Table 17.2 provides estimates of the impact that changes in the birthweight distribution would have on subsequent CHD mortality. Estimates are based on the results of studies of the Hertfordshire cohort.[3] The relative risk for CHD associated with each birthweight category in Table 17.2 was estimated using the birthweight category 9–9.5 pounds (3969–4422 g because birthweights were rounded to the nearest half pound) as the reference category. Two approximate estimates of relative risk were made based on the published findings:[3] the ratio of crude rates of CHD mortality and the ratio of the standardized mortality ratios. Although neither method of relative risk calculation is ideal, the results are generally similar and likely represent fair approximations.

We calculated two hypothetical estimates of the proportion of CHD cases that can be attributed to low birthweight.[81–83] The first etiologic fraction estimate (EF1) expresses the proportion of CHD deaths attributable to each birthweight category, with birthweights between 9 and 9.5 pounds taken as the reference. These estimates identify the proportion of CHD deaths that could be potentially prevented if all live births in any particular birthweight category attained birthweights in the 9–9.5 pound range.

Table 17.2 Estimated proportion of coronary heart disease that would be prevented if all infants in any birthweight category had weights in the 9–9.5 lb range, based on results of the Hertfordshire studies[3]

Birthweight* (lb)	Women					Men				
	Number	SMR	Crude RR	SMR ratio	EF1† (%)	Number	SMR	Crude RR	SMR ratio	EF1† (%)
≤5.5	307	83	1.8	1.9	3.5	458	102	1.7	1.8	2.7
6–6.5	1068	72	1.6	1.7	8.7	1317	83	1.4	1.5	4.6
7–7.5	1956	67	1.5	1.6	13.2	2991	82	1.4	1.5	10.1
8–8.5	1532	59	1.4	1.4	6.9	3166	75	1.3	1.3	7.8
9–9.5	551	43	1.0	1.0	0.0	1505	56	1.0	1.0	0.0
≥10	171	49	1.1	1.1	0.3	704	66	1.2	1.2	0.9

SMR, standardized mortality ratio; RR, relative risk; EF1, first etiologic fraction estimate.

*Birthweight categories are the same as those defined in the Hertfordshire studies, with weights rounded to the nearest half-pound. This means that, for instance, the birthweight category 9–9.5 lb includes birthweights in the range 3969–4422 g.

†EF1, proportion of coronary heart disease deaths that could be potentially prevented if births in any birthweight category attained birthweights in the 9–9.5 lb range. The SMR ratio was used as the RR estimate in the calculation.

For instance, 3.5% of CHD deaths among women would be averted if babies in the ≤5.5 pounds (≤2606 g because birthweights were rounded to the nearest half pound) birthweight category attained birthweights between 9 and 9.5 pounds (Table 17.2). If all births weighed between 9 and 9.5 pounds, 33% and 26% of CHD deaths would be prevented among women and men, respectively. Most of the impact under this scenario would arise from increases in the birthweight category 7–8.5 pounds (3061–3968 g). We also estimated the proportion of CHD deaths that would be averted if babies within any birthweight category attained birthweights in the succeeding birthweight category (EF2). Such an increase in birthweight would lead to a decrease in CHD deaths of approximately 9%. These latter estimates assume a mean birthweight increase of approximately 1 pound (454 g). Calculations based on the findings of more recent fetal origins studies from Finland[9,10] also show that only a relatively small fraction of CHD would be prevented despite drastic increases in birthweight.[17]

The scenarios considered in Table 17.3 are more realistic, because available interventions cannot change birthweight distributions as dramatically as assumed in Table 17.2. The CHD death rate for the 1998 Canadian birth cohort (Ontario excluded due to concerns about data quality)[84] was obtained by applying the birthweight-specific rates of CHD death observed in Hertfordshire to the Canadian birth cohort. The overall rates of

Table 17.3 Expected rates of coronary heart disease mortality in the 1998 Canadian birth cohort (data provided courtesy of Shiliang Liu, Health Canada) and estimated preventive fractions, assuming the birthweight-specific rates of coronary heart disease death observed in the Hertfordshire cohort[3]

Cohort	Assumption	Coronary heart disease death rate (per 1000)	Preventive fraction (%)
Women			
Hertfordshire	None	15.8	
Canada 1998 (reference)	None	16.0	
Canada 1998	≤5.5 lb births shifted to 6–6.5 lbs	15.8	0.9
Canada 1998	100 g increase in birthweight	15.6	2.3
Canada 1998	200 g increase in birthweight	15.3	4.4
Canada 1998	300 g increase in birthweight	14.8	7.3
Men			
Hertfordshire	None	84.1	
Canada 1998 (reference)	None	85.4	
Canada 1998	≤5.5 lb births shifted to 6–6.5 lbs	83.9	1.8
Canada 1998	100 g increase in birthweight	83.8	1.9
Canada 1998	200 g increase in birthweight	82.4	3.6
Canada 1998	300 g increase in birthweight	80.6	5.7

CHD death for both the male and female Canadian birth cohorts are virtually identical to those observed in Hertfordshire. This is because the (categorized) birthweight distribution of the Hertfordshire cohort is similar to that of the 1998 Canadian birth cohort. This identity of birthweight distributions is partly due to selective follow-up in the Hertfordshire cohort; for instance, in the Hertfordshire cohort, multiple births and infant deaths (which were more likely to have a low birthweight) were excluded and those who were followed up weighed more than those who were not traced. Exclusion of very low birthweight babies from the Canadian birth cohort does not appreciably alter these estimates. Altering the birthweight distribution of the Canadian birth cohort (100, 200, or 300 g shifts to the right in the birthweight distribution) does not appreciably reduce the estimated CHD death rates (preventive fractions 2.3%, 4.4%, and 7.3%, respectively, for women and 1.9%, 3.6%, and 5.7%, respectively, for men).

The preventive fractions for some of the other diseases considered in the Hertfordshire studies may be somewhat higher than those estimated for CHD. If the association between infant weight and adult chronic obstructive lung disease (COLD) mortality[85] is causal, then increases in infant weight will have a slightly greater impact on COLD mortality than will increases in birthweight on CHD mortality.

Thus interventions in early life seem likely to have a small impact, if any, on adult chronic disease. It is useful to compare the magnitude of such an impact with those of alternative interventions currently advocated for reducing the burden of adult disease. For instance, 20-year follow-up results from the Framingham heart study[86] show that CHD mortality declined by 51% across the 50–59-year-old female cohorts of 1950 and 1970. The same estimate for the decline in CHD mortality in the male Framingham cohorts was 44%. More than one-half of the decline in CHD mortality observed in women and one-third to one half of the decline observed in men has been attributed to changes in risk factor status (that is, changes in levels of cigarette smoking, total cholesterol, systolic blood pressure, and diabetes mellitus).[86] Similar estimates have been obtained from other studies.[87,88] Table 17.4, which is based on data from the British Regional Heart Study, presents estimates of the magnitude of impact likely to result from three potential areas for adult intervention. These data show that 51% of CHD deaths would be prevented if the entire population consisted of never smokers. Similarly, 48% and 34% of CHD deaths, respectively, would be prevented if the entire population had cholesterol and systolic blood pressure values in the reference range (these estimates are independent but not mutually exclusive).[89] On the other hand, a single category shift towards the reference category in cholesterol, systolic blood pressure, and smoking status would result in an approximately 13%, 12%, and 24% decrease, respectively, in CHD deaths.

Studies such as the Framingham analysis cited above have not considered fetal growth determinants in modelling CHD etiology. For this reason, it may be more appropriate to consider the results of experimental studies for evaluating the effects of adult intervention (fetal determinants would be balanced in the treatment groups because of randomization). The largest of the randomized trials on smoking cessation, the Multiple Risk Factor Intervention Trial (MRFIT), showed a substantial and rapid benefit of smoking cessation on CHD mortality in both the usual care and intervention groups.[90,91] Participants who had quit smoking for 1 year after trial initiation experienced a 37% decrease in the risk of CHD mortality. The effect was greater

Table 17.4 Estimated proportion of coronary heart disease events and deaths that would be prevented by changes in risk factor status, based on results of the British regional heart study

Factor (category)	Number of participants	CHD events	RR (age-adjusted)	EF1*	CHD deaths	RR (age-adjusted)	EF1*
Cholesterol (mmol/l)							
≤5.4	1613	105	1.00	0.0	54	1.00	0.0
5.5–5.9	1384	143	1.59	5.5	89	1.93	8.7
6.0–6.4	1492	167	1.69	6.9	83	1.60	6.1
6.5–7.1	1703	249	2.21	13.8	132	2.20	13.8
≥7.2	1495	297	3.22	22.3	145	2.91	19.3
Systolic blood pressure (mm Hg)							
<128	1550	131	1.00	0.0	60	1.00	0.0
128–137	1542	151	1.17	2.4	73	1.23	3.0
138–147	1540	165	1.24	3.4	77	1.22	2.9
148–160	1550	238	1.74	10.4	134	1.99	13.1
≥161	1542	282	1.97	13.6	160	2.16	15.2
Smoking							
Never	1819	124	1.00	0.0	54	1.00	0.0
Ex	2714	336	1.66	12.9	179	1.89	15.4
Current	3183	508	2.37	31.4	271	2.76	35.6

CHD, coronary heart disease; RR, relative risk; EF1, first etiologic fraction estimate.

*EF1, proportion of CHD events/deaths that would be prevented if participants in any risk factor category attained values in the reference category range (≤5.4 mmol/l of cholesterol, <128 mm Hg systolic blood pressure, and never smokers were the three reference categories).

Estimates calculated using RRs adjusted for risk factors other than age yield similar results.

Data provided courtesy of F. Lampe and P. Whincup.

among those who had quit smoking for at least the first 3 years of the trial, with a 62% decrease in CHD mortality compared with persistent smokers.[90] These results are not based on an intention-to-treat analysis, however.

Another randomized trial of diet and antismoking advice showed a 47% reduction in the incidence of major CHD events, though the effect was attributed more to changes in serum cholesterol than to smoking cessation.[92] The only randomized trial of antismoking advice alone involved a subset of the Whitehall study of civil servants; it showed a 7%, 13%, and 11% decrease in total mortality, CHD mortality, and lung cancer, respectively.[93] The study investigators estimated that for every 100 men who had stopped smoking, between 6 and 10 were alive 20 years later as a result.

These estimates refer to the impact of changes in smoking status among smokers. Reductions in CHD mortality will be smaller in the overall population and will depend on the prevalence of smoking in the population.

17.5 Implications for public health policy and clinical practice

Birthweight is a confusing target for intervention because it reflects two largely independent processes: gestational duration and rate of fetal growth.[94,95] Most of the recent emphasis in developed country settings has been on efforts to prevent preterm birth, particularly extremely preterm birth, because of its disproportionate contribution to infant mortality and morbidity and long-term health.[96–98] Yet these efforts have thus far borne little fruit; with the possible exception of France,[99,100] preterm birth rates have not declined.[101–104]

Interventions to improve fetal growth as a result of the programming hypothesis would change the focus from preterm birth to term, normal-weight infants. Our estimates (Table 17.2) show that the greatest impact (in terms of subsequent CHD reduction) will accrue if birthweights among normal-weight, term babies are increased. In fact, countries such as the USA,[105–107] Canada,[107–109] and England and Wales[110] have witnessed an increase in size of infants born at term. The health benefits of such an increase have heretofore been considered marginal. If the fetal origins hypothesis proves correct, a continued trend in this direction may yield small long-term reductions in cardiovascular and other adult chronic diseases and marginal increases in the rates of some cancers. However, efforts to further this trend will entail a substantial shift in focus from the current emphasis on preventing preterm births.

In conclusion, we (and others who have examined these issues),[111] believe that intervening to improve fetal growth based solely on the programming hypothesis is not justified. The reasons include the marginal impact of available interventions, the possible short- and long-term unintended effects of such interventions, and the potentially adverse effects of shifting the current focus from preventing preterm birth to increasing the size of term infants.

Acknowledgements

Dr Joseph is supported by a Clinical Research Scholar award from the Dalhousie University Faculty of Medicine and a Peter Lougheed/Canadian Institutes of Health Research New Investigator award. Dr Kramer is a Senior Investigator of the Canadian Institutes of Health Research.

References

Those marked with an asterisk are especially recommended for further reading.

1 Barker DJ, Winter PD, Osmond C, Margetts B, Simmonds SJ. Weight in infancy and death from ischaemic heart disease. *Lancet* 1989;**2**:577–80.

2 Barker DJP, Bull AR, Osmond C, Simmonds SJ. Fetal and placental size and risk of hypertension in adult life. *Br Med J* 1990;**301**:259–63.

3 Osmond C, Barker DJ, Winter PD, Fall CH, Simmonds SJ. Early growth and death from cardiovascular disease in women. *Br Med J* 1993;**307**:1519–24.

4 Barker DJP, Osmond C, Simmonds SJ, Wield GA. The relation of small head circumference and thinness at birth to death from cardiovascular disease. *Br Med J* 1993;**306**:422–6.

5 Leon DA, Koupilova I, Lithell HO, Berglund L, Mohsen R, Vagero D *et al.* Failure to realise growth potential *in utero* and adult obesity in relation to blood pressure in 50 year old Swedish men. *Br Med J* 1996;**312**:401–6.

6 Curhan GC, Chertow GM, Willett WC, Spiegelman D, Colditz GA, Manson JE *et al.* Birthweight and adult hypertension and obesity in women. *Circulation* 1996;**94**:1310–5.

7 Rich-Edwards JW, Stampfer MJ, Manson JE, Rosner B, Hankinson SE, Colditz GA *et al.* Birthweight and risk of cardiovascular disease in a cohort of women followed up since 1976. *Br Med J* 1997;**315**:396–400.

8 Barker DJP. *Mothers babies and health in later life* (2nd edn). Edinburgh: Churchill Livingstone, 1998.

9 Forsén T, Eriksson JG, Tuomilehto J, Osmond C, Barker DJP. Growth *in utero* and during childhood among women who develop coronary heart disease: longitudinal study. *Br Med J* 1999;**319**:1403–7.

10 Eriksson JG, Forsén T, Tuomilehto J, Winter PD, Osmond C, Barker DJP. Catch-up growth in childhood and death from coronary heart disease: longitudinal study. *Br Med J* 1999;**318**:427–31.

*11 Osmond C, Barker DJP. Fetal, infant and childhood growth are predictors of coronary heart disease, diabetes, and hypertension in adult men and women. *Environ Health Perspect* 2000;**108(suppl)**:545–53.

*12 Barker DJP. *Fetal origins of cardiovascular and lung disease*. New York: Marcel Dekker, 2001.

13 Leon D, Ben-Shlomo Y. Development of disease risk throughout life: cardiovascular disease. In Kuh D, Ben-Shlomo Y, eds. *A life course approach to chronic disease epidemiology* (2nd edn). New York: Oxford Medical Publications, 2004.

14 Joseph KS, Kramer MS. Review of the evidence on fetal and early childhood antecedents of chronic disease. *Epidemiol Rev* 1996;**18**:158–74.

15 Kramer MS, Joseph KS. Enigma of fetal/infant-origins hypothesis. *Lancet* 1996;**348**:1254–5.

*16 Kramer MS. Association between restricted fetal growth and adult chronic disease: is it causal? Is it important? *Am J Epidemiol* 2000;**152**:605–8.

*17 Joseph KS. Validating the fetal origins hypothesis: an epidemiologic challenge. In Black R, Michaelsen KM, eds. *Public health issues in infant and child nutrition* (Nestlé Nutrition Workshop Series, Pediatric Program Volume 48). New York: Lippincott Williams and Wilkins, 2002:295–315.

*18 Kramer MS. Determinants of low birthweight: methodological assessment and meta-analysis. *Bull W Health Org* 1987;**65**:663–737.

19 Maternal anthropometry and pregnancy outcomes. A WHO collaborative study. *Bull W Health Org* 1995;**73(suppl)**:1–98.

20 Schieve LA, Cogswell ME, Scanlon KS. An empiric evaluation of the Institute of Medicine's pregnancy weight gain guidelines by race. *Obstet Gynecol* 1998;**91**:878–84.

21 Blackwell RQ, Chow BF, Chinn KSK, Blackwell BN, Hsu SC. Prospective maternal nutrition study in Taiwan: rationale, study design, feasibility and preliminary findings. *Nutr Rep Int* 1973;**7**:517–32.

22 McDonald EC, Pollitt E, Mueller WH, Hsueh AM, Sherwin R. The Bacon Chow study: maternal nutritional supplementation and birthweight of offspring. *Am J Clin Nutr* 1981;**34**:2133–44.

23 Kramer MS. Balanced protein/energy supplementation in pregnancy (Cochrane Review). In *The Cochrane Library*, Issue 2, 2002. Oxford: Update Software.

24 Stein Z, Susser M, Saenger G, Marolla F. *Famine and human development: the Dutch Hunger Winter of 1944–45*. New York: Oxford University Press, 1975.

25 Kramer MS. Nutritional advice in pregnancy (Cochrane Review). In *The Cochrane Library*, Issue 2, 2002. Oxford: Update Software.

26 Mahomed K. Iron supplementation in pregnancy (Cochrane Review). In *The Cochrane Library*, Issue 2, 2002. Oxford: Update Software.

27 **Mahomed K.** Folate supplementation in pregnancy (Cochrane Review). In *The Cochrane Library*, Issue 2, 2002. Oxford: Update Software.

28 **Mahomed K.** Zinc supplementation in pregnancy. (Cochrane Review). In *The Cochrane Library*, Issue 2, 2002. Oxford: Update Software.

29 **Lumley J, Oliver S, Waters E.** Interventions for promoting smoking cessation during pregnancy (Cochrane Review). In *The Cochrane Library*, Issue 2, 2002. Oxford: Update Software.

30 **Mueller-Heuback E, Reddick D, Barnett B, Bente R.** Preterm birth prevention: evaluation of a prospective controlled randomized trial. *Am J Obstet Gynecol* 1989;**160**:1172–8.

31 **Heins HC, Nance NW, McCarthy BJ, Efird CM.** A randomized trial of nurse-midwifery prenatal care to reduce low birthweight. *Obstet Gynecol* 1990;**75**:341–5.

32 **Collaborative Group on Preterm Birth Prevention.** Multicenter randomized, controlled trial of a preterm birth prevention program. *Am J Obstet Gynecol* 1993;**169**:352–66.

33 **Hodnett ED.** Support during pregnancy for women at increased risk of low birthweight babies (Cochrane Review). In *The Cochrane Library*, Issue 2, 2002. Oxford: Update Software.

34 **Knight M, Duley L, Henderson-Smart DJ, King JF.** Antiplatelet agents for preventing and treating pre-eclampsia (Cochrane Review). In *The Cochrane Library*, Issue 2, 2002. Oxford: Update Software.

35 **Habicht J-P, Martorell R, Rivera JA.** Nutritional impact of supplementation in the INCAP longitudinal study: analytic strategies and inferences. *J Nutr* 1995;**125**:1042S–50S.

36 **Shroeder DG, Martorell R, Rivera JA, Ruel MT, Habicht J-P.** Age differences in the impact of nutritional supplementation on growth. *J Nutr* 1995;**125**:1051S–9S.

37 **Lutter CK, Mora JO, Habicht J-P, Rasmussen KM, Robson DS, Herrera MG.** Age-specific responsiveness of weight and length to nutritional supplementation. *Am J Clin Nutr* 1990;**51**:359–64.

38 **Dewey KG, Peerson JM, Brown KH, Krebs NF, Michaelsen KF, Persson LA** *et al.* Growth of breast-fed infants deviates from current reference data: a pooled analysis of US, Canadian, and European data sets. *Pediatrics* 1995;**96**:495–503.

39 **Nielsen GA, Thomsen BL, Michaelsen KF.** Influence of breastfeeding and complementary food on growth betweeen 5 and 10 months. *Acta Paediatr* 1998;**87**:911–17.

40 **Haschke F, van't Hof MA, the Euro-Growth Study Group.** Euro-Growth references for breast-fed boys and girls: influence of breast feeding and solids on growth until 36 months of age. *J Pediat Gastroenterol Nutr* 2000;**31**:S60–71.

41 **Dewey KG, Heinig MJ, Nommsen LA, Peerson JM, Lonnerdal B.** Growth of breast-fed and formula-fed infants from 0 to 18 months: the DARLING study. *Pediatrics* 1992;**89**:1035–41.

42 **Cunningham AS, Jelliffe DB, Jelliffe EFP.** Breast-feeding and health in the 1980's: a global epidemiologic review. *J Pediat* 1991;**119**:659–66.

43 **Howie PW, Forsyth JS, Ogston SA, Clark A, Florey CV.** Protective effect of breast feeding against infection. *Br Med J* 1990;**300**:11–16.

44 **Kramer MS, Chalmers B, Hodnett ED, Sevkovskaya Z, Dzikovich I, Shapiro S** *et al.* Promotion of Breastfeeding Intervention Trial (PROBIT): a randomized trial in the Republic of Belarus. *J Am Med Assoc* 2001;**285**:413–20.

45 **Turner MJ, Rasmussen MJ, Boylan PC, MacDonald D, Stronge JM.** The influence of birthweight on labour in nulliparas. *Obstet Gynecol* 1990;**76**:159–63.

46 **Parrish KM, Holt VL, Easterling TR, Connell FA, LoGerfo JP.** Effect of changes in maternal age, parity, and birthweight distribution on primary cesarean delivery rates. *J Am Med Assoc* 1994;**271**:443–7.

47 **Oral E, Cağdaş A, Gezer A, Kaleli S, Aydinli K, Öçer F.** Perinatal and maternal outcomes of fetal macrosomia. *Eur J Obstet Gynecol Reprod Biol* 2001;**99**:167–71.

48 **Parham ES, Astrom MF, King SH.** The association of pregnancy weight gain with the mother's postpartum weight. *J Am Diet Assoc* 1990;**90**:550–4.

49 Scholl TO, Hediger ML, Schall JI, Ances IG, Smith WK. Gestational weight gain, pregnancy outcome, and postpartum weight retention. *Obstet Gynecol* 1995;**86**:423–7.

50 Boardley DJ, Sargent RG, Coker AL, Hussey JR, Sharpe PA. The relationship between diet, activity, and other factors, and postpartum weight change by race. *Obstet Gynecol* 1995;**86**:834–8.

51 Gunderson EP, Abrams B. Epidemiology of gestational weight gain and body weight changes after pregnancy. *Epidemiol Rev* 2000;**22**:261–74.

52 Barker DJP, Winter PD, Osmond C, Phillips DIW, Sultan HY. Weight gain in infancy and cancer of the ovary. *Lancet* 1995;**345**:1087–8.

53 Tibblin G, Eriksson M, Cnattingius S, Ekbom A. High birthweight as a predictor of prostate cancer risk. *Epidemiology* 1995;**6**:423–4.

54 Thompson JA, Janerich DT. Maternal age at birth and risk of breast cancer in daughters. *Epidemiology* 1990;**1**:101–6.

55 Ekbom A, Thurfjell E, Hsieh C-C, Trichopoulos D, Adami H-O. Perinatal characteristics and adult mammographic patterns. *Int J Cancer* 1995;**61**:177–80.

56 Ekbom A, Trichopoulos D, Adami H-O, Hsieh C-C, Lans S-J. Evidence of prenatal influences on breast cancer risk. *Lancet* 1992;**340**:1015–18.

57 Innes K, Byers T, Schymura M. Birth characteristics and subsquent risk for breast cancer in very young women. *Am J Epidemiol* 2000;**152**:1121–8.

58 Andersson SW, Bengtsson C, Hallberg L, Lapidus L, Niklasson A, Wallgren A *et al.* Cancer risk in Swedish women; the relation to size at birth. *Br J Cancer* 2001;**84**:1193–8.

59 Vatten LJ, Mæhle BO, Nilsen TIL, Tretli S, Hsieh C-C, Trichopoulos D *et al.* Birthweight as a predictor of breast cancer: a case control study in Norway. *Br J Cancer* 2002;**86**:89–91.

60 Ekbom A. Growing evidence that several human cancers may originate *in utero. Semin Cancer Biol* 1998;**8**:237–44.

61 De Stavola BL, Hardy R, Kuh D, Silva IS, Wadsworth M, Swerdlow AJ. Birthweight, childhood growth and risk of breast cancer in a British cohort. *Br J Cancer* 2000;**83**:964–8.

62 McCormack VA, dos Santos Silva I, De Stavola BL, Mohsen R, Leon DA, Lithell HO. Fetal growth and subsequent risk of breast cancer: results from long term follow up of Swedish cohort. *Br Med J* 2003;**326**:248–51.

63 Potischman N, Troisi R, Vatten L. Development of disease risk throughout life: cancers. In Kuh D, Ben-Shlomo Y, eds. *A life course approach to chronic disease epidemiology* (2nd edn). New York: Oxford Medical Publications, 2004.

64 Platz EA, Giovannucci E, Rimm EB, Curhan GC, Spiegelman D, Colditz GA *et al.* Retrospective analysis of birthweight and prostate cancer in the health professionals follow up study. *Am J Epidemiol* 1998;**147**:1140–4.

65 Ekbom A, Wuu J, Adami H-O, Lu C-M, Lagiou P, Trichopoulos D *et al.* Duration of gestation and prostate cancer risk in offspring. *Cancer Epidemiol Biomarkers Prev* 2000;**9**:221–3.

66 Titus-Ernstoff L, Egan KM, Newcomb PA, Ding J, Trentham-Dietz A, Greenberg ER *et al.* Early life factors in relation to breast cancer risk in postmenopausal women. *Cancer Epidemiol Biomarkers Prev* 2002;**11**:207–10.

67 Sanderson M, Shu XO, Jin F, Dai Q, Ruan Z, Gao Y-T *et al.* Weight at birth and adolescence and premenopausal breast cancer risk in a low-risk population. *Br J Cancer* 2002;**86**:84–8.

68 Godfrey KM, Barker DJP, Osmond C. Disproportionate fetal growth and raised IgE concentration in adult life. *Clin Exp Allergy* 1994;**24**:641–8.

69 Kaye SA, Robison LL, Smithson WA, Gunderson P, King FL, Neglia JP. Maternal reproductive history and birth characteristics in childhood acute lymphoblastic leukemia. *Cancer* 1991;**68**:1351–5.

70 Westergaard T, Anderson PK, Pedersen JB, Olsen JH, Frisch M, Sorensen HT *et al.* Birth characteristics, sibling patterns and acute leukemia risk in childhood: a population-based cohort study. *J Natl Cancer Inst* 1997;**89**:939–47.

71 Seidman DS, Laor A, Gale R, Stevenson DK, Danon YL. A longitudinal study of birthweight and being overweight in late adolescence. *Am J Dis Child* 1991;**145**:782–5.

72 Martorell R, Stein AD, Schroeder DG. Early nutrition and later adiposity. *J Nutr* 2001;**131**:874–80S.

73 Johansson C, Samuelsson U, Ludvigsson J. A high weight gain early in life is associated with an increased risk of Type I (insulin dependent) diabetes mellitus. *Diabetologia* 1994;**37**:91–4.

74 Dahlquist G, Bennich SS, Kallen B. Intrauterine growth pattern and risk of childhood onset insulin dependent (type I) diabetes: population based case-control study. *Br Med J* 1996;**313**:1174–7.

75 Hyppönen E, Kenward MG, Virtanen SM, Piitulainen A, Virta-Autio P, Tuomilehto J *et al.* Infant feeding, early weight gain and risk of type 1 diabetes. *Diabetes Care* 1999;**22**:1961–5.

76 Stene LC, Magnus P, Lie RT, Sovik O, Joner G. Birthweight and childhood onset type 1 diabetes: population based cohort study. *Br Med J* 2001;**322**:889–92.

77 Law CM, Shiell AW. Is blood pressure inversely related to birthweight? The strength of evidence from a systematic review of the literature. *J Hypertens* 1996;**14**:935–41.

78 Huxley R, Neil A, Collins R. Unravelling the fetal origins hypothesis: is there really an inverse association between birthweight and subsequent blood pressure? *Lancet* 2002;**360**:659–65.

79 MacMahon S, Peto R, Cutler J, Collins R, Sorlie P, Neaton J. Blood pressure, stroke, and coronary heart disease: Part 1, prolonged differences in blood pressure: prospective observational studies corrected for regression dilution bias. *Lancet* 1990;**335**:765–74.

80 Glynn RJ, Filed TS, Rosner B, Hebert PR, Taylor JO, Hennekens CH. Evidence of a positive linear relation between blood pressure and mortality in elderly people. *Lancet* 1995;**345**:825–9.

81 Kleinbaum DG, Kupper LL, Morgenstern H. *Epidemiologic research: principles and quantitative methods.* Belmont: Lifetime Learning Publications, 1982.

82 Rockhill B, Newman B, Weinberg C. Use and misuse of population attributable fractions. *Am J Pub Health* 1998;**88**:15–19.

83 Hanley JA. A heuristic approach to the formulas for population attributable fraction. *J Epidemiol Commun Health* 2001;**55**:508–14.

84 Joseph KS, Kramer MS. Recent trends in infant mortality rates and proportions of low-birth-weight live births in Canada. *Can Med Assoc J* 1997;**157**:535–41.

85 Barker DJP, Godfrey KM, Fall C, Osmond C, Winter PD, Shaheen SO. Relation of birthweight and childhood respiratory infection to adult lung function and death from chronic obstructive airways disease. *Br Med J* 1991;**303**:671–5.

86 Sytkowski PA, D'Agostino RB, Belanger A, Kannel WB. Sex and time trends in cardiovascular disease incidence and mortality: the Framingham heart study, 1950–1989. *Am J Epidemiol* 1996;**143**:338–50.

87 Goldman L, Cook EF. The decline in ischemic heart disease mortality rates. An analysis of the comparative effects of medical intervention and changes in lifestyle. *Ann Intern Med* 1984;**101**:825–36.

88 Sprafka JM, Burke GL, Folsom AR, Luepker RV, Blackburn H. Continued decline in cardiovascular disease risk factors: results of the Minnesota Heart Survey, 1980–1982 and 1985–1987. *Am J Epidemiol* 1990;**132**:489–500.

89 Rothman KJ, Greenland S. *Modern epidemiology* (2nd edn). Philadelphia: Lippincott-Raven Publishers, 1998.

90 Ockene JK, Kuller LH, Svendsen KH, Meilahn E. The relationship of smoking cessation to coronary heart disease and lung cancer in the Multiple Risk Factor Intervention Trial (MRFIT). *Am J Pub Health* 1990;**80**:954–8.

91 Kuller LH, Ockene JK, Meilahn E, Wentworth DN, Svendsen KH, Neaton JD. Cigarette smoking and mortality. *Prev Med* 1991;**20**:638–54.

92 Holme I, Hjermann I, Helgeland A, Leren P. The Oslo Study: diet and antismoking advice: additional results from a 5-year primary prevention trial in middle-aged men. *Prev Med* 1985;**14**:279–92.

93 Rose G, Colwell L. Randomized controlled trial of antismoking advice: final (20 year) results. *J Epidemiol Commun Health* 1992;**46**:75–7.

94 Kramer MS. Birthweight and infant mortality: perceptions and pitfalls. *Paediatr Perinat Epidemiol* 1990;**4**:381–90.

95 Kramer MS. Maternal nutrition, pregnancy outcome and public health policy. *Can Med Assoc J* 1998;**159**:663–5.

96 McCormick MC. The contribution of low birthweight to infant mortality and childhood morbidity. *N Engl J Med* 1985;**312**:82–90.

97 Morrison JC. Preterm birth: a puzzle worth solving. *Obstet Gynecol* 1990;**76**:5–12S.

98 Radetsky P. Stopping premature births before it's too late. *Science* 1994;**266**:1486–8.

99 Papiernik E, Bouyer J, Dreyfus J, Collin D, Winisdorffer G, Guegen S *et al.* Prevention of preterm births: a perinatal study in Haguenau, France. *Pediatrics* 1985;**76**:154–8.

100 Bréart G, Blondel B, Tuppin P, Grandjean H, Kaminski M. Did preterm deliveries continue to decrease in France in the 1980s? *Paediatr Perinat Epidemiol* 1995;**9**:296–306.

101 Division of Nutrition, National Center for Chronic Disease Prevention and Health Promotion. Increasing incidence of low birthweight—United States, 1981–1991. *Morb Mortal Wkly Rep* 1994;**43**:335–9.

102 Joseph KS, Kramer MS, Marcoux S, Ohlsson A, Wen SW, Allen A *et al.* Determinants of preterm birth rates in Canada from 1981 through 1983 and from 1992 through 1994. *New Engl J Med* 1998;**339**:1434–9.

103 Kramer MS, Platt R, Yang H, Joseph KS, Wen SW, Morin L *et al.* Secular trends in preterm birth: a hospital-based cohort study. *J Am Med Assoc* 1998;**280**:1849–54.

104 Demissie K, Rhoads GG, Ananth CV, Alexander GR, Kramer MS, Kogan MD *et al.* Trends in preterm birth and neonatal mortality among blacks and whites in the United States from 1989 to 1997. *Am J Epidemiol* 2001;**154**:307–15.

105 Kessel SS, Villar J, Berendes HW, Nugent RP. The changing pattern of low birthweight in the United States, 1970 to 1980. *J Am Med Assoc* 1984;**251**:1978–82.

106 Ventura SJ, Martin JA, Curtin SC, Menacker F, Hamilton BE. *Births: final data for 1999. National vital statisitcs reports; Vol. 49 No. 1.* Hyattsville, Maryland: National Centre for Health Statisitcs, 2001.

107 Ananth CV, Wen SW. Trends in fetal growth among singleton gestations in the United States and Canada, 1985 through 1998. *Semin Perinatol* 2002;**26**:260–7.

108 Arbuckle TE, Sherman GJ. An analysis of birthweight by gestational age in Canada. *Can Med Assoc J* 1989;**140**:157–65.

109 Health Canada. *Canadian perinatal health report, 2000.* Ottawa: Minister of Public Works and Government Services Canada, 2000. http://www.hc-sc.gc.ca/hpb/lcdc/ brch/reprod.html

110 Alberman E. Are our babies becoming bigger? *J Roy Soc Med* 1991;**84**:257–60.

111 Rasmussen KM. The fetal origins hypothesis: challenges and opportunities for maternal and child nutrition. *Ann Rev Nutr* 2001;**21**:73–95.

Chapter 18

Should we intervene to improve childhood circumstances?

W. Thomas Boyce and Daniel P. Keating

This chapter reviews epidemiological and developmental findings of relevance to the question, 'Should we intervene to improve childhood circumstances?' We begin with observations on the 'circumstances' of contemporary children in an international context, arguing that, despite major advances, there are reasons for continuing concern over the physical and social settings in which children are born and raised. The implications of such conditions, when considered within the framework of social disparities in mental and physical health, are disquieting. Social class gradients in morbidity are shown to be *pervasive*, in the sense that they involve multiple categories of disease within multiple developmental epochs, *convergent*, in that steeper national socioeconomic gradients in health are generally associated with lower average health outcomes, and *enduring*, in that socioeconomic-specific childhood experiences are carried forward into health effects in adult life. Further, the observed patterns of childhood socioeconomic status (SES) influences on later health suggest that such influences can be *cumulative*, in the sense that socioeconomic effects show gradual accretion over time, *pathway related*, in that SES may alter the trajectories in childhood from which adult health and well-being are derived, or *latent*, by virtue of experiences during critical developmental periods that have temporally distant consequences. Life course effects of socioeconomic and other adversities in childhood are rendered even more credible by evidence for plausible biological, social, and behavioural mediators of such effects. There is evidence from both human studies and animal experiments, for example, that experiences in early life are involved in the calibration of response characteristics within key neurobiological circuits activated under conditions of stress and adversity. Chronic or recurrent activation of such circuits may be one plausible pathway by which early hardships are transmuted into the disease processes of adult life. The chapter ends with a review of evidence supporting an affirmative answer to the target question and an argument, on both economic and moral grounds, for a societal imperative to protect and nurture the children of the world community.

18.1 **Introduction**

Children occupy a unique niche within the ecology of human populations. They are the demographic sector most likely both to benefit from a nation's advances and to be jeopardized by its indifferences and perils. As such, children constitute a subpopulation of disproportionate sensitivity to the social and environmental indiscretions of a society, a generation, or an era. Indeed, children can be usefully viewed as fulfilling a kind of 'signal detection' role in the adaptation of human groups, their environmental susceptibilities offering an early warning of threat or risk. Ensuring the environmental safety of *children*, it has been argued, guarantees the safety of an entire population. Countries and societies thus have moral and public health imperatives to protect children from the environmental hazards—both psychosocial and physical—that can impair health and undermine well-being, within childhood and over the human lifespan.

In many ways, posing the chapter's title question implies its own answer. Yes, we should intervene to improve the circumstances of children. Why would we not? In fact, rhetorical commitment to this affirmation is now represented among international conventions and government policies at many levels. In an ideal world, the simple affirmation might suffice. In the real world, efforts to advance childhood circumstances are challenged on many fronts. The costs associated with intervention are substantial and compete for priority not only with other items on the social agenda, but also with trends in the political economy to reduce social expenditures more generally. A rhetorical affirmative is thus nearly self-evident, but enacting a national or international policy far more challenging.

To argue for childhood interventions in this more complex policy arena requires substantive evidence and analyses, as well as precision with respect to the focal questions. In this chapter, we attempt both to parse the answer with respect to contemporary evidence and to offer detailed consideration of its critical components. Consider first the implied concluding phrase of the question, in the context of this volume: Should we intervene to improve childhood circumstances *in order to improve life course health*? An affirmative answer to this question implies a set of related questions, which we consider in detail. Is there evidence that experiences in early development have life course consequences for health? If so, are these consequences substantial enough (that is, account for enough variance in subsequent health outcomes) to warrant significant investment? If so, is there evidence that changes in childhood circumstances reap positive life course health benefits, suggesting that observed associations are more than merely correlational? If so, is there theory and evidence that affords an understanding of the underlying developmental mechanisms, such that interventions can be properly guided and unintended harm avoided? Finally, are the identified interventions feasible in current policy contexts, and what arguments can be made to make them more viable? Drawing on epidemiological, developmental, and biological evidence, we contend that provisionally affirmative answers can be given for each of these linked questions.

At a more fundamental level, there are classical as well as emerging ethical perspectives that give special attention to individuals in vulnerable periods of development, in part due to the inability of not yet mature individuals to argue on their own behalf. These developmental vulnerabilities interact with societal vulnerabilities, increasing risks during periods of high social stress.[1] We suggest that these ethical considerations serve as a crucial underpinning for the scientific and policy debates that are implied by the question that animates this chapter.

18.2 **What *are* the 'circumstances' of contemporary childhood?**

Acknowledging these special vulnerabilities, many nations of the world have adopted legislation, policies, and practices aimed at protecting the rights and well-being of children, ratifying trans-national agreements, such as the Convention on the Rights of the Child[2] and convening international meetings on children's interests, such as the 1990 World Summit for Children.[3]

Such rallying and focusing of international attention on issues of child health and welfare has resulted in public health practices that save millions of lives annually.[4] These efforts have led in recent years, for example, to the eradication of smallpox (at least in peacetime) and to the near-elimination of polio, two of childhood's most feared and destructive infectious diseases. Iodine deficiency, a leading preventable cause of mental retardation, may also soon disappear from the inventory of threats to healthy child development, and over 70% of children worldwide have been successfully immunized against measles, polio, diphtheria, pertussis, and tetanus.[4] As a consequence, disability and mortality under age 5 years has progressively declined since the 1960s, in all but a handful of nations.

Despite such advances, at least 600 million children continue to live in poverty, subsisting on less than US$ 1 per day. New infectious threats to the world's children have also emerged, to replace recently or imminently defeated morbidities. Each day, for example, 8500 children are newly infected with the human immunodeficiency virus (HIV) and 1.4 million children worldwide are living with HIV infection and acquired immunodeficiency syndrome (AIDS).[4] In 2000, 10.4 million children under 15 years of age were orphaned by the HIV epidemic, rendering them far more vulnerable to exploitation and more likely to become infected themselves. Further, as many as one million children are lured or forced into prostitution each year and more than half a billion children grow up in circumstances of national, local, or family violence,[5] resulting, for example, in two million war-related child deaths in the last 10 years.[6] Although an unprecedented 82% of children are now in school around the world, 130 million still have no access to education and among these girls are disproportionately deprived.[4] One-third of children from developing countries do not complete 5 years of elementary schooling, rendering them illiterate, disempowered, and susceptible to a generational cycle of poverty, resignation, and early death.

18.3 **Social disparities in health and well-being through the life course**

Beyond these well-documented global challenges to children's health and development, which create heavy burdens not only for individual children but also for the societies whose populations are most affected, there is substantial evidence for socioeconomic effects throughout the life course for both individuals and populations. Socioeconomic influences are dramatically apparent, for example, among indicators of child health status.[7] Despite anti-poverty programmes in place for more than 30 years, the number of poor US children has increased[8,9] and there is compelling evidence that mental and physical health in childhood are strongly tied to socioeconomic circumstances.[7,10] Lower SES children are at greater risk for most forms of childhood morbidity, from injuries and acute illnesses[11,12] to chronic medical conditions,[10,13,14] and behavioural disorders.[15] In the Great Smoky Mountains study, poverty was identified as the strongest demographic predictor of psychiatric diagnoses in urban and rural youth.[16] As noted by Keating and Hertzman,[17] these circumstances give rise to a central paradox: the existence of previously unimaginable material wealth and a concurrent deterioration of those human environments in which children grow and develop.

In circumstances where negative effects on child health are severe and widespread, as in the HIV/AIDS epidemic or war-related trauma, life course consequences—that is, childhood effects on the incidence or course of adult morbidities—are even more obvious and dramatic. Indeed, the evidence for life course health effects of early childhood circumstances, even in the absence of observed direct effects on child health, has been growing steadily. For example, numerous studies of the long-term effects associated with gradients in SES in the developed world have established a robust pattern linking childhood SES with adult health status.[18] Such patterns have been extensively reviewed elsewhere (see, for example, References 17–21) and in Chapters 4 and 16 in this volume. It is, however, important to examine these gradient effects more precisely, not only to sharpen the argument that improvement in childhood circumstances will have a beneficial impact on life course health, but also to identify potential mechanisms that govern the effect. Without an understanding of potential mechanisms, recommendations on improving childhood circumstances may be too general as a guide for policy and action.

18.3.1 Key elements of the childhood socioeconomic status and health gradient

As a first step, we can consider key elements of the SES gradient effect as it has been observed across a number of studies. The first element is the *pervasiveness* of the SES gradient effect.[22,23] It is observed not only for mortality data at all stages of life, but also for virtually all types of morbidity. Although disease-specific pathways exist, the SES gradient effect appears to function as a more general risk/resilience factor, extending even to measures of competence and behaviour,[24] from literacy[25] and mathematics[26] to emotional and behavioural problems.[27–29] Given the overall similarity of gradient effects for health and developmental outcomes, a full understanding of the impact of childhood circumstances must therefore accommodate their robust relationship with the broader construct of 'developmental health'.[17]

A second key element arises from cross-national or cross-regional comparisons of the shape of the SES gradient. A robust pattern is that societies with steeper SES gradients in health have generally lower average health outcomes, whereas societies with flatter gradients have generally higher average health outcomes.[30] Willms[31] has described this as a 'fan-*convergent*' pattern, such that cross-national or cross-regional differences are greatest at the lower end of SES and smallest at the higher end. Although the effects are starkest at the lower end of SES, there is little support for a specific poverty explanation; rather, the gradient effect operates similarly throughout the SES range.[29,30,32]

The third key element of the SES gradient is observed in longitudinal datasets, where the prospective impact of childhood circumstances can be directly observed. Where such evidence is available, it appears that SES of the family of origin bears a graded relationship to adult health similar in pattern and magnitude to that obtained when the individual's SES is the independent variable (see, for example, Reference 21). Although the generalizability of this finding is constrained by the availability of appropriate longitudinal datasets, the evidence to date is generally supportive.[18,30,33] The implications of these provisional but key findings are profound, in that they suggest that the SES gradient is both portable (as individuals, on average, carry that legacy into their adult lives) and *enduring* (as life course health effects). Thus, failure to attend to childhood circumstances may create, at the population level, a range of societal burdens that are hard to subsequently shift. Conversely, investments in early development may generate enduring societal opportunities.[34]

18.3.2 Patterns of childhood socioeconomic status influence

There are several hypothetical patterns of influence through which childhood circumstances may affect health outcomes over the life course and for both scientific and policy purposes, it is helpful to attempt a conceptual disaggregation of such patterns.[18,20,21] This book (especially Chapter 1), as well as other published and forthcoming work (for example, References 35 and 36), represents a substantive attempt to define these patterns of influence and the features by which they can be usefully differentiated. Thus, one pattern progresses through stability of socioeconomic circumstances from childhood to later life, with an *accumulation of risk*—via environmental exposures, social experience, or health-damaging behaviours—occurring over time.[18,33,35,36] This can be conceived as the product of an individual's 'health capital' over time, a construct with the two major components of environmental conditions and health-related habits.[19] These can be further disaggregated, with environmental effects arising from both living and working conditions and behavioural effects comprising a range of lifestyles and practices. The implication of this account is that broad societal differences in the quality of the social and physical environment play a major role in health outcomes, through the overall degree of social partitioning and the SES-related patterns that emerge in early life.

A related set of childhood influences may be thought of as *pathway effects*[18] or *chains of risk or protection*.[35,36] If we construe the previous set as representing the cumulative effects of contexts over time, this set focuses, in contrast, on the ways in which early circumstances constrain or enable trajectories of health and development. For example, educational attainment plays a substantial role in both subsequent health and social status (as measured by occupation, income, wealth, and so on). Beyond simple continuity of context, the early acquisition of competencies, skills, and dispositions likely affects directly the pathways leading towards future health, well-being, and developmental attainments. Analyses of data from the Dunedin Multidisciplinary Health and Development Study, for example, have demonstrated longitudinal associations between low childhood SES and poorer cardiovascular and oral health status (as well as certain aspects of mental health status), independent of socioeconomic circumstances in adulthood.[37] Such associations are likely attributable to sequences of linked exposures, in which early risk factors increase the likelihood of subsequent exposures, which in turn augment the probability of encountering others.

Another indicator of such pathway or linked effects is the phenomenon of resilience,[38] in which significant early disadvantage is surmounted. The developmental trajectories of many children growing up in adverse or suboptimal circumstances belie the expected declines in physical and mental health that are known to attend such conditions. Observations of anomalously good outcomes emerging from impoverished or unsupportive social settings are non-normative, but far from rare. In such accounts, resilience appears often derived from the establishment of chains of *protection*—individual characteristics and forms of individual support that predispose towards the pursuit of health-protective developmental trajectories.

The third type of influence can be thought of as *critical period*[36] or *latent* effects[18] (see Chapter 1). Even after removing the effects from other, later sources—adult SES, health habits, and so on—there is often a non-trivial impact of childhood circumstances on life course health outcomes. For example, the early instantiation of an overreactive stress response system (described further below) may affect developmental trajectories through success in selected environments (pathway effects), but in addition, may create a health risk that will become manifest only at a later stage in the life course as stressors accumulate or grow more intense. Note, in this example, that the early experiential calibration of stress-responsive neural circuitry might alternatively affect later health via *risk accumulation* (cumulative, long-term costs of repeated activation of biological circuits), *pathway effects* (exaggerated reactivity biasing developmental trajectories toward risk induction or away from risk protection), or *critical period effects* (early exposure in, for example, infancy alone results in biological response profiles that jeopardize adult health and adaptation).

Thus, consideration of the SES gradient effect (pervasive, convergent, and enduring) and patterns of transmission (cumulative, pathway, and critical period) leads toward a hypothesis of 'biological embedding', a process 'whereby systematic differences in psychosocial/material circumstances, from conception onward, embed themselves in human biology such that the characteristics of gradients in developmental health can be accounted for' (p11).[39] The term 'biological embedding' bears conceptual commonality, if not identity, with the alternate terms 'embodiment'[36,40] and 'experience-based brain development'.[41] All three refer to the processes by which differential social experiences establish functional and structural changes in the physiology, neurobiology, and gene expression of the individual, particularly in early life. Entertaining the biological embedding hypothesis therefore entails a detailed consideration of the biobehavioural mechanisms linking childhood circumstances and later developmental health gradients.

18.4 Biobehavioural mediators of socioeconomic risk

What are the biological pathways by which socioeconomic liabilities and supports are transmuted into the physical processes of disease and disorder? Are individual differences in the character or functioning of such pathways responsible for the broad variability in consequences of challenge, stress, and hardship? Advances in understanding the mechanisms involved in biological responses to adversity have shed new light on such questions by revealing how early exposures 'get into the body' and create vulnerabilities to acute and chronic disease processes. Equally important and compelling are more recent studies suggesting that individual differences in biological sensitivity to aspects of social context may offer an explanation for both disproportionate vulnerability and unexpected resilience. Processes of biological embedding may thus illuminate either the *mediating* pathways by which social disadvantages predispose to maladaptive outcomes or the *moderating* processes by which individual children are differentially affected by such disadvantages. As elucidated by Kraemer and colleagues,[42] mediators are variables, which, in this context, explain how or why SES inequalities affect developmental outcomes, while moderators specify in which subgroup or under what conditions such effects will hold. Although the moderation of SES effects is itself a topic of substantial importance for understanding life course development, our focus here is upon plausible mediators of socioeconomic adversity and the possibility that a richer understanding of SES mediation could lead to viable and effective interventions. We begin with a consideration of biological embedding as a possible mediating pathway for socioeconomic risk.

18.4.1 Biological embedding as a possible mediator of socioeconomic status risk

Accumulating advances in developmental neuroscience have produced an elegant and compelling picture of brain development and how early experience affects the character and complexity of central neural circuitry. Development of the fetal brain during prenatal life is characterized by profuse overgrowth of neurones and the synaptic junctions through which networks of neurones communicate. At the height of its prenatal growth, the brain adds 250 000 new neurones per minute, an exuberant neurogenesis resulting in a central nervous system of staggering complexity. At maturity, the brain comprises more than a 100 billion neurones, each with an average 10 000 synaptic connections to other neural units. All of the basic pathways involved in human emotion, volition, movement, and thought are already in place at birth, awaiting the experiential input that will propel latent pathways into the neural substrates of individual personalities, predispositions, talents, and failings. Over the course of the next several postnatal months, this rich neural network is progressively 'pruned', selectively eliminating neurones (through apoptosis, or programmed cell death) and synapses from the less utilized pathways and circuits. It appears that this process of neuronal elimination is as essential to the emergence of normal intelligence, behaviour, and mental functioning, as is the stage of neuronal proliferation that precedes it within fetal life.

Greenough and colleagues (for example, Reference 43) have proposed three distinct mechanisms for this 'sculpting' of brain circuitry through the sequential proliferation and elimination of synapses: experience-independent, experience-expectant, and experience-dependent processes. Experience-independent synaptogenesis refers to the formation of synapses without requirement for experiential input, such as the development of taste buds on the tongue. Experience-expectant and -dependent mechanisms, on the other hand, are the pathways through which aspects of social experience are transduced into the neural imprints of environmental experience. Experience-expectant processes reduce the amount of information the genome must carry by relying on information that is dependably present in the normal perinatal environments of the species. An example is the development of vision, in which normal visual input is both anticipated and necessary for the production of ocular neuronal columns in the visual cortex of the brain. These columnar structures fuse two retinal images, one from each eye, into a stereoscopic, three-dimensional representation and if one eye is occluded during the early, 'sensitive' developmental period, vision in that eye may not ever develop normally due to aberrations in the formation of ocular cortical columns. Experience-dependent induction, by contrast, optimizes adaptation to specific, possibly unique features of the environment by facilitating individual learning of new cognitive structures and information. It is known, for example, that animals raised in complex (rather than impoverished) laboratory environments are cognitively superior on motivated learning tasks due to greater synaptic density and efficiency in several regions of the dorsal neocortex.[44–46] Greenough and colleagues have thus argued that the neural substrate for the 'expectation' of postnatal environmental influences is the non-patterned, temporary over-production of synapses during an early sensitive period, with a subsequent purging of unessential or under-utilized synaptic linkages.

18.4.2 Experiential effects on stress response systems

Many features of emotional or social development likely depend on unique aspects of such interactions between environmental experience and the child's developing neurobiology.[47,48] Indeed, much of what we know as normative human behaviour and cognition is reliant upon this experiential shaping and calibrating of brain structures through the process of neural pruning. Among the neural structures and circuits modified by such early experience are the two principal brain systems involved in responses to adversity and challenge: the locus coeruleus–norepinephrine (LC–NE) system and the corticotropin-releasing hormone or hypothalamic–pituitary–adrenocortical (CRH–HPA) system. The LC-NE system triggers, through dopaminergic pathways from the dorsal pons to the hypothalamus, the activation of the sympathetic arm of the autonomic nervous system, which in turn mediates the so-called 'fight or flight' responses to threat. Such responses include the familiar behaviours and physiological changes that accompany stressors, that is, tremulousness, dry mouth, escalations in vigilance and arousal, and elevations in heart rate and blood pressure. Responses within the CRH–HPA axis—which begin with the activation of the arcuate and paraventricular nuclei of the hypothalamus—result in the production of CRH and cortisol, stress hormones responsible for the regulation of blood pressure, glucose and lipid metabolism, and immune competence.

In both experimental animals and humans, experiences in very early life appear to play an important role in defining and calibrating response characteristics of these two closely coordinated stress response systems, regulating parameters such as their trigger points, response intensities, and the rapidity of their recovery. The work of Meaney,[49] for example, has demonstrated the capacity of early maternal–infant separations in rodent pups to up- or down-regulate the reactivity of the CRH–HPA axis, depending upon the duration and disruptiveness of such separations. Low frequency, short-duration separations (known as 'handling'), for example, appear to alter central glucocorticoid receptor expression in such a way that the early experience dampens adrenocortical responses to stress for the remainder of the infant's life. More prolonged maternal–infant separations, on the other hand, have the opposite effect, producing adult animals that are systematically *over*-reactive to subsequent encounters with stressors. Meaney has further shown that the maternal behaviour that mediates these effects is the amount of licking and grooming of the rodent pup, a normative behaviour amplified by brief mother–infant separations and capable of altering the expression of genes for cortisol receptors in the hypothalamus.

The work of Suomi and colleagues[50,51] has similarly shown, in non-human primate species, that early rearing conditions can have regulatory effects on the activation of stress responsive neural systems. As in rodent models, maternal separations produce predictable changes in peripheral and central neural circuitry, altering functional immune competence,[52] up-regulating autonomic responses to physical stressors,[53] increasing CRH expression in cerebrospinal fluid,[54] and producing dysregulatory changes in CRH–HPA axis reactivity.[55] In one study,[56] for example, peer rearing (as opposed to mother rearing) of infant macaques was associated with blunted, down-regulatory changes in the circadian periodicity of cortisol secretion. The work of Sapolsky and Share,[57,58] among wild olive baboons, has also revealed associations between dominance status and adrenocortical activation, suggesting either that experiences related to social adeptness and dominant hierarchical status tend to lower cortisol levels or that constitutionally less reactive individuals occupy higher status positions. Thus, comparable to observations within rodent models of stress reactivity, studies of non-human primates offer further evidence for social contextual influences on the regulation of stress response systems.

Finally, there is evidence that early social experience—including both trauma and experiences of supportiveness and care—can have important, lasting effects on stress reactivity in the human child as well. Several studies suggest, for example, that disruptions in early attachment relationships are associated with regulatory influences on and disturbances in stress-responsive biological systems.[59–62] In a study of healthy women by Heim and colleagues,[63] participants with a history of abusive experiences in childhood had dramatically increased levels of CRH–HPA and autonomic reactivity to a standardized laboratory stress protocol. De Bellis and colleagues[64] similarly found increased 24 h urinary excretion of cortisol and norepinephrine among children with abuse-related post-traumatic stress disorder symptoms, in comparison to healthy control participants and Perry[65] reported diminished adrenergic receptors on platelets and increased heart rates in a group of severely abused children. A series of studies by Yehuda and coworkers[66–68] has further documented the psychobiological sequelae of early abusive experiences, including elevated 24 h urinary cortisol excretion,[67] increased density of lymphocyte glucocorticoid receptors, and enhanced suppression of plasma cortisol responses to dexamethasone,[69] each reflecting disturbances in the regulation of the CRH–HPA axis. In studies of broader societal influences on the development of stress responses, Lupien and colleagues[70] found that lower SES was associated with higher salivary cortisol levels in children as young as 6 years of age and Fernald and Grantham-McGregor[71] observed higher salivary cortisol levels and greater cardiovascular reactivity among growth-stunted children growing up in impoverished neighbourhoods in Jamaica. Steptoe and colleagues[72] have also shown that autonomic responses to laboratory stressors are differentially graded by social class membership.

Downstream from the CRH–HPA and LC–NE axes, the neurotransmitters and hormones that are the effector products of these systems have important influences—both acute and chronic—on a variety of target end organs. Such targets include the structures and cells that coordinate immune surveillance and response, the cardiovascular and neuroendocrine systems, organs involved in the regulation of metabolic activities, and the brain itself. The long-term consequences of repeated physiological reactivity, over years of stressful or traumatic experience, have been termed *allostatic load*, that is, the cumulative biological costs of achieving homeostatic stability through recurrent psychobiological changes.[73,74] As elucidated by McEwen and colleagues,[75–77] the price of persistent, recurrent stress responses triggered by environmental events is a broad array of more enduring physiological changes, including but likely not limited to, alterations in lipid metabolism and the accumulation of abdominal fat, loss of bone minerals, the development of hypertension, the atrophy of nerve cells in the hippocampus, and the development of insulin resistance, leading to increases in glycosylated hemoglobin and type II diabetes mellitus. Allostatic load across the life course is clearly cumulative, but it may also operate at various points during the life course to deflect or further solidify particular developmental pathways; moreover, the 'breaking point' of the stress response system, when effects become evident as specific health problems, may be partially set in early life. The acuity of stress reactivity, integrated over years of developmental time, may produce the chronic burdens of allostatic load and the repeated challenges of an adverse and difficult life may become the degenerative changes of aging and decline.

Taken together, rodent, non-human primate, and human research all suggest that, in addition to genetically derived individual differences in stress reactivity, environmental factors contribute to the attunement and calibration of biological stress response systems over the course of early development. These studies further suggest that, while stable individual differences in stress reactivity emerge with maturation, there is pronounced early plasticity in the neurobiological systems that subserve such reactivity.[78] There is also provisional evidence for a central developmental role of primary attachment relationships and maternal behaviour in shaping, constraining, and regulating psychobiological responses to experiences of future challenge and difficulty. The biological perturbations that reliably—but variably—accompany the social, economic, and psychological stresses of life may thus represent one credible mediating link between early adversity and health over the life course.

18.4.3 Socioemotional and behavioural mediators of social class disparities

Observations of social environmental influences on biological response characteristics are not surprising, however, given known disparities in the material and psychological resources of different SES groups and the deep influences of early childhood experience on social and biological development. As substantively reviewed in Chapters 4 and 16 of this book, children from lower SES backgrounds experience less adequate nutrition,[79] more conflictive and fewer positive communications with their families,[80] less warmth in parental relationships,[81] and (variably) both over- and under-control of their behaviour.[82] Lower SES may also undermine health through psychological mediators, such as hostility, hopelessness, or a diminished sense of control over life circumstances.[83] Children from impoverished homes enter adulthood with more hostility and hopelessness,[84] known risk factors for depression and heart disease[85,86] and an impaired sense of control, which predicts poorer overall health status in adults[87] and children.[88] Those experiencing early hardships—such as parental divorce, domestic violence, or a substance- or alcohol-abusing family member—are also at heightened risk for the acquisition of harmful health behaviours, such as smoking.[89] Higley and colleagues[90] have shown that early deprivation in infant macaques results in reduced serotonin turnover and a predisposition toward risk-taking behaviour and alcohol abuse. Though limited to experimental animals, these observations are important, because they identify the socioemotional and behavioural sequelae of the social, economic, and psychological challenges faced by low-SES families. Although lower childhood SES is demonstrably a risk factor for more frequent, accelerated, and severe morbidities in both childhood and adulthood, too little is currently known of the behavioural and interpersonal mediators and causal processes by which such risks are conveyed.

18.4.4 The role of social ordering *per se*: human and primate evidence

Another relatively unexplored, potentially mediating aspect of the SES–health association is the possibility that social ordering *per se* is a mechanism for socioeconomic influences on health. Resembling the dominance structures of primate troops,[91] human children as young as 2–3 years of age form stable, linearly transitive social hierarchies within weeks of their assembly into social groups.[92–94] Among possible reasons for the evolutionary preservation of such hierarchical organizations is the diminution in interpersonal aggression that follows development of stable, socially ordered relationships.[95] Pre-school social hierarchies become increasingly fixed as children develop and in older children, such structures appear less dependent upon agonistic behaviours, but are rather more reflective of peer friendships and affiliative interactions.[96] Dodge and colleagues have also shown that family SES may influence developmental outcomes through effects on parenting and child behaviour.[81] Lower class children, who are more likely to experience harsh discipline and punitive parent behaviour, display more aggression than higher SES peers and are therefore more often rejected and marginalized within their social groups.

The social positions of young children may also affect psychobiological and neuroanatomic features that can lead to specific disease processes. In primate animal models, Sapolsky and Share have shown that a subordinate social position is associated with chronically upregulated adrenocortical secretion, lower gonadal steroids, and impaired immune competence[57,58] and Kaplan and colleagues have demonstrated accelerated coronary atherogenesis among subordinate monkeys fed a high-cholesterol diet.[97]

Such social position-related differences in psychobiological arousal may have consequences for either the incidence or severity of disease. Summarizing three prospective studies of social status and host susceptibility to infection, Cohen[98] demonstrated that low SES and low perceived social status in humans, as well as subordinate social positions in monkeys, have in common a pattern of decreased host resistance to experimental inoculations with respiratory viral pathogens. In one study, low-SES volunteers exposed to rhinovirus were three times more likely to develop clinical infections than were higher-SES volunteers.[99] In a second paper, participants' self-assessments of low status relative to others in the same community were associated with increased rates of infection following exposure, independent of smoking status, sleep, alcohol consumption, or exercise.[100] In a third, chronically stressed, subordinate monkeys had a higher incidence of infection following nasal inoculation with virus.

The most direct evidence for the possible role of social ordering in child health outcomes, however, is derived from pilot studies recently completed at the Institute of Human Development, University of California, Berkeley. In a cross-sectional study examining social position, stress reactivity, and health problems in pre-school age children, Goldstein and colleagues[94] found that children in higher social positions in their pre-school groups showed lower heart rate reactivity, lower baseline salivary cortisol concentrations, lower parasympathetic and sympathetic reactivity, and fewer parent-reported chronic medical conditions. Notably, these results parallel findings by Lupien and colleagues,[70] showing that low-SES children have significantly higher salivary cortisol levels than high-SES children and by Steptoe and colleagues,[72] demonstrating poorer cardiovascular recoveries from stressors among lower-grade UK civil servants. Together, these findings indicate that social position is itself associated with illness and health risk factors in ways that are comparable to the health correlates of dominance in subhuman primates and to the effects of SES on health in human adults. The influence of SES on child health may be both analogous and partially attributable to the biologically mediated effects of low position within the 'pecking orders' of childhood social groups.

18.4.5 Childhood as critical period

As summarized above, early experiences of both trauma and protection may structurally alter the developing brain by their transcription into its evolving neural circuitry and by their other influences upon molecular systems of neurotransmission. These processes may also be time dependent, in two senses: (1) in that social experiences occurring within developmentally timed critical periods may have disproportionately large effects[101] or (2) in that the character of experiential effects may vary with developmental stage. In an example of the former, Essex and colleagues[102] found that exposures to maternal stress during infancy sensitized children's CRH–HPA axis, resulting in heightened cortisol responses to concurrent stressors, several years later, in the pre-school period. Similarly, studies of children born during the Dutch famine suggested that only exposures to maternal under-nutrition *early* in gestation affected lipid profiles and coronary disease risk,[103] while significant increases in rates of major affective disorders in adulthood were related only to exposures in the third trimester.[104] Parallel experimental work has shown that stress hormone administration in pregnant sheep produces increases in offspring blood pressure if given at a gestational age of 1 month, but not 2 months.[105,106] The biological substrate for such period-restricted developmental effects may be the capacity of certain social, nutritional, and biophysical exposures to turn on and off the expression of genes regulating aspects of growth, behaviour, and neuroendocrine functions.[107]

A literature review by Chen and colleagues,[7] summarizing how SES differences in children's health vary with age, demonstrated the second category of time-dependent experiential effects—in which the character or direction of the effect varies within developmental time. The review cited three possible developmental models of the relationship between SES and child health: (1) a *persistence* model in which SES differences in health are established early in life and remain relatively constant (as, for example, in severe asthma), (2) a *childhood-limited* model in which SES effects are initially large but gradually diminish over time (for example, incidence of injuries), and (3) an *adolescent-emergent* model in which SES differences are initially modest but increase with development, becoming most apparent in the teenage years (as in, for example, physical inactivity, a risk factor for heart disease). Among the prevalent sources of morbidity and mortality in childhood, different disorders and health conditions thus appeared to follow different models of SES–health associations over the course of development. The period of development in which children or adolescents are exposed to a particular risk factor is therefore capable of influencing the magnitude, and even the direction, of its health altering effects.

18.5 The case for intervention and experimentation: benefits to health

Despite the time-dependent effects of early experience on developmental outcomes, childhood is not destiny and there are thankfully few events so traumatic and prevalent as to alter irreversibly the health trajectories that originate, for most individuals, in the early years of life. There is also reason to believe that simple caretaking practices in the ordinary, day-to-day experiences of children can have disproportionately large effects on the direction and plasticity of such trajectories.[80] In a seminal theoretical paper comparing the determinants of morbidity in 'sick individuals and sick populations', Rose[108] pointed out that the disease risk factors most difficult to identify are always those with the highest prevalences in the population under study. Thus, in a population in which every individual smoked, lung cancer would be principally attributed to genetic variation, thereby overlooking the aetiologic role of smoking itself. In work examining 'hidden regulators' in the maternal behaviour of rats, Hofer[109] advanced a related argument, noting that some of the most prevalent behaviours and features involved in maternal–infant interactions play regulatory roles in the homeostasis and calibration of infant physiological systems. Just as highly prevalent risk factors are more difficult to detect, the preventive, health-promoting effects of the most ubiquitous and mundane aspects of parenting, even in human species, may prove difficult to discern. Aspects of the care and support of young children and families—routine in many societies, cultures, and human subgroups—may play essential, but often 'hidden', roles in the prevention of disorder and the preservation of health.

Indeed, evidence is now quite compelling that the experiences of childhood—those both extraordinary and mundane—have visible and enduring life course effects that are disproportionate in magnitude and, at times, anomalous in direction. Although substantial gaps remain in our knowledge of such effects, there is sufficient reason and justification to advance both research and policy agendas in parallel. As Keynes noted with respect to economic policy, it is better to be 'vaguely right than precisely wrong'. What is rather urgently needed is better articulation between the research and the policy agenda. There are also needs for a monitoring scheme to provide feedback on policy and programme successes and failures and a conceptual framework for evaluating which forms of intervention—universal, targeted, clinical—may be most effective.[34,110] Before interventions can be put into place, however, a prior necessity is knowledge of the salient dimensions of childhood social contexts on which policies and programmes might operate.

18.5.1 **Salient dimensions of childhood social contexts**

Such dimensions of context can be thought of as the social and experiential targets of intervention for improving childhood circumstances.[111] The focus here is on broader social contexts rather than on specific clinical interventions of an individual nature, because it is with respect to the former that social policies may conceivably alter circumstances. Three broad categories of context can be identified: national or regional *income inequities*, the availability of supportive *developmental opportunities*, and *social capital*—generally defined as those benefits derived from social relationships and affiliations—at the level of both society and community. Again, there is no a priori reason to assume that these categories of the broader social context operate independently or are mutually exclusive. Indeed, their natural covariation may complicate analytic efforts to disaggregate effects. Note also that the robustness of the evidence varies across categories. Because income data are relatively accessible and less prone to measurement error, the evidence for the first category is more robust. National and regional variations in policies that affect the provision of developmental opportunities can be readily identified, but quantifying their contribution to outcomes is more problematic. Finally, the social capital construct is perhaps the most susceptible to measurement error at this time and has accumulated less substantial evidence owing both to its recency and to challenges of measurement.

In considering any proposed intervention to improve childhood circumstances and developmental health outcomes, there are key questions to be asked, which together comprise a set of four criteria for intervention credibility. The first is whether there is evidence for a relationship between the target of intervention and health outcomes. More than the existence of a relationship, we should be interested in its magnitude or, more precisely, what percentage of the variance in health is attributable to the source in question. The second is whether the evidence is purely an association or whether there is reason to believe that a change in circumstances leads to a change in outcomes, whether through planned or naturally occurring experiments. For example, even if the magnitude of income inequality is associated with national or regional variations in health outcomes, it does not necessarily follow that change in the former will lead to change in the latter. Both may be governed by an unexamined third variable (social capital, for example). A third and more stringent test is whether there exists a hypothesized mechanism that can explain either association or correlated changes. While *post hoc* arguments for biological plausibility are often far too simple to construct, the possibility of unexamined, confounding variables or chance findings are more difficult to exclude in the absence of an evidence-based account of the underlying mechanisms. This is not an argument for inaction, because sensible policies can be and often are generated in the absence of a clear understanding of mediating processes. But the impact of successful interventions is enhanced and the risks of harm are reduced when the underlying mechanisms are well understood. Finally, it is important to consider the potential for meaningful change within the broader policy environment.[112] For example, flattening income inequities might be shown to have substantial impact with respect to all the identified criteria, but the prospects for enacting such a change also need to be considered from the perspective of political economy.

18.5.2 **Interventions on income inequality**

With respect to income inequalities, the evidence for impacts on health is substantial.[113–116] Recall that there are two gradients that should be kept conceptually separate. The first is the bivariate relation between SES and some developmental health outcome. The second is the gradient of income distribution, that is, the relative equality or inequality across different levels of a society. The latter can be measured in several different ways, such as a Gini coefficient (where 0 means every individual has an identical income and 1 indicates that all income is held by a single individual) or median share (or the proportion of total household income held by those below the median of income).

The general finding is that in both cross-national and cross-regional comparisons, there is a relationship between level of income inequality (a population indicator) and levels of health (most often indexed as life expectancy or age-adjusted mortality). Wilkinson's[116] comparison of Organization for Economic Cooperation and Development (OECD) countries showed a substantial association between the Gini coefficient and life expectancy, with the Scandinavian countries having the highest equality of income and greatest longevity. In a comparison of US states, Kaplan and colleagues[114] reported a strong correlation ($r=-0.62$) between age-adjusted mortality and median share of income. A comparison using major US metropolitan areas revealed a similar pattern, with 'the most economically divided metropolitan areas' showing excess mortality 'equivalent to the combined loss of life from lung cancer, diabetes, motor vehicle accidents, HIV infection, suicide and homicide during 1995'.[117] When Canadian metropolitan areas were included to comprise a US dataset, the same pattern was obtained, although there was not a significant relationship among the Canadian metropolitan areas analysed separately.[115]

Although evidence for an association between income inequality and health has been strongly supported and defended,[17,116,118] the field has not yet achieved unanimity and a number of investigators have raised questions regarding the association's authenticity. More specifically, dissenting voices have questioned the selection of countries from which data have been drawn and the quality of the national data from which the association has been inferred.[119–132] It has also been suggested that an association at the aggregate level could result from statistical artifact due to the curvilinear relationship between income inequality and health at the individual level, a variation on the ecological fallacy.[123] Clearly, testing the association within a broader set of national data would be valuable not only for generalizability but also to obtain more precise estimates of effect size. The substantial effect of income inequality for the US states (about 35% of variance) can be contrasted, for example, with the absence of an effect for comparisons of Canadian provinces and metropolitan areas. Beyond mere estimates of effect magnitude, multiple comparison points will generate more productive hypotheses about the possible sources of these effects. Evidence for correlated changes, mechanisms, or dynamics and opportunities for change in the broader policy environment, however, is sparse. There is a 'natural experiment' underway, at least in the USA, where income inequality has been sharply increasing for over a decade, affording the possibility of assessing correlated changes.

With respect to underlying dynamics, it is difficult to disaggregate income inequality *per se* from other societal differences, on the basis of evidence in hand. In the available datasets, the nations or regions with higher income equity and greater longevity tend also to be those with putatively higher social and human capital, such as the northern USA and Canada versus the southern USA or Scandinavia versus the USA, the UK, Canada, and Australia. Because these comparisons are at the 'flat of the (international wealth–health) curve', that is, among the wealthier societies, the distribution of material resources may be less important than the distribution of social status, educational and occupational pathways, or other less tangible factors. On the final criterion, the potential for policy change, it is noteworthy that current trends, at least in the USA and possibly globally, are tending in the opposite direction, towards greater rather than less income inequality.[113]

18.5.3 Interventions on developmental opportunities

A different picture emerges with respect to direct interventions through the provision of *developmental opportunities*. The efficacy of some specific interventions to improve various aspects of developmental health is well-established, as in interventions involving the augmentation of social support.[110,124,125] A 15-year follow-up of a randomized controlled trial (RCT) on prenatal and early childhood home visits by nurses showed significant and clinically important declines in subsequent pregnancies, use of welfare, substance abuse, criminality, and child abuse and neglect.[126] These are especially compelling results given that the women recruited for the study were consecutively recruited from a rural clinic offering free prenatal care (that is, they were extreme in neither the direction of abject poverty nor middle-class comfort) and that the intervention involved the provision of only developmental screening, free transportation to the clinic, and brief, supportive visits to the home. The same RCT had earlier shown that the intervention resulted, over the short-term, in a lower incidence of pregnancy-induced hypertension, fewer paediatric visits for injuries or ingestions, and fewer second pregnancies.[127]

Targeted programmes for children in disadvantaged or high-risk circumstances have also shown long-term benefits across a range of outcomes (see a review by Hertzman and Wiens[128]) and there are plausible if not fully identified developmental mechanisms through which these benefits may operate. The most successful interventions have been multisystemic, however, complicating the search for specific mechanisms. Nonetheless, pre-school, school, and community interventions have often yielded significant enhancements in behavioural and developmental outcomes among children receiving enriched early educational and care experiences. One of the largest and most successful national experiments to enhance child development is the Headstart program, based on the Perry Pre-school curriculum.[129,130] In the Ypsilanti/Perry Pre-school study, 3–6-year-old children received an intensive pre-school curriculum 5 days per week for a period of 30 weeks per year, along with parental involvement facilitated through teacher home visits. Long-term effects at age 27 included lower high school dropout rates, fewer teen pregnancies, better and more consistent employment, and reduced drug abuse. The Carolina Abecedarian Project, an RCT involving frequent home visits and year-round, high-quality, centre-based care beginning in infancy, found higher IQs in intervention group children at school entry, higher reading and maths scores at age 15 years, and better long-term educational achievements among the mothers of intervention children.[131] The Child Development Project, a quasi-experimental study, showed significant reductions in student drug use and delinquency following a school-based intervention designed to 'help schools become caring communities of learners—environments that are characterized by supportive social relationships, a common sense of purpose, and a commitment to prosocial values'.[132] The Infant Health and Development Project, among the most extensive and carefully planned educational interventions, included an intensive programme of post-partum parent education and home visiting. Results showed significant though modest effects on maternal child behavioural competence and adaptive functioning[133] and moderate effects on cognitive development.[134]

Another elementary school-based intervention involved the introduction of a violence prevention curriculum and produced a sustained decrement in physical aggression and an increase in prosocial behaviour.[135] The Ottawa Project, one of very few community-based child development studies, is a recreational programme focused on non-academic skill development for 5–15-year-old children from a subsidized housing complex.[136] The intervention group in this project has shown significant declines over control participants in the extent of ongoing anti-social behaviour, as well as positive effects on behavioural competence[133] and cognitive development.[134] Similarly, children participating in the Chicago Child–Parent Center Program—which provided education, social and health services, and pre-school to low-income families—had higher rates of high school completion and lower rates of arrest and school dropout.[137] Taken together, these and other studies suggest that targeted, early intervention programmes can produce sizeable, sustained effects on developmental outcomes such as IQ, academic achievement, grade retention, high school graduation, and social competence.

This body of work addressing interventions to augment developmental opportunities appears to meet at least two of the evidential criteria noted above. There is evidence that targeted changes in circumstances lead to changes in outcomes and there are plausible mechanisms to begin accounting for these changes. More difficult to answer, however, are the questions of population impact and the potential for changes in social policy. The targeted interventions for which evidence is strongest tend also to be those most extensive and costly. Treating substantial portions of the childhood population as potential targets of specific interventions raises difficult questions on both implementation costs and on broad public support for such an approach.[110] On the other hand, through monitoring mechanisms such as the UN Human Development Index, it has become clear that improvements in basic nutrition, health services, and education have strong and positive effects on developmental health. At a global level, extending provision of these basic developmental supports can be defended as among the highest international priorities.[138,139]

Although these general findings are useful as support for the broader notion that childhood circumstances matter, they provide little guidance for social policy in the developed world. Even though there is little variation in basic provisions—for example, elementary and secondary education is universal and generally available through public resources in these countries—there are identifiable differences in policies affecting the provision of developmental opportunities. Variation in the availability of early childhood education and learning opportunities, for example, is quite extensive.[140]

More generally, 'public goods' are unevenly distributed across regions and nations. These include not only programmes for children but also broader services (such as parks and recreation) that may be related to child development. Are the distributional patterns of these public goods, as they affect childhood circumstances, responsible for the observed variations in developmental health? Here again is the difficulty that distributional patterns covary with patterns of income inequality. Societies that have less income inequality tend also to have a greater supply of public goods, including those provided directly for children.[141] It is possible to imagine empirical probes into the relative influences of income inequality and lack of developmental opportunities and such investigations may be fruitful. One possible outcome of such investigation would be that relative income equality and provision of developmental opportunities are correlated for substantive reasons. Such an association could be direct (income inequality is reduced through more progressive taxation regimes, whose proceeds are used for developmental investments) or indirect, through the social capital function. Societies with higher social capital in the sense of greater coordination and collaboration (see for example, Reference 141) may make similar policy choices on income distribution and on developmental investments.

18.5.4 Interventions on social capital

To date, social capital literature has primarily focused on economic outcomes.[141] Where developmental health outcomes have been explored, it has been primarily in circumstances of significant deprivation. In these instances, the operating hypothesis is that social capital may act as a buffer against economic disadvantage for a variety of outcomes.[142,143] That is, are individuals in distressed circumstances better off if their neighbourhood possesses higher levels of social capital (social cohesion, interpersonal trust, collective efficacy, and so on)? Application of the intervention criteria above is least clear in the case of social capital, largely owing to the fact that evidence is only beginning to emerge. It is, however, potentially a very productive research agenda and not only as a buffering hypothesis.[144]

Even at this early point in such research, an important thought experiment is to consider the social policy implications of a major social capital effect. Assume that positive evidence on association, correlated changes, and underlying dynamics were obtained. Are there social policy tools that can reliably increase the social capital of a community or society? Case studies of successful community development efforts[145] lead more strongly toward a contrasting inference, that positive changes tend to be largely self-organizing at a local level, often with the catalyst of personal charisma. At a larger level, the cultural supports for changes in social capital may be quite complex and not easily amenable to policy interventions.

18.5.5 Summary

To summarize, there is robust evidence that variation in childhood circumstances shows substantial concurrent and longitudinal relationships with variation in a wide range of developmental health outcomes. There are plausible hypotheses on the underlying developmental mechanisms that may give rise to these patterns. The evidence on these potential biodevelopmental mediators suggests a substantial role of child development in life course developmental health and points towards a potentially productive research agenda that follows from current evidence. Three sources at the broader societal level have been considered in this section: income inequality, the provision of developmental opportunities, and social capital. There are credible arguments to be made within each category and a proposed evaluation scheme identifies four key criteria: the degree of association, the evidence for correlated changes, the plausibility of underlying developmental mechanisms, and the potential for change within the prevailing policy environment. In none of the categories have all the relevant questions been successfully addressed, but taken together the existing evidence supports an emerging research agenda on human development that may prove quite productive.

As opposed to the evident gaps in our knowledge of how best to proceed, the evidence for the potential benefits of thoughtful intervention is substantial.[34,110] As we expand our consideration of the contributors to and consequences of developmental health, it becomes clear that the issues have implications beyond health outcomes alone. In the following two sections, we briefly consider the overlap of these issues with the economic and the ethical arguments for intervention to improve childhood circumstances. In each case, space permits only an outline of the major issues that should be considered.

18.6 Economic arguments for intervention

By far the most common economic argument in favour of intervention to improve childhood circumstances is that future savings to society outweigh the initial investment. These savings have been identified in a wide range of areas (see, for example, Reference 40): lower special education services, lower use of social services, lower rates of arrest and incarceration, lower unemployment, and higher income and thus higher taxes paid. In the often cited Perry Pre-school Project, these savings over a two-decade period have been estimated to generate a 7:1 return on initial programme investment.[129,130] Other studies that have focused on universal programmes, such as high-quality day care, estimate more modest but still substantial returns on investment.[146] Not estimated in these models are the effects on physical and mental health across the life course. If there is indeed a link between developmental health gradients and early experience-based brain development, as argued above, it is likely that such savings to the health system could be substantial. Thus, there is a sound economic argument to be made on behalf of early intervention to improve childhood circumstances arising from the return on this investment from subsequent savings to social and health services across the life course.

Supporters of this argument in the public policy arena face three important challenges. The first is the generalizability and robustness of the econometric estimates that have been put forward. Clearly, these are contingent on a host of local circumstances and are not easily transferable across jurisdictions. On the other hand, the consistency, if not the magnitude, of cost–benefit analyses in a number of jurisdictions supports the argument that early intervention is properly viewed as a social investment rather than a social expenditure.[34] The second challenge is that the benefits (that is, the savings to future health and social services) rest on a premise that the services in the future will continue to be available in approximately similar fashion to the present. This is obviously not guaranteed. Cutbacks to the availability of such services due to changes in policies governing their administration could alter the cost–benefit ratios substantially.

The third challenge is the time horizon of the benefits (life course) relative to the costs (in early life). It is perhaps this factor more than any other—except perhaps the relative political weakness of the immediate beneficiaries, young children and their families, compared to claimants on, for example, health services—that has undermined the investment argument on behalf of early intervention. In short, current governments must bear the investment burden, whereas the benefits accrue to future, unknown governments.

There is a second category of economic arguments on behalf of improving childhood circumstances and this focuses on production rather than consumption. One version of this argument[39] takes note of the similar or overlapping pathways to health and competence that are denoted by the term 'developmental health'. From this observation, it is possible to identify a construct of population competence that shares many of the features and underlying dynamics of population health. Thus, a society's pool of human resources for economic growth and production is likely to be affected in similar ways. Assessing these competencies at a population level, especially for comparative purposes, is less advanced than our population health indicators.[112,147] But the available data (see, for example, Reference 25) offer considerable support for the argument that similar gradient effects—the bivariate SES/competence gradient, the comparative epidemiology associating steeper gradients with lower overall population competence, and the longitudinal effects of early experience—are observed. It is plausible that the similarity in gradient effects arises from common developmental pathways.

The importance of population competence is emphasized in light of contemporary economic theories that technological innovation lies at the centre of economic growth and that such innovation is endogenous to society, arising from numerous social innovations.[148–150] Across history, this feedback loop from technological to social innovation can be viewed as an 'innovation dynamic' that has the characteristics of a dynamic system with a positive feedback loop, leading to accelerative change.[39,151] The implication for the current historical moment, often characterized as the information or knowledge revolution, is that the cultivation of human resources may represent a society's most significant investment for future economic growth.[112,149,152]

It could be argued that such investments create an economic drag in the present and that policies to support future competence among elites alone will suffice,[160] rather than more costly investments in population developmental health. The future cannot, of course, be known, but the available evidence seems *not* to support a view that investments in childhood circumstances create an economic drag. In a recent analysis of the post-Second World War economic performance of OECD countries, Hall and Soskice[153] identify two major varieties of capitalism, coordinated market economies (for example, northern Europe and Scandinavia) and liberal market economies (for example, the UK, the USA, Canada, and Australia). The former tend also to be those countries with flatter and higher gradients in developmental health (although the degree of this association remains, thus far, unquantified). The long-term economic growth of both varieties is approximately the same, however, suggesting that a higher level of human development investment does not create a significant economic drag. Whether there is a major future benefit remains to be seen and is obviously dependent on a range of factors beyond population developmental health. Transformations of economic activity arising from advances in the organization of production (the 'learning organization') and technological breakthroughs (the world wide web and its associated features) may capitalize more effectively on the breadth and depth of population competence.[149,152]

To summarize, there are sound economic arguments to be made on behalf of investments to improve childhood circumstances. The first argument identifies the cost–benefit ratios from targeted interventions and such analyses typically yield positive returns on investment. The second argument is not yet quantified, but draws on contemporary economic growth theory to infer that future growth may be heavily dependent on population developmental health, which is in turn dependent on investments early in the life course. The combination of savings from services not consumed in later life and increased economic growth arising from higher competence and health, makes a strong case for the economic sense of such investments, given the proper time horizon.

18.7 Ethical arguments for intervention

Arguments based on the biological or economic consequences of intervening, or failing to intervene, to improve childhood circumstances are viewed by some as unnecessary or even inappropriate. From this perspective, justifications for the improvement of childhood circumstances based on future health or economic benefits undermine more fundamental ethical reasons to do so. In this chapter we have argued instead that a full understanding of the consequences arising from the circumstances of childhood is important for both science and policy. But societal utility (in terms of population health or economic prosperity) is clearly not the only basis for supporting the improvement of childhood circumstances. Identifying the fundamental ethical reasons for improving childhood circumstances is an essential complement, by elevating the issues beyond strictly utilitarian arguments.

We identify two major categories of ethical concern. The first is that the quality of life during childhood is itself a core issue, independent of life course consequences. In part, this is a reaction against excessive utilitarianism, in that children should be seen as valuable in their own right and not merely as cogs in some future political economy. This counterargument is somewhat tendentious, in that it down-plays the foreseeable interests of children in becoming healthy and productive adults. But there is a more positive version of the argument, drawing on Rawls'[154] notions of 'natural justice'. The core argument is that choices of fair social arrangements are inextricably influenced by one's perceptions of how these arrangements affect one's own personal circumstances. 'Haves' and 'have-nots', for example, view greater income equity differently. A thought experiment, the 'veil of ignorance', is proposed as a way to get beyond this. What social arrangements would individuals choose if they were unable to know what positions they would hold in the resulting society? This thought experiment has particular force with respect to children, because they are not in a position to influence such choices in reality. It is most likely that individuals would choose for children to have high-quality physical and social environments and equitable access to developmental opportunities.

The second category of ethical dilemma arises from the growing acceptance of the extension of fundamental human rights to children, as in the international conventions noted above. It is useful here to make a distinction that is often overlooked, though a distinction that adolescents and their parents are able to make.[155,156]

Much attention has been paid to rights of self-determination, to give children standing as individual people in legal and quasi-legal contexts. Considerable efforts have been made in many jurisdictions to accommodate this emerging understanding. Equally important, and perhaps more germane to the improvement of childhood circumstances, is the notion of nurturance rights. Because of their relative powerlessness not only in society at large but also within families, children are in a vulnerable position with regard to the meeting of basic needs. Asserting that they have rights to nurturance, as the relevant international conventions do, is an attempt to raise the profile of such expectations. There has been less societal activity to date to explicate and embody nurturance rights compared with self-determination rights and thus much remains to be done. This remains, however, a promising avenue towards supporting arguments for the improvement of childhood circumstances.

From a pragmatic perspective, it seems productive to deploy both utilitarian arguments (that is, life course consequences for health and economic consequences for society) and ethical arguments (that is, natural justice and fundamental rights), because both point in the same direction. If policy change to improve circumstances in childhood is the goal, then attracting the widest range of support is a sensible approach.

18.8 The promise of non-genomic intergenerational transmission of benefits

To the variable extent with which valid human inferences can be made from experimental evidence in animal models, the work of Meaney and Champagne[49,157] on non-genomic inheritance offers an illuminating and potentially encouraging additional perspective on the possibility of blunting or reversing developmental effects of early social inequities. As noted above, Meaney's work has demonstrated that aspects of early maternal behaviour—behaviour that can be effectively altered by manipulations within the infant-rearing environment—are capable of calibrating set points and response characteristics within key biological systems that are activated under conditions of adversity. Such calibration—at least in rodent pups—becomes a stable response disposition, enduring over the life course of the individual and producing an adult with diminished fearfulness and more modest HPA responses to stress. What is less universally appreciated within this body of work is the finding that alterations in maternal caring behaviour have biological effects not only on the next, most immediate generation, but on the temporally and genetically more distal third generation, as well. Pups reared by mothers whose caring behaviour is attentive, tactile, and sustained grow up to become mothers who are themselves less anxious, more attentive, and in turn more likely to produce infants with similar adult, maternal predispositions. If such findings proved transferable, even in part, to human populations, the implications for societal interventions would be profound. What results from the Meaney laboratory suggest is the possibility that intensive and effective efforts to promote caring, nurturant maternal behaviour in one generation could have positive developmental effects not just on the offspring of the mothers whose behaviour was changed, but on those of future generations, as well. The findings seem speculatively to suggest that altering the parenting experience of a generation of children could have more enduring influences, promoting the health and well-being of their children and grandchildren to come.

18.9 **Early intervention: ensuring the beneficence of childhood**

How might the world be changed by a generation of children carefully and protectively nurtured through hazards of childhood into the promises of adult life? Given the evidence reviewed above for both cumulative and critically timed effects of early experience on health over the life course, it is plausible to argue that a hypothetical society's commitment to a caring and protected childhood could have health effects as persistent and lasting as they would be pervasive and deep. Although developmental science has much yet to learn about the long-term consequences of early experience, there are a sufficient number and variety of observations now in place to argue that the biological, behavioural, and social implications of an *intentional childhood* might be vast indeed. Imagine a society in which children experienced, by virtue of a community's specific intent, sustained, caring, and supportive parenting, the presence, love, and encouragement of at least two generations of family members, the advantages of universal preparation for school and learning, vigilant and reflexive community protection from situations of abuse or neglect, commitment to a minimum standard of housing and nutrition, and the availability of richly evocative environments for play, imagination, and creativity. It is arguably the case that such a society would visibly bear the mark of its children's experiences and that a just and more egalitarian social order would emerge, dramatically distinguishing that society from its contemporary neighbours and peers.

Over the course of history,[158] childhood has been variably regarded as: a developmental phase of trivial activity and interest; the cauldron of immaturity from which emerge the passions, skills, and disorders of adult life; or an apprenticed preparation for the exigencies and serious business of adulthood. What has broadly emerged from the accumulating annals of developmental studies are two fundamental observations about the nature and significance of childhood and of children. First and perhaps most self-evident to twenty-first century sensibilities, children are fully intact and sentient human beings, invested of the full social, moral, and legal rights conferred upon adults within democratic societies. Neither the developmental anlage of an adult persona nor a primitive irrelevance on the road to legitimate maturity, a child is a *human being*, imbued with all of the same complexities, pains, sensitivities, and capacities for nuanced social interchange that characterize their parents and their future selves. As such, children are deserving of the same protection, opportunities, and advantages that we would more readily and easily grant their senior counterparts. Childhood is thus distinctive as a developmental period but indistinguishable in its moral and ethical substance.

Although this first observation alone would be sufficient basis for protecting and ensuring the beneficence of childhood, this chapter has argued, we hope persuasively, that the implications of children's experience for health and well-being in adult life are likely profound. Even on economic grounds, it is to every society's advantage to nurture and tend its youngest and most vulnerable members. We are finally learning, in the construction of social policy, what was long ago encoded in the evolutionary history of our species, that 'the growing good of the world is partly dependent on unhistoric acts'[159] and the flourishing of a human society partly contingent upon acts of protection and care toward its children, who are—collectively—the legacy, promise, and future of every earthly nation.

References

Those marked with an asterisk are especially recommended for further reading.

1. **Keating DP, Mustard JF.** Social economic factors and human development. In Ross D, ed. *Family security in insecure times: National forum on family security.* Ottawa: ,1993: 87–105.

2. **Convention on the Rights of the Child, 20 November 1989.** *Annu Rev Popul Law* 1989;**16**:95, 485–501.

3. **Black M.** World summit for children. *Lancet* 1990;**336**:1586.

4. **Bellamy C.** *The state of the world's children 2002.* New York: UNICEF, 2002.

5. **Bellamy C.** *The state of the world's children 2000.* New York: UNICEF, 2000.

6. **Lachman P, Poblete X, Ebigbo PO, Nyandiya-Bundy S, Bundy RP, Killian B** *et al.* Challenges facing child protection. *Child Abuse Negl* 2002;**26**:587–617.

7. **Chen E, Matthews KA, Boyce WT.** Socioeconomic differences in children's health: how and why do these relationships change with age? *Psychol Bull* 2002;**128**:295–329.

8. **National Center for Children in Poverty.** *One in four: America's youngest poor.* New York: Columbia University School of Public Health, 1996.

9. **St Pierre RG, Layzer JI.** Improving the life chances of children in poverty: assumptions and what we have learned. *Social Policy Report of the Society for Research in Child Development* 1998;**12**:1–24.

10. **Aber JL, Bennett NG, Conley DC, Li J.** The effects of poverty on child health and development. *Annu Rev Pub Health* 1997;**18**:463–83.

11. **Egbuonu L, Starfield B.** Child health and social status. *Pediatrics* 1982;**69**:550–7.

12. **Nelson MD.** Socioeconomic status and childhood mortality in North Carolina. *Am J Pub Health* 1992;**82**:1131–3.

13. **Duncan GJ, Brooks-Gunn J, Klebanov PK.** Economic deprivation and early childhood development. *Child Dev* 1994;**65**:296–318.

14. **Newacheck PW.** Poverty and childhood chronic illness. *Arch Pediatr Adolesc Med* 1994;**148**:1143–9.

15. **Moss HB, Mezzich A, Yao JK, Gavaler J, Martin CS.** Aggressivity among sons of substance-abusing fathers: association with psychiatric disorder in the father and son, paternal personality, pubertal development, and socioeconomic status. *Am J Drug Alc Abuse* 1995;**21**:195–208.

16. **Costello EJ, Angold A, Burns BJ, Stangl DK, Tweed DL, Erkanli A** *et al.* The Great Smoky Mountains Study of Youth: Goals, design, methods, and the prevalence of DSM-III-R disorders. *Arch Gen Psychiat* 1996;**53**:1129–36.

*17. **Keating DP, Hertzman C.** *Developmental health and the wealth of nations: social, biological, and educational dynamics.* New York: Guilford Press, 1999.

18. **Hertzman C.** Population health and human development. In Keating DP, Hertzman C, eds. *Developmental health and the wealth of nations: social, biological, and educational dynamics.* New York: Guilford Press, 1999:21–40.

19. **Kuh D, Ben-Shlomo Y, eds.** *A life course approach to chronic disease epidemiology.* Oxford: Oxford University Press, 1997.

20. **Kuh D, Power C, Blane D, Bartley M.** Social pathways between childhood and adult health. In Kuh D, Ben-Shlomo Y, eds. *A life course approach to chronic disease epidemiology.* Oxford: Oxford University Press, 1997:169–98.

21. **Power C, Hertzman C.** Health, well-being, and coping skills. In Keating DP, Hertzman C, eds. *Developmental health and the wealth of nations: Social, biological, and educational dynamics.* New York: Guilford Press, 1999:41–54.

22. **Kaplan GA, Lynch JW.** Whither studies on the socioeconomic foundations of population health? *Am J Pub Health* 1997;**87**:1409–11.

23. **Evans RG, Barer ML, Marmor TR.** Why are some people healthy and others not? The determinants of health of populations. New York: Aldine DeGruyter, 1994.

24. **Brooks-Gunn J, Duncan GJ, Britto PR.** Are socioeconomic gradients for children similar to those for adults? Achievement and health of children in the United States. In Keating DP, Hertzman C, eds. *Developmental health and the wealth of nations: Social, biological, and educational dynamics.* New York: Guilford Press, 1999:94–124.

25. **Willms JD.** Quality and inequality in children's literacy: The effects of families, schools, and communities. In Keating DP, Hertzman C, eds. *Developmental health and the wealth of nations: Social, biological, and educational dynamics.* New York: Guilford Press, 1999:72–93.

26. **Case R, Griffin S, Kelly WM.** Socioeconomic gradients in mathematical ability and their responsiveness to intervention during early childhood. In Keating DP, Hertzman C, eds. *Developmental health and the wealth of nations: Social, biological, and educational dynamics.* New York: Guilford Press, 1999:125–49.

27. **Miller FK, Jenkins J, Keating DP.** Parenting and children's behavior problems. In Willms JD, ed. *Vulnerable children: findings from Canada's National Longitudinal Survey of Children and Youth.* Edmonton: University of Alberta Press, 2002:167–82.

28. **Tremblay RE.** When children's social development fails. In Keating DP, Hertzman C, eds. *Developmental health and the wealth of nations: Social, biological, and educational dynamics.* New York: Guilford Press, 1999:55–71.

29. **Willms JD.** Vulnerable children: findings from the National Longitudinal Study of Children and Youth. Edmonton: University of Alberta Press, 2002.

30. **Hertzman C.** Health and human society. *Am Sci* 2001;**89**:538–45.

31. **Willms JD.** *Ten hypotheses about gradients.* Ottawa: Human Resources Development Canada (in press).

*32. **Adler NE, Boyce WT, Chesney MA, Cohen S, Folkman S, Kahn RL** *et al.* Socioeconomic status and health: the challenge of the gradient. *Am Psychol* 1994;**49**:15–24.

33. **Kuh D, Hardy R, Langenberg C, Richards M, Wadsworth ME.** Mortality in adults aged 26–54 years related to socioeconomic conditions in childhood and adulthood: post war birth cohort study. *Br Med J* 2002;**325**:1076–80.

34. **Keating DP.** Developmental health as the wealth of nations. In Keating DP, Hertzman C, eds. *Developmental health and the wealth of nations: Social, biological, and educational dynamics.* New York: Guilford, 1999:337–47.

35. **Kuh D, Ben-Shlomo Y, Lynch JW, Hallqvist J, Power C.** Glossary of life course epidemiology. *J Epidemiol Commun Health* 2003;**57**:778–83.

36. **Ben-Shlomo Y, Kuh D.** A life course approach to chronic disease epidemiology: conceptual models, empirical challenges, and interdisciplinary perspectives. *Int J Epidemiol* 2002;**31**:285–93.

37. **Poulton R, Caspi A, Milne BJ, Thomson WM, Taylor A, Sears MR** *et al.* Association between children's experience of socioeconomic disadvantage and adult health: A life-course study. *Lancet* 2002;**360**:1640–5.

38. **Masten AS.** Ordinary magic. Resilience processes in development. *Am Psychol* 2001;**56**:227–38.

39. **Keating DP, Hertzman C.** Modernity's paradox. In Keating DP, Hertzman C, eds. *Developmental health and the wealth of nations: Social, biological, and educational dynamics.* New York: Guilford Press, 1999:1–17.

40. **Krieger N.** Theories for social epidemiology in the 21st century: An ecosocial perspective. *Int J Epidemiol* 2001;**30**:668–77.

41. **Barr RG, Mustard JF.** *Experience-based brain and biological development.* Toronto, Canada: Canadian Institute for Advanced Research, 2003.

42. **Kraemer HC, Stice E, Kazdin A, Offord D, Kupfer D.** How do risk factors work together? Mediators, moderators, independent, overlapping and proxy-risk factors. *Am J Psychiat* 2001;**158**:848–56.

43. **Greenough WT, Black JE.** Induction of brain structure by experience: substrates for cognitive development. In Gunnar MRR, Nelson CA, eds. *Developmental behavioral neuroscience.* New Jersey: Lawrence Erlbaum, 1992.

44. **Black JE, Sirevaag AM, Wallace CS, Savin MH, Greenough WT.** Effects of complex experience on somatic growth and organ development in rats. *Dev Psychobiol* 1989;**22**:727–52.

45. **Greenough WT, Juraska JM, Volkmar FR.** Maze training effects on dendritic branching in occipital cortex of adult rats. *Behav Neural Biol* 1979;**26**:287–97.

46. **Greenough WT, Madden TC, Fleischmann TB.** Effects of isolation, dailing handling, and enriched rearing on maze learning. *Psychonomic Sci* 1972;**27**:279–80.

*47. **Caspi A, McClay J, Moffitt TE, Mill J, Martin J, Craig IW** *et al.* Role of genotype in the cycle of violence in maltreated children. *Science* 2002;**297**:851–4.

48. **Bennett AJ, Lesch KP, Heils A, Long JC, Lorenz JG, Shoaf SE** *et al.* Early experience and serotonin transporter gene variation interact to influence primate CNS function. *Mol Psychiat* 2002;**7**:118–22.

*49. **Meaney MJ.** Maternal care, gene expression, and the transmission of individual differences in stress reactivity across generations. *Annu Rev Neurosci* 2001;**24**:1161–92.

50. **Suomi SJ.** Early determinants of behaviour: evidence from primate studies. *Br Med Bull* 1997;**53**:170–84.

51. **Champoux M, Boyce WT, Suomi SJ.** Biobehavioral comparisons between adopted and nonadopted rhesus monkey infants. *J Dev Behav Pediatr* 1995;**16**:6–13.

52. **Lubach GR, Coe CL, Ershler WB.** Effects of early rearing environment on immune responses of infant rhesus monkeys. *Brain Behav Immun* 1995;**9**:31–46.

53. **Martin RE, Sackett GP, Gunderson VM, Goodlin-Jones BL.** Auditory evoked heart rate responses in pigtailed macaques (*Macaca nemestrina*) raised in isolation. *Dev Psychobiol* 1988;**21**:251–60.

54. **Coplan JD, Andrews MW, Rosenblum LA, Owens MJ, Friedman S, Gorman JM** *et al.* Persistent elevations of cerebrospinal fluid concentrations of corticotropin-releasing factor in adult non-human primates exposed to early-life stressors: implications for the pathophysiology of mood and anxiety disorders. *Proc Natl Acad Sci USA* 1996;**93**:1619–23.

55. **Shannon C, Champoux M, Suomi SJ.** Rearing condition and plasma cortisol in rhesus monkey infants. *Am J Primatol* 1998;**46**:311–21.

56. **Boyce WT, Champoux M, Suomi SJ, Gunnar MRR.** Salivary cortisol in nursery-reared rhesus monkeys: Reactivity to peer interactions and altered circadian activity. *Dev Psychobiol* 1995;**28**:257–67.

57. **Sapolsky R.** Adrenocortical function, social rank, and personality among wild baboons. *Biol Psychiat* 1990;**28**:862–85.

58. **Sapolsky RM, Share LJ.** Rank-related differences in cardiovascular function among wild baboons: role of sensitivity to glucocorticoids. *Am J Primatol* 1994;**32**:261–75.

59. **Hertsgaard L, Gunnar MR, Erickson MF, Nachmias M.** Adrenocortical responses to the strange situation in infants with disorganized/disoriented attachment relationships. *Child Dev* 1995;**66**:1100–6.

60. **Meyer SE, Chrousos GP, Gold PW.** Major depression and the stress system: a life span perspective. *Dev Psychopathol* 2001;**13**:565–80.

61. **Nachmias M, Gunnar MR, Mangelsdorf S, Parritz RH, Buss K.** Behavioral inhibition and stress reactivity: The moderating role of attachment security. *Child Dev* 1996;**67**:508–22.

62. Willemsen-Swinkels SH, Bakermans-Kranenburg MJ, Buitelaar JK, van IJzendoorn MH, van Engeland H. Insecure and disorganised attachment in children with a pervasive developmental disorder: relationship with social interaction and heart rate. *J Child Psychol Psychiat* 2000;**41**:759–67.

63. Heim C, Newport DJ, Heit S, Graham YP, Wilcox M, Bonsall R *et al.* Pituitary–adrenal and autonomic responses to stress in women after sexual and physical abuse in childhood. *J Am Med Assoc 2000*;**284**:592–7.

64. De Bellis MD, Baum AS, Birmaher B, Keshavan MS, Eccard CH, Boring AM *et al.* AE Bennett Research Award. Developmental traumatology. Part I: Biological stress systems. *Biol Psychiat* 1999;**45**:1259–70.

65. Perry B. Neurobiological sequelae of childhood trauma: PTSD in children. In Murburg M, ed. *Catecholamine function in post-traumatic stress disorder: emerging concepts.* Washington, DC: American Psychiatric Press, 1994:233–55.

66. Yehuda R, Halligan SL, Bierer LM. Relationship of parental trauma exposure and PTSD to PTSD, depressive and anxiety disorders in offspring. *J Psychiat Res* 2001;**35**:261–70.

67. Yehuda R, Halligan SL, Grossman R. Childhood trauma and risk for PTSD: relationship to intergenerational effects of trauma, parental PTSD, and cortisol excretion. *Dev Psychopathol* 2001;**13**:733–53.

68. Yehuda R. Post-traumatic stress disorder. *N Engl J Med* 2002;**346**:108–14.

69. Stein MB, Yehuda R, Koverola C, Hanna C. Enhanced dexamethasone suppression of plasma cortisol in adult women traumatized by childhood sexual abuse. *Biol Psychiat* 1997;**42**:680–6.

*70. Lupien SJ, King S, Meaney MJ, McEwen BS. Child's stress hormone levels correlate with mother's socioeconomic status and depressive state. *Biol Psychiat* 2000;**48**:976–80.

71. Fernald LC, Grantham-McGregor SM. Stress response in school-age children who have been growth retarded since early childhood. *Am J Clin Nutr* 1998;**68**:691–8.

72. Steptoe A, Feldman PJ, Kunz S, Owen N, Willemsen G, Marmot M. Stress responsivity and socioeconomic status: A mechanism for increased cardiovascular disease risk? *Eur Heart J* 2002;**23**:1757–63.

*73. McEwen BS. Sex, stress and the hippocampus: allostasis, allostatic load and the aging process. *Neurobiol Aging* 2002;**23**:921–39.

74. McEwen BS. Protective and damaging effects of stress mediators. *New Engl J Med* 1998;**338**:171–9.

75. Galea LAM, McEwen BS, Tanapat P, Deak T, Spencer RL, Dhabhar FS. Sex differences in dendritic atrophy of CA3 pyramidal neurons in response to chronic restraint stress. *Neuroscience* 1997;**81**:689–97.

76. McEwen BS. The neurobiology of stress: from serendipity to clinical relevance. *Brain Res* 2000;**886**:172–89.

77. Karlamangla AS, Singer BH, McEwen BS, Rowe JW, Seeman TE. Allostatic load as a predictor of functional decline. MacArthur studies of successful aging. *J Clin Epidemiol* 2002;**55**:696–710.

78. Davidson RJ, Jackson DC, Kalin NH. Emotion, plasticity, context, and regulation: perspectives from affective neuroscience. *Psychol Bull* 2000;**126**:890–909.

79. Barker DJP. The fetal origins of coronary heart disease. *Acta Paediatr* 1997;**422**(**suppl**):78–82.

*80. Hart T, Risley TR. *Meaningful differences in the everyday experience of young American children.* Baltimore: Paul H Brookes, 1995.

81. Dodge KA, Pettit GS, Bates JE. Socialization mediators of the relation between socioeconomic status and child conduct problems. *Child Dev* 1994;**65**:649–65.

82. Bates JE, Pettit GS, Dodge KA, Ridge B. Interaction of temperamental resistance to control and restrictive parenting in the development of externalizing behavior. *Dev Psychol* 1998;**34**:982–95.

83. **Bosma H, van de Mheen HD, Mackenbach JP.** Social class in childhood and general health in adulthood: questionnaire study of contribution of psychological attributes. *Br Med J* 1999;**318**:12–22.

84. **Lynch JW, Kaplan GA, Salonen JT.** Why do poor people behavior poorly? Variation in adult health behaviours and psychosocial characteristics by stages of the socioeconomic lifecourse. *Soc Sci Med* 1997;**44**:809–19.

85. **Chesney MA, Rosenman RH, eds.** *Anger and hostility in cardiovascular and behavioral disorders.* Washington: Hemisphere, 1985.

86. **Kazdin AE, French NH, Unis AS, Esveldt-Dawson K, Sherick RB.** Hopelessness, depression, and suicidal intent among psychiatrically disturbed children. *J Consult Clin Psychol* 1983;**51**:504–10.

87. **Marmot MG, Bosma H, Hemingway H, Brunner E, Stansfeld S.** Contribution of job control and other risk factors to social variations in coronary heart disease incidence (see comments). *Lancet* 1997;**350**:235–9.

88. **Weigel C, Wertlieb D, Feldstein M.** Perceptions of control, competence, and contingency as influences on the stress-behavior symptom relation in school-age children. *J Pers Soc Psychol* 1989;**56**:456–64.

89. **Anda RF, Croft JB, Felitti VJ, Nordenberg D, Giles WH, Williamson DF** *et al.* Adverse childhood experiences and smoking during adolescence and adulthood. *J Am Med Assoc* 1999;**282**:1652–8.

90. **Higley JD, Thompson WW, Champoux M, Goldman D, Hasert MF, Kraemer GW** *et al.* Paternal and maternal genetic and environmental contributions to cerebrospinal fluid monoamine metabolites in rhesus monkeys (*Macaca mulatta*). *Arch Gen Psychiat* 1993;**50**:615–23.

91. **Bernstein IS.** Dominance, aggression and reproduction in primate societies. *J Theor Biol* 1976;**60**:459–72.

92. **Vaughn B, Waters E.** Social organization among preschooler peers: dominance, attention and sociometric correlates. In Omark DR, Strayer FF, Freedman D, eds. *Dominance relations: An ethological view of human conflict and social interaction.* New York: Garland STPM Press, 1978:359–80.

93. **Strayer FF, Trudel M.** Developmental changes in the nature and function of social dominance among young children. *Ethol Sociobiol* 1984;**5**:279–95.

94. **Goldstein LH, Trancik A, Bensadoun J, Boyce WT, Adler NE.** Social dominance and cardiovascular reactivity in preschoolers: Associations with SES and health. *Ann NY Acad Sci* 1999;**896**:363–6.

95. **La Frenière PJ, Charlesworth WR.** Dominance, attention, and affiliation in a preschool group: A nine-month longitudinal study. *Ethol Sociobiol* 1983;**4**:55–67.

96. **Strayer FF.** Co-adaptation within the early peer group: A psychobiological study of social competence. In Schneider BH, ed. *Social competence in developmental perspective.* Boston: Kluwer, 1989:145–172.

97. **Kaplan JR, Manuck SB, Clarkson TB, Lusso FM, Taub DM.** Social status, environment, and atherosclerosis in cynomolgus monkeys. *Arteriosclerosis* 1982;**2**:359–68.

98. **Cohen S.** Social status and susceptibility to respiratory infections. *Ann NY Acad Sci* 1999;**896**:246–53.

99. **Cohen S, Frank E, Doyle WJ, Skoner DP, Rabin BS, Gwaltney JM Jr.** Types of stressors that increase susceptibility to the common cold in healthy adults (see comments). *Health Psychol* 1998;**17**:214–23.

100. **Cohen S, Line S, Manuck SB, Rabin BS, Heise ER, Kaplan JR.** Chronic social stress, social status, and susceptibility to upper respiratory infections in nonhuman primates (see comments). *Psychosom Med* 1997;**59**:213–21.

101. **Bornstein MH.** Sensitive periods in development: structural characteristics and causal interpretations. *Psychol Bull* 1989;**105**:179–97.

*102. **Essex MJ, Klein MH, Cho E, Kalin NH.** Maternal stress beginning in infancy may sensitize children to later stress exposure: Effects on cortisol and behavior. *Biol Psychiat* 2002;**52**:776–84.

103. **Roseboom TJ, van der Meulen JH, Osmond C, Barker DJ, Ravelli ACJM, van Montfrans GA** *et al.* Coronary heart disease after prenatal exposure to the Dutch famine, 1944–45. *Heart* 2000;**84**:595–8.

104. **Brown AS, van Os J, Driessens C, Hoek HW, Susser ES.** Further evidence of relation between prenatal famine and major affective disorder. *Am J Psychiat* 2000;**157**:190–5.

105. **Dodic M, Wintour EM, Whitworth JA, Coghlan JP.** Effect of steroid hormones on blood pressure. *Clin Exp Pharmacol Physiol* 1999;**26**:550–2.

106. **Gatford KL, Wintour EM, De Blasio MJ, Owens JA, Dodic M.** Differential timing for programming of glucose homoeostasis, sensitivity to insulin and blood pressure by *in utero* exposure to dexamethasone in sheep. *Clin Sci (Lond)* 2000;**98**:553–60.

107. **Kandel ER.** A new intellectual framework for psychiatry. *Am J Psychiat* 1998;**155**:457–69.

108. **Rose G.** Sick individuals and sick populations. *Int J Epidemiol* 1985;**14**:32–8.

109. **Hofer MA.** Hidden regulators in attachment, separation, and loss. *Monogr Soc Res Child Dev* 1994;**59**:192–207.

110. **Offord DR, Kraemer HC, Kazdin AE, Jensen PS, Harrington R, Gardner SJ.** Lowering the burden of suffering: Monitoring the benefits of clinical, targeted, and universal approaches. In Keating DP, Hertzman C, eds. *Developmental health and the wealth of nations: Social, biological, and educational dynamics.* New York: Guilford Press, 1999: 293–310.

*111. **Boyce WT, Frank E, Jensen PS, Kessler RC, Nelson CA, Steinberg L** *et al.* Social context in developmental psychopathology: recommendations from the MacArthur Network on Psychopathology and Development. *Dev Psychopathol* 1998;**10**:143–64.

112. **Keating DP.** Definition and selection of competencies from a human development perspective. In Organization for Economic Co-operation and Development, ed. *Additional DeSeCo expert opinions.* Paris: 2001:1–44.

113. **Dunn J.** *Are widening income inequalities making Canadians less healthy.* Ottawa: Health Determinants Partnership Making Connections Project, 2002.

114. **Kaplan GA, Pamuk ER, Lynch JW, Cohen RD, Balfour JL.** Inequality in income and mortality in the United States: analysis of mortality and potential pathways. *Br Med J* 1996;**312**:999–1003.

115. **Ross NA, Wolfson MC, Dunn JR, Berthelot JM, Kaplan GA, Lynch JW.** Relation between income inequality and mortality in Canada and in the United States: cross sectional assessment using census data and vital statistics. *Br Med J* 2000;**320**:898–902.

116. **Wilkinson RG.** *Unhealthy societies: the afflictions of inequality.* London: Routledge, 1996.

*117. **Lynch JW, Everson SA, Kaplan GA, Salonen R, Salonen JT.** Does low socioeconomic status potentiate the effects of heightened cardiovascular responses to stress on the progression of carotid atherosclerosis? *Am J Pub Health* 1998;**88**:389–94.

118. **Marmot M, Wilkinson RG.** Psychosocial and material pathways in the relation between income and health: A response to Lynch *et al.* *Br Med J* 2001;**322**:1233–6.

119. **Wagstaff A, van Doorslaer E.** Income inequality and health: what does the literature tell us? *Annu Rev Pub Health* 2000;**21**:543–67.

120. **Lynch JW, Davey Smith G, Kaplan GA, House JS.** Income inequality and mortality: importance to health of individual income, psychosocial environment, or material conditions. *Br Med J* 2000;**320**:1200–4.

121. Lynch J, Davey Smith G, Hillemeier M, Shaw M, Raghunathan T, Kaplan G. Income inequality, the psychosocial environment, and health: comparisons of wealthy nations. *Lancet* 2001;**358**:194–200.

122. Judge K. Income distribution and life expectancy: a critical appraisal. *Br Med J* 1995;**311**:1282–5 and discussion 1285–7.

123. Gravelle H. How much of the relation between population mortality and unequal distribution of income is a statistical artefact? *Br Med J* 1998;**316**:382–5.

124. Regalado M, Halfon N. Primary care services promoting optimal child development from birth to age 3 years: review of the literature. *Arch Pediatr Adolesc Med* 2001;**155**:1311–22.

125. McCain M, Mustard JF, Reference Group. *Early years study: reversing the real brain drain.* Toronto: Canadian Institute for Advanced Research, 1999.

126. Olds DL, Eckenrode J, Henderson CR, Kitzman H, Powers J, Cole R *et al.* Long-term effects of home visitation on maternal life course and child abuse and neglect: Fifteen-year follow-up of a randomized trial. *J Am Med Assoc* 1997;**278**:637–43.

127. Kitzman H, Olds DL, Henderson CR, Hanks C, Cole R, Tatelbaum R *et al.* Effect of prenatal and infancy home visitation by nurses on pregnancy outcomes, childhood injuries, and repeated childbearing. *J Am Med Assoc* 1997;**278**:644–52.

128. Hertzman C, Wiens M. Child development and long-term outcomes: A population health perspective and summary of successful interventions. *Soc Sci Med* 1996;**43**:1083–95.

129. Berrueta-Clement JR, Schweinhart LJ, Barnett WS, Epstein AS, Weikart DP. *Changed lives: the effects of the Perry Preschool Program on youths through age 19.* Ypsilanti, Michigan: High Scope Press, 1984.

130. Schweinhart L, Barnes H, Weikart D. *Significant benefits: the High/Scope Perry Preschool Study through age 27* (Report No. 10). Ypsilanti, Michigan: High Scope Educational Research Foundation, 1993.

131. Campbell F, Ramey C. Effects of early intervention on intellectual and academic achievement: a follow-up study of children from low-income families. *Child Dev* 1994;**65**:684–98.

132. Battistich V, Schaps E, Watson M, Solomon D. Prevention effects of the Child Development Project: early findings from an ongoing multisite demonstration trial. *J Adoles Res* 1996;**11**:12–35.

133. Spiker D, Ferguson J, Brooks-Gunn J. Enhancing maternal interactive behavior and child social competence in low birth weight, premature infants. *Child Dev* 1993;**64**:754–68.

134. McCormick MC, McCarton C, Brooks-Gunn J, Belt P, Gross RT. The Infant Health and Development Program: interim summary. *J Dev Behav Pediatr* 1998;**19**:359–70.

135. Grossman DC, Neckerman HJ, Koepsell TD, Liu P-Y, Asher KN, Beland K *et al.* Effectiveness of a violence prevention curriculum among children in elementary school: a randomized controlled trial. *J Am Med Assoc* 1997;**277**:1605–11.

136. Offord D, Jones MB. *Skill development: A community intervention program for the prevention of antisocial behaviour.* New York: Raven Press, 1983.

137. Reynolds AJ, Temple JA, Robertson DL, Mann EA. Long-term effects of an early childhood intervention on educational achievement and juvenile arrest: a 15-year follow-up of low-income children in public schools. *J Am Med Assoc* 2001;**285**:2339–46.

138. van der Gaag J. From child development to human development. In Young ME, ed. *From early child development to human development.* Washington, DC: The World Bank, 2002:63–78.

139. Young ME. *From early child development to human development.* Washington, DC: The World Bank, 2002.

140. Organization for Economic Co-operation and Development. *Starting strong: Early childhood education and care.* Paris, 2001.

141. **Putnam RD.** *Making democracy work: civic traditions in modern Italy.* Princeton: Princeton University Press, 1992.

142. **Kohen D, Hertzman C, Willms JD.** The importance of quality child care. In Willms JD, ed. *Vulnerable children: findings from Canada's National Longitudinal Survey of Children and Youth.* Edmonton: University of Alberta Press and Applied Research Branch, Human Resources Development Canada, 2002:261–76.

143. **Sampson RJ, Morenoff JD, Gannon-Rowley T.** Assessing 'neighbourhood effects': Social processes and new directions in research. *Annu Rev Sociol* 2002;**28**:443–78.

144. **Keating DP.** Social capital and developmental health: making the connection. *J Dev Behav Pediatr* 2000;**21**:50–2.

145. **Schorr LB.** *Common purpose: Strengthening families and neighborhoods to rebuild America.* New York: Anchor Books, 1997.

146. **Cleveland G, Krashinsky M.** *The benefits and costs of good child care: The economic rationale for public investment in young children—a policy study.* Toronto: University of Toronto, Childcare Resource and Research Unit, 1998.

147. **Rychen DS, Salganik LH.** *Defining and selecting key competencies.* Seattle: Hogrefe and Huber, 2001.

148. **Dudley L.** *The word and the sword.* Cambridge, Massachusetts: Basil Blackwell, 1991.

149. **Rohlen TP.** Social software for a learning society: Relating school and work. In Keating DP, Hertzman C, eds. *Developmental health and the wealth of nations: social, biological, and educational dynamics.* New York: Guilford Press, 1999:251–73.

150. **Rosenberg N, Birdzell LE.** *How the West grew rich: the economic transformation of the industrial world.* New York: Basic Books, 1986.

151. **Fogel RW.** *The fourth great awakening and the future of egalitarianism.* Chicago: University of Chicago Press, 2000.

152. **Keating DP.** The learning society: A human development agenda. In Keating DP, Hertzman C, eds. *Developmental health and the wealth of nations: social, biological, and educational dynamics.* New York: Guilford, 1999:237–50.

153. **Hall PA, Soskice DW.** *Varieties of capitalism: the institutional foundations of comparative advantage.* New York: Oxford University Press, 2001.

154. **Rawls J.** *A theory of justice.* Cambridge, Massachusetts: Belknap/Harvard University Press, 1971.

155. **Ruck MD, Keating DP, Abramovitch R, Koegl C.** Adolescents' and children's knowledge about rights: Some evidence for how young people view rights in their own lives. *J Adolesc* 1998;**21**:275–89.

156. **Ruck MD, Abramovitch R, Keating DP.** Children's and adolescents' understanding of rights: balancing nurturance and self-determination. *Child Dev* 1998;**69**:404–17.

157. **Champagne F, Meaney MJ.** Like mother, like daughter: evidence for non-genomic transmission of parental behavior and stress responsivity. *Prog Brain Res* 2001;**133**:287–302.

158. **DeMause L.** *The history of childhood.* New York: Psychohistory Press, 1974.

159. **Eliot G.** *Middlemarch.* Toronto, New York: Bantam Books, 1985.

Chapter 19

Conclusions

Yoav Ben-Shlomo and Diana Kuh

There is a growing body of evidence that life course exposures may play a role in the development of many of the adult chronic diseases that form the major public health problems in both developed and developing countries. Until recently most of the research on the early life origins of adult disease focused on intrauterine growth and development but there is growing evidence of the importance of postnatal growth and developmental trajectories in the development of adult disease risk. The relative influence of early as compared with later life factors is yet to be fully determined and is likely to differ by disease outcome and by time and place. Cumulative and interactive effects of exposures across the life course have both been described. The extent to which socioeconomic differentials in adult health and disease are explained by socially patterned exposures acting earlier in the life course is a growing and active area of research. Several emerging research themes are identified and include understanding heterogeneity between exposures and outcomes and going beyond simple temporal exposure associations to model lifetime trajectories of environmental exposures, behaviours, and physiological function with cause-specific outcomes. They also include elucidating the role of neurodevelopmental and genetic factors in early life and adult disease associations, understanding the embodiment of social phenomena through biological intermediaries, and the reciprocal role of biological capital in mediating social trajectories. Historical cohorts continue to provide important aetiological clues to the origins of adult disease. Prospective studies beginning at birth or in childhood are increasingly providing evidence, as they mature, about the importance of social and biological factors acting across the life course and can use more sophisticated measures of exposure as well as early pre-clinical manifestations of disease or functional status. Most of these longitudinal studies are in developed countries and there is a great need to collect data from developing countries so that consistency between exposure–disease associations can be examined in different contexts. Systematic reviews and meta-regression may help identify heterogeneity and the degree to which this is explained by temporal and geographical factors. A life course perspective encourages health service providers to place healthy development as well as disease management on their agenda and to offer longitudinal integration of services across the life course. Even where evidence on long-term health outcomes from high-quality intervention studies is limited, there are strong ethical and economic reasons for policy makers to consider social and behavioural interventions in childhood a priority. To be successful, policy must not only target high-risk groups but also tackle macro-level determinants that influence population health.

19.1 **Introduction**

The purpose of this book has been to review the scientific literature on possible factors acting at different stages of the life course, which, via biological or social processes, affect the development of chronic disease risk in individuals and populations. Most of the chapters have focused disproportionately on pre-adult exposures, as this is the area where there have been the most exciting epidemiological developments over the last few years.

The strong revival of a life course approach in epidemiology and public health in the last decade has been shaped by two influences. The work of David Barker and colleagues at the Medical Research Council Environmental Epidemiology Unit in Southampton, UK,[1] acted as a catalyst in reawakening epidemiologists to the importance of early life factors on adult chronic disease, establishing the concept of programming firmly within the domain of chronic disease epidemiology and revitalizing the historical cohort design. Their original focus on the fetal origins of adult disease has been recognized as too narrow and this frame of reference has recently been extended to include postnatal growth and development. The development of life course epidemiology was also influenced by the growing use made of a life course perspective in psychology, sociology, anthropology, and demography and the concurrent revival in interdisciplinary developmental science with its more recent focus on heterogeneity, discontinuity, and context-specific development (Chapter 2). The observations emanating from life course epidemiology have, in turn, attracted the attention of researchers in a wide number of disciplines. For example, from the beginning, infant mortality and birthweight were seen as mere proxy measures for more complex physiological phenomena. The clear demonstration of how much more there is to discover about the determinants of fetal and infant growth and development acted as an important trigger for work by experimental physiologists, embryologists, neonatologists, and others. Similarly, measures of socio-economic position in childhood or adulthood are crude markers of underlying biological and social processes. Understanding how social factors across the life course are embodied physiologically requires an interdisciplinary research effort, yet to be fully realized.

19.2 **What can we conclude?**

The contributors to this book demonstrated that there is evidence that early life factors affect the subsequent development of cardiovascular diseases, diabetes, hypertension and obesity, respiratory and allergic diseases, some cancers such as breast and testicular cancer, neuropsychiatric disorders, and disorders associated with musculoskeletal ageing. This is not to deny the importance of adult risk factors; indeed, Whincup and colleagues conclude (in Chapter 9) that adult rather than fetal factors are more important in the development of hypertension. What is clear is that factors acting independently, cumulatively, or interactively throughout the life course need to be considered; Strachan and Sheikh's chapter on respiratory diseases (Chapter 10) remains an eloquent expression of such an approach.

The idea that early life may determine one's future health trajectory is not new, yet until the 1990s chronic disease epidemiology, particularly cardiovascular epidemiology, followed a logical but narrow path that chose to ignore these ideas (Chapter 2). The inclusion of early life factors enriches our understanding of the development of adult chronic disease both because of the additional independent risk they may confer and because of the *interactive* nature of factors acting at different stages of the life course. For example, the evidence that overweight adults with the lowest birthweight have the highest risk of hypertension or diabetes helps further to explain the variation that occurs in the relationship between adult exposure and outcome and to target the most at-risk group.

While the broad direction of change in early life circumstances this century is congruent with declining all-cause adult mortality rates, early life factors seem to play a less important role than adult factors in accounting for trends in cardiorespiratory outcomes (see Chapters 4, 9, and 10); although, as Davey Smith and Lynch (Chapter 4) and dos Santos Silva (Chapter 12) point out, the interaction of exposures at different points of the life course renders the explanation of trends rather problematic. Trends in proximal risk factors such as cigarette smoking, blood pressure, cholesterol, and insulin resistance provide a better explanation than trends in early life factors for the increasing social class differentials in coronary heart disease (CHD). Migrant studies also support the relative importance of the adult environment over early life for CHD and blood pressure (Chapter 6). The cohort-related rise and fall in chronic obstructive pulmonary diseases is clearly related to the uptake of cigarette smoking (Chapter 10). Several authors concur in concluding that, despite evidence for early life factors, control of obesity and the cessation of smoking are still the most effective means of reducing individual and population chronic disease risk. However, for some health behaviours, intervening in adult life may be less effective than interventions in childhood or adolescence before these behaviours become more engrained (Chapters 8 and 9).

19.3 Emerging and common themes in life course research

Several common themes have emerged across different contributors and topics, which we believe are particularly relevant to any future life course research agenda. Not all of these ideas are new or specific to life course epidemiology. However, they lie at the heart of developing more elaborate life course models. Our ability to apply more powerful and novel methodological and analytical techniques will enable us to advance our understanding further than previous generations of researchers.

19.3.1 The importance of heterogeneity

Epidemiologists all too often shudder at the inconsistencies observed between exposure and disease when systematically comparing observational studies. Such heterogeneity is usually assigned to random variation, variations in study design, or differences in adjustment for confounding. Rarely do they consider that such heterogeneity may be real and informative as highlighted by Davey Smith and Lynch (Chapter 4). As they point out, understanding the 'heterogeneity of associations across outcomes, place, and time' should be 'the departure point for a more complete understanding of socioeconomic health differentials … '. For example, the stronger association between childhood social conditions, discordant secular patterns of risk, and ethnic differences in risk for haemorrhagic as compared to ischaemic stroke, suggest that risk factors acting in early life are relatively more important for the former than latter disease (Chapters 3 and 4).

Heterogeneity of exposure associations even within the same disease may highlight important biological clues as well as have policy relevance. For example, the evidence linking birthweight with breast cancer consistently shows positive associations with premenopausal disease and little if any association with postmenopausal breast cancer (see Chapter 11). This suggests that the different phenotypic expressions of this disease, in this case relating to age at presentation, are linked to different biological pathways where genetic and environmental factors have different degrees of importance.

Those whose focus has been the fetal origins of adult disease also increasingly acknowledge the heterogeneity of pathways linking early life exposures to later outcomes. For example, a multiplicity of triggers and intermediate mechanisms are assumed to be involved in the creation of the survival phenotype that is associated with the programming of insulin resistance and other components of the metabolic syndrome.[2,3]

19.3.2 Going beyond repeat measures to understand trajectories

Unless historical records are extensive (for example, in the Helsinki cohorts[4,5]), only prospective longitudinal studies collect sufficient repeat measures to enable researchers to model an individual's trajectory rather than simply treating such measures as a series of cross-sectional observations. Such observations have generally been limited to developmental indices such as height or weight, but may also include other exposures or outcomes such as blood pressure,[6] lung function, serum cholesterol, or adult weight gain.[7] It is likely that using more complex data on growth trajectories will help better identify key variables, the potential timing of key exposures, and high-risk groups. For example, whilst adult height shows little association with systolic blood pressure, early puberty, as indicated by age at peak height velocity, is positively associated with systolic blood pressure.[8] In this case children entering puberty at different ages may reach a similar final height, but have different adult blood pressures because of the timing of puberty and its hormonal correlates.[9]

The apparent paradox that both early menarche and tall adult stature, usually associated with later menarche, are both associated with increased breast cancer risk (Chapter 11) highlights the role of two different growth trajectories with their own probably different biological pathways for cancer risk.[10] To mask such heterogeneity by simply comparing average patterns of growth will result in a failure to understand the complex multifactorial nature of disease aetiology.

With respect to adult obesity, several critical or sensitive periods have been identified—prenatal, infancy, time of the adiposity rebound, and adolescence (see Chapter 8). The trajectory that each individual follows during these four periods may leave an imprint on later body size.

Finally, it is important to appreciate that the trajectory of some risk factors may be less important in terms of intervention than for aetiology. As Whincup and colleagues remark (Chapter 9), earlier weight (in childhood or adult life) is not an independent predictor of blood pressure after adjusting for current weight. In addition, weight loss in adulthood shows that its effects on blood pressure are reversible and not permanent. However, it is unclear whether the success in reducing adult weight or the degree of blood pressure decline subsequent to weight loss is dependent on the duration of obesity across the life course.

19.3.3 The role of accelerated postnatal weight and height gain

One area of considerable interest is the growth trajectories of infants who exhibit centile crossing in the immediate postnatal period usually referred to as catch-up or catch-down growth. One of the most striking epidemiological findings to emerge in the last few years is that the general finding that those most at risk of developing a number of chronic conditions have a pattern of growth characterized by small body size at birth followed by rapid postnatal weight gain. The precise nature of postnatal trajectories varies across outcomes. For CHD in the Helsinki II cohort, centile crossing in height and weight was not observed in the initial postnatal year but only in later childhood and different patterns were seen for boys and girls (Chapter 3). It is important to iden-tify subgroups with different growth trajectories at heightened risk of later disease who may be obscured by a comparison of average growth trajectories. For example, the postnatal trajectory associated with type 2 diabetes may be modified by birth size.[11] Both children who are thin and children who are obese may both have a higher risk of later diabetes (Chapter 7) or CHD (Chapter 3).

The interpretation of these data is an active area of debate. Does allowance for post-natal weight or height change better characterize those small babies exposed to various prenatal exposures with a long-term effect on health? This would locate the underlying mechanism in the prenatal period. Alternatively, postnatal growth may identify a different mechanism, such as the thrifty phenotype, that is dependent upon environ-mental factors operating during both fetal and postnatal periods. The role of postnatal growth may also explain the discordant findings in long-term outcomes between those exposed to the Dutch famine and the Leningrad famine (Chapter 7). In the latter pop-ulation, the prolonged duration of the famine may have modified any prenatal effects so that the survivors did not show any increased risk. Studying the genetic and envi-ronmental factors in the prenatal and postnatal periods that distinguish between these different growth trajectories should provide further clues to aetiology.

19.3.4 Neurodevelopment and adult function and disease

Early biological and social risk factors may impair childhood neurodevelopment. There is growing evidence, for example, that early social experiences can have lasting effects on stress reactivity in children and that this may mediate the link between early adversity and later poor health (Chapter 18). Other evidence points to associations between subtle deficits in thyroid hormone exposure prenatally or in the early postnatal period and subsequent neurodevelopmental deficits in childhood (Chapter 14). The extent to which these childhood deficits continue into adulthood with possible implications for neuropsychiatric outcomes in later life forms a dynamic research agenda (Chapter 14). There may also be implications for adult physical function and chronic disease. Observed relationships between cognitive impairment or dementia and cardiovascular disease, lung function, grip strength, and functional decline in adult life[12–17] are usually attributed to common adult risk factors and ageing processes,[15] but they may also reflect common developmental processes and early risk factors.

One way of investigating the link between neurodevelopment and adult physical function and chronic disease is to study childhood cognitive ability and this information is available in a number of cohort studies. Early cognitive ability may provide a window on brain development, for example, acting as an indicator of the efficiency of information processing in the central nervous system.[18] Numerous neuroendocrine, neuroanatomical, and neurochemical systems are involved in cognitive function and in the control of physical organ systems, some of which may have their origins in early life. There is growing evidence of an association between childhood cognitive ability and longevity.[18–21] As yet, it is unclear whether the association is accounted for primarily by neurodevelopmental pathways or social pathways given that early cognitive ability is also associated with safer adult environments and healthy adult behaviours.[18,20] Neurodevelopmental deficits may also mediate the effects of early poverty and adversity on adult socioeconomic outcomes (Chapter 16) with implications for long-term health. An emerging area of life course research is extending these studies of childhood cognitive ability and mortality to disease-specific outcomes[21] and adult function.[22,23]

19.3.5 Determining biological mechanisms

The advocates of the programming hypothesis have not hesitated to speculate on the potential biological mechanisms that may account for the link between proxy measures of fetal development and later disease. Inevitably, the theoretical framework underpinning the fetal origins hypothesis has been adapted, as evidence has emerged to support some potential mechanisms over others. The original framework highlighted how long-term effects of fetal undernutrition might vary depending on the trimester of pregnancy.[24] This is being replaced with a more complex framework that recognizes the importance of the maternal and fetal genotype, the maternal prenatal and perinatal environment, the maternal prepregnancy nutritional status, metabolism, and physiology, the hormonal, metabolic, and circulatory milieu, and the infant's postnatal environment (Chapter 15). Such mechanisms may not only influence an individual's own disease risk but may also explain intergenerational patterns. The observation that relatively small perturbations of the intrauterine environment could affect oocyte development is a potential mechanism for long-term consequences across generations.[25] In Chapter 15, Perry and Lumey succinctly observe that we are moving away from a simple critical model based on nutritional deficits *in utero* towards a broader life course model of programming involving interactions between a range of early life factors acting at different levels.

The biological mechanisms put forward to explain programming have drawn heavily on animal research and, by indicating its possible relevance for the development of chronic disease in humans, have helped to rebuild a valuable bridge between scientific disciplines. In the last 5 years there has been an enormous growth of animal studies to test programming hypotheses, as evidenced by the abstracts to the Second Congress on Fetal Origins of Adult Disease (see *Pediatric Research* 2003; **53**(2)). The generalizability of findings from animal to human populations remains an area of active scientific debate.[26]

Linking physiological parameters such as growth with metabolic, endocrine, or cellular events is perhaps less daunting than understanding the biobehavioural consequences of social phenomena such as social hierarchies[27] or early stress (Chapter 18). Progress has been made in understanding the role of the central nervous system, the neuro-endocrine system, and the neuroimmune system.[28–30] Understanding these biological mechanisms may elucidate potential interactions between earlier and later exposures.[31]

19.3.6 Genetic and early environmental effects on adult disease

The ability of genetic explanations to account for the observed associations between early life factors and adult disease has been a growth area of research in recent years. The degree to which fetal programming or growth trajectories in general may reflect genetic rather than environmental factors still remains unclear. Genetic influences on birthweight variability may have been previously underestimated (Chapter 7). A single twin study examining the birthweight CHD association failed to find an association amongst monozygotic twins, consistent with a genetic explanation (Chapter 3). However, the centagenerian debate over the relative importance of nature or nurture is as futile in this area of research as in others.[32] The weaker but consistent association between paternal CHD risk and offspring birthweight supports a genetic role for the birthweight and CHD association but does not exclude the additional importance of either maternal programming or some other epigenetic phenomenon triggered by a perinatal exposure (Chapter 3). Similarly, neonatal bone mass is associated with both paternal and maternal birthweight, through a possible genetic mechanism, but is also clearly influenced by maternal smoking and nutritional status in pregnancy (Chapter 13). Both genetic and programming models, particularly those that test interactions between the two, are likely to be useful in understanding these observed epidemiological associations.

19.3.7 Duration and timing of exposures

Epidemiologists are familiar with and consider the importance of exposure duration. This is usually tested for by examining a dose–response relationship. For example, risk of lung cancer is strongly associated with increasing smoking pack years.[33,34] Better characterization of duration of exposure leads to higher estimates of the contribution of the classic adult risk factors for CHD.[35] The same is true for the effects of cumulative socioeconomic deprivation on poor self-reported health (Chapter 16). It is far harder to examine the specific effects of timing, to distinguish the presence or absence of critical or sensitive periods. In contrast to self-rated health, where cumulative disadvantage is important irrespective of its timing, the risk of stomach cancer and haemorrhagic stroke may be more sensitive to adverse social conditions in early than in adult life (Chapter 4). Certain developmental phases may be particularly sensitive to environmental exposures due to the rapid development of tissue and these are not necessarily limited to the first few years of life. For example, a recent study suggested that smoking increased the risk of premenopausal breast cancer only if it was within 5 years of onset of menarche.[36]

19.3.8 The development of unequal health

The extent to which socioeconomic differentials in adult health and disease are explained by socially patterned exposures acting earlier in the life course has become a dynamic and growing area of life course epidemiology, particularly in relation to cardiovascular disease. A growing number of studies have shown that indicators of the childhood socioeconomic environment are associated with a range of measures of adult health (Chapters 4 and 16). Generally these effects are independent of the later socioeconomic environment and do not explain the adult socioeconomic differentials. This suggests that factors acting across the life course impact on later health and that better characterization of lifetime socioeconomic circumstances provides evidence that the differential is larger than observed from studies limited to a single life stage.[37,38] An obvious question is whether early life exposures can explain the child or adult socioeconomic differentials in adult disease risk but as Kuh and colleagues point out in Chapter 16 there are few studies that have both detailed biological and social measures across the life course. Davey Smith and Lynch (Chapter 4) explore to what degree adult differentials in cardiovascular disease risk can be explained by socioeconomic patterning of adult risk factors. Whilst arguing that much of the socioeconomic gradient in cardiovascular disease can be explained by the social patterning of proximal adult risk factors, they remain open minded as to how much of the latter effect is itself determined by childhood socioeconomic status. As childhood socioeconomic position is generally associated with cardiovascular disease independently of adult socioeconomic position, it remains unclear whether this effect is also abolished after adjustment for adult risk factors. It is also unclear whether the same pattern holds for other diseases. Both childhood and adult factors appear to be important for explaining socioeconomic differentials in adult psychological distress and self-reported morbidity in the 1958 cohort.[39,40] Clarifying the ways in which socially patterned early environmental exposures leave enduring imprints on physical growth or other aspects of health capital or on the development of personal capital and the extent to which these account for socioeconomic differentials in adult physiological function, behaviour, and specific diseases will continue to be a challenging area of life course research.

19.3.9 Life course influences on biological and personal capital

Most of the chapters in this book have focused on disease end-points but several highlight the value of a life course approach for other outcomes of function and behaviour. Such outcomes present particular challenges with assessing the temporal sequence for any hypothesized causal pathway. For example, the various models proposed in Chapter 10 highlight the difficulty in disentangling whether an exposure such as childhood infection results in poor lung function or vice versa so that poor lung function now acts as an exposure and increases the risk of childhood infection. Functional measures such as muscle strength, cognitive function, and bone density of relevance for successful ageing are particularly interesting from a life course perspective. Performance at any one time will be the outcome of the balance between mechanisms inducing damage or loss of function and those inducing repair, compensation, and growth (Chapter 13). Early life factors may contribute to peak levels of performance through developmental pathways as well as influence age related decline.[41] Adult exposures in mid-life can only effect the latter pathway but may be as or more important than early exposures.

Social scientists have frequently studied the determinants of personal capital (such as social and cognitive skills, self esteem, and coping strategies) or adult social circumstances in relation to parental education, early social conditions, education and employment history, and other life course transitions (Chapter 16). The role of an individual's personal capital in shaping the subsequent environment is increasingly acknowledged. Rarely, however, is the role of biological capital as exposures for social trajectories examined. This reciprocity between biological and personal capital and the environment is important if we are to synthezise both sociobiological as well as biosocial pathways across the life course.[41] Examples of such research include examining the mediating role of the child's physical and cognitive development in explaining the effect of childhood poverty on adult economic outcomes and the role of overweight and obesity in predicting a women's social and economic trajectory (Chapter 16).

19.4 Methodological challenges: study designs

19.4.1 Further use of life course and historical cohorts

The research on prenatal and postnatal growth in relation to hard chronic disease endpoints has been limited to a few cohorts from developed countries. There is a need to replicate these findings by assembling other cohorts from different populations living under different conditions. In particular, as highlighted in Chapter 3, few studies using such clinical end-points are available for developing countries. These would provide a further test of the consistency of the research findings and, where possible, disentangle the usual confounding nature between early and later life exposures.[42]

Prospective longitudinal studies beginning at birth[43–47] or in childhood[48–52] have been able to fill some of the gaps that are missing in the life course of historical cohorts. These studies can more readily test hypothesized 'chains of risk' by examining the sequence of events and assess whether later exposures are a direct consequence of earlier events or simply related through a common third factor (Chapter 8). While some are still relatively 'immature' in terms of the age of their participants, others have already transformed into studies of ageing, linking mid-life morbidity,[53,54] function,[6,55] disease,[10,56] and mortality[37] to social and biological factors across the life course. These studies provide a rich source of material for testing new hypotheses at different stages of the life course. More complex models that deal correctly with missing and hierarchical data are needed to study repeat exposures and outcomes and are becoming essential tools for the analysis of studies of the life course.

Other cohorts with better indicators of maternal characteristics such as prepregnancy nutritional status or aspects of metabolism and physiology during pregnancy, such as glucose tolerance, blood pressure, and preeclampsia provide greater insights into the underlying biological mechanisms behind programming offspring's future health and disease risk (Chapters 7, 11, and 15).

More detailed clinical outcomes of children and adults in cohort studies are enhancing our understanding of the underlying biological mechanisms. For example, one study, described in Chapter 7, has already shown that thinness at birth predicts defects in muscle fuel utilization. New birth cohorts also provide the opportunity for better measures of early life exposures. For example, the importance of abnormal placental development for fetal nutrition and growth can be examined with modern ultrasound techniques.[57] Maternal measures of insulin-like growth factors may also help differentiate inappropriately small babies from those who should be at the lower end of the birthweight distribution. In childhood, measurement of early precursors of atherosclerosis, such as endothelial dysfunction,[14] currently being undertaken in the Avon Longitudinal Study of Parents and Children (ALSPAC) birth cohort (www.alspac.bristol.ac.uk) will enable researchers to detect subclinical abnormalities at a younger age, when confounding by later adult factors may be unimportant. This same group of researchers are using dual X-ray absorptiometry (DEXA) scans rather than body mass index, which is acknowledged to be a poor measure of obesity in childhood, so that they can determine life course influences on both fat and lean mass.

The ability to examine tracking of biological measures is useful in determining not only the timing of an effect related to an exposure but also its reversibility by later life influences. For example, children in the upper decile of the blood pressure distribution may shift downwards because of alterations in either diet or weight.

19.4.2 Less conventional study designs

Studies on twins, half-siblings, adoptees, and genetically admixed populations with similar environmental exposures will help disentangle the relative contribution of genetic and environmental factors (Chapters 3 and 7). These designs have a long history within genetic epidemiology but they have only been recently applied to examine the association between birth size and disease outcome (Chapter 3). Studies of sibling pairs discordant for birthweight can help to tease out the relative importance of pregnancy specific characteristics and fixed maternal characteristics that underlie biological programming.[58] Intergenerational studies have been used to link birthweight to parental disease risk. As uterine programming can only be influenced by maternal factors, associations between offspring birthweight and paternal cardiovascular disease or diabetes risk support the role of paternal genes either through conventional Mendelian inheritance or paternal imprinting (Chapter 3). Studies of parent–offspring trios can examine whether there are stronger associations between either parent with their child and directly test maternal, paternal, and offspring genotypes. Another novel approach is to examine the non-diabetic offspring of mothers with type 1 diabetes (exposed) as compared to similar offspring whose fathers had type 1 diabetes (control participants). In both cases the offspring would have a greater genetic predisposition for diabetes in later life but the observation that impaired glucose tolerance and impaired insulin secretion was greater for exposed participants suggests that an intrauterine mechanism is more likely to explain these observations.[59]

19.4.3 Intervention studies

Ultimately, the clearest evidence regarding the causality, reversibility, and public health importance of early life factors will come from studies that first test the effectiveness of interventions to modify the pattern of human fetal growth and then follow up whether these interventions have the expected effect on measures of postnatal growth and development and markers of disease risk. Few studies exist that meet these criteria, though examples have been published in relation to diet and calcium intake during pregnancy[60,61] and postnatal nutrition.[62]

As well as randomized controlled trials, two natural experiments of extreme dietary deprivation during the Second World War, with marked effects on fetal development, have also been discussed (Chapters 3, 7, and 8). The interpretation of all these studies is difficult as there is frequently no opportunity to replicate their results, the interventions are idiosyncratic or extreme, and the study populations may not be generalizable to the general population. However, despite these limitations, they may provide the most powerful evidence as regards exposure timing, biological pathways, and potential mechanisms.

One new and particularly promising approach is to use Mendelian randomization as an ethically acceptable alternative in large-scale population-based cohorts.[63] Mendelian randomization makes use of the observation that a child's genotype is a function of the distribution of polymorphisms across both alleles inherited from their parents. This is unlikely to be confounded by the usual environmental exposures and hence is equivalent to a randomized controlled trial where genotype is allocated at random depending on prior parental genotypes. If the genotype is of known functional importance equivalent to an environmental exposure, then the presence of none, one, or two such alleles will confer a lifelong increased exposure to such a risk factor.

19.4.4 The role of meta-analyses

Systematic reviews and meta-analysis have had a major impact on clinical evidence for intervention studies. Meta-analysis of observational datasets remains more controversial especially in relation to the validity of any 'pooled estimate'.[64] A growing number of meta-analyses are now being published, synthesizing the ever-expanding number of studies that have examined associations between early life exposures and later disease or risk factors.[65–67] Such reviews are useful as they are less likely to present biased or selective results and have far greater power to examine potential subgroups or interactions.[68] More importantly they have the ability to explicitly test for heterogeneity of effect estimates across studies using meta-regression. In this way they can examine whether time period or geographical location, that is, developed or developing world countries, alter the association between exposure and outcome hence embedding exposure within its relative social and temporal context.

19.5 Policy implications

If early life factors affect later disease risk, either through programming or other mechanisms, there are implications for current preventive health policies. As yet, there has been relatively little discussion of what these might be. Both the English and Scottish Departments of Health have long recognized the potential importance of programming for policy[69,70] but fall short of any specific recommendations. Similarly, other UK Government reports acknowledge the importance for social inequalities in health of factors of a life course approach to aetiology.[71,72] For example, the working group on variations in health explicitly included biological programming as well as 'cumulative exposure to social advantage or disadvantage, and variation in behaviours, over the lifespan' (p. 18).[71]

In the ideal world policy makers would wait for the results of intervention trials before recommending a course of action to promote population health. However, putting aside the difficulties in undertaking such studies, the long time period before results become available force policy makers to consider action based on weaker or other circumstantial evidence. Strong adverse secular trends in risk factors such as childhood or adult obesity that have interactive effects with early life exposures in the development of disease risk prompt action before we necessarily have a full understanding of underlying processes. Several of our contributors have highlighted potential areas for intervention. First, we should not forget the importance of trying to reduce conventional adult risk factors such as smoking, lack of physical activity, high blood pressure, obesity, and raised cholesterol.[73] However, it is important to appreciate that health promotion approaches used in developed countries may simply be inapplicable in other contexts.[74]

A focus on primary prevention in adulthood has been highlighted by a recent suggestion that all adults aged over 55 years should receive a combination drug ('polypill') to lower blood pressure, cholesterol, and homocysteine and to improve platelet function, which could potentially reduce cardiovascular disease by 80% and add 11 years of life from an ischaemic heart disease event or stroke.[75] However, even assuming that the relative benefits are the same regardless of an individual's life history, absolute risks for cardiovascular disease will still be greater for those who have experienced cumulative life course disadvantage. Such a 'magic bullet' may be used inappropriately to avoid improving adverse early life circumstances despite the ethical and economic arguments for such an approach (Chapter 18).

Similarly, a life course approach would caution against 'magic bullet' policies based on biological programming. In Chapter 17, Joseph and Kramer concluded that intervening to improve fetal growth based solely on the programming hypothesis could not be justified, even if the reported associations are assumed to be causal. They argue that interventions designed to improve fetal and infant growth would lead to only marginal reductions in the occurrence of CHD and may have other adverse effects. However, the need to reduce fetal exposure to maternal diabetes, through better detection and management of gestational diabetes (discussed in Chapters 7 and 15), is one area that may be important and achievable, at least in developed world countries. The issue of postnatal catch-up growth remains contentious particularly within a developing world context where short-term benefits may outweigh any long-term harm. There is less controversy over the importance of controlling obesity in childhood as noted by Gillman (Chapter 8) and Forouhi and colleagues (Chapter 7). Whether strategies to prevent or reduce obesity in childhood are more cost effective at this stage of life than in later life remains unclear.

Health prevention based on a life course approach to adult health and disease would target infants, children, and adults. This may require a major reconfiguration of current health delivery structures, one that emphasizes the longitudinal integration of services over time, not just their integration at a particular life stage.[76,77] Current health monitoring is mainly based on measuring disease or risk factor outcomes rather than developmental health trajectories. Managed health care, which integrates primary, secondary, and tertiary care, will need to consider a longitudinal service with fiscal incentives to promote the development as well as the maintenance of long-term health.

Boyce and Keating (Chapter 18) make cogent and forceful arguments that investment in childhood is a key stage for intervention. Their evidence stems from preschool, school, and community sociobehavioural interventions with developmental and social rather than health outcomes. To support their sound ethical and economic justification for childhood interventions, they provide supportive biological data that such interventions may have important influences on neural and endocrine development, with long-term implications for adult health and chronic disease. The accompanying evidence from other contributors also highlights the relative importance of adverse childhood circumstance for a number of health outcomes. As well as targeting high-risk groups, discussion also focuses on the important issue of macro-level upstream interventions that influence the whole population, through income redistribution.

Besides childhood interventions, a life course approach alerts us to the need to identify opportunities to break adverse social and biological chains of risk at other life stages. Particularly during key life transitions, for example, from late adolescence to early adulthood, we need to provide not just safety nets but springboards[78] to alter life course trajectories with benefits for subsequent health.

Tackling health inequalities through a life course approach (Chapter 4) may also be an attractive option to social policy makers. Graham, in her case study, argues that different welfare systems have various strategies to tackle social disparities in living standards across the life course.[79] In particular, taxation, cash benefits, and welfare services can have major beneficial effects on reducing the proportion of households with children below 50% of average income.

Given the interdisciplinary nature of life course research, it is unsurprising that policy initiatives must at least straddle health promotion, educational, occupational, and fiscal domains. This need for 'joined-up thinking' as well as the long time frame for measuring success is unattractive to politicians unless the growing research base on early life determinants is used as part of a wider social problem.[80] It is almost a hundred years since the physical condition of children become a social problem and resulted in what were considered to be radical social reforms for mothers, infants, and children.[81–83] It is 50 years since Bowlby's work helped to create the conditions under which the emotional health of children came to be a social problem and led to a major change of direction in welfare services.[84,85] Both these developments occurred because the time was ripe politically for change, not least because they followed periods of considerable social upheaval. Today anxiety is growing again about the state of children in a number of countries (see Chapter 18 and References 86 and 87).

19.6 The future of a life course approach to chronic disease epidemiology

Interest in programming and early life factors in the development of chronic disease arose from a dissatisfaction with the conventional adult lifestyle model. This model, developed during the postwar period, forms part of what Susser[88] calls 'black box' epidemiology or conventional risk factor epidemiology; the main purpose is to relate individual exposure and outcome in statistical models with little or no attention to the underlying biological mechanisms or the wider social context. Some critics of this approach have advocated the need for further scientific reductionism, '... a purpose-built chain of necessary causes—with each link of evidence well tested, and cemented to its neighbours by bonds of strong inference' (p. 106).[89] Other critics have pointed to the current neglect of socioeconomic factors and the population perspective and called for an 'eco-social' model, which conceptualizes the 'determinants of disease distribution as economic and social relationships forged by a society's political and economic structure'.[90] Susser and Susser have suggested that a synthesis of both macro and micro levels of analysis is required, replacing the 'black box' with 'chinese boxes' where one box sits within another and hence integrates both 'causal pathways at the societal level ... with pathogenesis and causality at the molecular level'.[88]

We have advocated in this book a life course approach to chronic disease aetiology that studies the interaction of social and biological processes that have long-term effects on disease risk. These chains of risk may arise from programming at critical periods during gestation and infancy or accumulate more incrementally throughout life. A life course approach responds to the critics of 'black box' epidemiology because it incorporates various different spatial levels, from the molecular to the global, thereby weaving both longitudinal as well as hierarchical influences on health.[41,91] It argues that to understand the pattern of current exposures and their impact on adult chronic disease requires knowledge of how past events have shaped the risk of subsequent exposure, the responsiveness of physiological systems, and behavioural patterns.

A life course approach to chronic disease aetiology was in its infancy when we published the first edition of this book. Healthy growth and development during childhood and adolescence have given this dynamic field a strong base on which to build further research. It is insufficient to glibly state that all health and social outcomes are due to life course influences. This is analogous to stating that all health is a function of genetic and environmental exposures. Whilst factually correct, it does not further our understanding of aetiology or help policy formulation. We note, even amongst our contributors, dissent over the relative importance of early life or contemporary circumstances on adult obesity (see Chapters 7 and 8). Further epidemiological evidence will come from imaginative historical cohort studies, maturing longitudinal studies, newer cohorts using more sophisticated exposure and outcome measures, special study designs, developments in genomics and statistical methods, and further elaboration of testable life course models. These developments will lead to greater understanding of, and a wider interest in, the ways that experiences throughout the life course affect the development of many of the adult chronic diseases that are prevalent in developed countries and which are becoming increasingly prevalent in the developing world.

References

Those marked with an asterisk are especially recommended for further reading.

*1 Barker DJP. *Mothers, babies and health in later life*. Edinburgh: Churchill Livingstone, 1998.

2 Gluckman P. The early origins of health and disease—a biomedical and clinical perspective on an epidemiological hypothesis. *Pediatr Res* 2003;**53**:1A.

3 Barker DJP. Fetal origins: biological basis and size of effects. *Pediatr Res* 2003;**53**:1A.

4 Cooper C, Eriksson JG, Forsen T, Osmond C, Tuomilehto J, Barker DJP. Maternal height, childhood growth and risk of hip fracture in later life: a longitudinal study. *Osteoporosis Int* 2001;**12**:623–9.

*5 Eriksson JG, Forsen T, Tuomilehto J, Osmond C, Barker DJP. Early growth and coronary heart disease in later life: longitudinal study. *Br Med J* 2001;**322**:949–53.

*6 Hardy R, Kuh D, Langenberg C, Wadsworth MEJ. Birth weight, childhood social class and change in adult blood pressure in the 1946 British birth cohort. *Lancet* 2003;**362**:1178–83.

7 Hardy R, Wadsworth MEJ, Kuh D. The influence of childhood weight and socioeconomic status on change in adult body mass index in a British national birth cohort. *Int J Obesity* 2000;**24**:1–10.

8 Sandhu J, Ben-Shlomo Y, Cole TJ, Davey Smith G. Life course influence of anthropometry on components of insulin resistance. *Am J Epidemiol* 2003;**157(suppl. 11)**:528.

9 Lever AF, Harrap SB. Essential hypertension: a disorder of growth with origins in childhood? *J Hypertens* 1992;**10**:101–20.

10 De Stavola BL, dos Santos Silva I, McCormack V, Hardy R, Kuh D, Wadsworth M. Childhood growth and breast cancer. *Am J Epidemiol* (in press).

11 Eriksson JG, Forsen T, Tuomilehto J, Osmond C, Barker DJP. Early adiposity rebound in childhood and risk of Type 2 diabetes in adult life. *Diabetologia* 2003;**46**:190–4.

12 Albert MS, Jones K, Savage CR, Berkman L, Seeman T, Blazer D *et al*. Predictors of cognitive change in older persons: MacArthur Studies of Successful Aging. *Psychol Aging* 1995;**10**:578–89.

13 Schaub RT, Munzberg H, Borchelt M, Nieczaj R, Hillen T, Reischies FM *et al*. Ventilatory capacity and risk for dementia. *J Gerontol* 2000;**55A**:M677–83.

14 Vermeer SE, Prins ND, den Heijer T, Hofman A, Koudstaal PJ, Breteler MMB. Silent infarcts and the risk of dementia and cognitive decline. *N Engl J Med* 2003;**348**:1215–22.

15 Christensen H, Mackinnon AJ, Korten A, Jorm AF. The "Common Cause Hypothesis" of cognitive aging: evidence for not only a common factor but also specific associations of age with vision and grip strength in a cross-sectional analysis. *Psychol Aging* 2001;**16**:588–99.

16 Nourhashémi F, Andrieu S, Gillette-Guyonnet S, Reynish E, Albarède J-L, Grandjean H *et al*. Is there a relationship between fat-free soft tissue mass and low cognitive function? Results from a study of 7,105 women. *J Am Geriatrics Assoc* 2002;**50**:1796–801.

17 Black SA, Rush RD. Cognitive and functional decline in adults aged 75 and older. *J Am Geriatrics Assoc* 2002;**50**:1978–86.

*18 Whalley LJ, Deary IJ. Longitudinal cohort study of childhood IQ and survival up to age 76. *Br Med J* 2001;**322**:1–5.

19 Batty GD, Clark H, Morton SMB, Campbell D, MacIntyre S, Hall M *et al*. Intelligence in childhood and mortality, migration, questionnaire response rate, and self-reported morbidity and risk factor levels in adulthood—preliminary findings from the Aberdeen 'Children of the 1950s' study. *J Epidemiol Commun Health* 2002;**56(suppl 2)**:A1.

20 Kuh D, Richards M, Hardy R, Butterworth S, Wadsworth MEJ. Childhood cognitive function and deaths up until middle age. *Int J Epidemiol* (in press).

21 Hart CL, Taylor MD, Davey Smith G, Whalley IJ, Starr JM, Hole DJ *et al*. Childhood IQ, social class, deprivation and their relationships with mortality and morbidity risk in later life: prospective observational study linking the Scottish Mental Survey 1932 and the Midspan studies. *Psychosomatic Med* 2003;**65**:877–83.

22 Starr JM, Deary IJ, Lemmon H, Whalley LJ. Mental ability age 11 years and health status age 77 years. *Age Ageing* 2000;**29**:523–8.

23 Richards M, Kuh DL, Hardy R, Wadsworth MEJ. Lifetime cognitive function and timing of natural menopause. *Neurology* 1999;**53**:308–14.

24 Barker DJP. *Mothers, babies, and disease in later life.* London: British Medical Journal Publishing Group, 1994.

25 Eppig J. Oocyte origin of adult disease. *Pediatr Res* 2003;**53**:1A.

*26 Harding JE. The nutritional basis of the fetal origins of adult disease. *Int J Epidemiol* 2001;**30**:15–23.

27 Sapolsky RM. *Stress, the ageing brain and the mechanism of neuron death.* Cambridge, Massachusetts: MIT Press, 1992.

28 Suomi SJ. Developmental trajectories, early experiences, and community consequences: lessons from studies with rhesus monkeys. In Keating D, Hertzman C, eds. *Developmental health and the wealth of nations: social, biological and educational dynamics.* New York: Guildford Press, 1999:185–200.

29 Coe CL. Psychosocial factors and psychoneuroimmunology within a lifespan perspective. In Keating D, Hertzman C, eds. *Developmental health and the wealth of nations: social, biological and educational dynamics,* New York: Guildford Press, 1999:201–19.

30 Kiecolt-Glaser JK, Glaser R. Psychoneuroimmunology and cancer: fact or fiction? *Eur J Cancer* 1999;**35**:1603–7.

31 Jacobs JR, Bovasso GB. Early and chronic stress and their relation to breast cancer. *Psychol Med* 2000;**30**:669–78.

32 Ridley M. *Nature via nurture.* London: Fourth Estate, 2003.

33 Ben-Shlomo Y, Davey Smith G, Shipley MJ, Marmot MG. What determines mortality risk in male former cigarette smokers? *Am J Pub Health* 1994;**84**:1235–42.

34 Doll R, Peto R, Wheatley K, Gray R, Sutherland I. Mortality in relation to smoking: 40 years' observations on male British doctors. *Br Med J* 1994;**309**:901–11.

35 Magnus P, Beaglehole R, Rodgers A, Bennett S. The real contribution of the major risk factors to the coronary epidemics—time to end the "only-50%" myth. *Arch Int Med* 2001;**161**:2657–60.

36 Band PR, Le ND, Fang R, Deschamps M. Carcinogenic and endocrine disrupting effects of cigarette smoke and risk of breast cancer. *Lancet* 2002;**360**:1044–9.

*37 Kuh D, Hardy R, Langenberg C, Richards M, Wadsworth MEJ. Mortality in adults aged 26–54 years related to socioeconomic conditions in childhood and adulthood: a post war birth cohort study. *Br Med J* 2002;**325**:1076–80.

38 Power C, Manor O, Matthews S. The duration and timing of exposure: effects of socioeconomic environment on adult health. *Am J Pub Health* 1999;**89**:1059–65.

39 Power C, Matthews S, Manor O. Inequalities in self-rated health: explanations from different stages of life. *Lancet* 1998;**351**:1009–14.

40 Power C, Stansfeld SA, Matthews S, Manor O, Hope S. Childhood and adulthood risk factors for socio-economic differentials in psychological distress: evidence from the 1958 British birth cohort. *Soc Sci Med* 2002;**55**:1989–2004.

41 Ben-Shlomo Y, Kuh D. A life course approach to chronic disease epidemiology: conceptual models, empirical challenges, and interdisciplinary perspectives. *Int J Epidemiol* 2002;**31**:285–93.

42 Davey Smith G, Phillips A. Declaring independence: why we should be cautious. *J Epidemiol Commun Health* 1990;**44**:257–8.

43 Wadsworth MEJ, Kuh DJL. Childhood influences on adult health: a review of recent work in the British 1946 national birth cohort study, the MRC National Survey of Health and Development. *Paediat Perinat Epidemiol* 1997;**11**:2–20.

44 Power C. A review of child health in the 1958 cohort: National Child Development Study. *Paediat Perinat Epidemiol* 1992;**6**:91–110.

45 Strauss RS. Adult functional outcome of those born small for gestational age: twenty-six-year follow-up of the 1970 British Birth Cohort. *J Am Med Assoc* 2000;**283**:625–32.

46 Poulton R, Caspi A, Milne BJ, Thomson WM, Taylor A, Sears MR *et al.* Association between children's experience of socioeconomic disadvantage and adult health: a life-course study. *Lancet* 2002;**360**:1640–5.

47 Ong K, Kratzsch J, Kiess W, Dunger D. Circulating IGF-1 levels in childhood are related to both current body composition and early postnatal growth rate. *J Clin Endocrinol Metab* 2002;**87**:1041–4.

48 Whincup PJ, Cook DG, Adshead F, Taylor SJC, Walker M, Papacosta O *et al.* Childhood size is more strongly related than size at birth to glucose and insulin levels in 10–11-year-old children. *Diabetologia* 1997;**40**:319–26.

49 Davis PH, Dawson JD, Riley WA, Lauer RM. Carotid intimal-medial thickness is related to cardiovascular risk factors measured from childhood through middle age: The Muscatine Study. *Circulation* 2001;**104**:2815–9.

50 Must A, Jacques PF, Dallal GE, Bajema CJ, Dietz WH. Long-term morbidity and mortality of overweight adolescents. A follow-up of the Harvard Growth Study of 1922 to 1935. *N Engl J Med* 1992;**327**:1350–5.

51 Vaillant GE. *Aging well.* Boston: Little, Brown and Company, 2002.

52 Twisk JWR, Kemper HCG, van Mechelen W, Post GB. Tracking of risk factors for coronary heart disease over a 14-year period: a comparison between lifestyle and biologic risk factors with data from the Amsterdam Growth and Health Study. *Am J Epidemiol* 1997;**145**:888–98.

53 Kuh D, Hardy R, Rodgers B, Wadsworth MEJ. Lifetime risk factors for women's psychological distress in midlife. *Soc Sci Med* 2002;**55**:1957–73.

54 Kuh D, Cardozo L, Hardy R. The pattern and predictors of incontinence in women during middle life. *J Epidemiol Commun Health* 1999;**53**:453–8.

55 Richards M, Sacker A. Predicting midlife cognitive function: effects of parental socioeconomic status, childhood cognition, and educational and occupational attainment. *J Clin Exp Neuropsychol* 2003;**25**:614–24.

56 Aihie Sayer A, Poole J, Kuh D, Hardy R, Wadsworth, MEJ. Weight from birth to 53 years: a longitudinal study of the influence on hand osteoarthritis. *Arthr Rheumat* 2003;**48**:1030–3.

57 Jauniaux E, Ramsay B, Campbell S. Ultrasonographic investigation of placental morphologic characteristics and size during the second trimester of pregnancy. *Am J Obstet Gynecol* 1994;**170**:130–7.

58 Leon D, Mann V, Koupilova I, Tuvemo T, Lindmark G, Mohsen R *et al.* Parental, foetal and developmental influences on childhood blood pressure in 600 sib pairs: the Uppsala Family Study. *Paediatrics* 2003;**53**:9A.

59 Sobngwi E, Boudou P, Mauvais-Jarvis F, Leblanc H, Velho G, Vexiau P. Effect of a diabetic environment *in utero* on predisposition to type 2 diabetes. *Lancet* 2003;**361**:1861–5.

60 Campbell DM, Hall MH, Barker DJP, Cross J, Shiell AW, Godfrey KM. Diet in pregnancy and the offspring's blood pressure 40 years later. *Br J Obstet Gynaecol* 1996;**103**:273–80.

61 Belizan JM, Villar J, Bergel E, del Pino A, Di Fulvio S, Galliano SV *et al.* Long-term effect of calcium supplementation during pregnancy on the blood pressure of offspring: follow up of a randomised controlled trial. *Br Med J* 1997;**315**:281–5.

62 Singhal A, Cole TJ, Lucas A. Early nutrition in preterm infants and later blood pressure: two cohorts after randomised trials. *Lancet* 2001;**357**:413–9.

63 Davey Smith G, Ebrahim S. 'Mendelian randomization': can genetic epidemiology contribute to understanding environmental determinants of disease? *Int J Epidemiol* 2003;**32**:1–22.

64 Egger M, Davey Smith G, Altman DG, eds. *Systematic reviews in health care: meta analysis in context.* London: British Medical Journal Publishing Group, 2001.

65 Huxley R, Neil A, Collins R. Unravelling the fetal origins hypothesis: is there really an inverse association between birthweight and subsequent blood pressure? *Lancet* 2002;**360**:659–65.

66 Newsome CA, Shiell AW, Fall CHD, Phillips DIW, Shier R, Law CM. Is birth weight related to later glucose and insulin metabolism?—a systematic review. *Diabet Med* 2003;**20**:339–48.

67 Owen CG, Whincup PH, Odoki K, Gilg JA, Cook DG. Birth weight and blood cholesterol level: a study in adolescents and systematic review. *Pediatrics* 2003;**111**:1081–9.

68 **Lawlor DA, Ebrahim S, Davey Smith G.** Is there a sex difference in the association between birth weight and systolic blood pressure in later life? Findings from a meta-regression analysis. *Am J Epidemiol* 2003;**156**:1100–4.

69 **Department of Health.** *The health of the nation—a strategy for health in England.* London: Her Majesty's Stationery Office, 1992.

70 **Kendall R.** From the Chief Medical Officer. *Health Bull* 1993;**51**:351–2.

71 **Department of Health.** *Variations in health: what can the Department of Health and the NHS do?* London: Department of Health, 1995.

72 *Report of the Independent Inquiry into inequalities in health.* London: The Stationery Office, 1998.

73 **Aboderin I, Kalache A, Ben-Shlomo Y, Lynch JW, Yajnik CS, Kuh D et al.** *Life course perspectives on coronary heart disease, stroke and diabetes: key issues and implications for policy and research.* Geneva: World Health Organization, 2002.

74 **Ebrahim S, Davey Smith G.** Exporting failure? Coronary heart disease in developing countries. *Int J Epidemiol* 2001;**30**:201–5.

75 **Wald NJ, Law MR.** A strategy to reduce cardiovascular disease by more than 80%. *Br Med J* 2003;**326**:1419–23.

76 **Halfon N, Hochstein M.** Life course health development: an integrated framework for developing health, policy, and research. *Milbank Q* 2002;**80**:433–79.

77 **Halfon N, Inkelas M, Hochstein M.** The Health Development Organization: an organizational approach to achieving child health development. *Milbank Q* 2000;**78**:447–96.

78 **Bartley M, Blane D, Montgomery S.** Health and the life course: why safety nets matter. *Br Med J* 1997;**314**:1194–6.

*79 **Graham H.** Building an inter-disciplinary science of health inequalities: the example of life-course research. *Soc Sci Med* 2002;**55**:2005–16.

80 **Bartley M.** *Authorities and partisans.* Edinburgh: Edinburgh University Press, 1992.

81 **Kuh D, Davey Smith G.** When is mortality risk determined? Historical insights into a current debate. *Soc Hist Med* 1993;**6**:101–23.

82 **Dwork D.** *War is good for babies and other young children. A history of the infant and child welfare movement in England 1989–1918.* London, Tavistock Publications, 1987.

83 **Lewis J.** *The politics of motherhood: child and maternal welfare in England 1900–1939.* London: Croom Helm, 1980.

84 **Bowlby J.** *Maternal care and mental health* (World Health Organization Monograph Series No. 2). Geneva: World Health Organization, 1951.

85 **Bowlby J.** *Child care and the growth of love.* Harmondsworth: Penguin, 1953.

86 **Keating D, Hertzman C.** *Developmental health and the wealth of nations: social, biological and educational dynamics.* New York: Guilford Press, 1999.

*87 **Bradbury B, Jenkins SP, Micklewright J.** *The dynamics of child poverty in industrialised countries.* Cambridge: Cambridge University Press, 2001.

88 **Susser M, Susser E.** Choosing a future for epidemiology: II. From black box to Chinese boxes and eco-epidemiology. *Am J Pub Health* 1996;**86**:674–7.

89 **Charlton BG.** Attribution of causation in epidemiology: chain or mosaic? *J Clin Epidemiol* 1996;**49**:105–7.

90 **Krieger N, Zierler S.** What explains the public's health? A call for epidemiologic theory. *Epidemiology* 1996;**7**:107–9.

91 **Hertzman C, Power C, Matthews S, Manor O.** Using an interactive framework of society and lifecourse to explain self-rated health in early adulthood. *Soc Sci Med* 2001;**53**:1575–85.

Index